EIGHT EDITION

Primary Preventive Dentistry

Norman O. Harris, DDS, MSD, FACD

Professor Emeritus,
Department of Community Dentistry
University of Texas Health Science Center
at San Antonio

Franklin Garcia-Godoy, DDS, MS, PhD

Professor & Senior Executive Associate Dean for Research,
College of Dentistry
The University of Tennessee Health Science Center
Memphis, Tennessee

Christine Nielsen Nathe, RDH, MS

Professor and Chief,
Division of Dental Hygiene
Vice Chair,
Department of Dental Medicine
University of New Mexico

PEARSON

Boston   Columbus   Indianapolis   New York   San Francisco   Upper Saddle River
Amsterdam   Cape Town   Dubai   London   Madrid   Milan   Munich   Paris   Montréal   Toronto
Delhi   Mexico City   São Paulo   Sydney   Hong Kong   Seoul   Singapore   Taipei   Tokyo

Publisher: Julie Levin Alexander
Assistant to Publisher: Regina Bruno
Editor-in-Chief: Marlene Pratt
Executive Editor: John Goucher
Program Manager: Nicole Ragonese
Editorial Assistant: Erica Viviani
Senior Media Producer: Amy Peltier
Media Project Manager: Lorena Cerisano
Production Managing Editor: Patrick Walsh
Project Manager: Christina Zingone-Luethje

Full Service Production: John Shannon/Jouve North America
Operations Specialist: Lisa McDowell
Art Director: Maria Guglielmo
Cover Designer: Bruce Kenselaar
Director of Marketing: David Gesell
Executive Marketing Manager: Katrin Beacom
Marketing Specialist: Alicia Wozniak
Printer/Binder: RR Donnelley & Sons Company
Cover Printer: Phoenix Color Corporation
Cover Image: Olga Miltsova/Shutterstock.com

Notice: The authors and the publisher of this volume have taken care that the information and technical recommendations contained herein are based on research and expert consultation, and are accurate and compatible with the standards generally accepted at the time of publication. Nevertheless, as new information becomes available, changes in clinical and technical practices become necessary. The reader is advised to carefully consult manufacturers' instructions and information material for all supplies and equipment before use, and to consult with a healthcare professional as necessary. This advice is especially important when using new supplies or equipment for clinical purposes. The authors and publisher disclaim all responsibility for any liability, loss, injury, or damage incurred as a consequence, directly or indirectly, of the use and application of any of the contents of this volume.

Credits and acknowledgments borrowed from other sources and reproduced, with permission, in this textbook appear on the appropriate page within text.

Library of Congress Cataloging-in-Publication Data

Primary preventive dentistry / [edited by] Norman O. Harris,
Franklin Garcia-Godoy, Christine Nielsen Nathe. — 7th ed.
     p. ; cm.
  Includes bibliographical references and index.
  ISBN-13: 978-0-13-284570-0
  ISBN-10: 0-13-284570-9
  1. Preventive dentistry.   2. Preventive dentistry— Examinations,
questions, etc. I. Harris, Norman O.   II. García-Godoy, Franklin.
III. Nathe, Christine Nielsen.
  [DNLM: 1. Preventive Dentistry—methods. 2. Dental Plaque—prevention
& control. 3. Primary Prevention—methods.   WU 113 P9522 2009]
  RK60.7.H37 2009
  617.6'01—dc22

                              2008031941

10 9 8 7 6 4 3 2 1

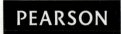

ISBN-13:   978-0-13-284570-0
ISBN-10:   0-13-284570-9

This 8th edition of *Primary Preventive Dentistry* is dedicated to the memory of Norman O. Harris, for his vision and efforts in the practice and evolution of primary preventive dentistry. His passion for preventing dental disease has been instilled in the preventive practices of multitudes of dentists and dental hygienists worldwide.

Contents

Chapter 9   Host Defense Mechanisms in the Oral Cavity ■ *Beth E. McKinney*   122

UNIT 3   Preventive Strategies   134

Chapter 10   Toothbrushes and Toothbrushing Methods ■ *Christine N. Nathe*   134

Chapter 11   Dentifrices, Mouthrinses, and Chewing Gums ■ *Meg Horst Zayan*   147

Chapter 19   Health Education and Promotion Theories ■ *Mary Catherine Hollister*   324

Chapter 27   Medically Compromised Populations ■ *Diana Burnham Aboytes*   434

Preface

The guiding principles that have sustained *Primary Preventive Dentistry* throughout the last several decades remain consistent. *Primary Preventive Dentistry* comprehensively presents the science and practice of assessment and treatment modalities of preventive dental care. This eighth edition strives to enhance the readability of this book for dental hygiene and dental students. Moreover, the Web site has been enhanced to provide additional opportunities for student study at www.myhealthprofessionskit.com.

The book is sequenced in units to organize the material for reader understanding and comprehension. The beginning unit focuses on a comprehensive discussion on preventive dental concepts with an emphasis on the historical perspective and creation of prevention in health care today. The relationship between prevention and urgent and restorative care is presented to help dental providers understand *all* facets of dental care delivery. A thorough discussion of assessment, diagnostic, and therapeutic sciences of dental care is presented.

The second unit focuses on oral disease etiology and contributing risk factors. This unit includes chapters on plaque, dental caries, periodontal disease, oral cancer, dental trauma, and host mechanisms. The etiology of all diseases is discussed comprehensively so that students completely understand the disease before prevention is discussed. The third unit addresses strategies to prevent these diseases/conditions and to maintain health. Chapters in this unit include discussion of toothbrushing, dentifrices, toothpastes and mouthrinses, oral hygiene aids, fluorides, dental sealants, nutrition, mouthguards, tobacco cessation, and health education and promotion theories.

The final unit includes chapters on target populations and approaches to preventing disease and maintaining health in these populations, which include infants, children, individuals with medical conditions and/or diseases, older adults, and hospitalized individuals.

NEW TO THIS EDITION

Primary Preventive Dentistry has been revised so that it provides for an even more valuable teaching and learning experience. Here are the enhancements we have made:

- New full color design with color photos and illustrations to capture the attention of students and enhance their overall learning experience.
- Additional images have been included to help learners better visualize the concepts presented in the text.
- New chapter on cultural health influences (chapter 2) which will allow students to be informed about how cultural differences may affect dental hygiene care.
- Table of contents has been reorganized so the material will flow in a more logical progression.

Christine Nielsen Nathe

Contributors

Diana Burnham Aboytes, RDH, MS
Assistant Professor, Division of Dental Hygiene
University of New Mexico
Albuquerque, New Mexico

Christine French Beatty, RDH, PhD
Professor Emeritus, Dental Hygiene
Texas Woman's University
Denton, Texas

Linda D. Boyd, RDH, RD, EdD
Dean, Forsyth School of Dental Hygiene
Massachusetts College of Pharmacy and Health
Sciences
Boston Massachusetts

Gary Cuttrell, DDS, JD
Associate Professor and Chief, Division of Dental
Services
Chair, Department of Dental Medicine
University of New Mexico
Albuquerque, New Mexico

Joan M. Davis, RDH, PhD
Professor, Dental Hygiene
Southern Illinois University
Carbondale, Illinois

Vicky Gianopoulos Pizanis, RDH, MS
Assistant Professor, Division of Dental Hygiene
University of New Mexico
Albuquerque, New Mexico

Maria Perno Goldie, RDH, BA, MS
President, International Federation of Dental
Hygienists
San Carlos, California

Elmer E. Gonzalez, RDH, MS
Lecturer, Division of Dental Hygiene
University of New Mexico
Albuquerque, New Mexico

Kathleen O. Hodges, RDH, MS
Professor, Department of Dental Hygiene
Office of Medical and Oral Health
Idaho State University
Pocatello, Idaho

Mary Catherine Hollister, RDH, MS, PhD
U.S. Public Health Service
United South and Eastern Tribes, Inc.
Nashville, Tennessee

Elizabeth Locke, PhD, MS, PT
Director of Clinical Education and Senior
Lecturer, School of Physical Therapy and Athletic
Training
College of Health Sciences
Old Dominion University
Norfolk, Virginia

Sandra J. Maurizio, RDH, PhD
Associate Professor, Dental Hygiene
Southern Illinois University
Carbondale, Illinois

Beth E. McKinney, RDH, MS
Public Health Dental Hygienist
Montgomery County Government
Rockville, Maryland

William J. Niendorff, DDS, MPH, MEd
Dental Educator
Board Certified Dental Public Health
Specialist
Albuquerque, New Mexico

Carole A. Palmer, RD, Ed.D
Professor and Head, Nutrition and Oral Health
Promotion
Department of Public Health and Community
Service
Tufts University School of Dental Medicine
Boston, Massachusetts

Sharon G. Peterson, RDH, MEd
Professor and Director, Dental Hygiene
Programs
College of Southern Nevada
Las Vegas, Nevada

Howard F. Pollick, BDS, MPH
Clinical Professor, Preventive and Restorative
Dental Sciences
University of California, San Francisco
San Francisco, California

Michelle L. Sensat, BSDH, MS
Adjunct Assistant Professor, Dental Hygiene
School of Dentistry
University of Minnesota
Minneapolis, Minnesota

Deanne Shuman, BSDH, MS, PhD
Interim Chair, School of Community &
Environmental Health
Professor & Program Director
PhD Health Services Research
College of Health Sciences
Old Dominion University
Norfolk, Virginia

Jill L. Stoltenberg, RDH, MA, RF
Associate Professor, Dental Hygiene
School of Dentistry
University of Minnesota
Minneapolis, Minnesota

Charles D. Tatlock, DDS, MPH
Professor, Division of Dental Services
University of New Mexico
Albuquerque, New Mexico

Amy Teague, RDH, MS
Clinical Assistant Professor
Texas Woman's University
Denton, TX

Meg Horst Zayan, RDH, MPH, EdD
Associate Professor and Dean
Fones School of Dental Hygiene
University of Bridgeport
Bridgeport, Connecticut

Reviewers

Mary D. Cooper, RDH, MSEd
College of Health and Human Services
Fort Wayne, Indiana

Jeanie L. Elliott, RDH, BS
Brevard Community College
Cocoa, Florida

Jeri Farmer, RDH, AAS, BAAS, MEd
Howard College
Big Spring, Texas

Monica M. Franklin, RDH, DHSc
Florida State College at Jacksonville
Jacksonville, Florida

Jan Hillis, RDH, MA
Iowa Western Community College
Council Bluffs, Iowa

Kay Jukes CDA, RDA, BS
Houston Community College
Houston Texas

Trina J. Morgan RDH, BA
Missouri College
Brentwood, Missouri

Cindy A. O'Neal, RDH, MS
Tarrant County College, NE
Hurst, Texas

Rebecca Smith, RDH, MPH
Miami Dade College
Miami, Florida

Adele Spencer, RDH MS
Farmingdale State College
Farmingdale, New York

Pamela Wade, RDH, BS, MS, CFCS
Tyler Junior College
Tyler, Texas

Introduction to Primary Preventive Dentistry

Christine N. Nathe

OBJECTIVES

After studying this chapter, the student should be able to:

1. Define and apply the following key terms: *primary, secondary,* and *tertiary prevention*.
2. Describe the historical aspect of preventive dental care.
3. Describe the state of dental health in the United States.
4. Describe categories that aid in classifying diseases.
5. Describe risk assessment in dental care delivery.

KEY TERMS

Craniofacial disorders, 8
Demineralization, 8
Diagnostic modality, 5
Health disparities, 4
In situ, 8
Incipient lesions, 6
Noninvasive caries, 8
Opportunistic infections, 7
Overt cavitation, 8
Periodontal debridement, 6
Plaque diseases, 8
Preventive dentistry, 5
Primary prevention, 5
Primary preventive care, 5
Remineralization, 6
Secondary prevention, 5
Self-care, 6
Sequelae, 10
Sugar discipline, 6
Tertiary prevention, 5
Therapeutic modality, 5

INTRODUCTION

The mission of dental care focuses on the ability to help individuals achieve and maintain maximum oral health throughout their lives. Success in attaining this mission is highlighted by the dramatic reduction in tooth loss among adults in the United States. This progress has been attributed mainly to the prevention of dental disease by the use of fluoride, the introduction of dental hygienists into the workforce, and the subsequent acceptance and practice of primary preventive care.

This textbook will discuss effective strategies that can reduce the number of carious (decayed) teeth, better control periodontal diseases, prevent the devastating effects of trauma caused by accidents, increase the early detection of oral cancer, and increase healthy behaviors. The U.S. Surgeon General has stated that mouth and throat diseases, which range from dental caries to cancer, cause pain and disability for millions of Americans, even though most oral diseases can be prevented.[1] In dental health, lack of preventive dental care results in the further progression of disease and in the increased number of restorations, extractions, surgeries, and dentures.

HISTORICAL ASPECT OF PREVENTIVE DENTAL CARE

Dr. Alfred C. Fones (Figure 1–1 ■), the founder of dental hygiene and preventive dentistry, eloquently stated in 1916 that hundreds of millions of dollars in public and private funds are expended to restore the sick to health, but only a relatively small portion of this amount is spent to maintain the health of well people, even though it is definitely known that the most common physical defects and illnesses are preventable.[2] He envisioned the tremendous effect of prevention before it was routinely practiced and promoted in health care.

The first college textbook on preventive dentistry, written by Fones, states that the mouth is the show window in which the body displays its physical wares.[2] This statement is similar to the 2000 report of oral health in America, in which the Surgeon General states that, indeed, the phrase "the mouth is the mirror," has been used to illustrate the wealth of information that can be derived from examining oral tissues.[1]

Fones continued to discuss the need for preventive dentistry departments in dental schools and the need to further enhance the dental hygienist movement.[2] See Figure 1–2 ■ for a list of the topics covered in this first college textbook on preventive dentistry. Moreover, Fones stated that the research field in preventive dental care was broadening into a study of constitutional causes, that is, causes related to systemic diseases, which affect one or more organs, or the whole body; these diseases are believed to have an influence on the general health and, consequently, on dental health.[2–6] In addition, this statement is similar to the Surgeon General's recommendation that dental providers need to help change perceptions regarding oral health and ideas so that oral health becomes an accepted component of general health.[1]

Preventive dentistry is flourishing as a science and practice. The majority of U.S. dentists who own their own practices

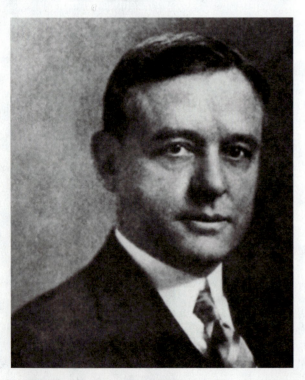

FIGURE ■ 1–1 Alfred C. Fones, DDS, founder of dental hygiene.
(*Source:* American Dental Hygienists' Association.)

TEXTBOOK TABLE OF CONTENTS

Fones, AC. *Preventive Dentistry for Dental Students.*

Philadelphia: Lea & Febiger. 1925.

The Normal Histology of Dental Tissues

The Alveolar Process

The Enamel and the Saliva

Normal Occlusion

Brief Pathology of the Dental Tissues

Dental Caries: Immunity and Susceptibility

Dietetics: Elements of the Human Body

The Unnatural Dietary Habits of Civilized Nations

Modern Methods of Preparing and Cooking Food

Principles of Dental Prophylaxis

The Prophylactic Treatment

Prevention Through Public Education

FIGURE ■ 1–2 Topics covered in the first book on preventive dentistry.
(*Source:* Lea & Febiger, 1925.)

employ a dental hygienist. Most dental insurance companies routinely cover preventive care because of the long-term benefit and cost effectiveness of prevention in dental health. Moreover, many communities voluntarily add fluoride to their water supplies as a method of preventing dental disease. And most recently, to aid in the prevention of dental disease, school systems in many areas of the country offer their students dental sealants through dental health providers.

Although many individuals studied and practiced preventive dental measures, it was Fones who actually initiated the practice of dental hygiene, which began the prevention movement in dental care witnessed today. Some may propose that the creation of dental hygiene, a preventive-based science and practice, truly was the primary component of the prevention movement in health care. A decade after dental hygiene began, Fones stated that it was no longer a theory that the service of the dental hygienist improved dental and overall health in the community and that those who were initially skeptical were finding it difficult indeed to suggest any other means by which similar positive results can be accomplished for the community.[4] Interestingly, skeptics at the time could not dispute the effectiveness of primary preventive dentistry delivered by dental hygienists.

DID YOU KNOW ?

A few years ago it was reported that two molar teeth of a Neanderthal were found to have grooves formed by the passage of a pointed object, which suggests the use of a small stick for cleaning the teeth.

Many interesting issues were addressed in the 2000 Surgeon General's oral health report and are included in Table 1–1 ■. This report provided more details on the meaning of oral health

---

TABLE ■ 1–1 The Burden of Oral Diseases and Disorders

Oral diseases are progressive and cumulative, and become more complex over time. They can affect our ability to eat, the foods we choose, how we look, and the way we communicate. These diseases can affect economic productivity and compromise our ability to work at home, at school, or on the job. Health disparities exist across population groups at all ages. Over one third of the U.S. population (100 million people) has no access to community water fluoridation. Over 108 million children and adults lack dental insurance, which is over 2.5 times the number who lack [*sic*] medical insurance.

The following are highlights of oral health data for children, adults, and the elderly. [Refer to the full report for details of these data and their sources.]

Children

- Cleft lip/palate, one of the most common birth defects, is estimated to affect 1 of 600 live births for whites and 1 of 1,850 live births for African Americans.
- Other birth defects, such as hereditary ectodermal dysplasias[a] where all or most teeth are missing or misshapen, cause lifetime problems that can be devastating to children and adults.
- Dental caries (tooth decay) is the single most common chronic childhood disease—5 times more common than asthma and 7 times more common than hay fever.
- Over 50 percent of 5- to 9-year-old children have at least one cavity or filling, and that proportion increases to 78 percent among 17-year-olds. Nevertheless, these figures represent improvements in the oral health of children compared to a generation ago.
- There are striking disparities in dental disease by income. Poor children suffer twice as much dental caries as their more affluent peers, and their disease is more likely to be untreated. These poor–nonpoor differences continue into adolescence. One out of four children in America is born into poverty, and children living below the poverty line (annual income of $17,000 for a family of four) have more severe and untreated decay.
- Unintentional injuries, many of which include head, mouth, and neck injuries, are common in children.
- Intentional injuries commonly affect the craniofacial tissues.
- Tobacco-related oral lesions are prevalent in adolescents who currently use smokeless (chewing) tobacco.
- Professional care is necessary for maintaining oral health, yet 25percent of poor children have not seen a dentist before entering kindergarten.
- Medical insurance is a strong predictor of access to dental care. Uninsured children are 2.5 times less likely than insured children to receive dental care. Children from families without dental insurance are 3 times more likely to have dental needs than children with either public or private insurance. For each child without medical insurance, there are at least 2.6 children without dental insurance.
- Medicaid has not been able to fill the gap in providing dental care to poor children. Fewer than one in five Medicaid-covered children received a single dental visit in a recent yearlong study period. Although new programs such as the State Children's Health Insurance Program (SCHIP) may increase the number of insured children, many will still be left without effective dental coverage.
- The social impact of oral diseases in children is substantial. More than 51 million school hours are lost each year to dental-related illness. Poor children suffer nearly 12 times more restricted-activity days than children from higher-income families. Pain and suffering due to untreated diseases can lead to problems in eating, speaking, and attending to learning.

---

[a]*Ectodermal dysplasia* is the abnormal development of the outer layer of cells in an embryo.

Source: U.S. Department of Health and Human Services. (2000). *Oral health in America: A report of the Surgeon General—Executive summary*. Rockville, MD: U.S. Department of Health and Human Services, National Institute of Dental and Craniofacial Research, National Institutes of Health, 2–3.

and explained why oral health is essential to general health and well-being. The major themes included:

- Oral health means much more than healthy teeth.
- Oral health is essential to general health.
- Safe and effective disease prevention measures exist so that everyone can voluntarily decide to improve oral health and prevent disease.

Major findings and a framework for action from the report are listed in Tables 1–2 ■ and 1–3 ■.[1] The Surgeon General published a subsequent document, *A National Call to Action to Promote Oral Health: A Public-Private Partnership under the Leadership of the Surgeon General*. This publication was an invitation to expand plans, activities, and programs designed to promote oral health, prevent disease, and emphasize the need to reduce **health disparities**, that is, the marked difference in quality of health status among populations. These disparities usually affect members of racial and ethnic groups, lower-income populations, many who are geographically isolated, and others who are vulnerable because of oral health care needs.[7] Prevention is the common thread within these documents, spotlighting the importance of prevention in dental health.

DENTAL DISEASES AND SYSTEMIC HEALTH

Although dental diseases are preventable, dental health in the United States remains an issue. In fact, frequently it is claimed that oral health is a major unmet need in this country. And although the majority of children have experienced dental decay, the burden of this disease is not evenly distributed.[8,9] Children who experience the majority of the decay are from lower-income households or ethnic minorities, and many times they have special needs.

The consequences of this widespread problem are disheartening. People who have the least access to preventive services and dental treatment have higher rates of oral diseases.[10] Untreated dental disease results in individuals who have constant pain, difficulty eating and speaking, chronic infections, increased use of pain medicine, and embarrassment over the appearance of their teeth. Unfortunately, emergency room and operating room staffs regularly see large numbers of children presenting with unrelenting toothaches and caries that cannot be managed in the dental office.[11,12] One study suggested that when Medicaid policy eliminated dental reimbursement, use of emergency rooms for the treatment of dental problems increased.[13] Emergency visits usually consist of providing antibiotic therapies and can require hospitalization if the problem is not treated in an effective manner.

DID YOU KNOW ?

The cost of dental visits to the hospital emergency room as opposed to a dental clinic are 10 times as higher, and many times emergency rooms treat only the symptoms. Simply put, the emergency room does not provide comprehensive dental care.

TABLE ■ 1–2   Major Findings from the Surgeon General's Report

- Oral diseases and disorders in and of themselves affect health and well-being throughout life.
- Safe and effective measures exist to prevent the most common dental diseases: dental caries and periodontal diseases.
- Lifestyle behaviors that affect general health, such as tobacco use, excessive alcohol use, and poor dietary choices, affect oral and craniofacial health as well.
- There are profound and consequential oral health disparities within the U.S. population.
- More information is needed to improve America's oral health and eliminate health disparities.
- The mouth reflects general health and well-being.
- Oral diseases and conditions are associated with other health problems.
- Scientific research is the key to further reduction in the burden of diseases and disorders that affect the face, mouth, and teeth.

Source: U.S. Department of Health and Human Services. (2000). *Oral health in America: A report of the Surgeon General—Executive summary*. Rockville, MD: U.S. Department of Health and Human Services, National Institute of Dental and Craniofacial Research, National Institutes of Health, 10-11.

TABLE ■ 1–3   Framework for Action

- Change perceptions regarding oral health and disease, so that oral health becomes an accepted component of general health.
- Accelerate the building of the science and evidence base, and apply science effectively to improve oral health.
- Build an effective health infrastructure that meets the oral health needs of all Americans and integrates oral health effectively into overall health.
- Remove known barriers between people and oral health services.
- Use public-private partnerships to improve the oral health of those who still suffer disproportionately from oral diseases.

Source: U.S. Department of Health and Human Services. (2000). *Oral health in America: A report of the Surgeon General—Executive summary*. Rockville, MD: U.S. Department of Health and Human Services, National Institute of Dental and Craniofacial Research, National Institutes of Health.

Moreover, oral health and its relationship to total health underscore the need for preventive dental care. Research has linked periodontal diseases to systemic diseases, such as cardiovascular and respiratory diseases, diabetes, cancer, premature and low-birth-weight babies, and a number of other systemic diseases.[1] Oral health is not a minor health concern; it affects overall health and well-being throughout life.

HEALTH DEFINED AND PRIMARY PREVENTIVE CARE

Although *health* can be defined as the period of time that an individual is not ill, it truly is much more expansive. The wellness scale defines a continuum from a state of health to a state of illness and death, with areas in between for quality-of-life indicators (Figure 1–3 ■). Quality-of-life indicators define those areas between total health and death when illness, injury, conditions, and diseases can affect the quality of life. For instance, an individual who broke a tooth while playing basketball would not be experiencing total health, even though the individual may not be close to fatal illness or death. Prevention focuses on maintaining quality of life by actively focusing on healthy behaviors that prevent diseases and maintain health.

Furthermore, it has been accepted that the individual is a multidimensional being who consists of five dimensions (see Figure 1–4 ■). This model shows the physical, mental, and social aspects of the first model and adds the spiritual and emotional aspects.[14] By accepting the concept of multidimensional health, health care providers believe that to experience total health, an individual must attain each dimension of health. This theory focuses on the need to address more than the physical dimension of health that previously defined health. Preventive strategies need to be focused on all multidisciplinary dimensions of health, realizing that all facets affect overall health.

DID YOU KNOW ?

It is becoming much more common for oral health to be publicized as a necessary entity for overall health. Flossing is being promoted as a way to increase one's life span.

The World Health Organization (WHO) defines *health* as the state of complete physical, mental, and social well-being, not merely the absence of disease or infirmity.[15] The WHO definition and other definitions are not without criticism; some

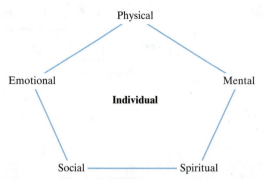

FIGURE ■ 1–4 Five-dimensional health model.

(*Source:* From R. Eberst (1984). Defining health: A multidimensional model. *Journal of School Health,* 54:99–104. Blackwell Publishing. Reprinted with permission from American School Health Association.)

argue that health cannot be defined as a state at all but must be seen as a process of continuous adjustment to the changing demands of living and of the changing meanings individuals give to life. If health is not described as merely the absence of disease, prevention then becomes an essential component of health and its definition. For instance, some individuals may actually be in excellent health but believe, for some reason logical to them, that they have oral cancer. These individuals do not have optimum mental well-being and will continue to worry until they are somehow convinced that they are indeed healthy. Another person may be functionally healthy but physically disfigured and consequently shunned socially throughout life. Thus, health can, at times, be what the patient thinks, not the actual condition of the body.

Even the terminology **preventive dentistry** has different meanings to different people. **Primary preventive care** focuses on the preventive aspects of the dental hygiene sciences and emphasizes the use of diagnostic and therapeutic modalities to prevent disease. A **therapeutic modality** is a method of applying or using any therapeutic agent, whereas a **diagnostic modality** is a method used to diagnose a condition. Preventive care can be defined and classified into three different levels.

1. **Primary prevention** uses strategies and agents to prevent the onset of disease, reverse the progress of disease, or arrest the disease process before secondary preventive treatment becomes necessary. This level is sometimes thought of as dental hygiene.

2. **Secondary prevention** uses routine treatment methods to terminate a disease process and/or restore tissues to as nearly normal as possible. This level can be termed *restorative care.*

3. **Tertiary prevention** uses measures necessary to replace lost tissues and rehabilitate patients to as nearly normal as possible. This level can be termed *reconstructive care.*

Some examples of each stage of prevention in dental care are described in Table 1–4 ■.

Health ➡ Death

FIGURE ■ 1–3 Health wellness scale.

TABLE ■ 1–4   Levels of Dental Preventive Care

Levels of Prevention	Therapies and Services
Primary prevention	Oral evaluation
	Dental prophylaxis
	Fluoride as a preventive agent
	Dental sealants
	Health education
	Health promotion
Secondary prevention	Dental restorations
	Periodontal debridement
	Fluoride use on incipient caries
	Dental sealants on incipient caries
	ART, alternative restorative treatment
	Endodontics
Tertiary prevention	Prosthodontics
	Implants
	Oromaxillofacial surgery

Primary Prevention

The general approaches to the primary prevention of dental caries and periodontal diseases involve the following measures:

- Professional oral assessments.
- Patient involvement in the control of plaque, a naturally acquired bacterial biofilm that develops on the teeth. This process is called **self-care** and is accomplished by brushing and flossing teeth and using other preventive products.
- Professional **periodontal debridement** (removal of soft and hard deposits from the teeth using manual or ultrasonic dental instruments).
- Community water fluoridation (addition of fluoride to a water supply).
- Use of products for self-care and for professionally initiated **remineralization** procedures (i.e., replacement of lost minerals in teeth).
- Use of antimicrobial agents to reduce plaque biofilm.
- Use of dental sealants.
- Practice of nutritionally healthy habits including **sugar discipline** (limitation of amount of sugar in the diet to prevent a nutrient source for oral bacteria).

See Table 1–5 ■ for a list of the responsibilities of the dental practitioner and the patient in implementing these preventive strategies. The information obtained from the clinical and radiographic oral examination, dietary analysis, patient history, and laboratory tests indicates the comprehensiveness with which these preventive measures should be prescribed and used.

At the time of the clinical and radiographic examinations, the first step should be to look for **incipient lesions**—the initial stage of tooth decay—and gingivitis (infection and subsequent inflammation of the gingiva). Then preventive strategies that would result in a reversal or control of either or both of these diseases caused by plaque could be applied. It is essential for the profession and the public to realize that biologic repair of incipient lesions and cure of gingivitis are preferred alternatives to restorations or periodontal treatment.

Even if these primary preventive dental modalities fail, tooth loss can still be avoided. In practice, the early identification and expeditious treatment of caries and periodontal diseases greatly minimizes the loss of teeth. When an annual dental examination that includes routine diagnostic and treatment services are linked with an effective dental hygiene program recommends an appropriate recall appointment based on risk assessment, tooth loss can realistically be reduced to zero or nearly zero.

Secondary and Tertiary Prevention

When prevention is not practiced, disease and infection frequently cause the undesirable effects of pain and discomfort. Furthermore, the shift from primary to tertiary prevention results in an extremely rapid increase in the cost of health care, with a proportional decrease in patient satisfaction.

An excellent example of the comparative cost of secondary and tertiary prevention is the treatment of an individual with poliomyelitis. The use of the polio vaccine to prevent the onset of the disease was highly effective and costs only a few dollars; however, for someone who was not adequately immunized, the

TABLE ■ 1–5   Preventive Strategies for the Reduction of Dental Caries and Periodontal Diseases (Associated with Plaque Biofilm)

Preventive Strategy	Dental Provider Treatment	Patient Tools
Mechanical reduction of plaque biofilm	Periodontal debridement	Toothbrush, dental floss, supplemental aids
Chemical reduction of plaque biofilm	Antibiotic therapies	Antimicrobial mouthrinses
Demineralization and remineralization of dental caries	Professionally applied fluoride, prescription fluoride, fabrication of fluoride custom trays	Toothpaste with fluoride, mouthrinse with fluoride, fluoridated water, products with ACP[a]
Prevention of a host surface	Dental sealants	Chewing gums and lozenges with xylitol
Diet	Nutritional counseling	Sugar discipline
Knowledge	Dental health education and promotion	Seeking information and care

[a]ACP, amorphous calcium phosphate

cost of treatment for poliomyelitis and subsequent rehabilitation was extremely expensive. Yet the individual receiving the expensive and difficult tertiary preventive treatment and who became disabled as a result certainly was not as happy as the one who benefited from only a few dollars' worth of primary preventive care.[16]

A dentally related example is the fluoridation of drinking water. This process costs approximately $0.50 per year per individual, yet it reduces the incidence of dental caries in the community by more than 20%.[17,18] If this primary preventive measure is not available, the necessary restorative dentistry (secondary prevention) can cost at least approximately $38 per restoration.[19] Finally, if secondary prevention fails, as it often does, dentures can be constructed at even higher costs.

Preventive Care

Possibly the most important benefit of preventive dental care is the fulfillment of the moral commitment to the Hippocratic oath, which health providers take upon graduation: "To render help to those in need, and to do no harm." Dental providers should derive a deep sense of satisfaction by helping individuals maintain their oral structures in a state of maximum function, comfort, and esthetics. Comprehensive dental care actively seeks to prevent disease and care for those individuals for whom prevention has failed. Furthermore, comprehensive preventive care involves the collaboration of dental hygienists providing assessment, primary preventive services, and referral to dentists who provide secondary and tertiary services and referrals to other health care providers as needed. Comprehensive preventive care must become a vital component in the health care delivery system to enhance the population's overall health and well-being.

Moreover, for the individual who thinks in terms of economic benefits and enjoyment of life, prevention is tremendously effective. Many studies document prevalence of dental diseases, which is the number of people in a population affected with a dental disease at the time of an epidemiology survey. Although dental disease prevalence is quantified, few studies define and describe the adverse effects on humans caused by dental neglect. One study suggests that 51% of dentate patients (those who have teeth) have been affected in some way by their oral health, and for 8% of them, the impact was sufficient to have reduced their quality of life.[20] If an individual (or the parents/guardians) starts preventive programs early, long-range freedom from diseases caused by plaque is possible. It is a sound cost–benefit investment. Teeth are essential for many dimensions of total health. In contrast, as stated earlier in this chapter, the absence of teeth or presence of broken-down teeth often results in pain, infection, disfigured appearance, and subsequent loss of self-esteem. These effects may minimize employment opportunities and often reduce social interaction.

Another example of prevention is of the ordinary seat belt in a car. This strategy illustrates how a simple preventive measure can greatly reduce facial injuries suffered in car accidents. Looming in the not-too-distant future is the very real possibility that many acquired health problems will be corrected or improved for total populations by the use of vaccines, genetic engineering, or specifically targeted drugs ("magic bullets"), which will be discussed in Chapter 22.

CATEGORIES OF ORAL DISEASES

Oral diseases and abnormalities can be conveniently grouped into three categories:

1. Dental caries and periodontal disease, both of which are acquired conditions.
2. Acquired oral conditions other than dental caries and periodontal diseases such as oral cancer, HIV/AIDS, and **opportunistic infections**, which are infections caused by a usually harmless microorganism that can become capable of causing disease when the host's resistance is impaired.

3. **Craniofacial disorders**, or disorders that involve both the cranium (portion of the skull that encases the brain) and the face, which would include a wide variety of conditions ranging from heredity to accidents.[21,22]

Preventive services costs approximately $172 per person in 2004 compared to restorative services, which costs approximately $217–$354 per person depending on the procedure.[23] The presence of pathogenic dental plaque on the surfaces of the teeth cause both caries and periodontal diseases and therefore are known as the **plaque diseases**. Any major reduction in the incidence of caries and periodontal disease will release resources for the investigation and treatment of conditions included in the acquired and craniofacial category. *Incidence* is defined as the number of new cases that occurs between two epidemiology surveys conducted over an agreed-upon time period. In contrast, *prevalence* is a measurement of the number of existing cases at the time of a survey.

Plaque Biofilm Prevention

The ideal or long-range planning objectives for coping with both dental caries and periodontal diseases should be the development of a preventive delivery system and methods to eventually attain a zero or near-zero disease incidence for the target population. However, a more realistic and feasible short-term goal is the attainment of a zero or near-zero rate of tooth loss from these diseases through integrated preventive and treatment procedures. Because of the varied etiology (cause) of acquired conditions other than caries and periodontal diseases, and of craniofacial malformations and diseases, the planning for the control of each of these problem areas must be individually addressed and placed within the priorities of any overall health plan.

In the quest for a zero or nearly zero incidence of the plaque diseases, it is critical that dental professionals identify the signs and symptoms of disease at a time when progression to more advanced stages can be prevented, arrested, or reversed. Examples are progression of an incipient caries lesion to **overt cavitation** (i.e., when undermined tooth enamel has demineralized into a carious lesion) and the progression of gingivitis to periodontitis and subsequent bone loss. Three notable factors make this preventive objective feasible:

1. Both dental caries and periodontitis are the result of a prolonged presence of pathogenic plaques affecting the enamel, cementum (a specialized bony layer of connective tissue that covers the root), and/or contiguous gingiva (gingiva in contact with the tooth).
2. In most cases, both diseases can be controlled by mechanical and chemical plaque control regimens.
3. Both of the plaque diseases must go through a continuum of two reversible interim stages from histological normalcy (i.e., having normal tissue structure or organization) to clinical pathology (structural and functional deviations from the normal that constitute disease or characterize a particular disease).

The earliest stage of the plaque diseases is **in situ** involvement, or involvement that does not extend beyond the site of origin. For caries, this stage is marked by the microscopic **demineralization** (loss of minerals) of the components that make up the tooth enamel.[24] For periodontal disease, initial involvement is the early infiltration of inflammatory cells beneath the sulcular epithelium, the tissue that lines the shallow space between the gingiva and the root of the tooth; this space is called the *gingival sulcus*.[25] Neither the early demineralization of caries nor the early cellular infiltration of gingivitis can be directly seen. Although these microscopic beginnings of plaque disease are not visible to the eye, they can be *suspected* on the basis of **noninvasive caries** (decay that has not penetrated tooth enamel) as well as periodontal risk assessment tests and indices that are *now* available to dental providers.

An in situ involvement, unless arrested or reversed, merges into the next stage of progression of the caries process, the incipient lesion. In caries, the lesion's clinical appearance is that of a "white spot" on the enamel, which is due to a more extensive subsurface demineralization of enamel.[26] Incipient lesions can occur on any surface as a precaries lesion. They may occur on the following areas of the tooth:

- Interproximally (on the contact areas of adjacent teeth; i.e., between teeth).
- Apical to the contact point (i.e., toward the area near the end of the root).
- On the cervical part of the tooth (i.e., near the junction of the crown and root).
- On the walls of the deep occlusal fissures, which are grooves on chewing surfaces of posterior teeth; the grooves developed during formation of the teeth.
- On buccal surfaces (surfaces located adjacent to the inside of the cheek).
- On lingual surfaces (surfaces located adjacent to the tongue).

Incipient lesions are found basically wherever there is plaque stagnation. These precaries lesions can be easily seen on dry, well-lighted buccal, lingual, and gingival enamel surfaces.[27] They are more difficult to detect on the occlusal surface where "sticky" pits and fissures should always be evaluated for having incipient carious lesions or even early undetected carious lesions.[28] The presence of white spots on the smooth interproximal surfaces can usually be identified first in radiographs.[29,30] In periodontal disease, the incipient lesion is gingivitis, with gingival bleeding being one of the first noticeable manifestations.[31] The incipient lesions of *both* caries and gingivitis can be reversed to histological normality, which by definition represents a cure.

The third and final stage of the plaque diseases is the overt, or clinically evident, lesion. In caries development, the overt lesion is characterized by cavitation with bacterial infiltration. For periodontal disease, an overt lesion is characterized by *irreversible* changes in the periodontium (tissue that surrounds the tooth) such as an apical migration of the epithelial attachment, which

Rev 8- 3

CRA FORM
First name: _____ Last name: _____ Date: _____

Adults and Children Age 6+

Due to new research on cavities and what causes them, we know everyone is at risk of developing decay at some point during their lifetime. The goal of this assessment form and the bacterial screening test is to determine your likelihood of experiencing new decay in the next 12 months. Please fill out the "Patient Use" section of this form to the best of your ability. These items will be discussed with your dental professional during your appointment today. Questions about this form? See the back for Q&A.

PATIENT USE

	yes		no
Would you like a free bacterial screening test to help determine your risk for cavities? (The test is a quick, painless swab of your teeth.)	yes		no
If diagnosed at risk for cavities today, would you be interested in discussing treatment options?	yes	maybe	no
If needed, are you willing to modify your dietary habits?	yes	maybe	no

RISK FACTORS

Do you notice plaque build-up on your teeth between brushings?	no	yes
Do you take medications daily? If yes, how many? (#____)	no	yes
Do you feel like you have a dry mouth at any time of the day or night?	no	yes
Do you drink liquids other than water more than 2 times daily between meals?	no	yes
Do you snack daily between meals?	no	yes
Do you have oral appliances present?	no	yes
Do any of these other health concerns apply to you? (check all that apply) ☐ Frequent tobacco use ☐ Other drug use ☐ Acid reflux ☐ Bulimia ☐ Diabetes ☐ Sjogren's Syndrome ☐ Head/neck radiation therapy	no	yes

CLINICIAN USE ONLY

DISEASE INDICATORS

	no	yes
New/Progressing Visible Cavitations	no	yes
New/Progressing Approximal Radiographic Radiolucencies	no	yes
New/Active White Spot Lesions	no	yes
Decay History is a Concern	no	yes

BIOFILM CHALLENGE

	low	high
CariScreen Bacterial Assessment (0-1500 low, 1501-9999 high)	low	high

PROFESSIONAL ASSESSMENT SUMMARY

	no	yes
Risk Factors are a Concern	no	yes
Disease Indicators are a Concern	no	yes
Biofilm Challenge is a Concern	no	yes

RISK IDENTIFICATION Transfer information above to boxes below to determine risk.

N Y	N Y	N Y	N Y	N Y
☐☐ Risk Factors ☐☐ Disease Indicators ☐☐ Biofilm Challenge	☐☐ Risk Factors ☐☐ Disease Indicators ☐☐ Biofilm Challenge	☐☐ Risk Factors ☐☐ Disease Indicators ☐☐ Biofilm Challenge	☐☐ Risk Factors ☐☐ Disease Indicators ☐☐ Biofilm Challenge	☐☐ Risk Factors ☐☐ Disease Indicators ☐☐ Biofilm Challenge
LOW RISK	**MODERATE RISK**	**HIGH RISK**	**HIGH RISK**	**HIGH/EXTREME RISK**
1	**2**	**3**	**4**	**5**

☐RECOMMENDED ☐PROVISIONAL ☐DECLINE

PATENT-PENDING
©CariFree

FIGURE ■ 1–5 CRA Form

(*Source:* Provided courtesy of Carifree.com.)

involves movement of the zone of soft tissue normally attached to the tooth toward the apex of the tooth root (i.e., area near the end of the root). If still untreated, the disease will usually progress to bone loss. At the overt lesion stage of the plaque diseases, treatment is usually indicated. However, two noninvasive preventive regimens may reverse overt caries: the use of antibacterial agents and/or remineralization therapy to arrest root decay and the use of sealants to arrest early pit-and-fissure caries.[32,33]

Not all in situ lesions progress to the incipient stage, nor do all incipient lesions progress to the overt stage of caries and/or periodontitis.[34] However, it is extremely important to note that no overt plaque disease lesion occurs at any site without first beginning as an in situ manifestation and then progressing to an incipient lesion before becoming overt. Thus, any prevention program must focus on identifying and reversing the in situ and incipient stages of the plaque diseases with the same, or greater, diligence that is now given to searching for and treating overt disease. Achievement of primary prevention will allow the profession to move from a traditional emphasis on secondary and tertiary preventive dentistry to a primary preventive focus and commitment.

RISK ASSESSMENT

Risk assessment is the procedure of determining the likelihood that an individual or population will experience specific diseases or conditions. Risk assessment can help predict a patient's risk of disease and improve clinical decision making. In turn, patient adherence to a self-care oral health regimen is a key component to successful periodontal disease management.[35]

Risk assessment is predicated on the assumption that dental providers should be individualizing treatment plans based on an individual's or populations' actual risk for developing disease as opposed to treating all individuals or populations the same, regardless of risk. An example could be a dental hygienist providing the same oral hygiene instruction that focused on dental flossing daily on Patient A, an adult female with gingival inflammation and bleeding in the interproximal areas, and on Patient B, a 3-year-old boy who exhibits early childhood decay when presenting to the clinic. It is readily apparent that flossing instructions could be helpful to Patient A but not to Patient B.

When assessing an individual's risk of caries, the Caries Risk Assessment (CRA Form) can be used. (Figure 1–5 ■) This assessment tool first assess an individual's caries disease indicators, risk factors, and protective factors and then determines the level of caries risk that the sum of these factors indicates (low, moderate, high, or extreme).[36] Based on the risk, a treatment plan is developed to prevent and manage dental caries.

A dental provider can also identify risks that may determine an individual's susceptibility to periodontal diseases.[35] The clinical practice of risk assessment may reduce the need for complex periodontal therapy, improve patient outcomes, and ultimately reduce oral health care costs.[35] Risk factors for periodontal diseases such as smoking, diabetes mellitus, poor oral hygiene, stress, or osteoporosis and nonmodifiable risk factors such as history of periodontitis, age, gender, race, genetic disorders may be modifiable (changed).

SUMMARY

This text emphasizes and specifically focuses on primary prevention as it applies to oral health. Each year billions of dollars are spent in the United States for dental care, mainly for the treatment of dental caries, periodontal disease, or their **sequelae**. Yet strategies now exist that, with patient knowledge and cooperation, could greatly aid in preventing, arresting, or reversing the onset of caries or periodontal disease.

This introductory chapter has briefly pointed out some problems of dental care and the means by which the dental and dental hygiene professions can make primary preventive dental care its hallmark. The remaining chapters provide the detailed background that can make this challenge become a reality.

PRACTICE CONSIDERATIONS

One of the greatest advances of modern dentistry has been the integration of preventive modalities into the daily practice of dental care in the United States. The advent of dental hygiene can be considered a milestone of dental science. All dental team members understand the inherently preventive measures of many common dental procedures and work to increase the values patients have on preventive dentistry. Furthermore, the common role of all dental providers is to maintain a prevention focus throughout the delivery of dental care.

SELF-STUDY QUESTIONS

1. Primary prevention uses strategies and agents to prevent the onset of disease, reverse the progress of disease, or arrest the disease process before secondary preventive treatment becomes necessary whereas secondary prevention uses routine treatment methods to terminate a disease process and/or restore tissues to as nearly normal as possible.

   a. Both statements are true.
   b. Both statements are false.
   c. The first statement is true; the second statement is false.
   d. The first statement is false.

   Rationale: *Primary prevention* uses strategies and agents to prevent the onset of disease, reverse the progress of disease, or arrest the disease process before secondary preventive treatment becomes necessary. This level is sometimes thought of as dental hygiene. *Secondary prevention* uses routine treatment methods to terminate a disease process and/or restore tissues to as nearly normal as possible. This level can be termed *restorative care.* *Tertiary prevention* uses measures necessary to replace lost tissues and rehabilitate patients to as nearly normal as possible. This level can be termed *reconstructive care.*

2. Initial demineralized tooth structure is referred to as which type of lesion?

   a. Frank

   b. Incipient

   c. Coronal

   d. Pulpal

   Rationale: *Incipient decay* is the initial demineralization that will continue to progress into tooth decay. Incipient lesions are found basically wherever there is plaque stagnation. These precaries lesions can be easily seen on dry, well-lighted buccal, lingual, and gingival enamel surfaces. They are more difficult to detect on the occlusal surface where "sticky" pits and fissures should always be highly suspect as having incipient carious lesions or even early undetected carious lesions.

3. Oral diseases are common in society and are progressive and _____, and become more complex over time.

   a. irreversible

   b. simple

   c. cumulative

   d. nonthreatening

   Rationale: Oral diseases are common in society and are progressive and cumulative, and become more complex over time.

4. Which of the following is a factor in both periodontal diseases and dental decay?

   a. Plaque

   b. Demineralization

   c. Incipient lesions

   Rationale: Bacterial plaque is a major factor in both tooth demineralization and gingival infection.

5. Which methods could reduce the occurrence of dental decay and periodontal diseases?

   a. Oral cancer screenings

   b. Brush biopsies

   c. Plaque removal interventions

   d. Athletic mouthguards

   Rationale: Because plaque is a major factor in both dental diseases, plaque removal interventions are needed to reduce dental diseases.

REFERENCES

1. U.S. Department of Health and Human Services. (2000). *Oral health in America: A report of the Surgeon General.* Rockville, MD: U.S. Department of Health and Human Services, National Institute of Dental and Craniofacial Research, National Institutes of Health.
2. Fones, A. C. (1916). *Mouth hygiene.* Philadelphia: Lea & Febiger.
3. Fones, A. C. (1921). *Mouth hygiene* (2nd ed.). Philadelphia: Lea & Febiger.
4. Fones, A. C. (1927). *Mouth hygiene* (3rd ed.). Philadelphia: Lea & Febiger.
5. Fones, A. C. (1934). *Mouth hygiene* (4th ed.). Philadelphia: Lea & Febiger.
6. Fones, A. C. (1925). *Preventive dentistry.* Philadelphia: Lea & Febiger.
7. U.S. Department of Health and Human Services. (May 2003). *A national call to action to promote oral health* (NIH Publication No. 03-5303). Rockville, MD: U.S. Department of Health and Human Services, Public Health Service, Centers for Disease Control and Prevention and the National Institutes of Health, & National Institute of Dental and Craniofacial Research.
8. Beltrán-Aguilar, E. D., Barker, L. K., Canto, M. T., Dye, B. A., Gooch, B. F., Griffin, S. O., Hyman, J., Jaramillo, F., Kingman, A., Nowjack-Raymer, R., Selwitz, R. H., & Wu, T. (2005). Surveillance for dental caries, dental sealants, tooth retention, edentulism, and enamel fluorosis—United States, 1988–1994 and 1999–2002. *MMWR, Surveillance Summaries,* 54:1–44.
9. Kaste, L. M., Selwitz, R. J., Oldakowski, R. J., Brunelle, J. A., Winn, D. M., & Brown, L. J. (1996). Coronal caries in the primary and permanent dentition of children and adolescents 1–17 years of age. *J Dent Res,* 75:631–41.
10. U.S. Department of Health and Human Services & Centers for Disease Control and Prevention (CDC). (March 2010). *Oral health: Preventing cavities, gum disease, tooth loss, and oral cancers: At a glance 2010.* Atlanta: CDC. Retrieved November 21, 2011, from http://www.cdc.gov/chronicdisease/resources/publications.
11. Wilson, S., Smith, G. A., Preish, J., & Casamassimo, P. S. (1997). Nontraumatic dental emergencies in a pediatric emergency department. *Clin Ped,* 36:333–37.
12. Sheller, B., Williams, B. J., & Lombardi, S. M. (1997). Diagnosis and treatment of dental caries-related emergencies in children's hospital. *Ped Dent,* 19:470–75.
13. Cohen, L. A., Manski, R. J., Magder, L. S., & Mullins, C. D. (2002). Dental visits to hospital emergency departments by adults receiving Medicaid. *J Am Dent Assoc,* 133:715–24.
14. Eberst, R. (1984). Defining health: A multidimensional model. *J School Health,* 54:99–104.
15. World Health Organization. (1948). Health Definition. Geneva, Switzerland: World Health Organization. Retrieved November 21, 2011, from http://www.who.int/suggestions/faq/en/index.html.

16. Thompson, K. M., & Duintjer, T. (2006). Retrospective cost-effectiveness analyses for polio vaccination. *Risk Anal,* 26: 1423–40. PDF.

17. CDC Fact Sheet: Cost savings of community water fluoridation fact sheet. September 1, 2009. Retrieved November 21, 2011, from http://www.cdc.gov/fluoridation/fact_sheets/cost. htm.

18. Griffin S. O., Gooch, B. F., Lockwood, S. A., & Tomar, S. L. (April 2001). Quantifying the diffused benefit from water fluoridation in the United States. *Community Dent Oral Epidemiol,* 29:120–29.

19. Griffin, S. O., Jones, K., & Tomar, S. L. (Spring 2001). An economic evaluation of community water fluoridation. *J Public Health Dent,* 61:78–86.

20. Nuttal, N. M., Steele, J. G., Pine, C. M., White, D., & Pitts, N. B. (2001). The impact of oral health on people in the UK in 1998. *Brit Dent J,* 190:121–26.

21. Mouradian, W. E. (1995). Who decides? Patients, parents or gatekeeper: Pediatric decisions in the craniofacial setting. *Cleft Palate Craniofac J,* 32:510–14.

22. Haug, R. H., & Foss, J. (2000). Maxillofacial injuries in the pediatric patient. *Oral Surg, Oral Med, Oral Path and Oral Radiol Endod,* 90:126–34.

23. Manski, R. J. and Brown, E. Dental Use, Expenses, Private Dental Coverage, and Changes, 1996 and 2004. Rockville (MD): Agency for Healthcare Research and Quality; 2007. MEPS Chartbook No.17. http://www.meps.ahrq.gov/mepsweb/data_files/publications/cb17/cb17.pdf

24. Barakow, F., Imfeld, T., & Lutz, F. (1991). Enamel re-mineralization: How to explain it to the patients. *Quint Int,* 22:141–47.

25. Brecx, M. C., Schlegel, K., Gehr, P., & Lang, N. P. (1987). Comparison between histological and clinic parameters during human experimental gingivitis. *J Periodontol Res,* 22:52–57.

26. Von der Fehr, F. R., Löe, H., & Theilade, E. (1970). Experimental caries in man. *Caries Res,* 4:131–48.

27. Nelson, A., & Pitts, N. B. (1991). The clinical behavior of free smooth surface carious lesions monitored over 2 years in a group of Scottish children. *Br Dent J.,* 171:313–18.

28. Konig, K. G. (1963). Dental morphology in relation to caries resistance with special reference to fissures in susceptible areas. *J Dent Res,* 42:461–76.

29. Wenzel, A., Pitts, N., Verdonschot, E. H., & Kalsbeck, H. (1993). Developments in radiographic diagnosis. *J Dent Res,* 21:131–40.

30. Espolid, I., & Tveit, A. B. (1984). Radiographic diagnosis of mineral loss in approximal enamel. *Car Res,* 18:141–48.

31. Lang, N. P., Adler, A., Joss, A., & Nyman, S. (1990). Absence of bleeding on probing: An indicator of periodontal stability. *J Clin Periodontol,* 7:714–21.

32. Malhotra, N., & Rao, A. (July–August 2011). The role of reminerlizing agents in dentistry: A review. *Compend Contin Educ Dent,* 32:26–33; quiz, 34, 36.

33. Peters, M. C. (July 2010). Strategies for noninvasive demineralized tissue repair. *Dent Clin North Am,* 54:507–25.

34. Silverstone, L. M. (1984). The significance of demineralization in caries prevention. *J Canad Dent Assoc,* 50:157–67.

35. Douglass, C. W. (2007). Risk assessment and management of periodontal disease. *J Am Dent Assoc,* 137(Suppl 3): 27S–32S.

36. Steinberg, S. (October 2009). Adding caries diagnosis to caries risk assessment: The next step in caries management by risk assessment (CAMBRA). *Compend Contin Educ Dent,* 30:522.

37. Page, R. A., Krall, E. Z., Martin, J., Mancl, L., & Garcia, R. I. (May 2002). Validity and accuracy of a risk calculator in predicting periodontal disease. *J Am Dent Asso,* 133:569–76.

Cultural Health Influences

Deanne Shuman
Elizabeth Locke

LEARNING OBJECTIVES

After reading this chapter, the student should be able to:

1. Define *culture* and explain its relevance to the contemporary healthcare professions.

2. Describe influences of culture on aspects of U.S. society that impact preventive healthcare to underserved populations.

3. Identify health beliefs among different cultural groups.

4. Describe how cultural beliefs influence preventive dental care.

5. Explain the relationship between cultural competence and health outcomes.

INTRODUCTION

...rectly influences how healthcare professionals relate ...nts, and, ultimately, impact health outcomes. A culturally ...petent health professional is one who is sensitive to cultural differences and makes a lifetime commitment to develop the beliefs, attitudes, values, and skills necessary to interrelate with people of all cultures, races, religions, and ethnic backgrounds with respect and empathy. This chapter will examine the influence of culture on health beliefs and the provision of healthcare services to different cultural groups including underserved populations. This chapter will explore culture, diversity, inclusiveness, and their collective influence on the provision of healthcare services to different cultural groups including underserved populations. Discussion will focus on health beliefs that exist between and among different cultural groups and discuss how these beliefs influence preventive dental care. **Cultural competence** facilitates effective patient-centered interactions, more involvement of patients in their own preventive healthcare, and improved health outcomes for all cultural groups.

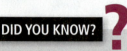

DID YOU KNOW?

A major challenge in dentistry is how to effectively address the health disparities that exist among various ethnic and racial groups in the American population.

OWNING CULTURE

Culture is a conceptual framework that has relevance in health professions research, education, and practice. All individuals, groups, and organizations have culture. Just as it is possible to be affiliated with several professional groups or organizations at one time, so it is possible to belong to several cultural groups at the same time. *Culture* may be operationally defined according to its characteristics or specific behaviors associated with individuals, groups, or organizations. Although no singular definition fully describes the *ethos* (characteristics) of an entire profession, a functional definition of *culture* as it relates to a profession may need to incorporate constructs such as custom, belief, cognition, perception, communication, interpretation, identification, and

differentiation, to name a few. **Culture**, then, may be defined functionally as "integrated patterns of human behavior that include the language, thoughts, communications, actions, customs, beliefs, values, and institutions of racial, ethnic, religious or social groups."[1] One such social group is a profession.

This operational definition declares that the professions of dentistry and dental hygiene are contractually accountable to society and that this declaration is sealed by a commitment to competence. The obligation to engage in the process of cultural competence,[2] therefore, is a professional responsibility grounded in societal expectation. Professional responsibility is reflected in the American Dental Education Association's 2009 Statement of Professionalism. This statement acknowledges respect as one of the six tenets of professionalism in dental education and is closely aligned with the codes of ethics of the American Dental Hygienists' Association (ADHA) and the American Student Dental Association. Students can demonstrate respect for cultural differences by acknowledging that a patient's beliefs and values on preventive care may be different from their own. The American Dental Education Association (ADEA) section on Dental Hygiene Education's Competencies for Entry into the Profession of Dental Hygiene stipulates the need for dental hygiene professionals to engage in culturally sensitive communication that respects individualized patient preferences.[3] Within the context of a profession, clinical cultural competence involves the profession's responsibility to recognize and understand the factors that influence the health beliefs of *different* individuals and communities.[4] As such, clinical cultural competence occurs within the context of diversity.

CULTURAL GROUP REPRESENTATION

According to the U.S. Census Bureau, **cultural diversity** will continue to increase through 2050.[5] Minorities will become the new majority population in 2042 and is projected to make up 54% of the U.S. population in 2050. The slowest projected population growth through 2050 will be in the non-Hispanic White group. See Table 2–1 ■ for U.S. census projections for **cultural group representation** through 2050.[6] The significance of cultural diversity shifts in the U.S. demographic lies in the fact that health profession programs are responsible for preparing graduates to meet the needs of an increasingly diverse population. This is accomplished by producing a culturally

TABLE ■ 2–1 Projected Increase in U.S. Cultural Diversity, 2008–2050

Cultural Group	U.S. Population in 2008 (in millions)	Projected U.S. Population in 2050 (in millions)	Population Change, 2008–2050 (in millions)
Aged 65+	38.7	88.5	49.8↑
Aged 85+	5.4	19.0	13.6↑
Asian	15.5	40.6	25.1↑
Black	41.1	65.7	24.6↑
Hispanic	46.7	132.8	86.1↑
Non-Hispanic White	199.8	203.3	3.5↑

(*Source:* U.S. Census Bureau.)

diverse educational environment that produces a culturally diverse workforce. However, diversity in health profession programs have not kept pace with the current and projected U.S. demographic shifts.[7] These workforce disparities are problematic because the 18-to-64-year working age group is projected to decline by 6% between 2008 and 2050.[6] To bridge these gaps, educational institutions and healthcare organizations are challenged to increase diversity while fostering cultural **inclusiveness**.[8,9]

Underrepresentation of minorities in dental hygiene programs persist despite projected increases in the U.S. population.[5,10] Similar to U.S. projected demographics, minorities are disproportionately represented in dental hygiene programs and subsequently the dental hygiene profession. The resultant workforce disparities stem from the lack of faculty and student diversity in dental hygiene programs across the country.[10] An increase in cultural diversity in dental hygiene education programs is needed to reduce and eliminate the increasing disparity between the dental hygiene profession and the increasingly diverse U.S. demographic served by this profession.

MOVING BEYOND DIVERSITY TO INCLUSIVENESS

Based on the information provided in Table 2–1 ■, we know that cultural groups are not equally represented nor are they expected to be through 2050.[6] However, numerically equivalent groups are not a prerequisite for a meaningful and helpful professional relationship to exist. The desire to progress toward cultural competence is prerequisite to an effective clinical encounter that ultimately leads to a trusting professional relationship between patient and provider. Providers are encouraged to engage in meaningful clinical encounters with and include all relevant aspects of patient care in the process of cultural competence.[2] This can be achieved by facilitating inclusion of patients in their own care. When providers demonstrate inclusiveness, they encourage full participation of patients in their own care while valuing and understanding the unique cultural differences among and between groups regardless of the size of those groups.

DID YOU KNOW? **?**

Barriers to access may include cultural values and language barriers.

CULTURAL BELIEFS AND PREVENTIVE DENTAL CARE

The notion of preventive oral healthcare is challenging for individuals regardless of their culture. If there is no pain or loss of function, few may value preventive measures. Many individuals do not seek healthcare unless they define the condition as seriously "wrong" even when they experience pain. The belief that healthy gums bleed is widespread, and many a story has been told of individuals who have pulled their own teeth when they became loose due to advanced periodontal disease. The health professional is challenged to deal with cultural beliefs related to preventive oral healthcare.

The U.S. healthcare system is closely related to the heritage of immigrants who settled North America to avoid religious persecution.[11] The class system depended on family status, and individualism, self-worth, hard work to succeed, and ability to earn money were valued characteristics. Large families provided more workers, which frequently translated to attaining success. Those who prospered were those who, in effect, "controlled nature." With industrialization, the ability to be mobile to obtain work became more important than dependence on the family. Collectively, these characteristics influenced the notions of how to treat illness as reflected by the development of innovations to prolong life (organ transplants, fetal monitoring, stem cell applications, etc.) and the view that with enough money, there is a cure for any illness. The ethnocentric values of individualism and freedom motivate the practice of giving health information directly to the patient, not the family or family head, and to expect patients to make their own healthcare decisions. The concept of self-care conceivably is a product of the notion of individualism.[11]

The theoretical perspective of adaptation theory helps us to understand the relationship between culture and health beliefs. In short, the theory proffers that people develop traditions for success that adapt to the larger environment in which they live.[11] For example, because Japanese view themselves in the context of the family unit, the delivery of health information to the family rather than the patient is desirable. Outside the family unit, esteem for the hierarchy might lead a patient to agree with the dentist or dental hygienist, out of respect, even if he or she has no intention to comply with given recommendations. The health professional who is not culturally sensitive may choose to view this patient in a negative way. Miscommunication then can influence trust and create stress and uncertainty on both sides.[11,12,13] If the health professional becomes frustrated or angry, the patient could become fearful of the dental experience and avoid visits altogether. Situations that cause tension and discomfort arise when different health belief systems clash. Responses under these conditions can include anxiety, anger, fear, and wariness. In any cross-cultural encounter, both parties need to acknowledge and respect health concepts and practices that differ from their own.[14] Lastly, consideration must be given to the balance between an individual's autonomy and freedom to practice personal beliefs versus the right of a community to be protected from harm. For example, allowing the use of open flame for ceremonial rites would be highly dangerous to people and the physical structure in a dental environment because of the presence of flammable liquids, gases, and other materials.

Providers who understand cultural behaviors of others will be better equipped to offer effective, individualized care and avoid cross-cultural misunderstanding. Focused consideration needs to be given to core cultural issues related to authority, physical contact, time orientation, communication styles, gender, sexuality, and family, among others. One must keep in mind that although such issues might have a cultural basis, they can be influenced by a patient's own beliefs and/or preferences.[15] On the other hand, the provider's personal biases and beliefs can be a hindrance to providing quality patient care.[16]

Cultural beliefs can shape one's views of illness/concepts of sickness and physical, mental, and spiritual well-being. A patient's understanding of the cause of illness, what is the expected treatment, the role of the sick individual, and how the illness affects his or her life is described as the **patient's explanatory model**.[15] The biomedical model of Western medicine posits that germs cause disease. The American Navajo culture believes that simply mentioning an illness will cause it.[17] Other cultures emphasize the disturbance of balance in the body, spirit possession, soul loss, or breach of taboos as the basis for illness and disease. Upset of body balance has its origins in China and has as its premise that a healthy body is in a state of balance and illness results when disruption occurs in this balance. In Asia, this balance is believed to exist in everything in the universe and is translated as hot (*yin*) and cold (*yang*). These terms refer to qualities, not temperature, and have nothing to do with the nature of good or bad. The balance between yin and yang is considered the ideal state.[18] Factors such as the improper balance of foods and sudden, strong emotional states influence yin and yang. Treatment for illness consists of restoring balance by using what are defined as "cold" foods, drinks, and herbs to cure a "hot" illness, and vice versa for a "cold" illness. To prevent disease, one would maintain a neutral diet and avoid extremes in daily living habits, such as drinking ice water.[18] Healthcare practitioners must exercise caution with generalities in health beliefs, which can lead a practitioner to demonstrate stereotypical beliefs that are inconsistent with clients' health beliefs. For example, hot food in one culture can be considered cold in another.[11]

DID YOU KNOW? ?

Communication is one of the most important attributes of a dental provider and is always an important component of successful interaction with all patients.

The explanatory model for the common cold is another example of understanding varying beliefs about illness. Clients might consider a cold to be caused by "being out in the cold" and will worsen to other illnesses such as pneumonia if not treated with antibiotics. Many Americans believe that they have not received appropriate care if they do not receive antibiotics for illnesses caused by viruses when in fact antibiotics are effective only against bacteria. In some cases, the patient's explanatory model may actually be a folk illness that does not fit well into the biomedical model of illness.[11,14] Although the beliefs about the causes of a cold are seemingly simple, more complex illnesses present greater challenges, particularly if the healthcare professional is not familiar with patients' sociocultural backgrounds. For any individual, it would be impossible to understand all cultural health beliefs, so the key to the successful care of a culturally diverse patient is to take into account the health beliefs of illness and disease when planning care.[19] A patient who believes an illness is caused by a spirit will not be cured by any amounts of antibiotics. Studies on placebo effects have shown that the mind is a very powerful aspect of human health and well-being. Adapting care to be congruent to the client's culture is central to the provision of culturally sensitive healthcare.[20]

DID YOU KNOW? ?

In America, cultural norms do not include taking infants to the dental provider for an assessment, rather many children do not visit a dental provider until they are three or older.

Another maxim for healthcare professionals is to be open to the health beliefs of other cultures and resist judging them.[20,21] Westerners may believe that germs cause disease because their mothers told them so even if they have never actually seen a germ. People who believe disease is caused by soul loss or spirit possession believe this because their mothers and healing experts told them so. Scientific evidence is not infallible, and most of us will believe what we see when others become ill and are healed when treated by whatever measure. Paradoxically, China is increasingly adopting Western medicine practices while Americans are embracing traditional Chinese medicine, such as tai chi (for exercise), the use of herbs, and acupuncture for pain relief. Certainly, the concept of balance (yin and yang) is not so dissimilar to the growing body of knowledge about stress and disease. Being open to the merits of other healing practices might uncover new areas for research investigations in efficacy and effectiveness.

CULTURAL COMPETENCE AND HEALTH OUTCOMES

Health professionals should examine their own cultural heritage, health beliefs, and biases to better understand cultural differences between themselves and their clients.[22,23,24] Health professionals should not assume that their own health beliefs and values are the same as those of their clients. Health professionals should become comfortable with cultural encounters and should refrain from making value judgments.[20] Recognizing and affirming the values and worth of individuals, family, and community are parts of being an accountable health professional based on professional ethnics and competencies for entry into the profession.[24,25]

Gaining knowledge of culturally driven health attitudes and practices is an important action measure to take before the first cultural encounter with a client. Whether these client attitudes and practices are based on the role of charms, potions, spells, herbs, tribal healers, or evil spirits, treating disease includes considering nutritional or dietary practices and food restrictions, such as for vegetarians or persons who fast for religious purposes or health beliefs. Oral health professionals can and should obtain as much knowledge as possible about the beliefs of the patient populations with which they interact in their community.[13,26] Gaining a knowledge of folk ways and alternative medical beliefs and behaviors also helps to inform healthcare recommendations.[13,26,27]

According to the 2010 Census, 18% of the U.S. population speaks a language other than English at home.[30] This percentage is higher in states whose population is most affected by immigration such as New Mexico, California, Arizona, Texas, Hawaii, New Jersey, and New York.[30] Clients with limited English proficiency encounter obstacles in obtaining adequate healthcare including these:

- Difficulty using the telephone to schedule appointments.
- Asking for and understanding directions to the healthcare facility.
- Providing incomplete or inaccurate information during the medical interview and when completing a health history that can lead to incorrect diagnosis and treatment.
- Being unable to understand implications for informed consent.
- Misunderstanding the need for follow-up care due to problems in understanding instructions.
- Having problems complying with specialized instructions for medications or chemotherapeutic agents.
- Misunderstanding details for referral appointments that decrease the likelihood of follow-up care.[11,14,28,29,31,32]

Culturally competent care is patient-centered care. Every patient encounter is a cultural encounter. In the healthcare setting, cultural competence suggests the ability to effectively interact with clients to work together in creating positive health outcomes. To this end, effective, understandable, and respectful care needs to be compatible with a patient's cultural health beliefs, practices, and language. Showing respect and care for another's beliefs will foster a client's trust.[21,22] This ability begins by learning to ask the right questions.

A useful model that healthcare providers can incorporate into their encounter is the LEARN model.[19] The primary focus is a suggested process for improving communication and has been shown to heighten awareness of cultural issues and achieve client acceptance of treatment plans. Guidelines for health practitioners in LEARN are:

L *Listen* with sympathy and understanding.

E *Explain* your perception of the problem.

A *Acknowledge* and discuss the differences and similarities.

R *Recommend* treatment.

N *Negotiate* agreement.

The LEARN model is intended to supplement the dental interview process, not to replace it. Relevant cultural, social, and personal information can be elicited and discussed to achieve appropriate communication between the provider and the client.[19]

Taking the time to question the client about his or her understanding of consent, a plan of care, or instructions for home care communicates care and interest. Using an appropriate interpreter, such as using phone interpreters if live interpreters are not available, is essential.[20,24,25] Avoiding hand gestures is critical because different gestures have different meanings in various cultures and can be quite offensive. Eliminating idioms in speech is a necessity because they have a basis in U.S. culture, but are not universally understood. Avoiding "yes" and "no" questions and encouraging clients to ask questions is a basic tenet for all health communication. Some clients may be very forthright, but others need some coaxing.[11] Taking time to ask clients if they have any questions is important because health professionals might believe themselves to be approachable and open to discussing concerns, but their clients might not view them in the same way.[11]

Results from the National Adult Literacy Survey reveal that some 90 million adults in the United States demonstrate literacy skills at the lowest levels of writing abilities.[32] Many factors help to explain why so many adults perform at this level. About two-thirds of the survey participants are either individuals who:

- May be learning to speak English.
- Did not complete high school or are of age 65 or older.
- Had physical, mental, or health conditions that kept them from actively participating in school, work, or other activities.
- Have visual difficulties that affect their ability to read print.

These individuals fail to perceive themselves to be "at risk" because of low literacy, yet they are less likely to respond correctly to literacy tasks requiring higher-level reading and problem-solving skills. They also experience difficulty in performing tasks that require them to integrate and synthesize information from complex or lengthy texts.[32] In dental care settings, patients might experience a problem reading and understanding medical/dental history forms, consent documents, or detailed written instructions. Low literacy has been associated with a number of adverse health outcomes such as "low health knowledge, increased incidence of chronic illness, higher risk of hospitalization, and less than optimal use of preventive health services."[33]

From a legal perspective, culturally competent care on the part of the oral healthcare provider can decrease the likelihood of liability or malpractice claims. A lack of awareness of cultural differences and the failure to provide culturally appropriate care may result, under the principles of tort law, in liability for breach of professional standards of care. Providing effective communication (both verbal and written) in other languages and addressing the need of individuals

with low or no literacy have been shown effective in reducing malpractice claims.[30]

SUMMARY

Achieving cultural competency is a lifelong commitment to become aware of one's biases and differences in one's own background to that of the client's cultural background. Effective communication skills, knowledge of disease incidence and prevalence, and treatment efficacy are essential to providing culturally competent care. One caveat is that healthcare professionals cannot rely solely on books, websites, or expert opinions for cultural knowledge, but must develop the

skills and ability to obtain cultural knowledge directly from each patient. Beyond awareness, the healthcare professional's journey is to develop beliefs, attitudes, values, skills, and policies that convey respect and empathy to people of all cultures, races, religions, and ethnic backgrounds. Advancing the body of knowledge through research that addresses new approaches and disseminates findings to achieve culturally competent practice is an ongoing goal.

PRACTICE CONSIDERATIONS

The U.S. population continues to increase in ethnic diversity. However, the oral health workforce has lagged behind these population trends.[34] Employers should focus close attention on hiring practices to achieve a diverse workforce whose staff members and leadership represent service area demographics.[35] Healthcare providers need specialized training in cross-cultural skills to care for patients of different sociocultural backgrounds.[13,22] The competency statements from the national associations representing oral healthcare providers and educators underscore the importance of an oral healthcare workforce that can meet diverse needs of underserved populations' healthcare.[3] Competencies describe the abilities of oral health professionals as they enter their respective professions. Keeping this in mind, oral health professionals are responsible for incorporating cultural and religious sensitivity in all professional interactions.[3,36,38]

Gaining competency is a process, a lifelong commitment to develop beliefs, attitudes, values, skills, and policies to respond with respect and empathy to people of all cultural, racial, religious, and ethnic backgrounds.[14,27,37,38,39] The best strategy to increase awareness of cultural diversity is through real-world experiences of interacting with and providing care for people of different cultures and ethnicities.[23,39,40] Participating in continuing education by reading, attending conferences and workshops, interacting with experts, and taking language classes are some formal ways to pursue the process of cultural competency.[13,37]

Assessing personal cultural competency by using standardized tools such as the Cross-Cultural Adaptability Inventory (CCAI) is one way to become aware of one's cultural values. This inventory assesses strengths and weaknesses in four skill areas: emotional resilience, flexibility/openness, perceptual acuity, and personal autonomy.[41] Another tool is the student

version of the Inventory for Assessing the Process of Cultural Competence Among Healthcare Professionals—Revised (IAPCC-SV©).[22] Identifying one's strengths and weaknesses in cross-cultural effectiveness, particularly when a student, may increase the person's motivation to improve skills when she or he is exposed to patient experiences and learning materials promoting cross-cultural effectiveness.[38,40] Furthermore, research has shown that college students who learn about intercultural communication have higher self-esteem and confidence when facing uncertainty and change.[43] Certainly, positive outcomes such as these are important to health professionals who experience uncertainty with every patient encounter.

Demonstrating sensitivity to differences that people will have in their dental experiences and responses to previous care based on their heritage, socioeconomic situation, ethnicity, and cultural background can be accomplished in verbal and nonverbal communications.[44] Asking patients how they would like to be addressed is important in the initial conversation because using a patient's first name may be quite offensive to some people. Many individuals prefer that their title (Mr., Mrs., Ms.) and last name be used as a sign of respect. Some cultures relate to authority figures by physical distancing themselves from others in comparison to close physical proximity. Observing the client and family members is one way to judge comfort zones. Maintaining professional proximity without unnecessary touching of the client respects the client's values about touching.[11,12,20]

If a patient does not establish eye contact, the professional should not become upset or offended by this behavior. In many cultures, making eye contact is considered impolite. Lastly, utilizing tools, such as the BELIEF instrument, to elicit patients' health beliefs can contribute to the oral health professional's understanding.[45]

SELF-STUDY QUESTIONS

1. What term describes a conceptual framework that has relevance in health, education, and practice that all individuals, groups, and organizations have?

   a. Diversity issues

   b. Health customs

   c. Culture

   d. Sensitivity

   Rationale: Culture is a conceptual framework that has relevance in health professions' research, education, and practice. All individuals, groups, and organizations have a culture.

2. The obligation to engage in the process of cultural competence is a professional responsibility grounded in societal expectation. Dental providers can demonstrate respect for cultural differences by acknowledging that a patient's beliefs and values on preventive care may be different from their own.

   a. The first statement is true; the second statement is false.

   b. The first statement is false; the second statement is true.

   c. Both statements are true.

   d. Both statements are false.

   Rationale: The obligation to engage in the process of cultural competence is a professional responsibility grounded in societal expectation. Dental providers can demonstrate respect for cultural differences by acknowledging that a patient's beliefs and values on preventive care may be different from their own.

3. From a legal perspective, culturally competent care on the part of the oral healthcare provider can decrease the likelihood of which of the following?

   a. Liability or malpractice claims

   b. Communication barriers

   c. Access to care

   d. Common health conditions

   Rationale: From a legal perspective, culturally competent care on the part of the oral healthcare provider can decrease the likelihood of liability or malpractice claims.

4. Which of the following describes the ability of oral health professionals as they enter their respective professions?

   a. Cultural diversity

   b. Cultural sensitivity

   c. Competency

   d. Morality

   Rationale: Competency describes the ability of oral health professionals as they enter their respective professions.

5. Which of these are ways to pursue cultural competency for a lifetime?

   a. Law school

   b. Continuing education

   c. Understanding one's self

   d. Competency education

   Rationale: Participating in continuing education by reading, attending conferences and workshops, interacting with experts, and taking language classes are some formal ways to pursue cultural competency.

REFERENCES

1. Cross, T., Bazron, B., Dennis, K., & Isaacs, M. (1989). *Towards a culturally competent system of care Volume I.* Washington, DC: Georgetown University Child Development Center, CASSP Technical Assistance Center.

2. Campinha-Bacote, J. (2003). *The process of cultural competence in the delivery of healthcare services: A culturally competent model of care.* Cincinnati, OH: Transcultural C.A.R.E. Associates.

3. American Dental Education Association. (2011). ADEA competencies for entry into the allied dental professions (As approved by the 2011 ADEA House of Delegates). *J Dent Educ,* 75:941–48.

4. Betancourt, J. R., Green, A. R., & Carrillo, J. E. (2002). *Cultural competence in health care: Emerging frameworks and practical approaches.* New York, NY: The Commonwealth Fund.

5. United States Census Bureau. State and County QuickFacts (2010). Retrieved January 27, 2012, http://quickfacts.census.gov/qfd/states/00000.html.

6. U.S. Census Bureau. (August 14, 2008). An older and more diverse nation by midcentury (news release). Public Information Office. Retrieved January 27, 2012 from http://www.census.gov/newsroom/releases/archives/population/cb08-123.html.

7. Giles, E. F. (2008). *Application of the interactional model of cultural diversity to identify diversity climate factors associated with organizational effectiveness in accredited U.S. physical therapist education programs.* Ph.D. dissertation. Old Dominion University, United States–Virginia. Retrieved January 27, 2012 from Dissertations & Theses: Full Text database. (Publication No. AAT 3338435).

8. Samuels, D. *Faculty preparedness to build cultural inclusiveness.* Ph.D. dissertation. University of Colorado at Colorado Springs, United States–Colorado. Retrieved January 27, 2012 from Dissertations & Theses: Full Text database. (Publication No. AAT 3406101).

9. Swanson, J. W. (2004). Diversity: Creating an environment of inclusiveness. *Nurs Admin Q,* 28:207–11.

10. Moore, T. A. (2012). The diversity dilemma: A national study of minorities in dental hygiene programs. Ed.D. dissertation. Wilmington University, United States—Delaware. Dissertations & Theses: Full Text database. Retrieved January 27, 2012, (Publication No. AAT 3491413).

11. Galanti, G. A. (2008). *Caring for patients from different cultures* (4th ed.). Philadelphia: University of Pennsylvania Press.

12. Spector, R. E. (2009). *Cultural diversity in health and illness* (7th ed.). Upper Saddle River, NJ: Pearson/Prentice Hall.

13. Kreps, G. L., & Kunimoto, E. N. (1994). *Effective communication in multicultural health care settings.* Thousand Oaks, CA: Sage Publications.

14. Charles, L. T., & Kennedy, D. B. (2001). Social and cultural influences on health. (Supercourse Lecture). Pittsburg, PA: WHO Collaborating Center, University of Pittsburg. Retrieved September 12, 2012, http://pitt.edu/~super1/lecture/lec4271/001.htm.

15. Carrillo, J. E., Green, A. R., & Betancourt, J. R. (1999). Cross-cultural primary care: A patient-based approach. *Ann Int Med,* 130:829–34.

16. Committee on Understanding and Eliminating Racial and Ethnic Disparities in Health Care. "Front Matter." (2003). Unequal treatment: Confronting racial and ethnic disparities in healthcare. Washington, DC: National Academies Press.

17. U.S. Department of Health & Human Services, Office of Minority Health. (2003). *A physician's practical guide to culturally competent care.* Washington, DC. Retrieved September 21, 2012, https://cccm.thinkculturalhealth.hhs.gov/default.asp?curcase=1.

18. Yuqun, L. (2010). *Traditional Chinese medicine: Understanding its principles and practice* (2nd ed.). Beijing, China: China Intercontinental Press.

19. Berlin, E. A., & Fowkes, W. C., Jr. (1983). A teaching framework for cross-cultural health care. *West J Med,* 139:934–38.

20. Purnell, L. D. (2009). *Guide to culturally competent health care* (2nd ed.). Philadelphia, PA: F. A. Davis Company.

21. Vaughn, E. J. (2008). Cultural competence and health education. In Pérez, M. A., & Luquis, R. R. *Cultural competence in health education and health promotion.* San Francisco, CA: Jossey-Bass, 43-62.

22. Campinha-Bacote, J. (2007). *The process of cultural competence in the delivery of healthcare services: The journey continues* (5th ed.). Cincinnati, OH: Transcultural C.A.R.E. Associates.

23. Fitch, P. (2004). Cultural competence and dental hygiene care delivery: Integrating cultural care into the dental hygiene process of care. *J Dent Hyg,* 78:11–21.

24. Spencer, A., & Trigilidas, J. (2008). Bridging the gap. *Dimensions Dent Hyg,* 6(12): 20–23.

25. American Dental Hygienists' Association. (March 2008). *Standards for clinical dental hygiene practice.* Chicago, IL: American Dental Hygienists' Association.

26. Luquis, R. R., & Pérez, M. A. (2008). Cultural competence and health education. In Pérez, M. A., & Luquis, R. R., Eds. *Cultural competence in health education and health promotion.* San Francisco, CA: Jossey-Bass, 231–44.

27. Connolly, I. (2011). Cultural competency. In Nathe, C. N., Ed. *Dental public health & research.* Upper Saddle River, NJ: Pearson, 156–67.

28. Prime®. (2009). *Cultural competency: A pocket guide for the health care professional.* Tamarc, FL: Prime®.

29. Gropper, R. C. (1996). *Culture and the clinical encounter: An intercultural sensitizer for the health professions.* Yarmouth, ME: Intercultural Press, Inc.

30. U.S. Census Bureau. (October 2003). *Language use and English-speaking ability: 2000.* Washington, DC: U.S. Department of Commerce, Economics and Statistics Administration.

31. Luciano, M., Overman, V. P., Fraiser, P. Y., & Platin, E. (2008). Survey of oral health practices among adults in a North Carolina Hispanic population. *J Dent Hyg,* 82:1–14.

32. Kirsch, I. S., Jungeblut, A., Jenkins, L., & Kolstad, A. (April 2002). *Adult literacy in America: A first look at the findings of the National Adult Literacy Survey* (3rd ed.). (NCES 1993-275). Washington, DC: U.S. Department of Education, Office of Educational Research and Improvement, National Center for Education Statistics.

33. Berkman, N. D., DeWalt, D. A., Pignone, M. P., Sheridan, S. L., Lohr, K. N., Sutton, S. F., Swinson, T., & Bonito, A. J. (January 2004). *Literacy and health outcomes.* Evidence report/Technology assessment No. 87. (AHRQ Publication No. 04-E007-h2). Rockville, MD: Agency for Healthcare Research and Quality.

34. Vemulakonda, V. M., & Sorensen, M. D. (2008). The current state of diversity and multicultural training in urology residency programs. *J Urol,* 180:687–672.

35. McKinnon, M., Luke, G., Bresch, J., Moss, M., & Valachovic, R. (2007). Emerging allied dental workforce models: Consideration for academic dental institutions. *J Dent Educ,* 71:1476–1491.

36. American Dental Hygienists Association. (2011). *ADHA bylaws and code of ethics for dental hygienists.* Retrieved September 21, 2012, http://www.adha.org/downloads/ADHA-Bylaws-Code-of-Ethics.pdf.

37. Wilson, A. H., Sanner, S., McAllister, L. E. (2010). A longitudinal study of cultural competence among health science faculty. *J Cult Diver,* 17:68–72.

38. Connolly, I. M., Darby, M. L., Tolle-Watts, L., & Thomson-Lakey, E. (2000). The cultural adaptability of health sciences faculty. *J Dent Hyg,* 74:102–9.

39. Aston-Brown, R. E., Branson, B., Cadbury-Amyot, C. C., & Bray, K. K. (2009). Utilizing public health clinics for service-learning rotations in dental hygiene: A four-year retrospective study. *J Dent Educ,* 73:358–74.

40. Gadbury-Amyot, C. C., Simmer-Beck, M., et al. (2006). Using a multifaceted approach including community-based service-learning to enrich formal ethics instruction in a dental school setting. *J Dent Educ,* 70:652–61.

41. Kelley, C., & Meyers, J. Cross-cultural adaptability inventory. (2012). Retrieved September 12, 2012, http://ccaiassess.com/Home_Page.html.

42. DeWald, J. P., & Solomon, E. S. (2009). Use of the Cross-Cultural Adaptability Inventory to measure cultural competence in a dental hygiene program. *J Dent Hyg,* 83:106–10.

43. Bolton, R. (1986). *People skills.* New York: Simon & Schuster.

44. Charbonneau, C. J., Neufeld, M. J., Craig, B. J., & Donnelly, L. R. (2009). Increasing cultural competence in the dental hygiene profession. *Can J Dent Hyg,* 43:297–305.

45. Dobbie, A. E., Medrano, M., Tysinger, J., & Olney, C. (2003). The BELIEF instrument: A preclinical teaching tool to elicit patients' health beliefs. *Fam Med,* 35:316–19.

46. U.S. Census Bureau. (2004). *US interim projections by age, sex, race and Hispanic origin 2000-2050*. Washington, D.C. Retrieved September 21, 2012, http://www.census.gov/population/www/projections/usinterimproj/

47. Randall-David, E. (1989). *Strategies for working with culturally diverse communities and clients*. Washington, DC: The Association for the Care of Children's Health.

48. Fadiman, A. (1997). *The spirit catches you and you fall down: A Hmong child, her American doctors, and the collision of two cultures*. New York, NY: Farrar, Straus and Giroux.

PEARSON myhealthprofessionskit™

Visit www.myhealthprofessionskit.com to access the interactive Companion Website for this textbook. Simply select "Dental Hygiene" from the choice of disciplines. Find this book and log in by using your user name and password to access additional learning tools.

For reference #8: Elizabeth Locke, contributor to this chapter, was previously Elizabeth Giles.

CHAPTER 3

Dental Hygiene Science

Christine N. Nathe
with contributions from
Christine French Beatty
Amy Teague
Kathleen O'Neill Smith
Carolyn Horton Ray

KEY TERMS

Assessment, 25
Comprehensive oral
  evaluation, 25
Dental hygiene, 23
Dental public health, 23
Diagnosis, 29
Implementation phase, 30
Periodic oral evaluation, 25
Planning phase, 29

OBJECTIVES

After studying this chapter, the student should be able to:

1. Describe the dental hygiene process of care.

2. Describe the integration of the dental hygiene process of care into the dental hygiene appointment.

3. Compare and contrast dental hygiene therapy for patients with and without attachment loss.

4. Describe the elements of the dental hygiene appointment.

5. Describe the use of the *CDT* in creating a dental hygiene care plan.

6. Define *dental public health*.

7. Describe community programs aimed at preventing diseases.

INTRODUCTION

Primary preventive dentistry emphasizes the science and practice of dental hygiene. The practice of dental hygiene is inherent in the primary prevention of dental diseases. **Dental hygiene** is defined as the practice of preventive oral health care and education. Comprehensive dental hygiene treatment includes assessment, dental hygiene diagnosis, planning, implementation with a focus on periodontal debridement and oral hygiene instruction, and evaluation, which a dental hygienist provides.

When defining dental hygiene, it is important to also define dental public health because of the interdependent relationship between the two disciplines in the provision of dental hygiene care. **Dental public health** is defined as the science and art of preventing and controlling dental diseases and promoting dental health through organized community efforts. Dental public health focuses on oral health care and education of a population, with an emphasis on the utilization of dental hygiene sciences. It is that form of dental practice that serves the community as patients rather than individuals. Dental public health is concerned with the dental health education of the public, with applied dental research and with the administration of group dental care programs as well as the prevention and control of dental diseases on a community basis.

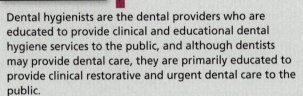

DID YOU KNOW

Dental hygienists are the dental providers who are educated to provide clinical and educational dental hygiene services to the public, and although dentists may provide dental care, they are primarily educated to provide clinical restorative and urgent dental care to the public.

DID YOU KNOW

Historically, dental hygiene was initiated as a public health profession developed to provide population-based preventive care and education to the masses.

EVIDENCE-BASED CARE

Providing care based upon scientific evidence should be inherent to primary dental care practice. There is frequently a gap between the published evidence and the evidence used by practitioners to make clinical decisions.[1] As researchers learn more about oral diseases, risk factors, and ways to prevent and control these diseases, clinicians will need to adjust their recommendations to match the new knowledge. The primary dental care provider needs to be informed of new evidence in relation to oral diseases, the efficacy and safety of self-care products,

and procedures to prevent oral diseases. Development of treatment and self-care plans should follow a systematic approach that incorporates prescribed techniques based on sound evidence in order to enhance plaque biofilm removal.

Preventive dental science should be based on known methods with predictable results rather than anecdotes. The concept of evidence-based care means that dental practice is based on independent research done by practitioners and scientists as reported in peer-reviewed journals. Evidence-based care also takes into account patient preferences. Commonly, dental providers will encounter patients who have selected an oral care product based on an advertisement or because the product worked for a friend; this highlights the importance of the provider being able to give advice supported by documented evidence.

Another reason that evidence-based care is important is the multifactorial nature of disease, which assumes that there are multiple causes of a disease or condition. Epidemiologists organize these factors—the host, the agent, and the environment—as the epidemiology triangle to demonstrate the interaction and interrelatedness of these factors over time in bringing about the disease or condition. In other words, the same anecdotal treatment that met with success on patient A does not guarantee the same results for patient B.

THE DENTAL HYGIENE PROCESS OF CARE

The process of care model is useful when determining the most appropriate products and practices in preventive dental care.[2] When providing care, the oral health professional must carefully assess numerous oral health and disease risk factors to be able to personalize recommendations for the most effective supplemental oral hygiene measures.

Having an understanding of risk for oral diseases is critical to being able to make decisions about treatment, prevention, and control of these conditions.[3] Identifying risk factors that relate to the development, progression, and maintenance of oral diseases and conditions is an essential aspect of dental hygiene care. These risk factors include current oral self-care practices as well as past and current oral health status in relation to all oral diseases and conditions.

Specifically, the dental hygiene process of care includes the assessment, dental hygiene diagnosis, planning, implementation, and evaluation of dental hygiene care of a target population.

The American Dental Hygienists' Association (ADHA) defines the process of care in the following policy definition as:

- **Assessment:** The systematic collection and analysis of data to identify patient needs.

- **Diagnosis:** The identification of patient strengths and oral health problems that dental hygiene intervention can improve.

- **Planning:** The establishment of realistic goals and the selection of dental hygiene interventions that can move the patient closer to optimal health.

TABLE ■ 3–1   Phases of the Process of Care Model

PHASES	ACTIVITIES
Assessment	Data of general and oral health status are systematically collected.
Diagnosis	Data are analyzed to formulate a diagnosis.
Planning	The evidence-based plan is derived and prioritized on the basis of mutually congruent goals.
Implementation	Delivery of preventive procedures to promote/maintain oral health and therapeutic procedures to control disease is performed to achieve oral health goals.
Evaluation	Attainment of oral health goals is mutually analyzed, and new care plan components are determined as necessary.

- **Implementation:** The act of carrying out the dental hygiene care plan.
- **Evaluation:** The measurement of the extent to which the patient has achieved the goals as specified in the plan as well as judgment to continue, discontinue, or modify the dental hygiene plan of care.[4]

DID YOU KNOW ❓

The process of care model can be applied to many facets of dental hygiene, including clinical care, education, and development of public health programs.

The process of dental hygiene care for the patient requires the application of biologic and psychosocial concepts of health and human functioning (Table 3–1 ■).

The dental hygiene appointment provides patient services that support total health through the promotion of optimal oral health. The dental hygiene appointment may include assessments, diagnoses, preventive oral prophylaxis, therapeutic scaling and root planing, periodontal debridement, education and counseling, preventive and therapeutic modalities, and/or supportive care. Formulation of a dental hygiene diagnosis may be necessary to direct the dental hygiene treatment during the appointment and to deliver quality oral health care. Several steps must occur before a dental hygiene diagnosis can be determined.

Dental hygienists frequently provide population-based dental health presentations to target populations but at times may operate a dental health program that entails more than just education. It also consists of providing dental hygiene education and treatment geared toward a population's needs. Population-based dental hygiene is a project designed to prevent disease in a target population. Prevention programs can occur in a wide range of settings, including communities, schools, long-term care facilities, health care support groups, and day care facilities. These programs involve the use of the dental hygiene process of care that encompasses the assessment, diagnosis, implementation, and evaluation stages of a dental public health program.

INDIVIDUALIZED DENTAL HYGIENE CARE

Assessment

The importance of this assessment phase cannot be overemphasized. Treatment plans and recommendations are always individualized based on the results of an assessment. Table 3–2 ■ presents the components of a comprehensive oral assessment that should be considered when making self-care recommendations.

These components reflect the human needs conceptual model.[5] This model focuses on the whole person rather than the disease and includes the concepts of the client, environment, health and oral health, and actions of the oral health care provider.[5]

Researchers have found that the assignment of risk scores for oral diseases varies among oral health practitioners. Computerized risk assessment tools have been developed to reduce the extent of variation and to increase the uniformity and accuracy of clinical decision making.[6]

The appointment begins with a thorough assessment of the patient. The systematic collection and analysis of data are necessary to identify patient needs. In the dental hygiene process, *patient* may refer to individuals, families, groups, or communities as defined in the ADHA Framework for Theory Development.[4]

Please note that the term *appointment* will be used to describe the integration of therapy used in the dental hygiene process of care. On the basis of the assessment, the dental hygienist can recognize deviation from health and intervene with appropriate therapy. The data collected during this process drive the treatment and care delivered to the patient. Assessment and analysis of risk factors provide information about a patient's periodontal disease susceptibility.[7–9] Recent evidence has identified certain risk factors that may make a patient more susceptible to periodontitis, and that may increase the extent and severity of the disease.[10]

The *CDT (Current Dental Terminology),* a manual published annually by the American Dental Association, provides a set of codes and accompanying definitions that reflect the commonly accepted dental procedures and can be used when billing dental insurance for procedures rendered. Although it is

TABLE ■ 3–2   Components of a Comprehensive Oral Assessment

Medical history

- Medical conditions
- Medications
- Allergies
- Physical/mental challenges
- Lifestyle, living circumstances, and social factors
- Mental health

Dental history

- Chief complaint
- Past periodontal treatment
- Past caries experience
- Exposure to fluoride
- Previous records and radiographs

Clinical examination

- Intraoral/extraoral soft tissues
- Temporomandibular joint (TMJ)
- Teeth and missing teeth
- Restorations
- Tooth mobility
- Tooth position
- Occlusal and interdental relationships
- Parafunctional habits[a]
- Periodontal soft tissues
- Probing depths, clinical attachment loss (CAL), and bleeding on probing
- Recession
- Mucogingival relationships
- Furcation involvement
- Hard and soft tissue trauma/lesions
- Flow and quality of saliva

Radiographs

- Caries
- Overhanging restorations and open margins
- Periodontal structures
- Furcation involvement
- Other pathology

Deposits

- Plaque
- Biofilm
- Calculus

Current self-care practices

- Use of products and devices
- Use of fluorides or other therapeutic agents
- Lifestyle (diet, tobacco, etc.)

Learning and compliance factors

- Coordination, dexterity, and ability
- Motivation and readiness
- Comprehension

[a]Parafunctional habit is the habitual use of a body part for other than the most common use, such as grinding teeth.

recognized that dental hygiene therapy is not driven by insurance codes, the dental provider must be aware of the utilization of the codes in treatment planning and implementation of therapy.

A **comprehensive oral evaluation** is always necessary to establish a baseline of medical and dental care. It is a thorough assessment of the extraoral and intraoral hard and soft tissues and may require interpretation of information acquired through additional diagnostic procedures. This **assessment** includes an evaluation for oral cancer, the patient's dental and medical history, and a general health assessment. "It includes the evaluation and recording of dental caries, missing or unerupted teeth, restorations, existing prostheses, occlusal relationships, periodontal conditions (including periodontal screening and/or charting), hard and soft tissue anomalies, etc." (D0150).[11]

If the patient is an established patient, a **periodic oral evaluation** is performed. The purpose of an evaluation performed on a patient of record is to determine any changes in the patient's dental and medical health status since a previous comprehensive or periodic evaluation. This procedure includes an oral cancer evaluation and a periodontal screening and/or charting when indicated and may require interpretation of information acquired through additional diagnostic procedures (D0120).[11]

Medical/Dental History

The concept that oral conditions can influence disease elsewhere in the body is not new; in fact, it can be dated back to the days of Hippocrates. Since the U.S. Surgeon General's report in 2000, awareness of the interaction between oral disease and systemic disease has increased.[12]

The mouth is no longer a separate entity from the body; what occurs in the mouth has disease implications for the entire body. Conditions such as cardiovascular disease, low-birth-weight infants and premature births, and respiratory tract infections have all been linked to periodontal disease.[13–18] Therefore, a thorough medical and family history must be taken and evaluated to identify predisposing conditions that may affect treatment, patient management, and outcomes. Such conditions include but are not limited to diabetes, hypertension, pregnancy, smoking, substance abuse, and medications, or other existing conditions that impact traditional dental therapy.[19] The dental provider must also thoroughly assess a patient's risk for certain oral diseases and conditions. A variety of health history forms that include health conditions to be considered before oral health care treatment (Figure 3–1 ■) is available.

Vital Signs

During a dental hygiene appointment, the following vital signs need to be measured: blood pressure, pulse, and/or respiration. *Respiration* is the fundamental process of life in which oxygen is used to oxidize organic fuel molecules, providing a source of energy as well as carbon dioxide and water.[20] Measurement of the patient's respiration involves observation of the depth of breath, rhythm, quality, and any sounds associated with breathing. The following steps are performed to measure respiratory rate: (1) count respirations so that the patient is not aware because the rate could be voluntarily or involuntarily altered, (2) maintain the finger over the radial pulse, (3) count respirations so that the patient is not aware because the rate could be voluntarily altered, and (4) count the number of times the chest rises in one clocked-minute.[21] All findings are recorded in the patient's record.

Extraoral/Intraoral Examination

An *examination* is any investigation or inspection made for the purpose of diagnosis, which is usually qualified by the method used.[22] Extraoral examination should include direct observation and palpation of the head, neck, skin, face, and gait. Intraoral examination should include screening and evaluating the oral mucosa, lips, floor of the mouth, tongue, salivary ducts, hard and soft palate, and oropharynx. The screening should also include detection of lesions and oral piercing.

Dental/Periodontal Examination

The *dental examination* will provide documentation of the exact location and condition of teeth, restorations, and dental caries.

UNM Health History

Date_____

_____
MEDICAL ALERT

Name_____

| Last | First | Initial | Soc. Sec. # | Home Phone | Business/Cell Phone |

| Address | City | State | Zipcode | Occupation | Employer |

Dr._____

| Birthdate | Sex | Height | Weight | Marital Status | Dentist's Name | Dentist's Phone |

Dr._____

| Physician's Name | Phone # | Person to contact in case of emergency | Phone # |

My last physical exam was on _____   Reason_____
                            Date

For the following questions check yes or no for the response that best applies. Your answers will be considered confidential. Please note that during your initial visit you will be asked some questions about your responses to this questionnaire and there may be additional questions concerning your health.

YES	NO	Patient Question	Provider's comments
		1. Are you in good health?	
		2. Are you now under the care of a physician?	
		3. Has there been any change in your general health within the past year?	
		4. Have you had any serious illness, operation, or been hospitalized in the past five years?	
		5. Have you had any problems with, or during, dental treatment?	
		6. Are you allergic, or had any reaction, to any medications, including local anesthetics?	
		7. Do you have any other allergies, such as metals, latex, food, pollen, etc.	
		Please check any of the following diseases or conditions you have experienced.	
		8. Damaged heart valves, artificial heart valves, shunts, heart murmur, or rheumatic fever	
		9. Cardiovascular disease such as heart trouble, heart attack, angina, high blood pressure, hardening of the arteries, stroke, etc.	
		10. Born with any heart problems	
		11. Sinus trouble, asthma, or hayfever	
		12. Fainting spells, seizures, epilepsy, or convulsions	
		13. Persistent diarrhea, weight loss, or vomiting	
		14. Diabetes	
		15. Hepatitis, yellow jaundice, cirrhosis, or liver disease	
		16. AIDS or HIV infection, Date of Diagnosis:_____ Current viral load count: _____ Current t-cell count or % _____	
		17. Thyroid problems (goiter)	
		18. Respiratory problems, emphysema, bronchitis, etc.	
		19. Arthritis or painful swollen joints	
		20. Stomach ulcer, hyperacidity, or other conditions	

FIGURE ■ 3–1 Sample health history form.

(*Source:* Reprinted by permission from Christine Nathe, University of New Mexico, Division of Dental Hygiene, Albuquerque, NM, 2008.)

	21 Kidney conditions or dialysis	
	22. Tuberculosis or positive TB skin test	
	23. Anemia or blood disorders	
	24. Gonorrhea, syphilis, herpes, or other similar diseases	
	25. Problems with mental health or nerves	
	26. Cancer	
	27. Prosthetic devices (joints, valves, hearing aid, implants) other than dentures	
	28. Use tobacco or snuff products	
	29. Diagnosed with alcoholism	
	30. Vision or hearing problems	
	31. Use recreational drugs	
	32. Pregnant or nursing a baby	
	33. Ever taken Redux or Ponimi "fen-phen"	
	Are you taking any medications, including any non-prescription medications or natural supplements? (birth control, calcium, ginseng, garlic, etc.)	

Medication Name:	Condition Used For	Dental Implications	Resource

I certify that I have read and understand the above questionnaire and that my medical condition may affect my dental health and treatment. I have answered the questions willingly, truthfully, and to the best of my ability.

_____   _____
Signature of Patient or Legal Guardian   Date

_____   _____
Signature of Student   Date

_____   _____
Signature of Dental Provider   Date

Vital Signs: Blood Pressure_____   Pulse_____   Respiration_____

FIGURE ■ 3–1 *(Continued)*

Date:_____

Please describe any changes in your health since you last completed this form and any medication you are taking. Write NONE if there has been no change.

_____
_____
_____
_____
_____

Vital Signs: Blood Pressure_____ Pulse_____ Respiration_____
Patient or Parent/Guardian Signature:_____
Student Signature _____ Faculty/Dentist Signature:_____

Date:_____

Please describe any changes in your health since you last completed this form and any medication you are taking. Write NONE if there has been no change.

_____
_____
_____
_____
_____

Vital Signs: Blood Pressure_____ Pulse_____ Respiration_____
Patient or Parent/Guardian Signature:_____
Student Signature _____ Faculty/Dentist Signature:_____

Date:_____

Please describe any changes in your health since you last completed this form and any medication you are taking. Write NONE if there has been no change.

_____
_____
_____
_____
_____

Vital Signs: Blood Pressure_____ Pulse_____ Respiration_____
Patient or Parent/Guardian Signature:_____
Student Signature _____ Faculty/Dentist Signature:_____

Date:_____

Please describe any changes in your health since you last completed this form and any medication you are taking. Write NONE if there has been no change.

_____
_____
_____
_____
_____

Vital Signs: Blood Pressure_____ Pulse_____ Respiration_____
Patient or Parent/Guardian Signature:_____
Student Signature _____ Faculty/Dentist Signature:_____

FIGURE ■ 3–1 *(Continued)*

The *periodontal examination* is the recognition of health, gingivitis, or periodontitis. This evaluation should include, but not be limited to, periodontal probing, loss of attachment calculations, presence of plaque biofilm and exudates, tooth mobility, and presence of clinical furcations and/or mucogingival defects.

Self-Care Evaluation

Review of current self-care practices and evaluation of the patient's skill levels and knowledge of hygiene practices should be investigated and recorded in the patient record. The effectiveness of self-care should also be documented. Many dental indices are available for the dental hygienist to incorporate in the patient's disease control monitoring; these aid in quantifying and evaluating disease and health.

Diagnostic Radiographs

Radiographs are used to confirm and diagnose the disease process. They should be of diagnostic quality and properly identified and dated. Information attained from the patient assessment is reviewed, and the findings are used in the dental hygiene diagnosis to establish realistic goals and treatment strategies.

Diagnosis

During the diagnosis and planning phases of the process of care model, appropriate preventive oral self-care practices and products to address the risks are jointly determined with the individual. Involvement of the patient in this decision-making process will increase the level of commitment and success of behavioral changes. A **diagnosis** is the determination of the nature of disease made from the study of the signs and symptoms.[23] Dental caries and periodontal disease are the two most common dental diagnoses.

S. Miller introduced dental hygiene diagnoses in 1982.[24] Miller suggested that the judgment and decision making of dental hygienists involved the formulation of a dental hygiene diagnosis. The ADHA published *dhdx* in 2005. The position paper recognizes the necessity of the dental hygiene diagnosis for the development, implementation, and evaluation of the dental hygiene treatment plan. To provide comprehensive quality oral health care, dental hygienists must fulfill the professional obligation of formulating a dental hygiene diagnosis.[25,26]

The assessment phase of the dental hygiene process of care provides the dental hygienist with an abundant amount of information to analyze, synthesize, and interpret. The hygienist uses information attained from the patient assessment to derive a dental hygiene diagnosis. This term has a specificity that implies the treatment is limited to that which can be accomplished by qualified and licensed hygienists.

Historically, dental hygienists have documented findings of the assessment phase in the patient's records along with the completed treatment notes. The dental hygiene diagnosis requires hygienists to take the process a step further by organizing the documentation to include probable cause and potential resolution that can be achieved by their intervention (Figure 3–2 ■).

In collaboration with the dental hygiene diagnosis, dental hygienists must determine the dental diagnoses. When clinical attachment loss is noted on the comprehensive periodontal evaluation, the dental diagnoses should use radiographs to confirm the degree of attachment loss. The extent and severity of gingival/periodontal disease can be determined with the criteria set forth by the American Academy of Periodontology.

A diagnosis and proposed treatment plan that is based on the results of the examination should be presented to the patient. Patients should be informed of the disease process, therapeutic alternatives, potential complications, the expected results, and their responsibilities in treatment. Consequences of no treatment should also be explained to the patient.[27]

Planning

During the **planning phase** of the dental hygiene process of care, dental hygiene therapy must be determined along with the establishment of realistic patient goals. The dental hygiene care plan serves as a component of the dental treatment plan (Figure 3–3 ■). It should be unique and customized on the basis of the findings of the assessment and diagnosis. The dental hygiene therapy, that is, self-care education, periodontal debridement, and so forth, includes all elements of the care plan.

Dental hygiene process of care.

Assessment Outcomes
Generalized bleeding on probing
50% plaque index
History of dental neglect
Localized 5- to 7-mm probing depths
30% attachment loss evident on x-rays

DHDX
Erythematous, enlarged marginal & papillary gingiva with BOP indicative of generalized, moderate gingivitis; localized areas of 5- to 7-mm attachment loss evident on radiographs, indicative of localized severe chronic periodontitis. Pt's hx would suggest inadequate plaque removal as 1° etiologic factor.

Possible DH Therapy
Periodontal debridement/periodontal scaling and root planing
Individualized oral hygiene instructions
Subgingival irrigation
Selective/coronal polishing
Appropriate periodontal maintenance appts.

DHDX, dental hygiene diagnosis; BOP, bleeding on probing; pt, patient; hx, history; 1°, first degree (primary); DH, dental hygiene; appts, appointments.

FIGURE ■ 3–2 Dental hygiene process of care.

(*Source:* Developed from the Commission on Dental Accreditation Standards 2008.)

The amount of time needed for the implementation of the therapy will guide the appointment planning. Elements to be considered in planning appointment times are number of appointments needed, allocation of time for dental hygiene interventions, and the sequencing of appointments. Patient involvement is essential to ensure informed consent and the setting of appropriate and realistic patient goals.

Implementation

During the implementation phase of the model, the oral health professional can then apply individualized, theory-based, and evidence-based educational and motivational strategies to facilitate behavioral change. This process should be accomplished during the appointments required for therapy.[28] Ensuring that recommended self-care plans are personalized and consistent with the lifestyle of the individual will increase the potential for long-term compliance. Monitoring and reinforcing at regular intervals will also increase compliance with

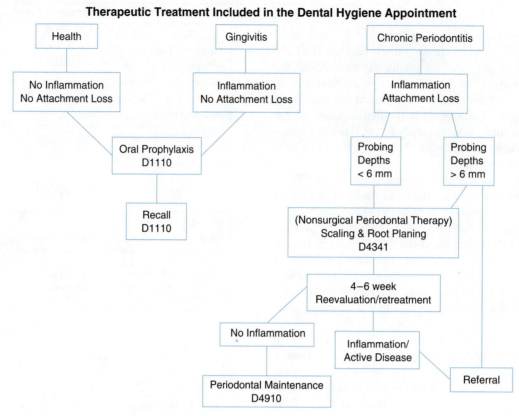

Therapeutic Treatment Included in the Dental Hygiene Appointment

FIGURE ■ 3–3 Dental hygiene care plan.

recommendations.[28] The self-care plan is documented in the dental chart and modified as needed at subsequent re-care or follow-up visits on the basis of the evaluation results. This type of documentation allows for continuity of care.

The **implementation phase** of the dental hygiene process of care occurs when treatment begins. Implementation begins with preparing the operatory for the treatment, using proper infection control procedures, and selecting the materials, instruments, and equipment to be utilized. The treatment is then performed by providing oral prophylaxis, pain management, periodontal debridement, patient instruction, selective coronal polishing, and/or other procedures identified in the planning phase (Figure 3–4 ■).

Even though the recall/maintenance dental hygiene appointment is typically an "hour," the dental hygienist really has only about 50 minutes for the patient. The appointment can be divided into segments[35]:

- Assessment (15 minutes)
  - Patient history (update with blood pressure)
  - Clinical data collection (intra- and extraoral exam), periodontal and dental charting
  - Radiographs
- Diagnosis/planning/implementation (30 minutes)
  - Diagnosis
  - Treatment planning

  - Informed consent
  - Patient instruction
  - Instrumentation (use of hand and/or ultrasonic instruments for removal of bacteria)
  - Selective coronal polishing
  - Fluoride application
- Evaluation/reevaluation (5 minutes).
  - Retreatment of localized active sites by instrumentation.
  - Application of chemotherapeutic agent as needed.
  - Dentist's examination if necessary.
- Disinfection (10 minutes).
  - Break down of unit.
  - Set up for next appointment.
  - Reschedule patient.

Table 3–3 ■ provides additional information about dental hygiene procedures and the process of diagnosis.

Evaluation

The evaluation phase of the process of care model focuses on outcomes to determine whether modifications to the oral hygiene strategies are indicated. The evaluation process is continuous over the patient's life span because the dentition and soft tissues may become altered with time, and the patient's abilities and dexterity change. Continuation or change of a self-care plan is based on outcomes such as current condition of the soft and hard tissues and changes made to the modifiable risk factors.[29] Involvement of the individual in these decisions will help to ensure long-term commitment to the oral self-care plan.[30]

Evaluation assesses the effectiveness and outcome of the completed treatment. The success of instrumentation is determined by evaluating the periodontal tissue after treatment and during the maintenance phase of therapy.[31] This evaluation will serve as the basis for determining whether the treatment was successful or if adjunct therapy is warranted.

Dental hygiene care plan.

Assessment	Appt. 1	Appt. 2	Appt. 3	Appt. 4	Appt. 5	Appt. 6
Chief complaint						
Medical/dental history						
Vital signs						
Intra- and extraoral examination						
Dental charting						
Periodontal examination						
Plaque indices						
Gingival assessment						
Risk assessment						
Radiographs						
Planning						
DH diagnosis						
Informed consent						
Implementation						
Pain management						
Periodontal debridement/scaling						
Ultrasonic debridement						
Hand scaling						
Subgingival irrigation						
Application of chemotherapeutic agents						
Selective/coronal polishing						
Application of pit-and-fissure sealants						
Fluoride application						
Health education/preventive						
Counseling						
Brushing						
Interdental aids						

FIGURE ■ 3–4 Therapeutic treatment included in the dental hygiene appointment.

(*Source:* Developed from the Commission on Dental Accreditation Standards.)

Nutritional counseling					
Infection control					
Desensitization					
Care of restorations					
Evaluation					
Reevaluation of oral/periodontal health					
Continuing care					
Recall					
Periodontal maintenance					
Referral(s)					

Note: DH, dental hygiene; appt., appointment.

FIGURE ■ 3–4 *(Continued)*

POPULATION-BASED DENTAL HYGIENE/DENTAL PUBLIC HEALTH ACTIVITIES

Dental health is a wide-reaching field of study, but it is grounded in distinct concepts within public health. The American Board of Dental Public Health (ABDPH) defines dental public health as:

> the science and art of preventing and controlling dental diseases and promoting dental health through organized community efforts. It is that form of dental practice that serves the community as a patient rather than the individual. It is concerned with the dental health education of the public, with applied dental research, and with the administration of group dental care programs, as well as the prevention and control of dental diseases on a community basis. Implicit in this definition is the requirement that the specialist have broad knowledge and skills in public health administration, research methodology, the prevention and control of oral diseases, and the delivery and financing of oral health care.[32]

Many times preventive dental care and education can be accomplished via dental public health activities. Public health is concerned with the health care of all. It focuses on the health of a population as a whole, rather than on the treatment of an individual. Thus, oftentimes, public health is focused on populations as opposed to individuals. The goal of public health is to protect and promote the health of the public across three essential domains: health protection, disease prevention and health promotion.[33] See Table 3–4 ■ for a comparison of individualized care (dental clinician) and population-based care (dental public health practitioner).

Assessment

As with other public health programs, effective programs for dental public health monitor the health of communities and populations at risk to identify health problems and priorities. Data needed to plan, monitor, and evaluate policies and programs for dental public health come from a number of sources.

Cancer Registries

State-based cancer registries are data systems that collect, manage, and analyze data about cancer cases and cancer deaths. In each state, medical facilities (including hospitals, physicians' offices, therapeutic radiation facilities, freestanding surgical centers, and pathology laboratories) report these data to a central cancer registry. These registries provide the ability to monitor trends in the number of new cases, oral cancer incidence rates (i.e., number of new cases per 100,000 population), oral cancer survival rates, and cancer stage at the time of diagnosis.

Vital Statistics

Vital statistics include data on birth, death, marriage, and divorce. One vital statistic of interest to dental public health is number of deaths from oral and pharyngeal cancer. The number of oral and pharyngeal cancer deaths and mortality rates (i.e., number of deaths from oral cancer per 100,000 population) are available for the nation, all 50 states, and the District of Columbia. Oral and pharyngeal cancer mortality statistics are from CDC's National Vital Statistics System.[34]

Clinical Surveys

The primary current source of national data on the most common oral health conditions is the National Health and Nutrition Examination Survey (NHANES), conducted by National Center for Health Statistics (NCHS). The survey is unique in that it combines interviews and physical examinations, including oral health examinations conducted by trained dental examiners. The most recent oral health data from NHANES were released in April 2007 and included data through 2004.[35]

At least 15 state dental programs have conducted statewide clinical surveys within the past six years, although none included adults.[36] Most states employed the Basic Screening Survey (BSS), which was developed by the Association of State and Territorial Dental Directors (ASTDD).[37] The BSS was developed as a simple training and data collection

TABLE ■ 3–3   Sample Treatment Options Based on Individual Dental Hygiene Diagnosis

Generalized moderate gingivitis (no attachment loss)

Procedures

Comprehensive oral examination (D0150)

Focused medical review (FMR) (D0210)

Oral hygiene instructions (OHI) (D1330)

Oral prophylaxis (D1110)

Selective polishing

Nutrition (D1310)

Smoking cessation (D1320)

Suitable maintenance interval

Generalized slight periodontitis (1- to 2-mm attachment loss)

Procedures (multiple appointments based on patient assessment and needs)

First appointment

Comprehensive oral health examination

FMR

OHI

Second appointment

Periodontal scale and root plane—4 quads (D4341)

Suitable periodontal maintenance appointment (D4910)

Generalized moderate periodontitis (3- to 4-mm attachment loss)

Procedures

First appointment

Comprehensive oral examination

FMR

OHI

Multiple appointments based on patient assessment and needs

Second appointment

Periodontal scale and root plane—2 quads (D4341)

Disease control/nutritional counseling (D1310)

Tobacco cessation (D1320)

Irrigation (D9630)

Suitable periodontal maintenance appointments (D4910)

Generalized severe periodontitis (5+-mm attachment loss)

Procedures

First appointment

Comprehensive oral examination

FMR

OHI

Multiple appointments based on patient assessment and needs

Second appointment

Periodontal scale and root plane (starting with worst quad)

Anesthesia

Disease control/nutritional counseling

Tobacco cessation

Irrigation (D9630)

(continued)

TABLE ■ 3–3 (Continued)

Third appointment

Periodontal scale and root plane quad

Anesthesia

Disease control/nutritional counseling

Irrigation

Fourth appointment

Periodontal scale and root plane quad

Anesthesia

Tobacco cessation

Irrigation

Fifth appointment

Periodontal scale and root plane quad

Anesthesia

Disease control/nutritional counseling

Tobacco cessation

Irrigation

Sixth appointment

Reevaluation

Coronal polishing

Localized chemotherapeutic agents (D4381)

Desensitizing medicament (D9910)/(D9911)

Referral for periodontal consult

TABLE ■ 3–4 Comparison of the Procedures Used by the Dental Clinician and the Dental Public Health Practitioner

DENTAL CLINICIAN	DENTAL PUBLIC HEALTH PRACTITIONER
Focuses on individual patient	**Focuses on community**
Conducts examination	Implements public health surveillance
Establishes diagnosis	Conducts analysis
Discusses findings with patient; develops treatment plan	Engages community partners; plans programs; develops policy
Provides treatment	Operates program
Receives payment for services	Obtains financing; conducts cost-effectiveness analysis
Schedules periodic follow-up visits	Conducts program evaluation

tool that could be used by screeners with or without dental backgrounds.

Nonclinical Oral Health Surveys

A wealth of information relevant to planning and monitoring oral health issues can be derived from nonclinical surveys. These surveys involve collection of data via telephone surveys, face-to-face interviews, or self-completed questionnaires, but they do not require clinical examination of participants. These types of surveys are often the most economically and logistically feasible way to reach adults, and valid data on many relevant oral health topics can be covered through self-reported surveys. The National Oral Health Surveillance System (NOHSS) is responsible for recognizing the need for uniform surveillance of key oral health indicators among the states. The NOHSS was developed as a collaborative effort between CDC's Division of Oral Health and the ASTDD[38] and is designed to monitor the burden of oral disease, use of the delivery system for oral health care, and the status of community water fluoridation on both a national and state level. It includes nine oral health indicators:

1. **Dental visit:** Adults aged 18+ who have visited a dentist or dental clinic in the past year.
2. **Teeth cleaning:** Adults aged 18+ who have had their teeth cleaned in the past year (among adults with natural teeth who have ever visited a dentist or dental clinic).

3. **Complete tooth loss:** Adults aged 65+ who have lost all of their natural teeth because of tooth decay or gum disease.

4. **Loss of six or more teeth:** Adults aged 65+ who have lost six or more teeth because of tooth decay or gum disease.

5. **Fluoridation status:** Percentage of people served by public water systems who receive fluoridated water.

6. **Dental sealants:** Percentage of third-grade students with dental sealants on at least one permanent molar tooth.

7. **Caries experience:** Percentage of third-grade students with caries experience, including treated and untreated tooth decay.

8. **Untreated tooth decay:** Percentage of third-grade students with untreated tooth decay.

9. **Cancer of the oral cavity and pharynx:** Incidence and mortality rates, survival rates, and stage at diagnosis for oral and pharyngeal cancer.

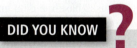

DID YOU KNOW

By accessing www.nohss.gov, a dental provider can review these oral health indicators for their respective state and compare their states to the national averages.

Diagnosis

When diagnosing for a population, the most common findings are generalized to determine need. The diagnosis is the natural conclusion to the assessment phase and focuses on those needs that can be fulfilled through dental hygiene care. The diagnosis will basically address the needs and be prioritized depending on importance.

Planning

After prioritizing the needs and deciding which direction the program will follow, the planner draws a dental program blueprint. This blueprint along with the methods to measure the program's effectiveness is created during the planning stage. A program's effectiveness can be measured both quantitatively and qualitatively. Pretest/posttest exams and dental indices can be developed to measure goals quantitatively. Surveys, interviews, and personal statements contribute to the qualitative measure of a program.

The planner first draws upon the assessment of the target population used in forming the diagnosis. Information regarding this population provides the basis for the formulation of program operations. The blueprint identifies the goals and objectives, activities planned and possible constraints that might be encountered and detailed strategies to overcome difficulties. In addition, alternative areas to develop resources should be addressed. The planning stage in dental public health often involves a variety of entities. Dental public health programs seek to provide these preventive services to whole communities (Table 3–5 ■) Many of the programs targeting children use school-based approaches, which are conducted in schools, or linked approaches, which are conducted in schools, private dental practices, and clinic settings outside of schools.

Implementation

At this stage, the program will actually begin operations. Revising the program and employing changes as necessary come into play during the implementation. A program planner should not be discouraged by difficulties evidenced at this stage. Most programs require revisions because of difficulties not forecasted or additional needs originally not assessed.

TABLE ■ 3–5   **Community Strategies for Prevention of Key Oral Diseases and Conditions**

Communitywide health promotion is an activity that includes educational, political, regulatory, and organizational interventions of the following:

Dental caries

- Fluoride use
- Community water fluoridation
- School water fluoridation
- Salt fluoridation[a]
- School-based dietary fluoride tablets
- School-based fluoride mouthrinse
- Fluoride varnish
- School-based and school-linked sealant programs
- School-based screening and referral

Periodontal diseases

- School-based personal hygiene, reinforcement of personal oral hygiene habits in Head Start or primary school classrooms
- School-linked screening and referral

(continued)

TABLE ■ 3–5 (Continued)

Oral and pharyngeal cancers
- Cancer screening programs

Inherited disorders
- Early detection programs

Trauma
- Mouth protector fittings for entire team

[a]Salt fluoridation is not currently used in the United States, but is used in several European and South American countries.
(*Source:* U.S. Department of Health and Human Services. (2000). *Oral health in America: A report of the Surgeon General.* Bethesda, MD: U.S. Department of Health and Human Services, National Institutes of Health, National Institute of Dental and Craniofacial Research, 156.)

Evaluation

Evaluation of the program is important and must be addressed to determine the program's success. Moreover, doing so aids in the ongoing revisions necessary to keep the program functioning at the optimum level. The methods used to evaluate the program are determined in the planning phase. Throughout the dental public health program and upon its completion, the dental provider uses scientific techniques to ascertain its effectiveness. Without evaluations, dental health programs cannot be promoted as effective tools in preventing and/or treating dental diseases.

The evaluation assesses the desired outcomes of the program and determines the strengths and weaknesses of the workforce, the strategies used, and the organization of the program itself.

To measure the goals, the provider uses baseline data and develops revisions to improve the outcomes. Evaluation of the program is an ongoing process. Moreover, it is important to provide qualitative and quantitative documentation of the program to the target population, administrators, funding agency, and public on an ongoing basis.

SUMMARY

As an oral health educator, it is the responsibility of every dental provider to teach the patient that oral disease is a disease like other ailments in the body and deserves treatment. The interrelationships exist between the oral environment and every other system in the body. Having a chronic infection is a serious problem that should not be ignored. Although treating periodontal disease will not guarantee patients a lifetime of health, it is one step they can take toward a healthier life overall.

Assessment, diagnosis, planning, implementation, and evaluation are the essential elements of the dental hygiene process of care. To meet each patient's distinct oral health care needs, the dental hygienist must formulate an individualized dental hygiene diagnosis and a comprehensive treatment plan. The dental hygiene process of care provides the criteria and mechanisms to establish such a plan.

Dental public health uses organized, interdisciplinary efforts to address the oral health concerns of communities and populations. A large part of the mission of dental public health is achieved through the application of health-promotion and disease-prevention technologies and interventions.

PRACTICAL CONSIDERATIONS

When providing dental treatment with an individual patient, it is always important to include preventive dental hygiene care or plan for dental hygiene intervention. Primary preventive dentistry can avert dental disease and the resulting systemic consequences. On a broad spectrum, dental hygiene should be incorporated into a public health model to provide preventive dental interventions and education to the masses. Dental public health activities will provide dental hygiene modalities to an increased number of people, thus benefitting many individuals who may not access dental care on their own accord.

SELF-STUDY QUESTIONS

1. Dental public health uses organized, interdisciplinary efforts to address the oral health concerns of communities and populations. A large part of the mission of dental public health is achieved through the application of health-promotion and disease-prevention technologies and interventions.

a. The first statement is true; the second statement is false.

b. The first statement is false; the second statement is true.

c. Both statements are true.

d. Both statements are false.

Rationale: Dental public health uses organized, interdisciplinary efforts to address the oral health concerns of communities and populations. A large part of the mission of dental public health is achieved through the application of health-promotion and disease-prevention technologies and interventions.

2. Health promotion is defined as

a. Health education

b. Health awareness

c. Healthy behaviors

d. Healthy habits

Rationale: Health promotion is a broader concept than health education and classically has been defined as any combination of educational, organizational, economic, and environmental supports for behavior conducive to health.

3. Which of the following are indicators of oral health?

a. Dental visits

b. Teeth cleanings

c. Dental hygienists to dentists ratios

d. Both A and B

Rationale: The nine oral health indicators include the following:

1. **Dental visit:** Adults aged 18+ who have visited a dentist or dental clinic in the past year.
2. **Teeth cleaning:** Adults aged 18+ who have had their teeth cleaned in the past year (among adults with natural teeth who have ever visited a dentist or dental clinic).
3. **Complete tooth loss:** Adults aged 65+ who have lost all of their natural teeth because of tooth decay or gum disease.
4. **Loss of six or more teeth:** Adults aged 65+ who have lost six or more teeth because of tooth decay or gum disease.
5. **Fluoridation status:** Percentage of people served by public water systems who receive fluoridated water.
6. **Dental sealants:** Percentage of third-grade students with dental sealants on at least one permanent molar tooth.
7. **Caries experience:** Percentage of third-grade students with caries experience, including treated and untreated tooth decay.
8. **Untreated tooth decay:** Percentage of third-grade students with untreated tooth decay.
9. **Cancer of the oral cavity and pharynx:** Incidence and mortality rates, survival rates, and stage at diagnosis for oral and pharyngeal cancer.

4. Which of the following is the correct order for the dental hygiene process of care?

a. Assessment, dental hygiene diagnosis, implementation, planning, evaluation

b. Assessment, planning dental hygiene diagnosis, implementation, evaluation

c. Assessment, evaluation, planning, implementation, evaluation

d. Assessment, dental hygiene diagnosis, planning, implementation, evaluation

Rationale: The dental hygiene process of care is as follows:

- **Assessment:** The systematic collection and analysis of data to identify client's (patient's) needs.
- **Dental hygiene diagnosis:** The identification of client (patient) strengths and oral health problems that dental hygiene intervention can improve.
- **Planning:** The establishment of realistic goals and the selection of dental hygiene interventions that can move the client (patient) closer to optimal health.
- **Implementation:** The act of carrying out the dental hygiene care plan.
- **Evaluation:** The measurement of the extent to which the client (patient) has achieved the goals as specified in the plan. Use judgment to continue, discontinue, or modify the dental hygiene plan of care.

5. Which of the following are dental hygiene community strategies?

a. School-based fluoride mouthrinse

b. Oral prophylaxis

c. Periodontal probing

d. Digital imaging

Rationale: The following are examples of dental hygiene community strategies: community water fluoridation, school water fluoridation and school-based fluoride mouthrinse, fluoride varnish, and school-based sealant programs.

REFERENCES

1. Pravikoff, D. S. (2004). The evidence-based practice dilemma. *CINAHLnews,* 23:6–7.
2. Nathe, C. N. (2011). *Dental public health and research* (3rd ed.). Upper Saddle River, NJ: Pearson, 131.
3. Anusavice, K. (2001). Clinical decision-making for coronal caries management in the permanent dentition. *J Dent Educ,* 65:1143–46.
4. American Dental Hygienists' Association. (1993). Policy 18–96, Glossary. Chicago: American Dental Hygienists' Association.

5. Darby, M. L., & Walsh, M. M. (2010). *Dental hygiene theory and practice* (3rd ed.). St. Louis, MO: Elsevier, 17.
6. Persson, G. R., Mancl, L. A., Martin, J., & Page, R. C. (2003). Assessing periodontal disease risk. A comparison of clinicians' assessment versus a computerized tool. *J Am Dent Assoc,* 134:575–82.
7. Page, R., & Beck, J. (1997). Risk assessment for periodontal disease. *Int Dent J,* 47:61.
8. Genco, R., et al. (1999). Overview of risk factors for periodontal disease and implications for diabetes and cardiovascular diseases. *Compendium,* 19 (Suppl):40.
9. Genco, R. J. (1996). Current view of risk factors for periodontal diseases. *J Periodontol,* 7:1041.
10. Newman, M. G., Korman, K. S., & Holtzman, S. (1994). Association of clinical risk factors with treatment outcomes. *J Periodontol,* 65:489–97.
11. American Dental Association. (2007). *CDT current dental terminology 2007–2008.* Chicago, IL: American Dental Association Health Foundation.
12. U.S. Department of Health and Human Services, Center for Disease Control and Prevention. (2001). *Healthy people 2000—Final review.* Retrieved September 5, 2012, from http://www.cdc.gov/nchs/data/hp2000/hp2k01.pdf.
13. Herzberg, M. C., & Meyer, M. W. (1996). Effects of oral flora on platelets: Possible consequences in cardiovascular disease. *J Periodontol,* 67: 1138–42.
14. Loesche, W. J. (1994). Periodontal disease as a risk factor for heart disease. *Compend Contin Edu Dent,* XV:976–91.
15. Loesche, W. J., Schork, A., Terpenning, M. D, et al. (1998). Relationship between dental disease and coronary heart disease in elderly U.S. veterans. *J Am Dent Assoc,* 129:301–11.
16. Slavkin, H. C. (1997). First encounters: Transmission of infectious oral disease from mother to child. *J Am Dent Assoc,* 128:773–78.
17. Gurenlian, J. R. (2006). Inflammation: The relationship between oral health and systemic disease. Retrieved September 5, 2012, from http://www.adha.org/ce_courses/course13/index.html.
18. Harfst, S. A., & Vick, V. C. (2008). Oral risk assessment and intervention planning. In Daniel, S. J., Harfst, S. A., & Wilder, R. S., Eds. *Mosby's dental hygiene concepts, cases, and competencies.* (2nd ed.). St. Louis. MO: Mosby Elsevier, 387–404.
19. American Academy of Periodontics. (2001). Treatment of plaque-induced gingivitis, chronic periodontitis, and other clinical conditions. (Position Paper). *J Periodontol,* 72:1790–800.
20. American Heart Association. (2007). What is high blood pressure. Retrieved March 2007, from http://www.americanheart.org/presenter.jhtml?identifier=2112.
21. Medical Economics. (1995). *PDR medical dictionary.* Montvale, NJ: Medical Economics, 1532.
22. Wilkins, E. M. (2009). *Clinical practice of the dental hygienist* (10th ed.). Philadelphia. PA: Lippincott, Williams and Wilkins, 182.
23. Medical Economics. (1995). *PDR Medical Dictionary.* Montvale, NJ: Medical Economics, 474.
24. Miller, S. (1982, July/August). Dental hygiene diagnoses. *RDH,* 46.
25. American Dental Hygienists' Association. (2005, June). Dental hygiene diagnosis: dhdx. (Position Paper). Chicago, IL: American Dental Hygienists' Association.
26. Wilkins, E. M. (2009). *Clinical practice of the dental hygienist.* (10th ed.). Philadelphia, PA: Lippincott, Williams and Wilkins, 353.
27. American Academy of Periodontology. (1999). International workshop for a classification of periodontal diseases and conditions. *Ann Periodontol,* 4:1.
28. Wolfe, H. F., & Hassell, T. M. (2006). *Color atlas of periodontology.* New York and Stuttgart: Thieme Medical Publishers.
29. American Academy of Periodontology. (2000). Parameters of care. *J Periodontol,* 71 (5 Suppl):847–83.
30. Kimbrough, V. J., & Henderson, K. (2006). *Oral health education.* Upper Saddle River, NJ: Pearson Prentice Hall.
31. American Academy of Periodontics. (2001). Treatment of plaque-induced gingivitis, chronic periodontitis, and other clinical conditions. (Position Paper). *J Periodontol,* 72:1790–800.
32. American Dental Association, Council on Access, Prevention and Interprofessional Relations. (1976). Definitions of recognized dental specialties: Dental public health. Retrieved June 1, 2007, from http://www.ada.org/prof/ed/specialties/definitions.asp.
33. World Health Organization Public Health Services. http://www.euro.who.int/publichealth/20070319_4. Retrieved May 8, 2008.
34. U.S. Cancer Statistics Working Group. (2006). *United States cancer statistics: 2003 incidence and mortality.* Atlanta, GA: U.S. Department of Health and Human Services, Centers for Disease Control and Prevention and National Cancer Institute.
35. Dye, B. A., Tan, S., Smith, V., Lewis, B. G., Barker, L. K., Thornton-Evans, G., Eke, P. I., Beltrán-Aguilar, E. D., Horowitz, A. M., & Li, C. H. (2007). *Trends in oral health status: United States, 1988–1994 and 1999–2004* (DHHS Publication No. [PHS] 2007–1698). [Vital Health Stat 11(248)]. Hyattsville, MD: U.S. Department of Health and Human Services, Centers for Disease Control and Prevention, National Center for Health Statistics.
36. Association of State and Territorial Dental Directors. (2007). State & territorial dental public health activities: A collection of descriptive summaries. Acquiring oral health data. Retrieved June 1, 2007, from http://www.astdd.org/index.php?template=sactnav_temp.php&topic=Acquiring%20Oral%20Health%20Data.
37. Association of State and Territorial Dental Directors. (2003). *Basic screening surveys: An approach to monitoring community oral health.* Columbus, OH: Association of State and Territorial Dental Directors.
38. Centers for Disease Control and Prevention. (2006). National Oral Health Surveillance System. Retrieved June 1, 2007, from http://www.cdc.gov/nohss/.

Dental Plaque Biofilm

Christine N. Nathe

OBJECTIVES

After studying this chapter, the student should be able to:

1. Differentiate between organic coatings of endogenous and exogenous (acquired) origin.

2. Explain why dental plaque is not unique among naturally occurring microbial layers.

3. Describe the mechanisms proposed to explain bacterial adhesion to the acquired pellicle.

4. Distinguish between primary and secondary bacterial colonizers in dental plaque, and cite examples of each.

5. Identify the primary sites of calculus formation, explain how calculus forms, and detail the differences between supragingival and subgingival calculus.

6. Describe the basis for the involvement of the acquired pellicle, bacterial dental plaque, and dental calculus in caries and the inflammatory periodontal diseases.

KEY TERMS

Acquired pellicle, 42
Bacterial biofilm, 40
Calculus, 40
Cocci, 44
Dental plaque, 40
Desquamated, 43
Ecologic niche, 45
Exogenous antimicrobial
 agents, 41
Fimbriae, 43
Hemidesmosomes, 42
Inflammatory exudate, 47
Materia alba, 43
Microbiota, 42
Palisades, 45
Perikymata, 48
Pilin, 43
Primary colonizers, 44
Secondary colonizers, 44
Subsurface pellicle, 41
Symbiosis, 45

INTRODUCTION

The dental professional comes into contact with two of the most widespread of all human maladies, dental caries and periodontal diseases (Figure 4–1 ■). Unlike typical infectious diseases, a single pathogenic microorganism does not cause dental caries and periodontal diseases. Rather, these oral diseases result from the accumulation of many different species of bacteria that form **dental plaque**, a naturally acquired **bacterial biofilm** that develops on the teeth (Figure 4–2 ■).[1,2] Given that dental plaque is a multi-species biofilm, it should be taken into account that some bacterial species may be of greater relevance in the development of caries and periodontal diseases. Bacterial species are found in the plaque in a healthy mouth, in the plaque associated with caries, and in the plaque of an individual with inflammatory periodontal disease.[3,4]

To understand the role of dental plaque in caries and inflammatory periodontal diseases, dental plaque formation will be discussed, and how changes in the proportions of different plaque bacteria can contribute to the development of oral diseases.[5,6]

DENTAL PLAQUE: A MICROBIAL BIOFILM

Most natural surfaces have their own coating of microorganisms, or biofilm, adapted to their individual habitats. The features of dental plaque formation are by no means unique; they merely reflect a single instance of a widespread and ancient natural phenomenon.

DID YOU KNOW?

One of the first known examples of life is mineralized bacteria, or algae, attached to rocks from the Precambrian era.[7,8] These organic organisms were converted into a mineral (i.e., inorganic) format.

Bacterial adhesion to surfaces, as seen with these mineralized organisms, primarily involves two types of reactions: physicochemical and biochemical. These same interactions occur in the formation of plaque and calculus on oral structures.[9–11] **Calculus** is a hard calcified deposit of plaque that has become mineralized. For example, all living cells in nature, including bacterial plaque cells, have a net-negative surface charge. The cells can, therefore, be attracted to oppositely charged surfaces on such items as rocks in a stream, skin, or, as in the case of bacterial plaque, the surfaces of cells, teeth, and soft tissues of the oral cavity. In an attempt to prolong the existence of biofilms, the microorganisms within bacterial plaque and in other environments can produce (extracellular coatings) such as slime layers; they can also produce a variety of surface fibrils, or appendages, that extend from their cell walls. These

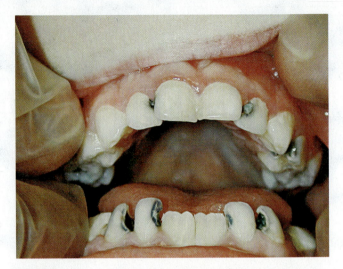

FIGURE ■ 4–1 A 13-year-old female with dental caries on the facial surface of the incisors in the maxilla and swollen, discolored gingival tissues around the mandibular incisors, which is characteristic of chronic gingivitis.

(*Source:* University of Kentucky College of Dentistry-OHRI.)

mechanisms mediate (indirectly cause) attachment of bacteria to a substrate by providing additional attachment structures between the tooth surface and the plaque, thus allowing the formation of adherent matrices.[9,12]

Because biofilm is composed of various species of organisms, interactions with other members of the multispecies community in the oral cavity can influence the behavior of dental bacterial plaque. The mixed-species bacteria engulfed within the biofilm population behave differently from planktonic, liquid-phase, mono-species cells. This difference in behavior has significant clinical implications.

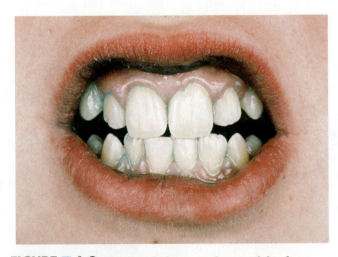

FIGURE ■ 4–2 The dental plaque on these teeth has been stained with a discoloring solution and rinsed. Note the presence of plaque interproximally and adjacent to the gingiva but relatively absent closer to the incisal edge.

(*Source:* Alex Bartel/Photo Researchers, Inc.)

Current research indicates that bacteria growing in biofilms are more resistant to the effects of host defense mechanisms and **exogenous antimicrobrial agents** (agents applied to the surface of the organism) when compared to the same cells in a liquid suspension.[13–15] This resistance could be attributed to the fact that biofilm communities house an assortment of microorganisms that have individual fluctuations in cellular structures. As a result, not all microorganisms within the biofilm population react uniformly to antimicrobial treatment at a given time. Thus, it is very important to include mechanical oral hygiene practices to disturb the attached biofilm in addition to using antimicrobial therapy.

BACTERIAL COLONIZATION OF THE MOUTH

Microorganisms found in the oral cavity are naturally acquired from the environment. Bacteria are acquired from the atmosphere, food, human contact, and even from contact with animals,

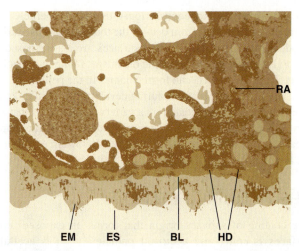

FIGURE ■ 4–4 Junction of reduced enamel epithelium and enamel. The reduced *ameloblasts* (RA) are attached to the enamel by hemidesmosomes (HD) and a basal lamina (BL). EM, enamel matrix remnants form a subsurface pellicle; ES, enamel space. Original magnification × 45,000.

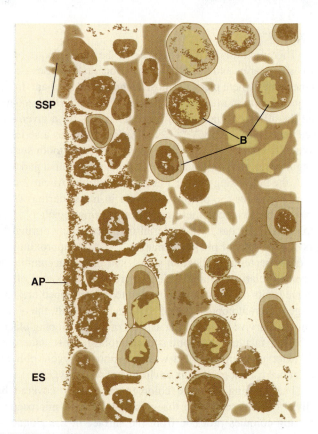

FIGURE ■ 4–3 This transmission electron micrograph demonstrates remnants of the subsurface pellicle (SSP) and the acquired pellicle (AP) between the enamel (ES) surface and the bacterial cells (B) of the dental plaque.

such as pets. The bacteria subsequently form colonies between saliva and oral soft tissues such as the gingiva, tongue, cheeks as well as alimentary tract. Bacteria also form colonies between saliva and hard tissues such as erupted teeth, and exposed root cementum and dentin. Cementum and dentin become exposed during a process called *gingival recession.* The tongue and tonsils are covered by a mucosal surface (a surface covered by a membrane that secretes mucus). Mucosal surfaces may serve as reservoirs for organisms that form dental plaque, including those related to disease.[16]

Prior to eruption, the external surface of tooth enamel is lined by remnants of the enamel-forming organ. These tissue remnants are the reduced enamel epithelium (REE) and the basal lamina. The basal lamina connects the epithelium to the enamel surface. The basal lamina is also continuous with organic material that fills the microscopic voids in the superficial enamel. This subsurface organic material appears as a fringelike structure attached to the basal lamina and is composed of residual enamel matrix proteins (Figures 4–3 ■ and 4–4 ■). This material is referred to as a **subsurface pellicle**. The pellicle originates from local cells during tooth formation; therefore, it is considered to be of endogenous origin. When the tooth emerges into the oral cavity, the remnants of the reduced enamel epithelium are worn off or digested by salivary and bacterial enzymes.[17]

A thin, microscopic coating of saliva materials immediately covers an erupted tooth. The salivary components become *ad*sorbed (the process in which a solid substance, such as tooth enamel, attracts and holds a liquid suspensions, such as the salivary components, to its surface whereas *ab*sorption involves the incorporations of a substance into the tooth) to the surface of the enamel within seconds. This coating is also referred to as a *pellicle.* Because it is acquired after eruption of teeth, it is said to have an exogenous origin—that is, the pellicle was formed by a substance from outside the tooth rather than during the development of teeth. Tooth surfaces are also exposed to the oral **microbiota** (microscopic organisms found in a specific area). The oral bacteria can form colonies in the pellicle.[17]

Thus, the tooth surface, during development or after eruption, is almost always coated by a variety of structures that are either of endogenous origin (derived from cells of the dental organ) or of exogenous origin (acquired following eruption of the teeth into the oral cavity).[17]

THE ACQUIRED PELLICLE

The coating of salivary origin that forms on exposed tooth surfaces is called the **acquired pellicle**.[18,19] It is acellular and consists primarily of glycoproteins (a glycoprotein is a protein molecule that includes an attached carbohydrate component) derived from saliva (Figure 4–3 ■). The pellicle also occupies the millions of microscopic voids in the erupted tooth caused by chemical and mechanical interactions of the tooth surface with the oral environment. Collectively, these organic fringelike projections form a subsurface pellicle, which is of exogenous, or acquired, origin. Oral fluids and small molecules can slowly diffuse through the acquired pellicle into the superficial enamel. If the pellicle is displaced, for example by a prophylaxis, the pellicle begins to reform immediately.[20,21] It takes about a week for the pellicle to develop its condensed, mature structure, which may also incorporate bacterial products.[22–24]

An acquired pellicle also forms on artificial surfaces, such as dental restorations and dental prosthetics (i.e., dentures and partials). These organic coatings are similar to the pellicles on natural teeth and may be colonized by bacteria.[25–27] Colonization of the acquired pellicle can be beneficial for the bacteria because the pellicle components can serve as nutrients.[28] For example, proline-rich salivary proteins may be degraded by bacterial collagenases. This action releases peptides, free amino acids, and salivary mucins that may enhance the growth of dental plaque organisms, such as actinomycetes and spirochetes.[29,30]

The carbohydrate components of certain pellicle glycoproteins may serve as receptors for proteins that bind bacteria to surfaces (e.g., adhesins), thereby contributing to bacterial adhesion to the tooth.[31–33] There is competition for the binding sites on the pellicle, not only by receptors on bacteria but also from host proteins, including immunoglobulins (i.e., antibodies), the enzyme lysozyme, and proteins of the complement system, which are found in the blood and help to support the body's immune defenses. These host proteins originate from saliva and gingival sulcus fluid.[34,35] Once a pellicle site is occupied by one of the competing entities, occupancy by another is inhibited.[36] Competition not only arises for occupancy of binding sites, but an antagonistic relationship also often exists between different types of bacteria competing for the binding sites. For example, it has been shown that some streptococci synthesize and release proteins called *bacteriocins,* which can inhibit some strains of *Actinomyces* and *Actinobacillus* species.[37,38]

DENTAL PLAQUE FORMATION

All bacteria that initiate plaque formation come in contact with the organically coated tooth surface by chance. Forces exist that tend either to allow bacteria to accumulate on teeth or to remove them. Shifts in these forces determine whether more or less plaque accumulates at a given site on a tooth. Many factors, ranging from simple to complex, influence the buildup of plaque. The simple factors include mechanical displacement, stagnation (colonization in a sheltered or undisturbed environment), and availability of nutrients. The complex factors include interactions between the microbes and the host's inflammatory–immune systems.[39] (Chapter 9 discusses these host defense mechanisms.) Bacteria tend to be removed from the teeth during mastication of foods, by the tongue, by toothbrushing, and by other oral hygiene activities. For this reason, bacteria tend to accumulate on teeth in sheltered, undisturbed environments, which basically are sites at risk. These sites include the occlusal fissures, the surfaces apical to the contact between adjacent teeth, and in the gingival sulcus.

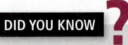

DID YOU KNOW ?

Plaque removal can help prevent both dental caries and periodontal diseases.

Therefore, it is no coincidence that the major plaque-based diseases—caries and inflammatory periodontal diseases—arise at these sites where plaque is most abundant and stagnant. Initial plaque formation may take as long as 2 hours.[40] Binding sites and the affinity of individual bacterial strains for a given surface vary considerably.[41,42] Colonization begins as a series of isolated colonies, often confined to microscopic tooth surface irregularities.[23] With the aid of nutrients from saliva and host food, the colonizing bacteria begin to multiply. About 2 days are required for the plaque to double in mass, during which time the bacterial colonies have been growing together.[43] The most dramatic change in bacterial numbers occurs during the first 4 or 5 days of plaque formation.[44,45] After approximately 21 days, bacterial replication slows, and plaque accumulation becomes relatively stable.[46] The increasing thickness of the plaque limits the diffusion of oxygen to the entrapped original, oxygen-tolerant populations of bacteria. As a result, the organisms that survive in the deeper aspects of the developing plaque are either facultative or obligate anaerobes. These anaerobes can exist in an environment with or without oxygen; obligate anaerobes cannot exist in an environment with oxygen.

The forming bacterial colonies are rapidly covered by saliva.[47] When seen with the scanning electron microscope, growing colonies protrude from the surface of the plaque as domes (**hemidesmosomes**), giving the appearance of a cluster of igloos beneath newly fallen snow (Figure 4–5 ■). In individuals with poor oral hygiene, superficial dental plaque may incorporate food debris and human cells such as epithelial cells

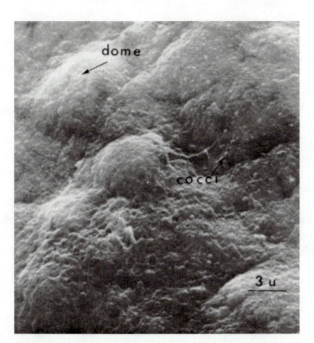

FIGURE ■ 4–5 Scanning electron micrograph of dome formation in the plaque.

(*Source:* J. M. Brady. (1973). *J Periodontol,* 44:416–28.)

shed by oral tissues (**desquamated** cells) and leukocytes. This debris is called **materia alba**, which literally means "white matter." Unlike plaque, it is usually removed easily by rinsing with water.[18] At times, the plaque demonstrates staining, which is caused by sources including coffee, tea, red wine, and tobacco and chromogenic bacteria, which produce a brown pigment.

MOLECULAR MECHANISMS OF BACTERIAL ADHESION

The initial bacterial attachment to the acquired pellicle (Figure 4–6 ■) is thought to involve physicochemical interactions (e.g., electrostatic forces and hydrophobic bonding) between molecules or portions of molecules, such as the side chains of the amino acids phenylalanine and leucine.[48–51] It has been suggested that the hydrophobicity of some streptococci, a major plaque group, is caused by cell wall–associated molecules including glucosyltransferase, an enzyme that converts the glucose portion of the sugar, sucrose, into extracellular polysaccharide. Some glucosyltransferases have been designated as hydrophobins.[52] These polysaccharides include "sticky" glucans that, through hydrogen bonding, are thought to contribute to the mediation of bacterial adhesion.[53] Once the bacteria adhere, they are often "entombed" as additional glucan is produced.[54]

Bacteria also have external cell-surface proteins termed *adhesins,* which have lectinlike activity (lectins are plant proteins with receptor sites that bind specific sugars) because they can bind to carbohydrate components of glycoproteins.[32,33,55,56] These molecules are believed to aid colonization of the acquired pellicle.[57,58] Some researchers have suggested the adhesins may be located on bacterial surface appendages, such as **fimbriae** (Figure 4–6D ■). Fimbria-associated adhesins probably mediate bacterial adhesion via ionic or hydrogen-bonding interactions. Adhesins and fimbria may function together to promote bacterial attachment to pellicle-coated surfaces.[59] For example, **pilin,** a structural protein that constitutes the bulk of some fimbria, is hydrophobic because of its amino acid content.[60] These

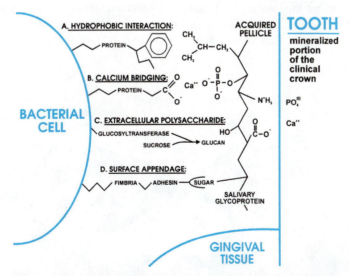

FIGURE ■ 4–6 This diagram illustrates some of the possible molecular mechanisms that mediate attachment of bacteria to teeth during dental plaque formation. **A.** A side chain of a phenylalanine component of a bacterial protein interacts via hydrophobic bonding with a side chain of a leucine component of a salivary glycoprotein in the acquired pellicle. **B.** The negatively charged carboxyl group of a bacterial protein is attracted to a positively charged calcium ion (i.e., electrostatic attraction), which in turn is attracted to a negatively charged phosphate group of a salivary phosphoprotein in the acquired pellicle. **C.** The host's dietary sucrose is converted by the bacterial enzyme, glucosyltransferase, to the extracellular polysaccharide, glucan, which has many hydrophobic groups and can interact with amino acid side-chain groups, such as serine, tyrosine, and threonine. **D.** The fimbrial surface appendage extends from the bacterial cell to permit the terminal adhesin portion to bind to a sugar component of a salivary glycoprotein in the acquired pellicle.

fibrillar surface appendages extend from the bacterial surface and may reduce or mask the repelling effect of the net-negative surface charges. Carbohydrate-binding adhesins have been shown to link actinomycetes to streptococci in early dental plaque formation.[61,62]

Another molecular mechanism of bacterial adhesion is calcium bridging. In this process, *positively* charged, divalent calcium ions in the saliva help to link the *negatively* charged cell surfaces of bacteria to the *negatively* charged acquired pellicle (Figure 4–6B ■).[63,64,65] Calcium bridging may be important in only early plaque formation because recently formed plaque is readily disrupted by exposure to a calcium-complexing (chelating) agent, such as ethylenediaminetetraacetic acid (EDTA).[66]

Although some or all of the previously described mechanisms may play a role in the attachment of bacteria to one another and to the tooth surface, the nature of the actual linking molecules in plaque, or between plaque and tooth surface coatings, is not known.

BACTERIA IN THE DENTAL PLAQUE

Within the mouth of any one individual, plaque bacteria vary in number and proportions from time to time and site to site. The diversity is even greater between individuals, between races, and between supragingival and subgingival plaques.[67–69] The only abundant bacteria found almost universally in the mouths of humans and animals are streptococci and actinomycetes.

The bacteria colonize the teeth in a reasonably predictable sequence. The first to adhere are **primary colonizers**, sometimes referred to as *pioneer species.* These are microorganisms that are able to stick directly to the acquired pellicle. Those that arrive later are **secondary colonizers**. They may be able to colonize an existing bacterial layer, but they are unable to act as primary colonizers. Generally speaking, the primary colonizers are not pathogenic. If the plaque is allowed to remain undisturbed, it eventually becomes populated with secondary colonizers that are the likely etiologic agents of dental caries and periodontal diseases. (Figure 4–7 ■)

The earliest colonizers are overwhelmingly **cocci** (spherical bacteria), especially streptococci, which constitute 47% to 85% of the cultivable cells found during the first 4 hours after professional tooth cleaning.[1,69–71] These organisms tend to be followed by short rods and filamentous bacteria. Because of stagnation, the most abundant colonization is on the proximal surfaces, in the fissures of teeth and in the gingival sulcus region.[72]

Cocci are probably the first to adhere because they are small and round and, therefore, have a smaller energy barrier to overcome than other bacterial forms.[73] The first or primary colonizers tend to be aerobic (oxygen-tolerant) bacteria including *Neisseria* and *Rothia*. The streptococci, the gram-positive facultative rods, and the actinomycetes are the main organisms in plaque found in early fissures and approximal plaque).[73–75] As plaque oxygen levels fall, the proportions of gram-negative rods (e.g., fusobacteria) and gram-negative cocci such as *Veillonella* tend to increase.

Of the early colonizers, *Streptococcus sanguis* often appears first, followed by *Streptococcus mutans* (*S. mutans*).[76] Both depend on a sheltered environment for growth and the presence of extracellular carbohydrate (e.g., sucrose). Sucrose is used to synthesize intracellular polysaccharides that serve as an internal source of energy as well as external polysaccharide coats.[77,78] The polysaccharide coating helps protect the cell from the osmotic effects of sucrose. In addition, the coating reduces the inhibitory effect of toxic metabolic end products, such as lactic acid, on bacterial survival.

Whereas nonmotile cells, including streptococci and actinomycetes, come into contact with the tooth randomly, motile cells such as the spirochetes are likely to be attracted by chemotactic factors (e.g., nutrients). Surface receptors probably

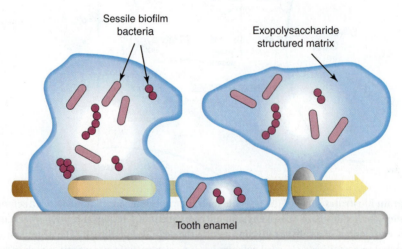

Structure of a polymicrobial biofilm. Dental plaque is an example of a polymicrobial biofilm in which *Streptococcus* species and other bacteria secrete a thick exopolysaccharide matrix and exist within this matrix in a dormant or sessile state of low metabolic activity. Biofilm bacteria have increased resistance to host immune clearance and antibiotic medicines.

FIGURE ■ 4–7 Polymicrobial biofilm structure.

provide a means of attachment for secondary colonizers onto the initial bacterial layer.[79] Bacteria that cannot adhere easily to the tooth initially via organic coatings can probably attach by strong lectinlike, cell-to-cell interactions with similar or dissimilar bacteria that are already attached (i.e., the primary colonizers).[33,80,81]

Gram-negative, anaerobic species such as *Treponema, Porphyromonas, Prevotella,* and *Fusobacterium* species predominate in the subgingival plaque during the later phases of plaque development, but they may also be present in early plaque.[82] There is evidence that oxygen does not penetrate more than 0.1 mm into the dental plaque, a fact that may explain the presence of anaerobic bacteria in early plaque.[83,84]

DENTAL PLAQUE MATRIX

A great variety of factors affects the colonization of bacteria on teeth. Dental plaque consists of different species of bacteria that are not uniformly distributed because different species colonize the tooth surface at different times and under different circumstances. The newly formed supragingival biofilm frequently exhibits **palisades** (columnar microcolonies of cells) made up of firmly attached cocci, rods, or filaments. The organisms are positioned perpendicular to the tooth surface as a result of competitive colonization. An intercellular plaque matrix surrounds the bacterial cells in the biofilm (Figure 4–8 ■).[1,56,69,85] The matrix is composed of both organic and inorganic components that originate primarily from the bacteria. Polysaccharides

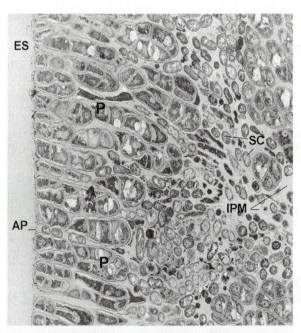

FIGURE ■ 4–8 An electron micrograph showing palisades (P) of bacteria perpendicular to the enamel surface (ES), bacterial cells that are probably secondary colonizers (SC), the intercellular plaque matrix (IPM), and the acquired pellicle (AP).

(*Source:* Courtesy of Dr. M. A Listgarten, University of Pennsylvania School of Dental Medicine, Philadelphia.)

derived from bacterial metabolism of carbohydrates are a major constituent of the matrix whereas salivary and serum proteins/glycoproteins represent minor components. The bacteria in the subgingival biofilm consist of several motile species that do not form distinctive microcolonies. They tend to be located on the surface of the adherent bacterial layer and are separated by an abundant intercellular matrix. Some bacteria on the surface of the biofilm aggregate into distinctive structures that include arrangements of cocci ("corn-cob" configurations) and rods ("test-tube brush" configurations)[1,2,69,86] radially arranged around a central filament (Figure 4–9 ■).

DENTAL PLAQUE METABOLISM

For metabolism to occur, a source of energy is required. For the caries-related *S. mutans* and many other acid-forming organisms, this energy source can be sucrose.[87] Almost immediately following exposure of these microorganisms to sucrose, they produce (1) acid, (2) intracellular polysaccharides, which provide a reserve source of energy for each bacterium, much like glycogen does for human cells,[88] and (3) extracellular polysaccharides including glucans (dextran)[89] and fructans (levan).[90] As mentioned previously, glucans can be viscid substances that help anchor the bacteria to the pellicle, as well as stabilize the plaque mass. Fructans can act as an energy source for any bacteria having the enzyme levanase.[91,92] Quantitatively, the glucans constitute up to approximately 20% of plaque dry weight, levans about 10%, and bacteria the remaining 70% to 80%. As stated earlier, the glucans and fructans are major contributors to the intercellular plaque matrix.[92]

Plaque organisms grow under adverse environmental conditions, which include varying pH, temperature, ionic strength, oxygen tension, nutrient levels, and antagonistic elements, such as competing organisms and the host inflammatory–immune response. The numerous fluctuations in the oral environment can influence many aspects of the initial colonization, maturation, and survival of microorganisms within oral plaque. Variations of the aforementioned conditions can affect the primary and extended adherence of microorganisms to the surface as well the diffusion of essential elements (i.e., oxygen and nutrients), all of which are required for the prolonged existence of bacterial biofilm. To cope with this hostile environment, the plaque organisms must find a safe haven in relation to their neighbors and the oral environment. Such a favorable location is termed an **ecologic niche**.[5] Normally, once the niches are established, the bacteria of the resident microbiota coexist with the host and the surrounding microcosm. This relationship is referred to as **symbiosis**, and it results in a resistance to colonization by subsequent nonindigenous organisms. In this manner, the resident microbiota can protect the host against infection by major primary pathogens (e.g., *Corynebacterium diphtheriae* and *Streptococcus pyogenes*).

With dietary sugars entering the plaque, anaerobic glycolysis results in acidogenesis (acid production) and accumulation of acid in the plaque.[5] If no acid-consuming organisms (e.g., *Veillonella*) are available to use the acids, the plaque pH drops rapidly from 7.0 to below 4.5. This drop is important because

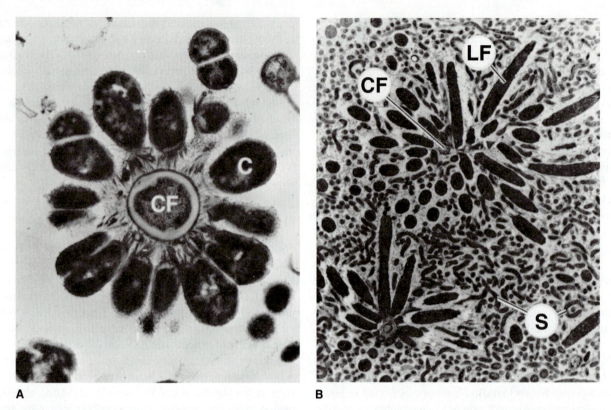

FIGURE ■ 4–9 **A.** Cross section of "corn cob" from 2-month-old plaque. A coarse fibrillar material attaches the cocci (C) to the central filament (CF). Original magnification × 22,500. (*Source:* M. A. Listgarten, H. E. Mayo, & R. Tremblay. (1975). *J Periodontol,* 46:10–26.) **B.** Coarse "test-tube brush" formations consisting of central filament (CF) surrounded by large, filamentous bacteria with flagella uniformly distributed over its body (LF). Background consists of a spirochete-rich microbiota (S). Original magnification × 4,300. (*Source:* M. A. Listgarten. (1976). *J Periodontol,* 47: 1–18.)

enamel begins to demineralize between pH 5.0 and 5.5. One possible outcome of the drop in pH may be the dissolution of the mineralized tooth surface adjacent to the plaque, resulting in carious cavitation of the tooth.[77] This process provides the bacteria access to the inorganic elements (e.g., calcium and phosphate) needed for their nutritional requirements. By adhering to the tooth surface via an organic layer of salivary origin, dental plaque bacteria can also gain access to a supply of organic nutrients, a widespread phenomenon.[47] The same search for nutrients may explain the extension of bacteria from the supragingival plaque into the gingival sulcus.[93,94] To prevent or reduce subgingival colonization, the host tissues defend against the bacterial challenge with antibacterial strategies, such as the passage of antibodies and the emigration of polymorphonuclear neutrophils from the adjacent connective tissue into the gingival sulcus. The continued metabolic activity of plaque in the subgingival environment initiates the inflammatory response of the gingival tissues (gingivitis) and also may eventually lead to progressive destruction of the periodontium (periodontitis).[95,96]

Until supragingival plaque mineralizes as dental calculus, it can be removed by mechanical debridement (e.g., toothbrushing, flossing, or use of interdental aids).[97] Dental plaque cannot be removed by rinsing alone. As the plaque matures, it becomes more resistant to removal with a toothbrush. In one study, at 24, 48, and 72 hours after formation, 5.5, 7.8, and 14.0 g/cm² of

pressure, respectively, were required to dislodge the plaque—almost 3 times as much pressure to remove it on the third day as on the first.[98] Once dental calculus is formed, use of professional instruments is necessary for its removal.

DENTAL CALCULUS

A last stage in the maturation of some dental plaques is characterized by the appearance of mineralization in the deeper portions of the plaque to form dental calculus.[99] The term *calculus* is derived from the Latin word meaning pebble or stone. The lay term *tartar* refers to an accumulated sediment or crust on the sides of a wine cask. Some people do not form calculus, others form only moderate amounts, and still others form heavy amounts.

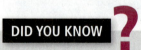

DID YOU KNOW

It formerly was thought that calculus formed to help stabilize teeth, thus decreasing mobility and eventual tooth loss.

Calculus itself is not harmful. However, a layer of unmineralized, viable, metabolically active bacteria that are closely

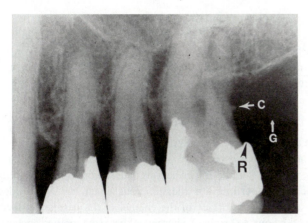

FIGURE ■ 4–10 Radiograph demonstrating a "spur"-shaped deposit of calculus (C) on the *distal* side of the left first molar in the maxilla. The calculus is apical to the overhanging metallic restoration (R). The arrow (G) marks the coronal level of the gingival tissues, which indicates that this is a subgingival deposit of calculus.

(*Source:* Courtesy of Dr. W. K. Grigsby, University of Iowa College of Dentistry, Iowa City.)

associated with the external calculus surface is potentially pathogenic. Calculus cannot be removed by brushing or flossing. It is often difficult to remove all the calculus, even professionally, without damaging the tooth, especially the softer root cementum. However, calculus needs to be removed because its presence makes routine oral hygiene more difficult or even impossible by forming calculus spurs (Figure 4–10 ■). These structures may contribute to plaque accumulation and stagnation. Calculus removal is also a prerequisite to regenerating lost or damaged periodontal tissues after treatment.

In addition to local factors, calculus formation may be affected by behavioral factors and systemic conditions. For example, smoking causes accelerated formation of calculus.[100] Children afflicted with asthma or cystic fibrosis form calculus at approximately twice the rate of other children.[101] Similarly, nonambulatory, individuals with disabilities, or those individuals tube-fed over long periods, may develop heavy calculus within 30 days, despite the fact that no food passes through the mouth.[102] Conversely, medications such as beta-blockers, diuretics, and anticholinergics can result in significantly reduced levels of calculus. The authors of the study that made this determination concluded that either the medications were excreted directly into the saliva, affecting the rate of crystallization, or altered the composition of the saliva and thus indirectly affected calculus formation.[103]

Calculus formation is related to the fact that saliva is saturated with respect to calcium and phosphate ions.[104] Precipitation of these elements leads to mineralization of dental plaque, which gives rise to calculus. The crystals in calculus include hydroxyapatite, brushite, and whitlockite, all of which have different proportions of calcium and phosphate in combination with other ions, such as magnesium, zinc, fluoride, and carbonate. Supragingival calculus forming on the tooth coronal to the gingival margin frequently develops opposite the duct orifices of the major salivary glands. It is often found where saliva

pools on the lingual surfaces of the mandibular incisors (Figure 4–11 ■). Supragingival calculus can also form in the fissures of teeth. Subgingival calculus forms from calcium phosphate and organic materials derived from blood serum, which contribute to mineralization of subgingival plaque.

DID YOU KNOW ?

Calculus can form on restorative materials.

One of the means by which formation and growth of calculus may be studied is by ligating thin plastic strips around the teeth and then removing the strips at various intervals.[105] Within 12 hours after placement, x-ray diffraction studies demonstrate mineral elements in the forming plaque. By 3 to 4 days, the concentration of calcium and phosphate is significantly higher in the plaque of those with heavy calculus formation than in the plaque of those with no calculus formation.

Subgingival calculus is about 60% mineralized whereas supragingival calculus is only about 30% mineralized.[106] Because subgingival calculus is harder, thinner, and more closely adapted to tooth surface imperfections, it can be more difficult to remove than supragingival calculus. The two types of calculus may differ in color. Supragingival calculus, which derives its mineral content from saliva, usually appears as a yellow to white mass with a chalky consistency. Subgingival calculus derives its minerals from the **inflammatory exudate** in the sulcus and periodontal pocket. Subgingival calculus appears gray to black in color and has a flintlike consistency. The dark coloration may be caused by bacterial degradation of components of the hemorrhagic exudate that accompanies gingival inflammation.

Alkaline conditions in dental plaque may be an important predisposing factor for calculus formation,[107] which is not restricted to one bacterial species or even to those growing at

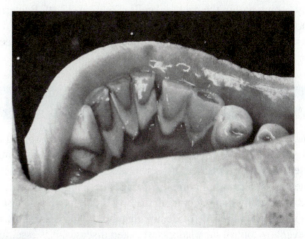

FIGURE ■ 4–11 Deposits of supragingival calculus on the *lingual* surface of incisors and canines that could not be removed by brushing.

(*Source:* Courtesy of Dr. W. K. Grigsby, University of Iowa College of Dentistry, Iowa City.)

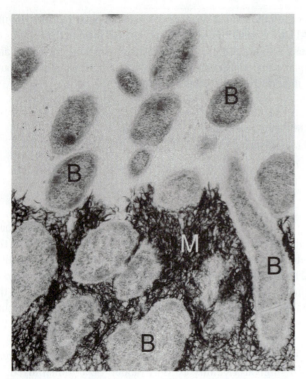

FIGURE ■ 4–12 **Typical pattern of dental plaque mineralization in which the initial mineralization occurs in the inter-bacterial plaque matrix (M) with bacterial cells (B) becoming mineralized secondarily. Original magnification ✕ 40,000.**

(*Source:* Courtesy of Dr. M. A. Listgarten, University of Pennsylvania School of Dental Medicine, Philadelphia.)

neutral or slightly acidic pHs. This is evidenced by the fact that caries-related streptococci may mineralize.[108] Not all plaques mineralize, but a plaque that is destined to mineralize begins to do so within a few days of its initial formation even though this early change is not detectable at a clinical level. Mineralization usually begins in the intercellular plaque matrix but eventually occurs within the bacterial cells (Figure 4–12 ■). Bacterial phospholipids and other cell-wall constituents may act as initiators of mineralization, in which case it may begin in the cell wall and subsequently extend to the rest of the cell and into the surrounding matrix.[109] Calculus may also form on the tooth surfaces of germ-free animals.[110] This type of calculus consists of an organic matrix of nonmicrobial origin, which becomes mineralized.

Attachment of Calculus to the Teeth

At the tooth interface with calculus, neither the enamel nor the root cementum is perfectly smooth, and invariably both contain a variety of surface imperfections. These normal irregularities, such as the **perikymata** (the numerous, small, transverse ridges on the exposed surface of the enamel of the permanent teeth) and the point of origin of Sharpey's fibers (the tooth is anchored by connective tissue fibers that extend between the cementum and the bone; the ends embedded in the cementum and bone are known as *Sharpey's fibers*) on the cementum, appear to aid calculus attachment. Other defects in the enamel and cementum, including areas of demineralization and cemental tears, may also contribute to a stronger attachment of calculus to the tooth.[111] Electron micrographs indicate a very close relationship between the matrix of the tooth surface and the matrix of calculus; the crystalline structures of both are also very similar.[112]

Inhibition of Calculus Formation

Several agents are currently available to reduce calculus formation, including dentifrices that contain pyrophosphate or metal ions such as zinc.[113,114] One dentifrice contains two soluble phosphates, tetrasodium pyrophosphate and disodium dihydrogen pyrophosphate, in addition to fluoride.[114,115] The pyrophosphate ion is an analog of the orthophosphate ion, which means that the former differs structurally from the parent compound (orthophosphate) by a single element but has many of the same functions. In the case of dental calculus, the pyrophosphate ion disrupts the formation of calcium phosphate crystals. This analog also inhibits some bacterial growth at concentrations significantly lower than the levels found in dentifrices without pyrophosphate. Pyrophosphates may cause adverse reactions inlcuding soft tissue ulcerations, sloughing, erythema, migratory glossitis, and a burning sensation.[116]

SUMMARY

Bacteria in dental plaque directly cause the most widespread of all human diseases: dental caries and inflammatory periodontal diseases. These diseases, however, are not classic infections. They arise because of complex changes in plaque ecology and are affected by many factors in the host's protective responses. To understand the role of dental plaque in disease and how to prevent or control the plaque-associated diseases, it is essential to understand the nature of dental plaque.

Plaque forms initially on the organic layer that coats the erupted tooth. This organic layer originates from salivary products that are deposited on the teeth, forming an acquired pellicle to which bacteria adhere. Adhesion is mediated by a variety of bonding mechanisms, including physicochemical and electrostatic interactions as well as stereo-chemical interactions between bacterial adhesins and receptors in the acquired pellicle and bacterial surfaces.

The earliest of the primary bacterial colonizers are mainly gram-positive facultative cocci. They are followed by a variety of gram-positive and gram-negative species—the secondary colonizers. Caries-related bacterial species have a greater ability than others to adapt to excess sugars and their metabolites.

Supragingival plaque is associated with caries and gingivitis whereas subgingival plaque is associated with gingivitis and periodontitis. With higher pH (i.e., less acidity), some plaques mineralize to form supragingival and subgingival dental calculus. In calculus formation, mineralization of dental plaque generally begins in the extracellular matrix and eventually spreads to include the bacteria. Rarely, mineralization may begin within the walls of bacterial cells and spread to the extracellular matrix. Calculus is generally covered by actively metabolizing bacteria, which can cause caries, gingivitis, and periodontitis.

Regular toothbrushing and flossing can remove dental plaque and control its formation. Once dental plaque mineralizes to form calculus, use of professional instruments is necessary for its removal. Although calculus does contribute to inflammatory periodontal diseases, it is stagnation of pathogenic bacteria at critical sites that leads to both dental caries and periodontal diseases.

PRACTICAL CONSIDERATIONS

It is important to note that plaque biofilm is a tremendous factor in both tooth demineralization and inflammatory gingival and periodontal diseases. One of the most important roles of the primary dental provider is to educate patients on the role of plaque in dental diseases so that patients understand disease etiology. Equipping patients with knowledge of plaque and its subsequent role in disease is the first step in the patients' understanding of plaque, dental disease, and, ultimately, the need to practice prevention.

SELF-STUDY QUESTIONS

1. Adhesion is mediated by a variety of bonding mechanisms that include
   a. Exogenous antimicrobial agents
   b. Etching agents
   c. Physiochemical interactions
   d. Antimicrobial interactions

   Rationale: Adhesion is mediated by a variety of bonding mechanisms, including physicochemical and electrostatic interactions as well as stereo-chemical interactions between bacterial adhesions and receptors in the acquired pellicle and bacterial surfaces.

2. Supragingival plaque is associated with gingivitis and periodontitis whereas subgingival plaque is associated with caries and gingivitis.
   a. The first statement is true; the second statement is false.
   b. The first statement is false; the second statement is true.
   c. Both statements are true.
   d. Both statements are false.

   Rationale: Supragingival plaque is associated with caries and gingivitis whereas subgingival plaque is associated with gingivitis and periodontitis.

3. What factors may affect the onset of periodontal diseases?
   a. Plaque
   b. Host defense mechanisms
   c. Exogenous antimicrobial agents
   d. All of the above

   Rationale: Periodontal diseases arise because of complex changes in plaque ecology and are affected by many factors in the host's protective responses. Current research indicates that bacteria growing in biofilms may be resistant to the effects of host defense mechanisms and exogenous antimicrobial agents.

4. Which of the following can be used to prevent the excess accumulation of plaque?
   a. Host defense mechanisms
   b. Effective toothbrushing
   c. Biofilm lozenges
   d. No prevention necessary

   Rationale: Regular toothbrushing and flossing can remove dental plaque and control its formation.

5. Subgingival calculus derives its minerals from which of the following that is found in the sulcus and periodontal pocket?
   a. Sulcular epithelium
   b. Mucogingival fluid
   c. Inflammatory exudate
   d. Endotoxins

   Rationale: Subgingival calculus derives its minerals from the inflammatory exudate in the sulcus and periodontal pocket.

REFERENCES

1. Listgarten, M. A. (1976). Structure of the microbial flora associated with periodontal health and disease in man. A light and electron microscopic study. *J Periodontol,* 47:1–17.
2. Listgarten, M. A. (1999). Formation of dental plaque and other oral biofilms. In Newman, H. N., & Wilson, M., Eds. *Dental plaque revisited—Oral biofilms in health and disease.* Cardiff, UK: BioLine, 187–210.
3. Wolinsky, L. E. (1994). Caries and cariology. In Nisengard, R. J., & Newman, M. G., Eds. *Oral microbiology and immunology* (2nd ed.). Philadelphia, PA: W. B. Saunders, 341–59.
4. Nisengard, R. J., Newman, M. G., & Zambon, J. J. (1994). Periodontal disease. In Nisengard, R. J., & Newman, M. G., Eds. *Oral microbiology and immunology* (2nd ed.). Philadelphia, PA: W. B. Saunders, 360–84.
5. Marsh, P. D. (1999). Microbiologic aspects of dental plaque and dental caries. *Dent Clin North Am,* 43:599–614.
6. Chen, C. (2001). Periodontitis as a biofilm infection. *J Calif Dent Assoc,* 29:362–67.
7. Schopf, J. W. (1974). The development and diversification of Precambrian life. *Orig Life,* 5:119–35.
8. Schopf, J. W. (1975). The age of microscopic life. *Endeavor,* 34:51–58.
9. Costerton, J. W., Cheng, K. J., Geesey, G. G., Ladd, T. I., Nickel, J. C., Dasgupta, M., & Marrie, T. J. (1987). Bacterial biofilms in nature and disease. *Ann Rev Microbiol,* 41:435–64.
10. Costerton, J. W., Lewandowski, Z., Caldwell, D. E., Korber, D. R., & Lappin-Scott, H. M. (1995). Microbial biofilms. *Ann Rev Microbiol,* 49:711–45.
11. Costerton, J. W., Cook, G., & Lamont, R. (1999). The community architecture of biofilms: Dynamic structures and mechanisms. In Newman, H. N., & Wilson, M., Eds. *Dental plaque revisited—Oral biofilms in health and disease.* Cardiff, UK: BioLine, 5–14.
12. Newman, H. N. (1974). Microbial films in nature. *Microbios,* 9:247–57.
13. Gilbert, P., Das, J., & Foley, I. (1997). Biofilm susceptibility to antimicrobials. *Adv Dent Res,* 11:160–67.
14. Bowden, G. H. W., & Hamilton, I. R. (1998). Survival of oral bacteria. *Crit Rev Oral Biol Med,* 9:54–85.
15. Socransky, S. S., & Haffajee, A. D. (2002). Dental biofilms: Difficult therapeutic targets. *Periodontol,* 2000, 28:12–55.
16. Van der Velden, U., Van Winkelhoff, A. J., & Abbas de Graf, J. (1986). The habitat of periodontopathic microorganisms. *J Clin Periodontol,* 13:243–48.
17. Listgarten, M. A. (1976). Structure of surface coatings of teeth. A review. *J Periodontol,* 47:139–47.
18. Ericson, T. (1967). Adsorption to hydroxyapatite of proteins and conjugated proteins from human saliva. *Caries Res,* 1:52–58.
19. Meckel, A. R. (1965). The formation of biological films. *Swed Dent J,* 10:585–99.
20. Leach, S. A., Critchley, P., Kolendo, A. B., & Saxton, C. A. (1967). Salivary glycoproteins as components of the enamel integuments. *Caries Res,* 1:104–11.
21. Mayhall, C. W. (1970). Concerning the composition and source of the acquired enamel pellicle on human teeth. *Arch Oral Biol,* 15:1327–41.
22. Hardie, J. M., & Bowden, G. H. (1976). The microbial flora of dental plaque: Bacterial succession and isolation considerations. In Stiles, H. M., Loesche, W. J., & O'Brien, T. C., Eds.

Proceedings microbial aspects of dental caries. *Microbiol Abstr,* 1 (Spec Suppl):63–87.
23. Lie, T., & Gusberti, F. (1979). Replica study of plaque formation on human tooth surfaces. *Acta Odontol Scand,* 79:65–72.
24. Baier, R. E. (1977). On the formation of biological films. *Swed Dent J,* 1:261–71.
25. Tullberg, A. (1986). An experimental study of the adhesion of bacterial layers to some restorative dental materials. *Scand J Dent Res,* 94:164–73.
26. Kawai, K., & Urano. M. (2001). Adherence of plaque components to different restorative materials. *Oper Dent,* 26:396–400.
27. Quirynen, M., De Soete, M., & van Steenberghe, D. (2002). Infectious risks for oral implants: A review of the literature. *Clin Oral Implant Res,* 13:1–19.
28. Leach, S. A., & Critchley, P. (1966). Bacterial degradation of glycoprotein sugars in human saliva. *Nature,* 209:506.
29. Hay, D. I., & Oppenheim, I. G. (1974). The isolation from human parotid saliva of a further group of proline-rich proteins. *Arch Oral Biol,* 19:627–32.
30. Glenister, D. A., Salamon, K. E., Smith, K., Beighton, D., & Keevil, C. W. Enhanced growth of complex communities of dental plaque bacteria in mucin-limited continuous culture. *Microbiol Ecol Health Dis,* 1:31–38.
31. Gibbons, R. J., & van Houte, J. (1975). Bacterial adherence in oral microbial ecology. *Ann Rev Microbiol,* 29:19–44.
32. Weerkamp, A. H., van der Mei, H. C., Engelen, D. P., et al. (1984). Adhesion receptors (adhesins) of oral streptococci. In ten Cate, J. M., Leach, S. A., & Arends, J., Eds. *Bacterial adhesion and preventive dentistry.* Oxford, UK: IRL Press, 85–97.
33. Rosan, B. R., & Lamont, R. J. (2000). Dental plaque formation. *Microbes Infect,* 2:1599–1607.
34. Kraus, F. W., Orstavik, D., Hurst, D. C., & Cook, C. H. (1973). The acquired pellicle: Variability and subject dependence of specific proteins. *J Oral Pathol Med,* 2:165–73.
35. Orstavik, D., & Kraus, F. W. (1973). The acquired pellicle: Immunofluorescent demonstration of specific proteins. *J Oral Pathol Med,* 2:68–76.
36. Williams, R. C., & Gibbons, R. J. (1975). Inhibition of streptococcal attachment to receptors or human buccal epithelial cells by antigenically similar salivary glycoproteins. *Infect Immun,* 11:711–18.
37. Rogers, A. H., van der Hoeven, J. S., & Mikx, F. (1978). Inhibition of *Actinomyces viscosus* by bacteriocin producing strains of *Streptococcus mutans* in the dental plaque of gnotobiotic rats. *Arch Oral Biol,* 23:477–83.
38. Hammond, B. F., Lillard, S. E., & Stevens, R. H. (1987). A bacteriocin of *Actinobacillus actinomycetemcomitans. Infect Immun,* 55:686–91.
39. Christersson, L. A., Grossi, S. G., Dunford, R. G., Nachtei, E. E., & Genco, R. J. (1992). Dental plaque and calculus: Risk indicators for their formation. *J Dent Res,* 71:1425–30.
40. Baier, R. E., & Glantz, P. O. (1979). Characterization of oral *in vivo* film formed on different types of solid surfaces. *Acta Odontol Scand,* 36:289–301.
41. Liljemark, W. F., & Schauer, S. V. (1977). Competitive binding among oral streptococci to hydroxyapatite. *J Dent Res,* 56:156–65.
42. Kuramitsu, H., & Ingersoll, L. (1977). Molecular basis for the different sucrose-dependent adherence properties of *Streptococcus mutans* and *Streptococcus sanguis. Infect Immun,* 17:330–37.

43. Tanzer, J. M., & Johnson, M. C. (1976). Gradients for growth within intact *Streptococcus mutans* plaque *in vitro* demonstrated by autoradiography. *Arch Oral Biol,* 21:555–59.

44. Bjorn, H., & Carlsson, J. (1964). Observations on a dental plaque morphogenesis. *Odontol Rev,* 15:23–28.

45. Furuichi, Y., Lindhe, J., Ramberg, P., & Volpe, A. R. (1992). Patterns of de novo plaque formation in the human dentition. *J Clin Periodontol,* 19:423–33.

46. Howell, A., Jr., Risso, A., & Paul, F. (1965). Cultivable bacteria in developing and mature human dental calculus. *Arch Oral Biol,* 10:307–13.

47. Rudney, J. D. (2000). Saliva and dental plaque. *Adv Dent Res,* 14:29–39.

48. Newman, H. N. (1974). Diet, attrition, plaque and dental disease. *Br Dent J,* 136:491–97.

49. Leach, S. A. (1979). On the nature of interactions associated with aggregation phenomena in the mouth. *J Dent,* 7:149–60.

50. Rosenberg, M., Judes, H., & Weiss, E. (1983). Cell surface hydrophobicity of dental plaque microorganisms. *Infect Immun,* 42:831–34.

51. Busscher, H. J., & van der Mei, H. C. (1997). Physico-chemical interactions in initial microbial adhesion and relevance for biofilm formation. *Adv Dent Res,* 11:24–32.

52. Doyle, R. J., Rosenberg, M., & Drake, D. (1990). Hydrophobicity of oral bacteria. In Doyle, R. J., Rosenberg, M., Eds. *Microbial cell surface hydrophobicity.* Washington, DC: American Society for Microbiology, 387–419.

53. Edgar, W. M. (1979). Studies of the role of calcium in plaque formation and cohesion. *J Dent,* 7:174–79.

54. Matsukubo, T., Katow, T., & Takazoe, I. (1978). Significance of Ca-binding activity of early plaque bacteria. *Bull Tokyo Dent Coll,* 19:53–57.

55. Rose, R. K., Dibdin, G. H., & Shellis, R. P. (1993). A quantitative study of calcium binding and aggregation in selected oral bacteria. *J Dent Res,* 72:78–84.

56. Newman, M. N., & Britton, A. B. (1974). Dental plaque ultrastructure as revealed by freeze-etching. *J Periodontol,* 45:478–88.

57. Germaine, G. R., Harlander, S. K., Leung, W.-L. S., & Schachtele, C. F. (1977). *Streptococcus mutans* dextran-sucrase: Functioning of primer dextran and endogenous dextransucrase in water-soluble and water-insoluble glucan synthesis. *Infect Immun,* 16:637–48.

58. Gibbons, R. J., & van Houte, J. (1980). Bacterial adherence and the formation of dental plaque. Receptors and recognition. In Beachey, E. H., Ed. *Bacterial adherence.* London, UK: Chapman and Hall, 6:63–104.

59. Ofek, I., & Perry, A. (1985). Molecular basis of bacterial adherence to tissues. In Mergenhagen, S. E., & Rosan, B., Eds. *Molecular basis of oral microbial adhesion.* Washington, DC: American Society for Microbiology, 7–13.

60. Gibbons, R. J. (1984). Adherent interactions which may affect microbial ecology in the mouth. *J Dent Res,* 63:378–85.

61. Clark, W. B., Wheeler, T. T., Lane, M. D., & Cisar, J. O. (1986). Actinomyces adsorption mediated by type-I fimbriae. *J Dent Res,* 65:1166–68.

62. Kolenbrander, P. E., & London, J. (1992). Ecological significance of coaggregation among oral bacteria. *Adv Microb Ecol,* 12:183–217.

63. Handley, P. S., McNab, R., & Jenkinson, H. F. (1999). Adhesive surface structures on oral bacteria. In Newman, H. N., & Wilson, M., Eds. *Dental plaque revisited—Oral biofilms in health and disease.* Cardiff, UK: BioLine, 145–70.

64. Irwin, R. T. (1990). Hydrophobicity of proteins and bacterial fimbriae. In Doyle, R. J., & Rosenberg, M., Eds. *Microbial cell surface hydrophobicity.* Washington, DC: American Society of Microbiology, 137–77.

65. Cisar, J. O., Brennan, M. J., & Sandberg, A. L. (1985). Lectin-specific interaction of *Actinomyces* fimbriae with oral streptococci. In Mergenhagen, S. E., & Rosan, B., Eds. *Molecular basis of oral microbial adhesion.* Washington, DC: American Society for Microbiology, 159–63.

66. Kolenbrander, P. E., & Andersen, R. N. (1985). Use of co-aggregation-defective mutants to study the relationship of cell-to-cell interactions and oral microbial ecology. In Mergenhagen, S. E., & Rosan, B., Eds. *Molecular basis of oral microbial adhesion.* Washington, DC: American Society for Microbiology, 164–66.

67. Rosenberg, E. S., Evian, C. I., & Listgarten, M. A. (1981). The composition of the subgingival microbiota after periodontal therapy. *J Periodontol,* 52:435–41.

68. Cao, C. F., Aeppli, D. M., Liljemark, W. F., Bloomquist, C. G., Brandt, C. L., & Wolff, L. F. (1990). Comparison of plaque microflora between Chinese and Caucasian population groups. *J Clin Periodontol,* 17:115–18.

69. Listgarten, M. A., Mayo, H. E., & Tremblay, R. (1975). Development of dental plaque on epoxy resin crowns in man. A light and electron microscopic study. *J Periodontol,* 46:10–26.

70. Lie, T. (1978). Ultrastructural study of early plaque formation. *J Periodont Res,* 13:391–409.

71. Kolenbrander, P. E., & London, J. (1993). Adhere today, here tomorrow: Oral bacterial adherence. *J Bacteriol,* 175:3247–52.

72. Theilade, J., Fejerskov, O., & Hørsted, M. (1976). A transmission electron microscopic study of 7-day-old bacterial plaque in human tooth fissures. *Arch Oral Biol,* 21:587–98.

73. Newman, H. N. (1980). Retention of bacteria on oral surfaces. In Bitton, G., & Marshall, K. C., Eds. *Adsorption of microorganisms to surfaces.* New York, NY: Wiley-Intersciences, 207–51.

74. Hardie, J. M., & Bowden, G. H. (1974). The normal microbial flora of the mouth. In Skinner, F. A., & Carr, J. G., Eds. *The normal microbial flora of man.* London, UK: Academic Press, 47–83.

75. Socransky, S. S. (1977). Microbiology of periodontal disease—Present status and future considerations. *J Periodontol,* 48:497–504.

76. van Houte, J., Gibbons, R. J., & Banghart, S. B. (1970). Adherence as a determinant of the presence of *Streptococcus salivarius* and *Streptococcus sanguis* on the human tooth surface. *Arch Oral Biol,* 15:1025–34.

77. Donoghue, H. D., & Newman, H. N. (1976). Effect of glucose and sucrose on survival in batch culture of *Streptococcus mutans* C67-1 and a non-cariogenic mutant, C67-25. *Infect Immun,* 13:16–21.

78. Kilian, M., & Rölla, G. (1976). Initial colonization of teeth in monkeys as related to diet. *Infect Immun,* 14:1022–27.

79. Weerkamp, A. H. (1985). Coaggregation of *Streptococcus salivarius* with gram-negative oral bacteria: Mechanism and ecological significance. In Mergenhagen, S. E., & Rosan, B., Eds. *Molecular basis of oral microbial adhesion.* Washington, DC: American Society for Microbiology, 177–83.

80. Ciardi, J. E., McCray, G. F. A., Kolenbrander, P. E., & Lau, A. (1987). Cell-to-cell interaction of *Streptococcus sanguis* and *Propionibacterium acnes* on saliva-coated hydroxyapatite. *Infect Immun,* 55:1441–46.

81. Lamont, R. J., & Rosan, B. (1990). Adherence of mutans streptococci to other oral bacteria. *Infect Immun,* 58:1738–43.

82. Shah, H. N., & Gharbia, S. E. (1991). Microbial factors in the aetiology of chronic inflammatory periodontal disease. In Newman, H. N., & Williams, D. N., Eds. *Inflammation and immunology in chronic inflammatory periodontal disease.* Northwood, UK: Science Reviews Limited, 1–32.

83. Van der Hoeven, J. S., de Jong, M. H., & Kolenbrander, P. D. (1985). *In vivo* studies of microbial adherence in dental plaque. In Mergenhagen, S. E., & Rosan, B., Eds. *Molecular basis of oral microbial adhesion.* Washington, DC: American Society for Microbiology, 220–27.

84. Globerman, D. Y., & Kleinberg, I. (1979). Intra-oral pO₂ and its relation to bacterial accumulation on the oral tissues. In Kleinberg, I., Ellison, S. A., & Mandel, I. D., Eds. *Proceedings: Saliva and dental caries.* (A special supplement for *Microbiol Abst*). New York, NY: Information Retrieval, 275–92.

85. Newman, H. N. (1973). The organic films on enamel surfaces. 2. The dental plaque. *Br Dent J*, 135:106–11.

86. Kolenbrander, P. E. (1991). Coaggregation: Adherence in the human oral microbial ecosystem. In Dworkin, M., Ed. *Microbial cell-cell interactions.* Washington, DC: American Society for Microbiology, 316.

87. Simmonds, R. S., Tompkins, G. R., & Goerge, R. J. (2000). Dental caries and the microbial ecology of dental plaque: A review of recent advances. *N Z Dent J*, 96:44–49.

88. Mattingly, S. J., Daneo-Moor, L., & Shockman, G. D. (1977). Factors regulating cell wall thickening and intracellular iodophilic polysaccharide storage in *Streptococcus mutans. Infect Immun*, 16:967–73.

89. Critchley, P., Wood, J. M., Saxton, C. A., & Leach, S. A. (1967). The polymerization of dietary sugars by dental plaque. *Caries Res*, 112–29.

90. McDougall, W. F. (1964). Studies on the dental plaque. IV. Levans and the dental plaque. *Aust Dent J*, 9:1–5.

91. Da Costa, T., & Gibbons, R. J. Hydrolysis of levan by human plaque streptococci. *Arch Oral Biol*, 13:609–17.

92. Manly, R. S., & Richardson, D. T. (1968). Metabolism of levan by oral samples. *J Dent Res*, 47:1080–86.

93. Newman, H. N. (1972). Structure of approximal human dental plaque as observed by scanning electron microscopy. *Arch Oral Biol*, 17:1445–53.

94. Soames, J. V., & Davies, R. M. (1975). The structure of subgingival plaque in a beagle dog. *J Periodont Res*, 9:333–41.

95. Löe, H., Theilade, E., & Jensen, S. B. (1965). Experimental gingivitis in man. *J Periodontol*, 36:177–87.

96. Kinane, D. F. (2001). Causation and pathogenesis of periodontal disease. *Periodontol 2000*, 25:8–20.

97. Petersilka, G. J., Ehmke, B., & Flemmig, T. F. (2002). Antimicrobial effects of mechanical debridement. *Periodontol 2000*, 28:56–71.

98. Mehrotra, K. K., Kapoor, K. K., Pradhan, B. P., & Bhushan, A. (1983). Assessment of plaque tenacity on enamel surface. *J Periodont Res*, 18:386–92.

99. White, D. J. (1997). Dental calculus: Recent insights into occurrence, formation, prevention, removal and oral health effects of supragingival and subgingival deposits. *Eur J Oral Sci*, 105:508–22.

100. Feldman, R. S., Bravacos, J. S., & Rose, C. L. (1983). Association between smoking different tobacco products and periodontal disease indexes. *J Periodontol*, 54:481–88.

101. Wotman, S., Mercadante, J., Mandel, I. D., Goldman, R. S., & Denning, C. (1973). The occurrence of calculus in normal children, children with cystic fibrosis, and children with asthma. *J Periodontol*, 44:278–80.

102. Klein, F. K., & Dicks, J. L. (1984). Evaluation of accumulation of calculus in tube-fed mentally handicapped patients. *J Am Dent Assoc*, 108:352–54.

103. Turesky, S., Breur, M., & Coffman, G. (1992). The effect of certain systemic medications on oral calculus formation. *J Periodontol*, 63:871–75.

104. ten Cate, J. M. (1988). *Recent advances in the study of dental calculus.* Oxford, UK: IRL Press, 143–259.

105. McDougall, W. A. (1985). Analytical transmission electron microscopy of the distribution of elements in human supragingival dental calculus. *Arch Oral Biol*, 30:603–608.

106. Galil, K. A., & Gwinnett, A. J. (1975). Human tooth-fissure contents and their progressive mineralization. *Arch Oral Biol*, 2:559–62.

107. Turesky, S., Renstrup, G., & Glickman, I. (1961). Histologic and histochemical observations regarding early calculus formation in children and adults. *J Periodontol*, 32:7–14, 69–100.

108. Sundberg, M., & Friskopp, J. (1985). Crystallograph of supragingival human dental calculus. *Scand J Dent Res*, 93:30–38.

109. Schroeder, H. E. (1969). *Formation and inhibition of dental calculus.* Bern, Switzerland: Hans Huber, 559–62.

110. Listgarten, M. A., & Heneghan, J. B. (1973). Observations on the periodontium and acquired pellicle of adult germfree dogs. *J Periodontol*, 44:85–91.

111. Moskow, B. S. (1969). Calculus attachment in cemental separations. *J Periodontol*, 4:1125–30.

112. Selvig, K. A. (1970). Attachment of plaque and calculus to tooth surfaces. *J Periodontol Res*, 5:8–18.

113. Zacherl, W. A., Pfeiffer, H. J., & Swancar, J. R. (1985). The effect of soluble pyrophosphates on dental calculus in adults. *J Am Dent Assoc*, 110:737–38.

114. Ciancio, S. G. (1995). Chemical agents: Plaque control, calculus reduction and treatment of dentinal hypersensitivity. *Periodontol 2000*, 8:75–86.

115. Drake, D. R., Chung, J., Grigsby, W., & Wu-Yuan, C. (1992). Synergistic effect of pyrophosphate and sodium dodecyl sulfate on periodontal pathogens. *J Periodontol*, 63:696–700.

116. Kowitz, G., Jacobson, J., Meng, Z., & Lucatorto, F. (1990, October). The effects of tartar-control toothpaste on the oral soft tissues. *Oral Surg Oral Med Oral Pathol*, 70:529–36.

Carious Lesions

William J. Niendorff

OBJECTIVES

After studying this chapter, the student should be able to:

1. Describe the four types of carious lesions that are found on the different surfaces of teeth.

2. Describe the histologic characteristics of enamel and dentin that facilitate fluid flow throughout a tooth.

3. Describe the four zones of an incipient caries lesion.

4. Describe the conduits (pores) that directly conduct acid from the bacterial plaque to the body of the lesion.

5. List the bacteria most often implicated in the caries process, and indicate when each is present in the highest number during the caries process.

6. Describe the series of events in a cariogenic plaque and subsurface lesion from the time of bacterial exposure to sugar until the pH returns to a resting state.

7. Describe the characteristics of root caries, and explain the differences and similarities to coronal caries.

8. Describe why the profession takes so much time in treating secondary caries.

9. Describe the relationship between pH and the saturation of calcium and phosphorus ions in caries development.

10. Describe the protective relationship of calcium fluoride to hydroxyapatite and fluorhydroxyapatite during an acidogenic attack.

KEY TERMS

Acidogenesis, 54
Aciduric, 60
CAMBRA, 55
Canaliculi, 61
Cariogenic, 54
Cavitation, 56
Chemicoparasitic theory, 54
Enamel rods, 58
Glass ionomers, 63
Glucans, 60
Caries risk factors, 54
Multifactorial disease process, 54
pH values, 58
Remineralization, 58
Reparative dentin, 62
Stimulated and resting salivary flow, 64
Stephan curve, 63
White spot lesion, 57

INTRODUCTION

Dental caries is one of the most common diseases among humans, causing pain and disability that can lead to acute infection and tooth loss at any age.[1,2] Research has also revealed connections between chronic oral infection and other chronic diseases such as diabetes, cardiovascular disease, osteoporosis, and obesity.[3]

One of the oldest theories of dental caries development was that a "tooth worm" allegedly lived in the center of the tooth.[4] Various therapies were used to eradicate the tooth worm, such as fumigation with henbane seeds, magical formulas, and oaths.[5] In the early 1700s, Pierre Fauchard, the father of modern dentistry, rejected the worm theory to describe caries as an erosion of tooth enamel. He recommended those areas be smoothed with the use of files. In 1881, two speakers at the International Medical Congress, Miles and Underwood, proposed that dental caries was caused by the presence and proliferation of microorganisms.[2]

In 1890, W. D. Miller, an American dentist teaching in Germany, published his **chemoparasitic theory** of caries whose concept is still accepted today.[6,7] As a result of his experimentation, Miller believed that extraction of the lime salts from the teeth was a result of bacterial acidogenesis and was the first step in dental decay. However, Miller's work failed to identify dental plaque as the source of bacteria and their acidic by-products. The chemoparasitic theory became more convincing when combined with the findings of later research including the work of G. V. Black, known as the father of dentistry in the United States, who described the gelatinous microbic plaque as the source of the acids.[8] Today, dental caries is viewed as a continuum spanning the initial bacterial infection followed by the acidic attack of tooth surfaces with continuous cycles of demineralization and remineralization, controlled by multiple **caries risk factors** that vary the activity of this disease among individuals.

It is important to note that the epidemiology and disease attack pattern of dental caries has changed since the advent of fluoridated water and various fluoride products, which have become widely used to prevent or arrest enamel and dentinal lesions. General trends indicate that caries declined during the later half of the 20th century due principally to the use of fluoride, yet recent data suggest dental caries can be rising among young children due to heavy use of fermentable carbohydrates.[9]

MULTIFACTORIAL DISEASE PROCESS

Dental caries is now understood as a **multifactorial disease process**, often represented by the interlocking circles and an arrow depicting the passage of time (Figure 5–1 ■). For caries to develop, four conditions must be present simultaneously: (1) a susceptible tooth and host, (2) **cariogenic** microorganisms in a sufficient quantity, (3) frequent oral consumption of refined sugars (carbohydrates), and (4) occurrence over a period of time. When a tooth covered by a film of cariogenic bacteria is exposed to a suitable carbohydrate substrate, the bacteria metabolize it, producing a weak acid as a by-product of fermentation. This **acidogenesis** produces a local environment that can

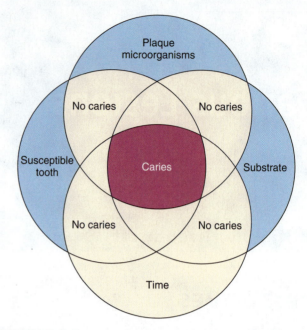

FIGURE ■ 5–1 Dental caries: multifactorial disease process.

demineralize (remove calcium from) tooth enamel and dentin. If these conditions persist over a sufficiently long period of time, an incipient carious lesion develops. An incipient lesion is the initial stage of tooth decay that has not penetrated (or cavitated) through the outer surface of the tooth. The lesion presents as a chalky white spot on the enamel surface (Figure 5–2 ■).

Each of the four main factors includes a number of secondary factors, which can either protect tooth structure or accelerate damage to it. For example, fluoride compounds added to drinking water or a dentifrice have been proven to increase dental enamel's resistance to decay. Conversely, a lack of normal salivary flow or buffering capacity (xerostomia) greatly increases the risk of dental caries, often seen in individuals taking medications or street drugs or undergoing radiotherapy, all of which reduce salivary flow. For example, "Meth mouth" is a rampant form of caries experienced by chronic abusers of methamphetamine (Figure 5–3 ■), a powerful anticholinergic drug.

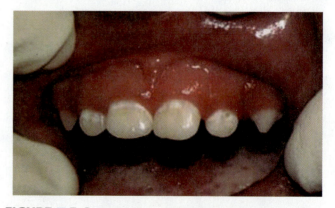

FIGURE ■ 5–2 White spot lesions (decalcifications) on labial surfaces.

(*Source:* Courtesy of Dr. Charles Tatlock, D.D.S., M.P.H.)

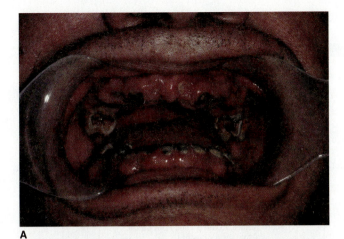

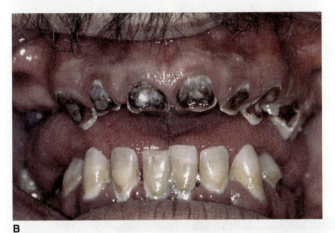

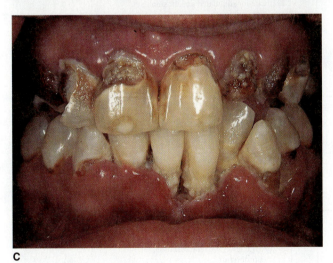

FIGURE ■ 5–3 "Meth mouth." Dental caries pattern due to drug induced xerostomia.

(*Source:* Courtesy of Dr. Charles Tatlock, D.D.S., M.P.H.)

DESCRIPTION OF CARIOUS LESIONS

Although lesions can form because of highly localized factors, *bilaterality* is the phenomenon in which carious lesions often occur on similar surfaces of paired teeth or tooth surfaces on the left and right sides of the mouth.[10,11] For example, patients with interproximal lesions on the distal surface of a left maxillary

DID YOU KNOW

Although many believe that sugar alone causes decay, it is really the acid production that caues decay. Acid is produced by certain bacteria when many types of carbohydrates are eaten and its production increases according to the length of time teeth are exposed. Because these risk factors vary by individual, the relative susceptibility of each patient to dental caries should be assessed prior to planning preventive services. This methodology for Caries Management by Risk Assessment (**CAMBRA**) is based on an understanding that both risk factors and the progression of carious lesions can be controlled using a variety of preventive modalities. CAMBRA is discussed in Chapter 1. A typical caries risk assessment and patient management protocol is shown in Figure 5–4 ■. This form depicts various conditions and risk factors that contribute to the development of carious lesions as well as preventive strategies to reduce the formation and progression of dental caries.

premolar often have a similar lesion on the right side for no clear reason (Figure 5–5 ■). Carious lesions occur in four general areas based on tooth anatomy as categorized as follows:

1. **Pit-and-fissure caries:** These are found on the occlusal surfaces of posterior teeth, in lingual pits of the maxillary incisors, and in buccal pits located on the surfaces of lower molars. Incomplete fusion or hypoplasia of the enamel in these pits (or grooves) during tooth development increases caries susceptibility. Resin sealants can be bonded to the surface of pits and fissures soon after tooth eruption to reduce the risk of caries in these areas.

2. **Smooth-surface caries:** These caries arise on intact smooth enamel surfaces other than at the location of the pits and fissures. Smooth-surface caries can be further divided into (1) caries that affect the buccal and lingual tooth surfaces and (2) interproximal caries, which affect the contact area of adjoining tooth surfaces (i.e., mesial or distal surfaces).

3. **Root-surface caries:** These might involve any surface of the root. Unlike coronal caries that begin in enamel, these lesions are initiated in dentin on root surfaces exposed to the oral environment. Thus, the risk of these lesions increases as gingival recession occurs in adults.

4. **Secondary/recurrent caries:** These occur on the tooth surface adjacent to an existing restoration. These lesions can occur when the initial treatment does not remove all active carious tissue that remains in contact with oral fluids over time.

PHYSICAL AND MICROSCOPIC FEATURES OF INCIPIENT CARIES

The development of a carious lesion occurs in three distinct stages (Figure 5–6 ■). The earliest stage is the incipient lesion, which is accompanied by histologic changes of the enamel. The changes include demineralization, which, simply put, is loss of

ORAL DISEASE RISK ASSESSMENT FOR ADULTS

RISK CATEGORY	EXISTING CONDITIONS		TREATMENT CONSIDERATIONS	CODE
Caries Risk	*Please use a check mark to indicate caries risk*	☑		

Low	No carious lesions in previous 3 years
	Adequately restored dentition
	Adequate oral hygiene
	Regular dental visits
	Diet History:
	    Consumes food/beverages<five times daily
	    Chews sugar-free gum
	    Avoids sweetened beverages between meals
	    Avoids refined sugars and/or fermentable
	        carbohydrates between meals
	    Drinks milk or eats cheese every day
			Review oral hygiene practices
			Review dietary factors
			Recommend fluoride dentifrice
			One year recall (repeat ODRA)
				1330
				1310
				
				0170

Moderate	One carious lesion in previous 3 years
	Exposed roots
	Fair oral hygiene
	Presence of white spots lesions (not fluorosis)
	Presence of interproximal radiolucencies (not into dentin)
	Irregular dental visits
	Orthodontic treatment (planned or in progress)
	Diet History:
	    Eats food or drinks beverages five or more times daily
	    Chews regular (non-sugar-free) gum
	    Drinks sweetened beverages between meals
	    Eats refined sugars and/or fermentable carbohydrates
	        between meals
	    Does not drink milk or eat cheese every day
			Pit and Fissure Caries:
			    Oral hygiene instructions
			    Nutritional counseling
			    Sealants
			    Preventive resins
			Smooth Surface, Recurrent and Root Caries:
			    Oral hygiene instructions
			    Nutritional counseling
			Professionally applies topical fluoride
			Recommend fluoride dentifrice
			Rx for self-applied fluoride
			Six month recall (repeat ODRA)
				1330
				1310
				1351
				2391
				
				1330
				1310
				1360
				
				1340
				0170

High	Two carious lesions in previous three years
	Previous root caries or numerous exposed roots
	Deep pits and fissures
	Poor oral hygiene
	Frequent sugar intake
	Inadequate use of topical fluoride
	Irregular dental visits
	Inadequate saliva flow
	Orthodontic treatment (planned or in progress)
	Diet History: (As described in moderate caries risk above)
			Pit and Fissure Caries:
			    Oral hygiene instructions
			    Nutritional counseling
			    Sealants
			    Preventive resins
			Smooth Surface, Recurrent and Root Caries:
			    Oral hygiene instructions
			    Nutritional counseling
			Professionally applies topical fluoride
			Recommend fluoride dentifrice
			Rx for self-applied fluoride
			3-6 month recall (repeat ODRA)
			Antimicrobial agents
				1330
				1310
				1351
				2391
				
				1330
				1310
				1360
				
				1340
				0170
				4381

Other Risks	*Please use Y (yes) or N (no) to indicate risk.*	Y/N		

Xerostomia	Patient's mouth dry when eating a meal
	Difficulty in swallowing food
	Liquid needed to aid swallowing
	"Too little" saliva in mouth most of the time
	Medications with potential to cause Xerostomia
	Head & neck radiation therapy
			Evaluate for stimulated and un-stimulated
			    flow reduction
			Evaluate contributing factors
			Fluoride therapy (see above)
			Oral hygiene instructions (special products)
			Select appropriate restorative materials
			Nutritional and hydration counseling
			Referral for salivary dysfunction evaluation
			    (unless medication - induced)
				
				0415

Regressive Alterations or Injury	Evidence of tooth erosion/abrasion Evidence of tooth attrition/bruxism Evidence of maladaptive oral habits Risk of oral injury (contact sport, no seatbelt use, physical abuse)		Oral hygiene instructions Occlusal guard Athletic mouth guard	1330 9940
Periodontal Risks	History of periodontitis Soft tissue disease Diabetes Genetics Tobacco or marijuana use		Follow periodontal treatment protocol Advise patient of potential risks	
Cancer Risks	HX of oral cancer Tobacco user past or present Heavy alcohol use Sunlight exposure/fair-skinned patient		Schedule intraoral/extraoral examination annually Teach patient oral self-examination Tobacco counseling to control/prevent oral disease: 5A program, RX nicotine cessation, refer as appropriate)	0120 1301 1320

FIGURE ■ 5–4 Dental caries risk assessment form for patients.

calcium, phosphorus, and other ions from the enamel. The second stage includes the progress of demineralization toward the dentinoenamel junction (DEJ), the boundary between the dentinal layer of the tooth and the enamel layer. Demineralization can then continue into the softer, less mineralized dentin toward the dental pulp. The final phase of caries development is the overt, or frank, lesion characterized by actual **cavitation** of the tooth surface—a "cavity"—or loss of the integrity of the outer enamel that is undermined by progressive slow or rapid demineralization. If the time between the onset of the incipient lesion and the development of cavitation is rapid and extensive, the condition is referred to as *rampant dental caries.*

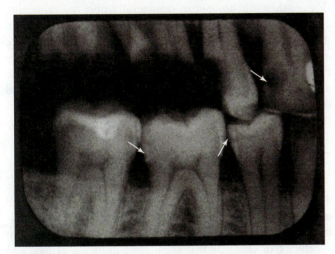

FIGURE ■ 5–5 Carious lesions on proximal surfaces revealed on radiographs.

(*Source:* Courtesy of Dr. Charles Tatlock, D.D.S., M.P.H.)

Clinically, recognizing and diagnosing the early lesion is often difficult; for this reason, recognizing its etiologic and histologic features is important.[12] Evidence of the incipient lesion is microscopically characterized by the appearance of an area of enamel opacity, the **white spot lesion**. At this earliest clinically visible stage, the subsurface demineralization at the microscopic level can be well established. Interestingly, the surface of the enamel appears intact although the electron microscope can show a surface that is more porous than sound enamel. On the buccal and lingual surface of a tooth, the white spot lesion can be localized, or it can extend along the entire gingival area of the tooth or along multiple teeth at places where plaque tends to accumulate and mature. Interproximally, the incipient lesion often can be detected on a periapical or bitewing radiograph. The lesion presents as a small radiolucency, darkened area, located immediately on the gingival side of the contact point and then gradually expands to a small kidney shape with the indentation of the kidney contour directed coronally.[13] In fissure caries, the initial lesion, comparable to white spot lesions on smooth surfaces, usually occurs bilaterally on the opposing surfaces of the fissure at its orifice. The lesion eventually coalesces at the base of the fissure (Figures 5–7 ■ and 5–8 ■).[14] Lesion formation can also begin in deep or poorly fused fissures well below the tooth surface along the wall of the fissure or at its base, either unilaterally or bilaterally. Adequate sealing of these fissures with a resin can be effective in arresting the carious process.

During early stages, the loss of outer enamel cannot be detected in the incipient lesion. Instead, the mature surface layer remains intact. If an explorer is used, the surface enamel could provide no indication of active demineralization. However,

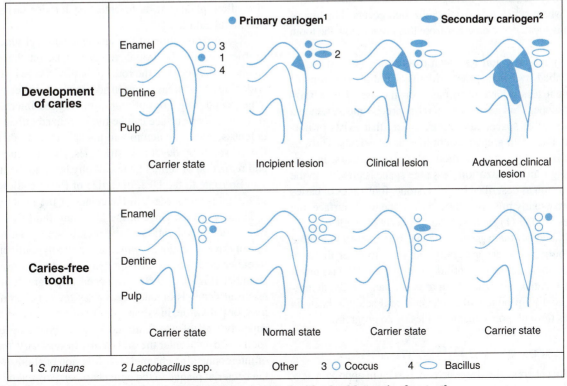

FIGURE ■ 5–6 Development of a carious lesion by stages compared with a healthy, caries-free tooth.

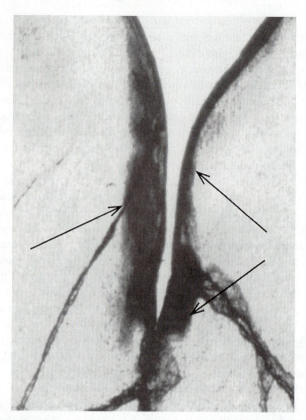

FIGURE ■ 5–7 Incipient caries in an occlusal fissure. The bilaterality of the lesion is evident in the microradiograph.

(*Source:* Courtesy of J. S. Wefel, University of Iowa College of Dentistry, Iowa City.)

microscopic pores extend through the mature surface layer to the point where subsurface demineralization occurs. The foci of the lesion is located and enlarges from this point below the tooth surface.

The incipient lesion has been extensively studied and is best described by Silverstone.[13] Many of the observations of the incipient lesion have been based on the use of a polarizing microscope. This instrument permits precise measurements of the amount of space, called pore space, that exists in normal enamel and to a greater extent in enamel defects. Thus, as demineralization progresses, more pore space occurs; in contrast, during **remineralization**, less pore space is present. In the incipient lesion as described by Silverstone, four zones of caries activity are usually present. Starting from the tooth surface, the four zones are the (1) surface zone, (2) body of the lesion, (3) dark zone, and (4) the translucent zone. It is important to note that microorganisms are generally too large to enter the pore zones of an incipient lesion until demineralization breaks down the enamel matrix, allowing them to penetrate. Yet, the demineralizing acid by-products of acidogenic and aciduric bacteria freely pass through pores enabling a lesion to progress.

Pore Spaces of the Different Zones

The translucent zone, the deepest zone, is seen in approximately 50% of the carious lesions examined.[13] In this zone, which is the advancing front of the lesion, slight demineralization occurs,

resulting in a 1% pore space, compared with 0.1% for intact enamel. In contrast, the dark zone occurs in approximately 95% of carious lesions and has a pore volume of 2% to 4%. When teeth showing no dark zone are placed in a remineralizing solution, the dark zone becomes visible in its expected position between the translucent zone and the body of the lesion.[15] On the basis of this finding, it is suggested that this dark zone is where remineralization can occur; and, that a wider dark zone requires a greater amount, or a longer period, of remineralization of the lesion.

Peripheral to the dark zone is the main body of the lesion. In this zone, pore volume ranges from approximately 5% on the fringes of the lesion to about 25% in the center.[13] Despite this considerable amount of demineralization, the remaining crystals still maintain their basic orientation on the protein matrix. Finally, the surface zone has a nearly normal pore space of approximately 1%. The surface zone and the dark zone are the remineralization zones of the incipient lesion. Thus, surface and subsurface remineralization of pore space with calcium and other minerals is possible until cavitation occurs with the complete breakdown of the enamel matrix.

Direct Connection of the Bacterial Biofilm to the Body of the Lesion

Tooth enamel is made up of interlocking structures called **enamel rods**, which contain billions of hydroxyapatite crystals. The pores present between the crystals and the rods form a network of channels that allow fluid diffusion of ions and small molecules found in the enamel cap. Other structures such as the *striae of Retzius* extend this network into deeper layers of the enamel. This diffusion network allows remineralization of the tooth throughout its life; however, the channels also allow plaque acids to enter the interior enamel, causing demineralization.

Demineralization of the surface enamel produces a ragged profile; in fact, the initial attack can be on the ends of the enamel rods, between the rods, or both.[16] There is a subsequent widening of the areas between adjacent rods (inter-rod space).[17] When conditions are optimum, this ragged interface between surface and subsurface can be remineralized either by the body defenses, such as calcium and phosphate and other ions from the saliva, or by developed strategies, such as fluoride therapy and reduction of fermentable carbohydrates in the diet.

En route to the DEJ, the striae of Retzius allow access out of the inter-rod space into the center of the intact or damaged rods and crystals. Once at the DEJ, any fluid flow, whether it causes demineralization or remineralization, can trichotomize (go in three directions), either along the hypomineralized DEJ in either direction or into the dentinal tubules toward the pulp chamber (Figure 5–9 ■). The speed of progression of the caries front depends on such factors as the concentration of acid ions, or **pH value**, in saliva, salivary flow rates and its buffering capacity—all of which are continually changing each day as food and drinks enter the oral cavity. In summary, there is a trail of interconnecting channels for diffusion of fluids moving from the bacterial plaque to the pulp chamber. Any chemical changes in the plaque (biofilm) are soon reflected throughout the enamel and dentin as part of the incipient lesion.

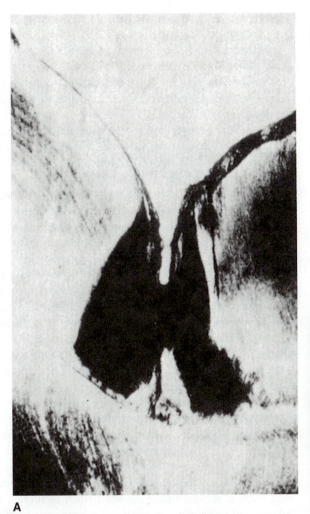

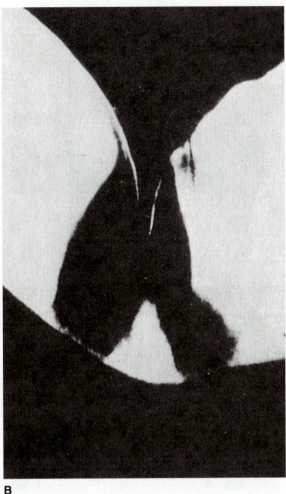

A

B

FIGURE ■ 5–8 The bilaterality of caries development. Note coalescence of two lateral carious areas at base of fissure.

(*Source:* From Konig, K. G. (1963). Dental Morphology in Relation to Carious Resistance with Special Reference to Fissures as Susceptible Areas. *J Dent Res,* 42:461–76.)

DID YOU KNOW?

The acidity of resting saliva (not stimulated by food/drink intake) varies with the species of microorganisms that populate the biofilm in various areas around teeth. When the oral pH (a measure of acidity) drops below 5.5, the environment shifts toward demineralization of teeth. When the pH of resting saliva (sampled from minor glands of the inner lip) approaches neutral acidity (7.0), less aciduric bacteria are favored, and the equilibrium toward natural remineralization is reestablished.

The pores allow plaque acids to exit directly to the subsurface region. The initial acid attack preferentially dissolves the magnesium and carbonate ions, followed by removal of the less soluble calcium, phosphate, and other ions that are part of the crystal.

Eventually, the undermined surface zone collapses. At the same time, the more soluble proteins are lost from the subsurface matrix. Once cavitation occurs, the zones of the incipient lesion become less clearly defined because of mineral loss and the presence of bacteria, bacterial end products, biofilm, and residual substrate, which can support further lesion development with cavitation. The lesion is no longer incipient but an overt caries one requiring operative intervention.

CARIOGENIC BACTERIA

Following Miller's works in the 1890s, fundamental experimental evidence proved that bacteria were the agents of acid production in 1954. Orland and colleagues demonstrated that gnotobiotic rats (grown in a germ-free environment) did not develop caries when fed a cariogenic diet that promotes tooth decay. However, they did develop caries when acidogenic bacteria and a cariogenic diet were introduced into the previous germ-free environment.[18]

Keyes's experiments later demonstrated the transmissible nature of caries in animals by finding that previously gnotobiotic hamsters that were caries inactive (i.e., had incipient lesions but no cavitation) developed caries after contact with the other animals.[19] Specific acidogenic organisms in dental

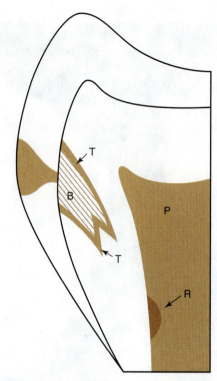

FIGURE ■ 5–9 Diagram of a trichotomized lesion attributable to diffusion of acids in both directions under the enamel and directly into the body of the lesion in the dentin. T, translucent zone; B, body of the lesion; R, reactionary dentin; P, pulp.

(*Source:* From Silverstone L. M., & Hicks, M. J. (1985). The structure and ultrastructure of the carious lesion in human dentin. *Gerodontics,* 1:185–93.)

plaque, notably the Mutans streptococcus (MS) group and some strains of *Lactobacillus* species, are those implicated most in dental caries. Recent research suggests that multiple strains of non-MS species can also play an important role in promoting caries by becoming more aciduric and acidogenic, thus lowering the acidity (pH) of resting saliva in the mouth.

Mutans Streptococci and Caries

For caries to develop, acidogenic bacteria must be present, and a means must exist to prevent the acid from being washed away from the point where the carious lesion is to develop. Dental plaque fulfills both of these functions. It helps protect the bacterial colonies from being flushed, neutralized (buffered), or affected by antimicrobial agents in the saliva by enveloping the colonies in a cocoon of gel-like glucan, an insoluble extracellular polysaccharide.

Of the 300 or more species of microorganisms inhabiting the plaque, the great majority are not directly involved in the caries process. Two bacterial genera are of special interest in cariogenesis: (1) the mutans streptococci and (2) the lactobacilli.[20,21] MS is a group of bacterial species characterized by the ability to produce extracellular glucans from sucrose and by their acid production in animal and human studies. One species in this group, *Streptococcus mutans,* received its name in 1924 when J. K. Clarke in England isolated organisms from human carious lesions. He noted that the organisms were more

oval than round and assumed them to be a mutant form of a streptococcus.[22]

Mutans streptococci are now considered the major pathogenic bacterial species involved in the caries process.[23–32] MS are usually found in relatively large numbers in the plaque that occurs immediately over developing smooth-surface lesions. In one study, specific sites were periodically sampled for the presence of MS, and the teeth were later examined for caries. Teeth destined to become carious exhibited a significant increase in the proportions of MS from 6 to 24 months before the eventual diagnosis of caries.[33] Similarly, dental plaques isolated from sites overlying most developing white spot lesions have a significantly higher proportion of MS than plaques sampled from sound enamel sites.[34] Increased numbers of MS in the saliva also parallel the development of the smooth-surface lesion. In another study, MS counts from the saliva of 200 children indicated that 93% with detectable caries were positive for MS whereas uninfected children were almost always caries free.[35]

Certain physiologic characteristics of the MS favor their reputation as a prime agent in caries. These traits include the ability to adhere to tooth surfaces, production of abundant **glucans** from sucrose, rapid production of lactic acid from a number of sugar substrates, acid tolerance, and the production of intracellular polysaccharide (energy) stores. These features help the MS survive in an unfriendly environment related to periods of very low availability of substrate (i.e., between meals and snacks). As a general rule, the cariogenic bacteria metabolize sugars to produce the energy required for their growth and reproduction. The by-products of this metabolism are acids and are released into the plaque fluid. MS mainly causes damage with lactic acid, although other acids, such as formic, acetic, butyric, and propionic, are present in a cariogenic biofilm and can have a pH range as low as 3.8 to 4.8.[36] These weak organic acids are small enough in molecule size to fit inside the diffusion channels of enamel and the subsurface layer causing demineralization (e.g., the white spot lesion).

Lactobacilli and Caries

Lactobacilli (LB) are cariogenic, acidogenic, and **aciduric**. From the early 1920s until the 1950s, LB were considered the essential bacteria that caused caries. Not until 1954 did the studies of Orland demonstrate that if rodents living in a germ-free environment were infected with lactic acid–producing enterococci, but no LB, they still developed caries.[18] This was the first knowledge that LB were not required for caries development. Often the number of LB isolated from either saliva or plaque was too low in number to be considered capable of producing the range of pH values required for the initiation of caries.[37] However, once a carious lesion develops, the stability of the immediate plaque population changes rapidly. The low pH environment of LB often eliminates, or at least suppresses, the continuity of colonization of MS (i.e., its formation of compact groups of bacteria).[38,39]

This phenomenon of a lowering pH causing MS to be displaced by LB is seen after irradiation therapy for head and neck cancer. During the treatment, multiple caries lesions develop rapidly because of the destruction of the salivary glands.[40]

During the initial phases of the developing carious lesions, large numbers of MS are involved only to decrease in number later as the LB population increases. This decrease is believed to be caused by LB creating a sufficiently low pH to establish a monopoly of the environment.

ADHERENCE OF BACTERIA TO TEETH

Continuous adherence to the solid tooth surface by MS is necessary both before and after initial colonization. The first bacteria must establish a hold on the acquired pellicle on the tooth surface and then maintain their positions while other bacteria continue to colonize in other protected areas offered by the interproximal spaces, along the gingiva, or in the pits and fissures. Otherwise the bacteria would be swept away by the saliva.

Children who consume little or no sucrose because of sucrase or fructase enzyme deficiencies have a less cariogenic plaque. Similarly, patients receiving long-term nourishment via a stomach tube have less plaque and fewer MS.[41] Individuals restricting their sucrose intake have a decreased proportion of MS in their plaque, but the MS increases when sucrose is reintroduced into the diet.[42] Dietary restriction of sugar has also been shown to reduce the acidogenicity of dental plaque.[43,44] There are multiple sources of acid in the oral biofilm ecology: bacterial, dietary (many nonsugary foods and drugs have an acidic pH), environmental, and intrinsic (e.g., bulimia, reflux), and they can all work in combination to maintain an acidic biofilm in local regions or in the entire oral cavity.

ECOLOGY OF CARIES DEVELOPMENT

Caries Transmission

Several studies support the possibility that the first bacteria to adhere to teeth (primary colonizers) can help determine the eventual pathogenicity of the plaque.[33] Once a species has established a haven safe from competing bacteria and saliva (i.e., its ecologic niche), other bacteria introduced at a later date appear to have a more difficult task in colonizing. Once established, a niche can last a long time. For instance, children with the highest number of MS for primary teeth usually experience a higher attack rate for the permanent teeth.[45]

Mutans streptococci require a solid surface for successful colonization. During the first year of life before eruption of the primary teeth, very few MS are found in the mouth.[46] When teething begins at approximately 8 months, MS often rapidly colonize the plaque of newly erupting teeth.[47] It has been shown that an important source of MS infection in infants is from the caregivers, usually the mother, by mouth-to-mouth transmission via kissing or by sharing a spoon during feeding.[48] Mothers with the highest MS counts often have infants with similarly high counts of caries lesions.[49] Because early infection by MS is associated with high decay rates, it has been strongly suggested that an effective means of preventing caries in young children would be to reduce the number of MS in the parents' and siblings' mouths before a child's birth.[50] A growing body of evidence suggests that mothers using xylitol gums or lozenges have decreased levels of

MS and do not transmit these cariogenic bacteria as readily to their children.[51] Xylitol is a sugar alcohol that has a sweet taste but is less cariogenic than sucrose because it acts as a selective factor favoring MS stains that are less acidogenic.

At the time of eruption, no populations of bacteria are entrenched on the tooth's surface; therefore, primary colonizers have little difficulty establishing their ecologic niches on the acquired pellicle and in the saliva. After tooth eruption, many bacteria already present in the mouth participate in the formation of plaque. Each firmly established niche can act as a "seeding" area for other areas of the mouth. Mutans streptococci decrease in number as teeth are lost throughout life and practically disappear after full-mouth extraction.[52] After dentures are inserted, MS reappear only to disappear again when the dentures are removed for an extended period. Thus, as a disease of the biofilm, dental caries is more complicated than previously thought because it involves multiple species of bacteria interacting as an ecosystem.

Coronal Dentin Caries

During the embryonic stage of the tooth, the ameloblasts and the odontoblasts are lined up at the location of the future DEJ.[53] Ameloblasts are responsible for the formation of enamel, which subsequently becomes the future surface of the tooth whereas odontoblasts are responsible for the formation of the dentin, which becomes the border of the dental pulp. The primary function of enamel is to protect the underlying dentin. In turn, the dentin forms a protective layer around the dental pulp. Dentin also contains a network of tubules that allows the transport of fluids to and from the dental pulp. The dental pulp is located at the center of the tooth and contains nerves and blood vessels, which provide nutrients to the tooth through the dentinal tubules. A detailed description of these processes follows.

During the period of tooth formation, each odontoblast lays down a trailing odontoblastic process. This is an extension of the odontoblast into the dentinal tubules. Between the tubules there is intertubular dentin, also called *mantle dentin*.[54] The tubules contain fluid that originates from the pulp chamber. There is intertubular communication and fluid transport via secondary tubules and smaller-sized **canaliculi**. All tubules act as channels for the convection flow of fluids outward from the pulp.[55] Dentinal fluid is constantly pumped into tubules by the forces of mastication with a return of the fluid to the pulp upon release of the pressure.[56] When bacterial toxins from caries arrive in the tubules, more fluid is forced into the tubule.[57,58] The pulp fluid also contains important calcium, phosphate, and secretory immunoglobulin A.[58,59]

When enamel caries reach the DEJ, many of the odontoblastic processes underlying the carious inter-rod areas of the enamel lose their vitality. These tubules become dead tracts and begin to partially or wholly calcify. Complete calcification results in a hard calcified group of tubules called **sclerotic dentin**. This acts as a protective barrier to the advancing caries. At the same time, the odontoblasts located on the periphery of the pulp are triggered to begin laying down increments of amorphous **reparative dentin** to further protect the pulp. This calcified dentin is often a feature in arrested carious lesions, which are no longer decalcifying.

In summary, the millions of diffusion and convection channels in the enamel and dentin, respectively, permit movement of fluid from the tooth surface to the pulp.[60,61] The intertubular secondary canals and the canaliculi provide permeability within the dentin whereas the DEJ allows acid to move laterally in these channels, undermining the enamel and aiding in its collapse, forming overt carious lesions. According to in vitro studies, if an x-ray shows a radiolucency that extends even into deep dentin, the entire precaries lesion can theoretically and slowly be remineralized *if* the surface zone where the caries began has not broken down into an overt cavity.[62] In other words, restorative treatment cannot be the treatment of choice until cavitation of the enamel has occurred.[63]

Root Caries

A general demographic shift is continually occurring in the United States with each successive generation living longer and retaining more of their natural dentition. This increase in tooth retention can be attributed to the success of dental hygiene in preventing and controlling infectious diseases during the last century as well as socioeconomic factors.[64,65] As older adults retain much of their natural dentition, chronic gingival recession exposes root surfaces that become at risk for root caries. In addition, this population is using an increasing number of medications (polypharmacy) that are known to reduce salivary flow (xerostomia).[66] Katz and colleagues estimated that individuals entering their thirties have about 1 in 100 surfaces with recession and root caries. When they enter their sixties, about 1 of 5 exposed surfaces is involved. The roots of the molars in the mandible are at greatest risk, whereas the mandibular incisors are at the least risk.[67]

The percentage of adults with root caries was higher with age: 9% of adults aged 20–39 years had root decay compared with 18% of adults aged 40–59 years and 32% of adults 60 years and older. The greatest disparities in the prevalence of root caries were seen for current smokers. Twice as many current smokers (28%) as nonsmokers (14%) had root caries.[64–68] A Canadian study concluded that the increase in the prevalence of root decay with age might not be due to aging per se; instead, the increase can be the result of neglect of oral health during the years of growing older. Older adults with continual good oral health still had low rates of root decay.[69] A study of 5,000 subjects in Finland found that men had 1.1 to 2.5 times more root caries than women. The greatest difference was in the group 60 to 69 years of age.[70]

A number of risk factors have been identified for root caries development, including age, gender, fluoride exposure, systemic illness, medications, oral hygiene, and diet.[71,72] In terms of the microbiology of root caries, despite early indications of a strong association between the *Actinomyces* species and progressive root lesions,[73,74,] more recent studies indicate that plaque and salivary concentrations of MS are correlated positively with the presence of root-surface caries.[73–76]

Root caries differs from coronal caries in several aspects. A critical difference is that the tissues affected, enamel versus cementum, are fundamentally dissimilar. Enamel on the tooth surface is more highly mineralized than the cementum, which covers the root surface, or the underlying dentin. Because of the lower mineral content and higher organic content of the cementum–dentin complex, root caries can progress both by acid demineralization of the inorganic structure and by proteolysis of the organic component.[77] In proteolysis, the organic components (proteins) are broken down into simpler substances, usually through the action of enzymes. These tissue differences determine variations in the rate of lesion formation, its histologic and visual appearance, and the potential for and rate of remineralization.[78] Clinically, the lesion is initially noncavitated. The carious material is soft and has a yellowish-brown coloration. The lesion can eventually assume any outline and can involve multiple root surfaces. When cavitation is evident, lesions tend to spread laterally, have a depth of approximately 0.5 to 1.0 mm, and have a dark brown appearance.[79] The lesions appear immediately below the cemento–enamel junction, undermining but not involving the enamel.

DID YOU KNOW ?

Dental caries is not just a child's disease, and decay among older adults has increased for a variety of reasons including increased tooth retention rates and increased use of medications that cause xerostomia.

Root caries differ from coronal caries in that bacterial invasion of cementum and dentin occurs quickly once the cariogenic process begins because there is no overlying enamel. At times in the carious invasion, columns of organisms appear between spikes of relatively intact cementum. At other times, a complete loss of cementum exposes the dentin. Similar to enamel caries, root caries are amenable to remineralization and/or arrest.[78] Arrested root caries demonstrate three physical characteristics: (1) an outer barrier of hypermineralized surface dentin, (2) a sclerotic inner barrier between carious and sound dentin, and (3) mineralization occurring within the dentinal tubules.[79] Clinically, such remineralized lesions can appear dark and hard; tactile examination with a dental explorer easily distinguishes the smooth, hard, and glassy feel of arrested lesions from the leathery feel of active root caries. Active root surface lesions have a relatively short penetration distance compared to that of coronal caries in order to reach the pulp tissues. These caries can also be difficult to restore or to remineralize effectively (particularly proximal lesions), thus posing a difficult management problem for clinicians and patients.

Secondary, or Recurrent, Caries

Secondary caries can result from imperfections in or around restorations, such as incomplete removal of active carious tissue, poor bonding of adhesive restorative materials, which allows marginal leakage, or overhangs that can exist between the proximal tooth surface and the gingival margins of a restoration.[80] Also, some tooth-colored fillings (composites) are more porous and have a higher affinity for plaque.[81] Bacteria are able to colonize and multiply at these vulnerable sites, sheltered from the protective effects of saliva and patients' self-care efforts. Secondary caries is a significant problem that is largely preventable, and these lesions are most likely to occur among high-risk caries patients.

Diagnosis of these lesions is difficult.[82,83] In one study, extracted teeth were cut so that the section included both a clinically sound amalgam margin and one defined as "ditched." A ditched margin means visible space exists between the tooth surface and the restoration due to wear or fracture. This defect creates a risk of recurrent caries. The prevalence of recurrent lesions in both sound and ditched restorations was close to 50%, although it is unknown whether these lesions were truly recurrent or due to residual caries left during a previous cavity preparation.[84] The magnitude of the problem of secondary decay is illustrated by studies indicating that the median survival time of restorations ranges from 5 to 10 years.[85] Prevention of the number of primary lesions is the best solution. One strategy to prevent recurrent caries is to apply materials that bond/fuse to the tooth tissue and slowly release fluoride. Fluoride-releasing materials include **glass ionomers** and the newer fluoride-releasing composites and amalgams.[86–88]

Measuring Plaque pH, the Stephan Curve

There is a pH value (acidity level) change in plaque each time a food or beverage is consumed. Even during sleep, the acidity of the mouth increases as salivary flow naturally diminishes during the night. Microelectrodes have been inserted in dental bridgework and telemonitored in numerous studies to determine these pH changes. There is an immediate drop in pH when any fermentable carbohydrate is consumed followed by a slower recovery period to a neutral pH than when other foods are eaten. This drop-and-recovery curve has been termed the **Stephan curve** after Dr. Robert Stephan, an officer in the United States Public Health Service, who first reported the cyclic change in pH that followed eating and drinking of

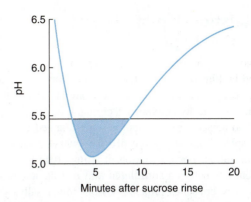

FIGURE ■ 5–10 Stephan curve after sucrose rinse.

different foods and beverages.[89] Plaque pH responses to simple sugar rinses performed by caries-free and caries-active individuals exhibited different drops in pH and different lengths of time to return to normal. Figure 5–10 ■ is a graph of the Stephan curve after a sucrose rinse. Figure 5–11 ■ graphs the variation in pH over a 24-hour period. Thus, different individuals have different capabilities to buffer acid production based on the frequency of dietary exposures over a typical day. Similar pH studies have identified foods that are not hazardous to the teeth as well as those that are accompanied by a drop past the critical pH of 5.5 to 5.0, such as dried fruits, white bread, cereals, carbonated soda, and starchy foods. These lists can be of considerable value when counseling caries active patients and parents or caregivers.[90]

Although food types are important in producing a cariogenic (low pH) environment, the frequency of the acid attack on enamel can be at least as important in creating a continuous environment for demineralization. Frequent between-meal snacks and drinks can maintain a low pH environment throughout the day, which shifts the demineralization/remineralization continuum toward caries formation.

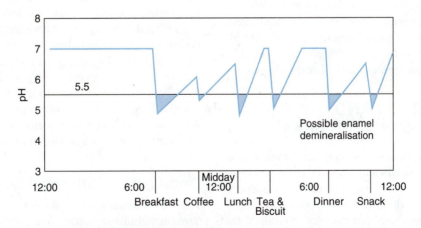

FIGURE ■ 5–11 Stephan curve during a normal day eating pattern.
Gradual return to resting values after about 40 minutes. Each curve represents the mean of 12 subjects; the pH was measured by sampling method and therefore is an average value for the whole-mouth plaque pH. In individual sites away from the salivary buffers, the pH values can fall close to 4.0. The upper curve was obtained from reconstituted skim milk and the lower one from an apple-flavored drink, showing a large difference in the acidogenicity of these two drinks.

(*Source:* Courtesy of M. W. J. Dodds, University of Texas Dental School, San Antonio.)

The Relationship of Mineral Saturation to pH

The concentration of calcium and phosphate ions in the salivary fluid and biofilm bathing the tooth at the plaque–tooth interface is extremely important because these are the same elements that compose the hydroxyapatite crystal found in the enamel. If the fluid adjacent to the tooth is supersaturated with calcium and phosphate ions at a given pH, the enamel cannot undergo demineralization. For this reason, it is important to understand the differences between **stimulated and resting saliva**. Resting salivary flow emanates principally from minor salivary glands throughout the mouth throughout the day. Its pH and buffering capacity are typically lower—more acidic—than stimulated salivary flow. During brief periods when food or drink are imbibed, salivary flow from major salivary glands (e.g., the parotid, submandibular, sublingual) is stimulated to lubricate the oral cavity. Stimulated saliva among most individuals is supersaturated with calcium and phosphate ions compared with the levels of these minerals in enamel.[85] The bacterial plaque can concentrate these ions to an even greater extent. For instance, the number of calcium and phosphate ions in plaque can be 3 times more than the number in the saliva.[91] This increased concentration of calcium and phosphate levels tends to be inversely related to the caries score.[50] As the pH drops below 5.5 in an acid attack, the level of mineral supersaturation also drops, and the risk of demineralization increases. Different plaques have various initial pHs, buffering potentials, and concentrations of calcium and phosphate in different parts of the mouth based on the ecology of localized microbial populations. Recent research has revealed that some non-MS bacteria, which are also aciduric and/or acidogenic, increase in numbers when an acidic environment prevails beyond the expected time period after eating based on the Stephan Curve. In other words, frequent eating of fermentable carbohydrates, particularly between meals, favors the population growth of acidogenic species, which then lowers the pH of resting saliva. Thus, the pH of resting saliva, which controls the nature of the oral environment during most of a 24-hour period, can becomes a more important a factor in controlling demineralization as is stimulated saliva. Some strategies in CAMBRA now involve trying to raise the pH of resting saliva by using self-applied alkaline rinses and other products, which that discourage the growth of acidic plaques.[92]

DEMINERALIZATION AND REMINERALIZATION PRINCIPLES

Throughout this chapter and others there are references to demineralization and remineralization of teeth, both as a pathologic and a therapeutic process. To review, demineralization is caused by plaque acids that dissolve the tooth minerals making up the basic calcium, phosphate, and hydroxyl crystals of the enamel, dentin, and cementum. Remineralization, on the other hand, requires the availability of the same ions, preferably with fluoride, which is a chemically stronger ion than calcium, as a catalyst to replace the missing or damaged enamel rods, a process that ten Cate aptly calls *nonrestorative repair*.[93] Recent studies have shown that products containing amorphous calcium phosphate (ACP) and calcium casein phosphopeptide (CCP) can stimulate remineralization of tooth enamel. Products containing ACP, or ingredients that form ACP, can be found in toothpastes, mouthrinses, artificial saliva, chewing gums, topically applied coatings, and other vehicles for topical use.[94–97]

There are many calcium and phosphate compounds in the body that vary in chemical composition and with changes in pH. The crystals and fluoride compound of most dental interest in the demineralization and remineralization process are hydroxyapatite (HAP), fluorhydroxyapatite (FHA), and calcium fluoride (CaF_2).

The long-term exposure of teeth to low concentrations of fluoride (as found in fluoridated water) results in the gradual incorporation of fluoride into the existing HAP crystals to form FHA, which is more resistant to acid damage. Conversely, a higher concentration of fluoride (as occurs with the use of professionally applied topical fluoride, fluoride dentifrices, rinses, and varnishes, etc.) results in the formation of surface globules of CaF_2 (as seen in electron microscope images). If phosphates and proteins of the saliva coat these globules, the globules become more insoluble.[98] When the fluoride is incorporated into HAP to form FHA, it is said to be firmly bound, whereas loosely bound fluoride is in the form of CaF_2, which is adsorbed onto the surface of HAP and FHA crystals.[99]

The Relationship between HAP, FHA, and CaF_2

After an attack by plaque acid(s), CaF_2 in enamel dissolves first, followed in sequence by HAP, and finally, FHA (with its fluoride substitutions). As the attack continues, the dissociated ions increase the saturation level of the immediate fluid sufficiently to slow crystal dissolution and eventually arrest further solution of the crystals. As the pH begins to return to normal, crystals begin to reform from the complex pool of dissolved ions, some as HAP, some as FHA (with many of the fluoride ions coming from the previous CaF_2). Finally, newly adsorbed CaF_2 is precipitated. Any deficiencies are subsequently replaced, in time, by calcium, phosphate, and fluoride from sources such as the saliva, water, and toothpastes. In observing this process, one must marvel at the body's defense system. Although components of the lymph system that provide cellular or humoral immunity are absent in the enamel, the body can use a chemical system to maintain a state of equilibrium (homeostasis)—one in which CaF_2 provides a reservoir for fluoride that is immediately available when and where it is needed.[100] The only time the system breaks down is when the attacks are too frequent and prolonged. (See Chapter 9 for further discussion of the oral cavity's defense system.)

Depth of Remineralization

There is little controversy about the success of topical procedures in stimulating surface remineralization and about the use of commercial fluoride products such as dentifrices, gels, and varnish to compensate for the daily wear and tear of demineralization. In the New Zealand School System, incipient lesions with x-ray lucencies that extend midway through the enamel are considered candidates for remineralization. An in vitro study performed by Cate showed that both the inner enamel and dentin could be remineralized, but very slowly. Only the outer part of the enamel appeared to be responsive to fluoride diffusion and remineralization.[94]

Some researchers believe that remineralization is a reasonable objective even for lesions reaching to the dentin. The test for remineralization in these cases is the lack of demonstrable caries progress for 2 to 3 years. However, an important fact is that no reported studies indicate whether deep remineralization is or is not successful.

SUMMARY

Dental caries is a multifactorial disease involving an interaction of bacteria, diet, host resistance, and time. These etiologic "risk" factors vary among individuals, and the management of caries (using CAMBRA) should take into account these risk factors with a careful assessment of patients and periodic evaluation based on their level of caries risk. Saliva is the most important natural protective factor against caries. Impaired salivary flow because of intrinsic factors (age) or extrinsic factors (various drugs) creates an extreme caries risk. Salivary flow, its buffering capacity and its acidity (pH) all play a crucial role in balancing the demineralization/remineralization continuum, which occurs in plaque. Stimulated saliva is released during eating and has a high buffering (remineralization) capacity and pH, but resting saliva can also play a large role in maintaining the homeostasis of tooth tissue. Frequent use of fermentable carbohydrates each day (between meals) can favor the growth of acideogenic bacterial colonies, thus lowering the pH (raising the acidity) of resting saliva. Several acidogenic bacteria can cause caries development with *Mutans streptococci* and *Lactobacilli* being the most studied, but species can play a role if the oral environment is compromised.

Silverstone[13] opened the possibility of nonrestorative repair of carious lesions when he described the demineralizing and remineralizing zones of an incipient lesion. Since that time, much research and effort by the dental care profession have been directed at ways to remineralize lesions. To simultaneously increase tooth resistance and the probability of remineralizing incipient lesions, individuals must still use an array of mechanical strategies for eliminating long-standing plaque formation, applying a fluoride dentifrice or rinses daily, using antimicrobial and neutralizing rinses, and adopting effective between-meal dietary controls.

PRACTICAL CONSIDERATIONS

Demineralization and remineralization of tooth are continuous processes. Cavitation can occur only when demineralization outstrips the body's defensive capability for remineralizations over a period of time. The enamel matrix and spacial relationships of rods, pores, and crystals allow fluids to diffuse throughout the enamel. Like the wick of an oil lamp, this network is available for the in-and-out movement of tooth-mineral ions and acids produced by bacteria in plaque. Even when an incipient lesion penetrates the enamel cap, it can often be remineralized without the need for an invasive restoration.

The use of fluoride compounds at home and in the dental office thus remain an essential tool of caries prevention, but strategies are broadening as research continues. At this point, community water fluoridation remains the most effective public health measure in preventing caries. Perhaps the most important role of dental care providers in modern caries control is to assess and to educate patients at all ages as to their caries risk factors. The early identification and treatment of risk factors rather than just treating lesions can prevent unnecessary restorative treatment or eventual tooth loss. Throughout this book, emphasis will be placed on the various strategies now available for preventing demineralization or enhancing remineralization of teeth.

SELF-STUDY QUESTIONS

1. For dental caries to develop, which conditions must occur simultaneously?

   a. There must be a susceptible tooth and host.

   b. Cariogenic microorganisms must be present in a sufficient quantity.

   c. There must be frequent oral consumption of refined carbohydrates.

   d. Only A and B.

   e. All of the above.

   Rationale: For caries to develop, four factors must occur simultaneously: (1) a susceptible tooth and host, (2) the presence of cariogenic microorganisms in a sufficient quantity, (3) frequent oral consumption of refined carbohydrates, and (4) this process must occur over a period of time.

2. Which areas can carious lesions occur?

   a. Gingival margin

   b. Periodontal dentin ligament

   c. Pit and fissures

   d. Gingival sulcus

   Rationale: Based on tooth anatomy as categorized here, carious lesions occur in four general areas. (1) Pit-and-fissure caries are found on the occlusal surfaces of posterior teeth, in lingual pits of the maxillary incisors, and in buccal pits located on the surfaces of lower molars. Incomplete fusion or hypoplasia of the enamel in these pits (or grooves) during tooth development increases caries susceptibility. Resin sealants can be bonded to the surface of pits and fissures soon after tooth eruption to reduce the risk of caries in these areas. (2) Smooth-surface caries arise on intact smooth enamel surfaces other than at the location of the pits and fissures. Smooth-surface caries can be further divided into (a) caries that affect the buccal and lingual tooth surfaces and (b) interproximal caries, which affect the contact area of adjoining tooth surfaces (i.e., mesial or distal surfaces). (3) Root-surface caries might involve any surface of the root. Unlike coronal caries that begin in enamel, these lesions are initiated in dentin on root surfaces exposed to the oral environment. Thus, the risk of these lesions increases as gingival recession occurs in adults. (4) Secondary/recurrent caries occur on the tooth surface adjacent to an existing restoration.

3. Which of the following is composed of tooth enamel?

   a. Enamel junctions

   b. Dentin

   c. Enamel rods

   d. Dentinal tubules

   Rationale: Tooth enamel is made up of interlocking structures called *enamel rods,* which contain billions of hydroxyapatite crystals.

4. When there is an immediate drop in pH after carbohydrate consumption, which returns to a normal pH, this is termed

   a. Stephan curve

   b. Liken curve

   c. Liken drop

   d. Strait of Reitz

   Rationale: There is an immediate drop in pH when any fermentable carbohydrate is consumed followed by a slower recovery period to a neutral pH than when other foods are eaten. This drop-and-recovery curve has been termed the *Stephan curve* after Dr. Robert Stephan, who first reported the continuous, cyclic change in pH that followed eating and drinking of different foods and beverages.

5. Although food types are important in producing a cariogenic (low pH) environment, frequent between-meal snacks and drinks can maintain a low pH environment throughout the day, which shifts the demineralization/remineralization continuum toward caries formation.

   a. The first statement is true; the second statement is false.

   b. The first statement is false; the second statement is true.

   c. Both statements are true.

   d. Both statements are false.

   Rationale: Though food types are important in producing a cariogenic (low pH) environment, the frequency of the acid attack on enamel can be at least as important in creating a continuous environment for demineralization. Frequent between-meal snacks and drinks can maintain a low pH environment throughout the day, which shifts the demineralization/remineralization continuum toward caries formation.

REFERENCES

1. Centers for Disease Control and Prevention. (2005). Surveillance for dental caries, dental sealants, retention, edentulism, and enamel fluorosis United States, 1988–1994 and 1999–2002. *MMWR Morb Mortal Wkly Rep,* 54(03):1–44.

2. Ismal, A. I., Hasson, H., & Sohn, W. (2001). Dental caries in the second millennium. *J Dent Ed,* 65:953–58.

3. The oral health and chronic disease connection. (2002). Retrieved February 29, 2008, from http://www.astho.org/docs/access/ohcd.htm.

4. Ring, M. E., Ed. (1985.) *Dentistry: An illustrated history.* New York: Harry N. Abrams.

5. Gerabek, W. E. (1999). The tooth-worm: Historical aspects of a popular medical belief. *Clin Oral Investig,* 3:1–6.

6. Ring, M. E., & W. E. Miller. (2002). The pioneer who laid the foundation for modern dental research. *N Y State Dent J,* 68:34–37.

7. Miller, W. D. (1973). *The microorganisms of the human mouth.* Philadelphia: SS White Dental Manufacturing Company; 1890. Reprinted Basel, Switzerland: Karger.

8. Black, G. V. (1898). Dr. Black's conclusions reviewed again. *Dental Cosmos,* 40:440–51.

9. Diagnosis and treatment of dental caries throughout life. Retrieved December 15, 2008, from http://concensus.nih.gov/2001/2001DentalCaries115html.htm.

10. Lu, K. H. 1965. A critical evaluation of the concept of bilaterality of caries and its statistical analysis. *J Dent Res,* 44:1227–1237.

11. Boffa J., Shwartz, M., Ash. A., Pliskin, J. S., & Grondahl, H. G. 1986. Bilateral dental caries from the individual perspective: A definition and a statistical test for its existence. *Caries Res,* 20:91–95.

12. Dodds, M. W. J. (1993). Dilemmas in caries diagnosis—Applications to current practice, and need for research. *J Dent Educ,* 57:433–38.

13. Silverstone, L. M. (1973). The structure of carious enamel, including the early lesion. *Oral Sci Rev,* 3:100–160.

14. Juhl, M. (1983). Localization of carious lesions in occlusal pits and fissures of human premolars. *Scand J Dent Res,* 91:251–55.

15. Silverstone, I. M. (1977). Remineralization phenomena. *Caries Res,* 11 (Suppl 1):59–84.

16. Johnson, N. W. (1967). Some aspects of the ultrastructure of early human enamel caries seen with the electron microscope. *Arch Oral Biol,* 12:1505–21.

17. Haikel, Y., Frank, R. M., & Voegel, J. C. (1983). Scanning electron microscopy of the human enamel surface layer of incipient enamel lesions. *Caries Res,* 17:1–13.

18. Orland, F. J., Blayney, J. R., Harrison, R. W., Reynzers, J. A., Trexler, P. C., Wagner, M., Gordon, H. A., & Luckey, T. D. (1954). Use of germ-free animal technic in the study of experimental dental caries. I. Basic observations on rats reared free of all microorganisms. *J Dent Res,* 33:147–74.

19. Keyes, P. H. (1960). The infections and transmissible nature of experimental dental caries—Findings and implications. *Arch Oral Biol,* 1:304–20.

20. Loesche, W. J. (1986). Role of *Streptococcus mutans* in human dental decay. *Microbiol Rev,* 50:353–80.

21. Tanzer, J. M. (1989). On changing the cariogenic chemistry of coronal plaque. *J Dent Res,* 68 (Spec Iss):1576–87.

22. Clarke, J. K. (1924). On the bacterial factor in the aetiology of dental caries. *Br J Exp Pathol,* 5:141–47.

23. Twetman, S., & Frostnec, N. (1991). Salivary mutans streptomutans and caries prevalence in 8-year-old Swedish schoolchildren. *Swed Dent J,* 15:145–51.

24. Keene, H. J., & Shklair, I. L. (1975). Relationship of *Streptococcus mutans* carrier status to the lesions in initially caries free recruits. *J Dent Res,* 53:1295.

25. Loesche, W. J., Rowan, J., Straffon, L. H., Loos, P. J. (1975). Association of Streptococcus mutans with human dental decay. *Infect Immun,* 11:1252–60.

26. Tenuta, L. M., Ricomini, F. A. P., Del Bel Cury, A. A., & Cury, J. A. (2006). Effect of sucrose on the selection of mutans streptococci and lactobacilli in dental biofilm formed in situ. *Caries Res,* 40:546–49.

27. Winston, A. E., & Bhaskar, S. N. (1998). Caries prevention in the 21st century. *J Am Dent Assoc,* 129:1579–87.

28. Thibodeau, E. A., & O'Sullivan, D. M. (1999). Salivary mutans streptococci and caries development in the primary and mixed dentitions of children. *Community Dent Oral Epidemiol,* 27:406–12.

29. Fure, S. (1998). Five-year incidence of caries, salivary and microbial conditions in 60-, 70-, and 80-year-old Swedish individuals. *Caries Res,* 32:166–74.

30. Kohler, B., Bjarnason, S., Care, R., Mackevica, I., & Pence, I. (1995). Mutans streptococci and dental caries prevalence in a group of Latvian preschool children. *Eur J Oral Sci,* 103:264–66.

31. Alaluusua, S., Kleemola-Jujala, E., Gronroos, L., & Evalahti, M. (1990). Salivary caries-related tests as predictors of future caries increment in teenagers. A three-year longitudinal study. *Oral Microbiol,* 5:77–81.

32. Shi, S., Liang, Q., Hayashi, Y., Yakushiji, M., & Achida, Y. (1998). The relationship between caries activity and the status of dental caries—Application of the Dentocult SM method. *Chin J Dent Res,* 1:52–55.

33. Loesche, W. J., Eklund, S., Earnest, R., & Burt, B. (1984). Longitudinal investigation of bacteriology of human fissure decay: Epidemiological studies in molars shortly after eruption. *Infect Immun,* 46:765–72.

34. Van Houte, J., Sansone, C., Joshipura, K., & Kent, R. (1991). *In vitro* acidogenic potential and mutans streptococci on human smooth-surface plaque associated with initial caries lesions and sound enamel. *J Dent Res,* 70:497–502.

35. Edelstein, B., & Tinanoff, N. (1989). Screening preschool children for dental caries using a microbial test. *Pediatr Dent,* 11:129–32.

36. Geddes, D. A. M. (1975). Acids produced by human dental plaque metabolism *in situ. Caries Res,* 9:98–109.

37. Gibbons, R. J. (1964). Bacteriology of dental caries. *J Dent Res,* 43:1021–28.

38. Burne, R. A. (1998). Oral streptococci ... Products of their environment. *J Dent Res,* 77:445–52.

39. Quivey, R. G., Kuhnert, W. L., & Hahan, K. (2001). Genetics of acid adaption in oral streptococci. *Crit Rev Oral Biol Med,* 12:301–14.

40. Brown, L. R., Dreizen, S., & Handler, S. (1976). Effects of elected caries regimens on microbial changes following radiation-induced xerostomia in cancer patients. In Stiles, H. M., Loesche, W. J., &

O'Brien, T. C., Eds. *Proceedings: Microbial aspects of dental caries.* Washington, DC: Information Retrieval, 275–90.

41. Littleton, N. W., McCabe, R. M., & Carter, C. H. (1967). Studies of oral health in persons nourished by stomach tube. II. Acidogenic properties and selected bacterial components of plaque material. *Arch Oral Biol,* 12:601–609.

42. De Stoppelar, S. D., van Houte, J. S., & Backer-Dirks, O. (1970). The effect of carbohydrate restriction on the presence of *Streptococcus mutans, Streptococcus sanguis* and iodophilic polysaccharide-producing bacteria in human dental plaque. *Caries Res,* 4:114–23.

43. Dodds, M. W. J., & Edgar, W. M. (1986). Effects of dietary sucrose levels on pH fall and acid–anion profile in human dental plaque after a starch mouthrinse. *Arch Oral Biol,* 31:509–12.

44. Sgan-Cohen, H. D., Newbrun, E., Huber, R., Tenebaum, G., & Sela, M. N. (1988). The effect of previous diet on plaque pH response to different foods. *J Dent Res,* 67:1434–37.

45. Zickert, I., Emilson, C.-G., & Krasse, B. (1982). Effect of caries preventive measures in children highly infected with the bacterium *Streptococcus mutans. Arch Oral Biol,* 27:861–68.

46. Carlsson, J., Grahnen, H., & Jonsson, G. (1975). Lactobacilli and streptococci in the mouth of children. *Caries Res,* 9:333–39.

47. Suhonen, J. (1992). Mutans streptococci and their specific oral target: New implications to prevent dental caries. *Schweiz Monafsschr Zahnmed,* 102:286–91.

48. Alaluusa, S. (1991). Transmission of mutans streptococci. *Proc Finn Dent Soc,* 87:443–47.

49. Köhler, B., & Bratthall, D. (1978). Intrafamilial levels of *Streptococcus mutans* and some aspects of the bacterial transmission. *Scand J Dent Res,* 86:35–42.

50. Zickert, I., Emilson, C.-G., & Krasse, B. (1983). Correlation of level and duration of *Streptococcus mutans* infection with incidence of dental caries. *Infect Immun,* 39:982–85.

51. Modesto, A. & Drake, D. R. (2006) Multiple exposures to chlorhexidine and Xylitol: Adhesion and biofilm formation by streptococcus mutans. *Curr Microbiol.*

52. Carlsson, J., Soderholm, G., & Almfedt, I. (1969). Prevalence of *Streptococcus sanguis* and *Streptococcus mutans* in the mouth of persons wearing full-dentures. *Arch Oral Biol,* 14:243–49.

53. Avery, J. K. (2000). *Essentials of oral histology and embryology: A clinical approach* (2nd ed.). St. Louis: C.V. Mosby, 94–106.

54. Silverstone, L. M., & Hicks, M. J. (1985). The structure and ultra structure of the carious lesion in human dentin. *Gerodontics,* 1:185–93.

55. Pashley, D. H., & Matthews, W. G. (1993). The affects of outward forced convective flow on inward diffusion in human dentine in vitro. *Arch Oral Biol,* 38:577–82.

56. Ciucchi, B., Bouillaguet, S., Holz, J., & Pashley, D. (1995). Dentinal fluid dynamics in human teeth, in vivo. *J Endod,* 21:191–94.

57. Heyeraas, K. J., & Berggreen, E. (1999). Interstitial fluid pressure in normal and inflamed puls. *Crit Rev Oral Biol Med,* 10:328–36.

58. Ahn, C. L., & Overton, B. (1997). The effects of immunoglobulins on the convective permeability of human dentine *in vitro. Arch Oral Biol Med,* 42:835–43.

59. Pashley, D. H. (1996). Dynamics of the pulpo-dentin complex. *Crit Rev Oral Biol Med,* 7:104–33.

60. Pashley, D. H. (1992). Dentin permeability and dentine sensitivity. *Proc Finn Dent Soc,* 88 (Suppl. 1):13–37.

61. Pashley, D. H. (1991). Clinical correlations of dentin structure and function. *J Prosthet Dent,* 66:777–81.

62. ten Cate, J. M. (2001). Remineralization of caries lesions extending into dentin. *J Dent Res,* 80:1407–11.

63. Tucker J., Barzel R., Holt K., & Siegal, M. 2009. *Caries prevention, risk assessment, diagnosis, and treatment.* Washington,

DC: National Maternal and Child Oral Health Resource Center. Retrieved December 1, 2011, from http://www.ohiodentalclinics.com/curricula/caries/.

64. Shay, K. (2004). The evolving impact of aging America on dental practice. *J Contemp Dent Pract,* 15:101–10.

65. Saunders, R. H., Jr., & Meyerowitz, C. (2005). Dental caries in older adults. *Dent Clin North Am,* 49:293–308.

66. Tugnait, A., & Clerehugh, V. (2001). Gingival recession—Its significance and management. *J Dent,* 29:381–94.

67. Katz, R. V., Hazen, S. P., Chilton, N. W., & Mumm, R. D., Jr. (1982). Prevalence and intraoral distribution of root caries in an adult population. *Caries Res,* 16:265–71.

68. Key Findings from NHANES 1999–2002. Surveillance for Dental Caries, Dental Sealants, Tooth Retention, Edentulism and Enamel Fluorosis—United States, 1988–1994 and 1999–2002. Retrieved November 30, 2011, from http://www.cdc.gov/oralhealth/publications/factsheets/nhanes_findings.htm.

69. Locker, D., Slade, G. D., & Leake, J. L. (1989). Prevalence of and factors associated with root decay in older adults in Canada. *J Dent Res,* 68:768–72.

70. Vehkalahti, M. M., & Paunlo, I. K. (1988). Occurrence of root caries in relation to dental health behavior. *J Dent Res,* 67:911–14.

71. Banting, D. W. (1986). Epidemiology of root caries. *Gerodontology,* 5:5–11.

72. Petersen, P. E. (2005). Sociobehavioural risk factors in dental caries—International perspectives. *Community Dent Oral Epidemiol,* 33:274–79.

73. Jordan, H. V., & Hammond, B. F. (1972). Filamentous bacteria isolated from human root surface caries. *Arch Oral Biol,* 17:1333–42.

74. Sumney, D., & Jordan, H. (1974). Characterization of bacteria isolated from human root surface carious lesions. *J Dent Res,* 63:343–51.

75. Van Houte, J., Jordan, H. V., Laraway, R., Kent, R., Sopark, P. M., & DePaula P. F. (1990). Association of the microbial flora of dental plaque and saliva with human root-surface caries. *J Dent Res,* 69:1463–68.

76. Bowden, G. H. W. (1990). Microbiology of root surface caries in humans. *J Dent Res,* 69:1205–10.

77. Dung, S. Z. (1999). Effects of mutans streptococci, *Actinomyces* species and *Porphyromona gingivalis* on collagen degenerations. *Chung Hua I, Hsueh Tsa Chihi* (Taipai), 62:764–74.

78. Mellberg, J. R. (1986). Demineralization and remineralization of root surface caries. *Gerodontology,* 5:25–31.

79. Nyvad, B., & Fejerskov, O. (1986). Active root surface caries converted into inactive caries as a response to oral hygiene. *Scand J Dent Res,* 94:281–84.

80. Wallman, C., & Krasse, B. (1992). Mutans streptococci on margins of fillings and crowns. *J Dent,* 20:163–66.

81. Lindquist, B., & Emlson, C. G. (1990). Distribution and prevalence of mutans streptococci in the human dentition. *J Dent Res,* 69:1160–66.

82. Kidd, E. A. M. (1990). Caries diagnosis within restored teeth. *Adv Dent Res,* 4:10–13.

83. Fontana, M., & Zero, D. (2006). Assessing patient's caries risk. *J Am Dent Assoc,* 137:1231–39.

84. Kidd, E. A. M., & O'Hara, J. W. (1990). The caries status of occlusal amalgam restorations with marginal defects. *J Dent Res,* 69:1275–77.

85. Elderton, R. J. (1983). Longitudinal study of dental treatment in the General Dental Service in Scotland. *Br Dent J,* 155:91–96.

86. Skartveit, L., Wefel, J. S., & Ekstrand, J. (1991). Effect of fluoride amalgams on artificial recurrent enamel and root caries. *Scand J Dent Res,* 99:287–94.

87. Dijkman, G. E. H. M., de Vries, J., Lodding, A., & Arenda, J. (1993). Long-term fluoride release of visible light-activated composites *in vitro:* A correlation with in situ demineralization data. *Caries Res,* 27:117–23.

88. Hudson, P. (2004). Conservative treatment of the Class I lesion: A new paradigm. *J Am Dent Assoc,* 135:1514, 1516.

89. Stephan, R. M. (1910). Changes in hydrogen–ion concentration on tooth surfaces and in carious lesions. *JADA,* 27:718–23.

90. Dodds, M. W. J., & Edgar, W. M. (1998). The relationship between plaque pH, plaque acid anion profiles and oral carbohydrate retention after ingestion of several "reference foods" by human subjects. *J Dent Res,* 67:861–65.

91. ten Cate, J. M. (1992). Saliva a physiological medium. *Ned Tijdschr Tandheelkr,* 99:82–84.

92. Takahashi N., & Nyvad, B. (2008). Caries ecology revisited: Microbial dynamics and the caries process. *Caries Res.* 42:409–18.

93. ten Cate, J. M. (2001). Remineralization of caries lesions extending into dentin. *J Dent Res,* 80:1407–11.

94. Tung, M. S., & Eichmiller, F. C. (2004). Amorphous calcium phosphates for tooth mineralization. *Compend Contin Educ Dent,* 25 (9 Suppl 1): 9–13.

95. Tung, M. S., Malerman, R., Huang, S., & McHale, W. A. (2005) Reactivity of prophylaxis paste containing calcium, phosphate and fluoride salts. *J Dental Res,* 84 (Spec Iss A), IADR Abstracts.

96. Ramalingam, L., Messer, L. B., & Reynolds, E. C. (2005). Adding casaein phosphopeptide-amorphous calcium phosphate to sports drinks to eliminate in vitro erosion. *Pediatr Dent,* 27:61–67.

97. Giniger, M., Spaid, M., MacDonald, J., & Felix, H. (2005) A 180-day clinical investigation of the tooth whitening efficacy of a bleaching gel with added amorphous calcium phosphate. *J Clin Dent,* 16:11–16.

98. Ogaard, B. (1999). The cariostatic mechanism of fluoride. *Comp Contin Educ Dent,* 20 (Suppl 1):10–17.

99. ten Cate, J. M., & Loveren, van C. (1999). Fluoride mechanisms. *Dent Clinics North Am,* 43:713–42.

100. Rosin-Grget, K., & Lincir, J. (2001). Current concept on the anticaries fluoride mechanism of the action. *Coll Antropol,* 25:703–12.

Periodontal Diseases

Kathleen O. Hodges

OBJECTIVES

After studying this chapter, the student will be able to:

1. Name and describe the functions of the four components of the periodontium.

2. Describe the normal gingival sulcus.

3. Differentiate between gingivitis and periodontitis.

4. Describe the role of clinical attachment loss in making the correct diagnosis between gingivitis and periodontitis.

5. Describe characteristic microflora associated with periodontal health, gingivitis, and periodontitis.

6. Starting with a healthy periodontium and ending with advanced periodontitis, describe how periodontal disease progresses.

7. Describe the relationship of supragingival plaque and subgingival plaque biofilm to periodontal diseases.

8. Describe the role of the host defenses involved in periodontal disease.

9. Discuss the purposes of a classification system for periodontal diseases.

10. Describe the classification system categories for gingivitis and periodontitis.

11. Define a "risk factor" for periodontal diseases.

12. List the risk factors associated with periodontal diseases.

KEY TERMS

Bidirectional synergism, 71
Col, 73
Free marginal groove, 71
Gingival crevice, 73
Gingival crevicular fluid (GCF), 75
Loss of attachment, 70
Mucogingival junction (MGJ), 73
Necrotizing disease, 80
Nonspecific plaque hypothesis, 75
Papillae, 73
Periodontal abscess, 80
Periodontal ligament, 74
Periodontal pockets, 71
Specific plaque hypothesis, 76
Sulcular epithelium, 73

INTRODUCTION

Periodontal diseases are induced by biofilm (dental plaque).[1] The mildest form of periodontal disease is characterized by slight inflammatory changes of the gingiva surrounding the teeth. The severest form is a massive loss of tooth-supporting structures, including alveolar bone and subsequently of tooth loss (Figure 6–1 ■). Early periodontal disease that is limited to the gingiva is referred to as *gingivitis,* a common clinical finding that affects nearly everyone at some time during the life cycle. It usually can be reversed by the use of primary preventive measures.

Periodontal disease that affects the tooth-supporting structures and alveolar bone is referred to as *periodontitis* as is gingival inflammation accompanied by a pathological loss of attachment.[2] Damage caused by periodontitis usually is not reversible with primary preventive measures; however, these procedures aid in the control of periodontitis. Loss of attachment is the primary clinical and diagnostic difference between gingivitis and periodontitis. Specifically, **loss of attachment** is the detachment of collagen fibers from the cementum and subsequent movement of the zone of soft tissue attached to the teeth (i.e., the junctional epithelium) toward the apex of the root. The presence of gingival inflammation without loss of attachment is gingivitis.

Periodontal disease is a broad term that encompasses multiple types of plaque-induced periodontal diseases. These diseases are infections associated with specific groups of bacteria. An individual's susceptibility to periodontal diseases depends on the person's host response to the oral bacteria. This host susceptibility explains why individuals present with varying clinical findings, types, and extent of the disease. The progression of periodontal disease also depends on risk factors that modify the host's susceptibility to the bacterial infection. Risk factors include medical or systemic conditions, environmental factors, and genetic diseases. Examples of risk factors that affect the progress of periodontal disease are the close relationship between the severity of periodontal disease and the severity of type 2 diabetes mellitus;[3,4] the strong relationship between periodontal disease and exposure to tobacco and tobacco products such as cigarettes and spit (chewing) tobacco, as well as the environmental exposure of nonsmokers to cigarette smoke;[5–8] and the less strong relationship between genetically influenced inflammatory mediators and periodontitis.[9]

Periodontal diseases are widespread and worldwide. Gingivitis is found in children, adolescents, and young adults, but

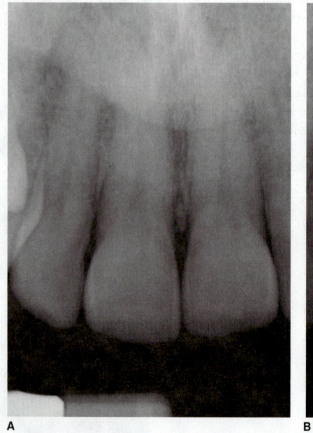

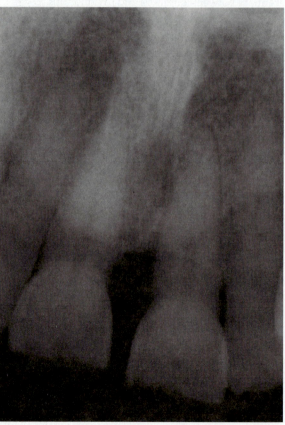

A

B

FIGURE ■ 6–1 Maxillary central incisors. Bone loss on radiographs. A. Slight interproximal bone loss. B. More bone loss is seen in advanced periodontal disease.

(*Source:* Courtesy of Christine N. Nathe.)

seems to decline in the older adult. In fact, gingivitis is almost universal in children and adolescents, but the prevalence of destructive forms of periodontal disease is lower in young adults than in adults.[10] Loss of attachment and bone are both rather uncommon in young individuals; however, incidence does increase in adolescents who are 12 to 17 years of age in comparison with children who are 5 to 11 years old.[10] The prevalence of severe attachment loss among children and young adults seems to be minimal; however, children, adolescents, and young adult patients should receive periodontal evaluation and relevant self-care education when seeking oral health care.[10]

Some form of periodontitis has been estimated to affect the majority of adults in the United States with severe generalized periodontitis affecting 5% to 15% of the overall population.[11] Periodontitis is age related; however, this statement can be misleading because it implies that periodontal disease is directly related to the aging process. Instead, studies have shown that the periodontal health of older adults is closely related to self-care and the cumulative effects of the disease process, rather than to age.

DID YOU KNOW ?

At one time, it was believed that the systemic disease and periodontal disease relationship was unidirectional, meaning that periodontitis could adversely affect a systemic disease but not vice versa.

The presence of certain systemic diseases affects the periodontal health and treatment outcomes of some patients. Systemic disease and periodontal diseases are related in three ways. First, systemic relationships might be suspected in individual situations in which periodontal disease appears to be disproportional to the local irritants.[12] The systemic disease itself affects the response to local irritants. Second, genetic (e.g., Down syndrome, Papillon-Lèfevre syndrome, Cohen syndrome) or hematologic diseases (e.g., acute leukemia or acquired neutropenia) can cause periodontitis. Third, a complex relationship also exists between periodontitis and systemic diseases such as cardiovascular diseases,[13,14] diabetes mellitus, pregnancy outcomes, and osteoporosis. This relationship has been referred to as **bidirectional synergism**, meaning that periodontal disease is a risk factor for adverse systemic diseases or conditions.[15] Periodontal medicine is an emerging discipline that strives to define the relationship between systemic disease and periodontal diseases through scientific inquiry.[16] Periodontal medicine focuses on periodontal disease as a risk factor for adverse systemic diseases or conditions.

The prevalence of periodontal diseases in the United States may increase in the future because longer life spans are increasing the time that teeth are at risk. Also, people are taking better care of their teeth and maintaining their teeth longer, which, in turn increases the number of teeth at risk. In addition, improved

diagnosis and detection of periodontal diseases by oral health professionals could, perhaps, increase the prevalence of periodontal diseases. On the other hand, the prevalence of periodontal disease in the United States might decrease because access to information about periodontal disease has exploded, making more people aware of preventive measures. Improvements in the early diagnosis and treatment of periodontal disease are still needed because some people may not have access to or choose not to access the personnel-intensive periodontal care needed for the repeated monitoring and treatment of this lifelong disease.

Although there are many scientific advances in the diagnosis and treatment of periodontal diseases, oral health care professionals still face challenges. It is not possible to predict periodontal disease risk accurately. The presence of **periodontal pockets** or clinical attachment loss is not an indicator of the actual activity of disease at the time of examination. Thus, some periodontal patients have frequent episodes of rapid disease progression that cannot be identified until an examination months or years later confirms that periodontal destruction has already occurred. Genetic research, however, is being conducted to find a marker that will help predict periods of disease activity, which might in turn lead to more efficacious treatment. The successful completion of the Human Genome Project to decode the DNA molecule offers the possibility of developing genetic approaches to prevention, diagnosis, nonsurgical treatment, prognosis and vaccination.[17,18]

THE PERIODONTIUM

Four anatomical structures support the teeth: (1) gingiva, (2) periodontal ligament, (3) cementum, and (4) alveolar bone (Figure 6–2 ■). Collectively, these structures compose the periodontium. The tissues of the periodontium attach the tooth to the alveolar process.

The gingiva covers the cervical and root portions of the teeth and the maxillary and mandibular alveolar processes. The gingiva consists of the free (or marginal) gingiva, interdental papillae, and attached gingiva (Figure 6–3 ■). The marginal gingiva surrounds each tooth in a "cufflike" fashion and is not attached to the tooth. The most coronal portion of the marginal gingiva is the edge of the gingiva that touches the tooth. Its most apical portion is the **free marginal groove**, which defines the boundary between the attached and marginal gingiva. In health, the gingival margin should be flat against the bone with scalloped coronal edges that follow the tooth contour. The marginal gingiva is about 1 mm wide on the facial and lingual surfaces.

The marginal gingiva is held firmly against the tooth by a complex arrangement of collagen fiber groups: circumferential, gingivodental, and transseptal. The gingival fibers aid the tissue in withstanding the forces of mastication, and connect the marginal gingiva with the cementum and the attached gingiva. These fibers, which are arranged in bundles, are divided into groups according to their orientation and insertion into the periodontal tissues. Fibers that encircle the tooth within the marginal gingiva are called *circular* or *circumferential fibers*. These fibers are attached to other collagen fibers much like those in

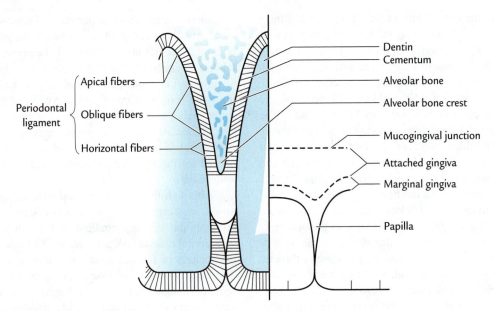

Periodontal ligament
- Apical fibers
- Oblique fibers
- Horizontal fibers

Dentin
Cementum
Alveolar bone
Alveolar bone crest
Mucogingival junction
Attached gingiva
Marginal gingiva
Papilla

FIGURE ■ 6–2 Parts of the periodontium.

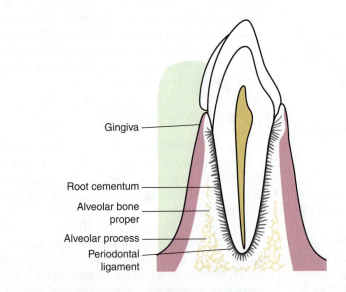

Gingiva
Root cementum
Alveolar bone proper
Alveolar process
Periodontal ligament

A

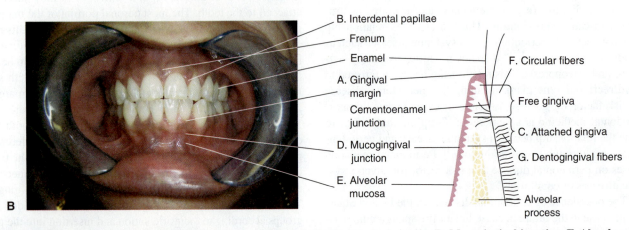

B

B. Interdental papillae
Frenum
Enamel
A. Gingival margin
Cementoenamel junction
D. Mucogingival junction
E. Alveolar mucosa

F. Circular fibers
Free gingiva
C. Attached gingiva
G. Dentogingival fibers
Alveolar process

FIGURE ■ 6–3 Gingiva. A. Marginal gingiva. B. Interdental papilla. C. Attached gingiva. D. Mucogingival junction. E. Alveolar mucosa. F. Circular fibers. G. Dentogingival fibers.

(*Source:* B. Courtesy of Vicki Gianopoulos.)

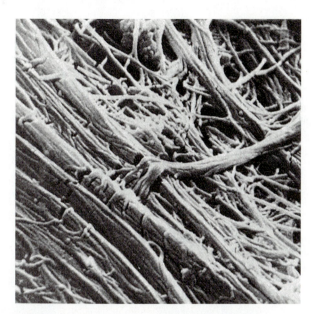

FIGURE ■ 6–4 Electron scanning microscopic view of collagen bundles in the periodontal ligament space. Note narrow bundle crossing thick bundle at right angle.

(*Source:* J. Svejda and M. Skach. (1973). The periodontium of the human teeth in the scanning electron microscope (stereoscan). *J Periodont,* 44:478–84.)

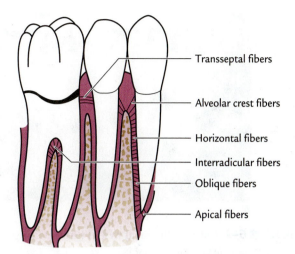

FIGURE ■ 6–5 Principal fibers of the periodontal ligament.

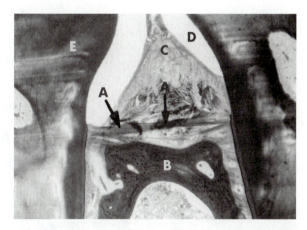

FIGURE ■ 6–6 Cross-sectional view of interdental papillae showing A. Transseptal fibers. B. Alveolar crest. C. Dental papilla. D. Enamel space. E. Dentin.

(*Source:* Courtesy of Dr. Don Willmann, University of Texas Dental School at San Antonio.)

Figure 6–4 ■. A second group of fibers, known as the *gingivo-dental* (or *dentogingival*) *fibers,* are inserted into the cementum and extend into the crest (upper ridge) and the periosteum (connective tissue surrounding the alveolar bone) of the alveolar bone just beneath the epithelium at the base of the gingival sulcus (Figure 6–3). These fibers are located in the facial, lingual, and interproximal surfaces. Also, two other fiber groups are present: the dentoperiosteal and the alveologingival groups; the dentoperiosteal fibers anchor the tooth to the bone whereas the alveologingival fibers extend from the alveolar crest to the marginal and attached gingiva (Figure 6–5 ■). Transseptal fibers are located interproximally and extend from the cementum of one tooth, over the alveolar crest of interproximal bone, and into the cementum of the adjacent teeth (Figures 6–5 and 6–6 ■). Together, these fibers serve to maintain the close, tight contact of the free marginal gingiva against the tooth.

The interdental gingiva is composed of two **papillae** (small protubernace of the gingiva), which fill the interproximal space between adjacent teeth and are also called *interdental papillae.* One papilla is located on the facial side of the teeth; the other is on the lingual side. The two papillae are connected beneath the tooth contact by a concave-shaped nonkeratinized tissue termed the **col** (Figure 6–7 ■). The attached gingiva is apical to the marginal gingiva and extends from the free marginal groove to the **mucogingival junction (MGJ)**, where it meets the loose and moveable alveolar mucosa (Figure 6–3). The alveolar mucosa is a thin, nonkeratinized mucosal layer that is loosely attached to the alveolar process and that extends into the cheek, lips, tongue, and palate. In contrast, the attached gingiva is firm, keratinized, and tightly attached to the periosteum of the alveolar bone.

The marginal gingiva attaches to the tooth at the base of the gingival sulcus (also called the **gingival crevice**), which is the shallow space around each tooth (Figure 6–8B ■ and 6–8C ■). The boundaries of the gingival sulcus are the cementum on one side, the **sulcular epithelium** of the marginal gingiva on the other side, and the epithelial attachment at the base or apical portion of the sulcus. The orifice of this sulcus opens into the oral cavity. The depth of the gingival sulcus is an important characteristic of health or disease; its depth is measured with a periodontal probe. The gingival sulcus measures 1 to 2 mm facially and lingually, and 1 to 3 mm proximally in health. In disease, edema or enlargement and/or erythema may create inflammation, increasing the depth of the sulcus more than 2 to 3 mm, or the gingival margin may recede below the cementoenamel junction. With disease, gingival bleeding might occur spontaneously or because of provocation (periodontal probing or patient self-care). Inflammation affects the interdental gingiva first, the marginal facial and lingual gingiva second, and the attached gingiva last.

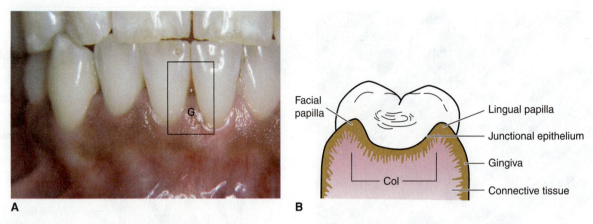

FIGURE ■ 6–7 Col area. Proximal view of tooth and gingiva. G, Interdental gingiva fills the gingival embrasure.
(*Source:* A. Courtesy of Vicki Gianopoulos.)

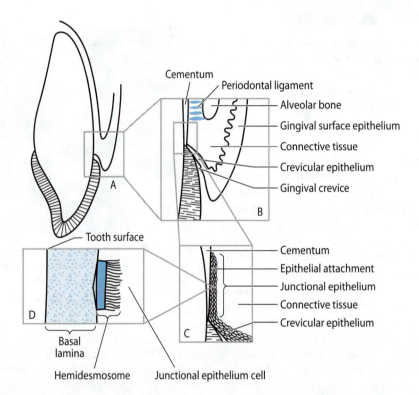

FIGURE ■ 6–8 Dentogingival junction: A. and B. The junction between the tooth and gingival soft tissues. C. This junction occurs where there are a few layers of junctional epithelial cells. D. The attachment mechanism for these cells consists of hemidesmosomes in each cell and a basal lamina between the cell body and tooth.

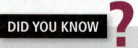

DID YOU KNOW

The five principal fibers of the periodontal ligament have different orientations and functions on the tooth root.

The **periodontal ligament** is a network of collagen fibers. This structure surrounds the tooth root and connects it with the alveolar bone (Figure 6–8B). Its collagen fibers embed into the cementum of the root on one side and into the alveolar bone on the other side. The five principal fibers of the periodontal ligament have different orientations and functions at various levels on the tooth root. They are arranged in bundles called *alveolar crest, horizontal, oblique, apical,* and *interradicular fiber groups* (Figure 6–5). The alveolar crest fibers extend obliquely from the cementum to the alveolar crest. They prevent lateral movement and extrusion of the tooth. The horizontal fibers are located at the cervical area and resist lateral forces. The oblique fibers extend in an oblique fashion from the alveolar bone to the cementum and bear the stress of chewing. The apical fibers form at the tooth apex and are generally parallel to the long axis of the tooth to help cushion the tooth from occlusal forces. The interradicular fibers are found in the furcation area of a multirooted tooth and connect the cementum and tooth. In addition, a network of blood vessels within the periodontal ligament protects the bone and periodontal fibers from excessive occlusal forces.

The junctional epithelium is found at the apical termination of the gingival sulcular/crevicular epithelium, which lines the gingival sulcus (Figure 6–8C). The junctional epithelium is attached to the tooth by gingival fibers that hold the marginal gingiva against the tooth as previously described. The junctional epithelium and the gingival fibers are considered a functional unit called the *dentogingival unit* or *dentogingival junction.* The junctional epithelium is several layers thick when it initially forms, and the number of layers increases with age. The length of the junctional epithelium ranges from 0.25 to 1.35 mm. This very special epithelium is actually attached to the enamel, forming a seal between the soft tissue and the tooth surface. This biologic seal functions to anchor the sulcular epithelium to the tooth surface and to protect the underlying periodontal fibers from the hostile oral environment (Figure 6–8). The junctional epithelium is one of the most important structures in the practice of periodontics. The junctional epithelial cells are joined to the tooth surface by hemidesmosomes, which consist of a few layers of epithelial cells that initially extend a short distance along the enamel surface at the cementoenamel junction[19] (Figure 6–8D ■). Inflammation, especially chronic inflammation such as in periodontitis, can result in apical migration of the cells, first over the cementoenamel junction, and then apically onto the cementum.

Each millimeter of apical migration of the attachment also has an accompanying loss of 1 mm of periodontal fibers attached between the cementum and bone. As the junctional epithelium migrates apically in more advanced disease, there is loss of alveolar bone and exposure of the cementum to which the fibers were originally attached. The migration also causes a deepening of the sulcus to form a periodontal pocket. This apical migration of the junctional epithelium and consequent loss of attachment (clinical attachment loss) is the hallmark sign for diagnosing periodontitis.

THE GINGIVAL SULCUS

In a longitudinal section of the free gingiva (Figure 6–8A ■), the tissues encountered from the sulcus to the oral vestibule or palate are (1) sulcular/crevicular epithelium, (2) connective tissue, and (3) attached gingiva surface epithelium. The sulcular and attached gingiva merge at the crest of the free gingival margin (Figure 6–3). The connective tissue between the sulcular and attached gingiva contains blood vessels, lymphatics, and nerves that supply both surfaces. The connective tissues immediately beneath the sulcular epithelium contain the oral cavity's (i.e., host) cellular and humoral defense system, which helps minimize the detrimental effects of bacteria in the plaque biofilm. (See Chapter 9 for discussion of host defense mechanisms.)

In an inflamed disease state, fluid flows from the depths of the gingival sulcus. This **gingival crevicular fluid (GCF)** is a

transudate, which contains a few cells and proteins as opposed to exudates, which are inflammatory in nature. Gingival crevicular fluid is derived from blood vessels in the connective tissue adjacent to the sulcus. An increase in GCF flow is one of the first detectable signs of impending gingivitis. Increased GCF flow is present prior to development of overt signs of inflammation, and the flow rate depends primarily on the severity of inflammation. After patients stop oral self-care, an increase of GCF can be observed as early as the ninth day.[20]

Gingival crevicular fluid serves several protective functions. It helps clear bacteria from the gingival sulcus, and it is the vehicle for leukocytes, complement, antibodies, and assorted enzymes that help protect the enamel and the periodontium from bacterial attack. Gingival crevicular fluid serves as one of the first lines of host defense against the bacteria that cause periodontal disease and the bacteria that cause caries. The presence of an increasing GCF flow has been related to the presence and increasing severity of gingivitis needed but not to the severity of periodontitis.

PERIODONTAL MICROFLORA

Historically, two hypotheses have guided thinking about periodontal microflora: the nonspecific plaque hypothesis and the specific plaque hypothesis. The **nonspecific plaque hypothesis** simply relates periodontal disease to the overall amount of plaque present. As the amount of plaque increases, inflammation and disease increase. In the 1960s, Löe and others recognized a causal relationship between bacterial plaque and gingivitis.[21] Gingivitis would result when plaque was not removed by self-care and would reverse when self-care was resumed. This landmark study seems to be the basis for the nonspecific plaque hypothesis. At that time, a single-disease concept was advocated, which said periodontal disease was caused by the transition from health to gingivitis to periodontitis in relation to the presence of bacterial plaque over time. All individuals were equally susceptible, gingivitis always progressed to periodontitis, and treatment was standard for each patient. This theory came into question, however, because clinical findings did not reflect this hypothesis. For example, some patients who had a vast accumulation of bacterial plaque had minimal disease.

When plaque bacteria could be cultured, researchers were able to differentiate between various bacterial species, and the specific plaque hypothesis became prevalent and accepted. The **specific plaque hypothesis** attributes the various demonstrations of signs or symptoms (manifestations) of the periodontal plaque-related diseases to "specific," although not necessarily known, bacteria. The quality of bacterial plaque biofilm is more important than the quantity. In other words, specific types and complexes of bacteria and their pathogenic potential are more important than the amount of plaque biofilm present. Also, not all plaque biofilm is associated with disease. Therefore, all individuals are not equally susceptible, gingivitis does not always progress to periodontitis, and treatment interventions vary depending on the type of disease.

Experimental gingivitis in children (i.e., versus adults) reveals increased subgingival levels of *Actinomyces* species, *Capnocytophaga* species, *Leptotrichia* species, and *Selenomonas* species. These species, therefore, might be important in the etiology and pathogenesis of gingivitis.[22,23] Periodontitis appears to conform to the specific plaque hypothesis because certain

bacterial species have been associated with the most destructive periodontal diseases.[24] Substantial evidence identifies certain microorganisms or combinations of organisms as etiologic factors. For example, the microbial species that appear to be associated with chronic periodontitis—the most common variety of periodontitis—are *Aggregatibacters actinomycetemcomitans* (AA), *Porphyromonas gingivalis, Prevotella intermedia, Bacteroides forsythus, Fusobacterium* species, *Campylobacter rectus, Treponema denticola,* and others. This list may seem long, but 300 to 500 different species of bacteria are estimated to inhabit the oral cavity. Despite this presumptive evidence of etiology, none of the suspected organisms has yet been successfully implanted into a test animal to duplicate the original disease.

As the status of the marginal gingiva deteriorates from health to gingivitis, a proportional shift begins to take place in the plaque biofilm bacteria, progressing first from aerobic, nonmotile, gram-positive cocci and rods[21,24,25] to facultative anaerobic bacteria, and then to anaerobic, gram-negative, motile species. This major shift in the plaque biofilm bacteria indicates the onset of gingivitis. Microscopic examination reveals an increase in

TABLE ■ 6–1   Inflammation in the Periodontal Lesion

Stages	Time Interval	Histologic Changes	Clinical Changes
I. Initial lesion • Initial response of tissues to bacterial plaque • Subclinical gingivitis	2–4 days	Brief vasoconstriction followed by vasodilation, margination, emigration, and migration of PMN[a] Slight alteration of junctional epithelium Increase in gingival crevicular fluid	None
II. Early lesion • Acute gingivitis	4–7 days	Continuation of initial lesion Macrophages and lymphocytes appear (chronic inflammatory cells) Junctional epithelium invaginates (folds in) with rete pegs Sulcular epithelium ulcerations Connective tissue fiber destruction	Erythema Bleeding upon probing Loss of tissue tone
III. Established lesion • Chronic gingivitis	14 or more days	Continuation of changes in early lesion Plasma cells predominate Chronic inflammation; blood vessels congested; blood flow impaired; increase in collagenase and other enzymes Elongated rete pegs in junctional epithelium extending deep into connective tissue; breakdown of connective fibers	Moderate-to-severe inflammation An underlying bluish hue might be present In addition to color, changes in consistency will be evident
IV. Advanced lesion • Transition from gingivitis to periodontitis	Dependent on host response	Continuation of changes in established lesion Inflammation extending into connective tissue attachment and alveolar bone Repair manifests as fibrotic tissue Bone resorption by osteoclasts and mononuclear cells; bone formation might occur	True periodontal pockets Attachment loss Bone loss

[a]Polymorphonuclear leukocyte.

numbers of both motile rods and between spirochetes with the two comprising approximately 20% of the microorganisms.[21,24]

THE DEVELOPING GINGIVAL LESION

The periodontal lesion has four stages of inflammation[26] (Table 6–1 ■). A sample of sulcular/crevicular fluid from healthy, tightly adapted marginal gingiva reveals only a few forms of bacteria in the sulcus. They include nonmotile coccal forms and motile vibrio. In a diseased gingival sulcus, the flora is markedly different and includes many motile bacteria.

The free margin of the gingiva constitutes the first line of defense for the periodontium, and it is usually the initial site of gingival disease. If plaque biofilm is allowed to accumulate on a tooth surface adjacent to the gingiva, inflammation of the free margin results. If self-care of a healthy mouth is stopped, gingivitis is observed clinically (i.e., changes in color, size, and/or texture) in only 9 to 21 days. Presumably, inflammation might manifest itself sooner in some cases.

With gingivitis, the extent of the gingival inflammation usually parallels the extent of plaque biofilm accumulation. Early gingival clinical changes include alterations in color, contour changes from knife-edge to rolled, and a consistency change from firm to spongy. The free margin often bleeds on gentle manipulation such as from toothbrushing or probing. In the early stages, the developing inflammatory process can be completely reversed by professional oral health care interventions and patient self-care strategies as shown in Figure 6–9 ■.

DID YOU KNOW?

Systemic conditions cause the tissues to react more readily to the bacterial insult and remind the patient that control of some conditions is a medical–dental responsibility.

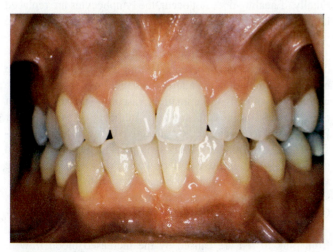

FIGURE ■ 6–9 Healthy periodontium.
(*Source:* University of Kentucky College of Dentistry-OHRI.)

Not all gingival pathology is caused solely by bacterial plaque biofilm. Systemic conditions such as pregnancy and other hormonal changes cause the tissues to react more readily to the bacterial insult. There can also be gingival changes caused by inherited diseases such as hereditary fibromatosis and by drug therapy such as phenytoin used to control seizure disorders.[27] Control of these conditions can be shared medical–dental responsibilities for the patient.

THE DEEPENING POCKET

All periodontitis is preceded by gingivitis, but not all untreated gingivitis progresses to periodontitis. For example, Ronderos completed a study of the indigenous people of the Amazon rain forest and found that most individuals had a loss of epithelial attachment. Despite poor oral hygiene and extensive gingival inflammation, they did not have severe periodontal destruction.[28]

DID YOU KNOW?

A diagnosis of periodontitis implies that the junctional epithelium has migrated apically 2, 3, or more millimeters from its original level at the cementoenamel junction.

A diagnosis of gingivitis implies that the actual level of the junctional epithelial attachment has migrated apically but is still on the enamel or on the cementoenamel junction. A diagnosis of periodontitis implies that the junctional epithelium has migrated apically 2, 3, or more millimeters from its original level at the cementoenamel junction. This migration creates a deeper gingival sulcus, which is a periodontal pocket. The formation of the periodontal pocket with its inaccessible subgingival plaque biofilm creates the need for periodontal treatment.

As the pocket deepens, subgingival plaque acquires new characteristics that differentiate it from the supragingival plaque. In the supragingival plaque, the bacteria and the interbacterial matrix are well confined to the enamel. This biofilm can easily be removed by oral prophylaxis, which is defined as the removal of plaque (biofilm), calculus, and stains from the exposed and unexposed surfaces of the teeth by scaling and polishing as a preventive measure for the control of local irritational factors.[29] (See Chapter 3 for discussion of dental hygiene science.) Oral prophylaxis maintains health or converts gingivitis to health. In the subgingival plaque, a two-compartment subgingival plaque system begins to evolve, and that system is made up of (1) tooth-associated subgingival plaque, a biofilm on the cementum, and (2) a more fluid environment referred to as *epithelium-associated plaque* that bathes the cementum. This fluid consists of purulent fluids (pus), food debris, body defense cells, and saliva confined under low-oxygen tension without circulation within the pocket.[30] Bacteroides and spirochetes are present in this fluid environment. The gram-negative organisms that extend deep into the pocket are believed to be the plaque biofilm responsible for the continued damage and migration of the epithelial attachment.

The tooth-associated subgingival plaque is initially an apical extension of the supragingival plaque into the deepening crevicular area. The bacterial population may still include some mutans streptococci, although their numbers decrease as the distance increases below the gingiva. Subgingival calculus complicates disease control by sheltering plaque bacteria from routine plaque control measures.

In the late 1970s, researchers also differentiated between adherent (attached) plaque and loosely adherent, unattached plaque as causative factors in periodontal disease.[31,32] It was suggested that the pathogenic potential of loosely adherent plaque was greater than that of adherent or attached plaque. The relationship of the specific periodontal pathogens and the host response was then explored. In the 1980s, the specific plaque hypothesis, as previously discussed, was studied, and periodontal diseases were reclassified to reflect bacteriologically and immunologically distinct forms of periodontal diseases. The result was the premise that the presence of pathogens is not enough to initiate disease; the host must also be susceptible to disease.

At this same time, researchers clarified similarities and differences between supragingival and subgingival plaque. It was clear that inflammation caused by supragingival plaque resulted in an altered relationship between the gingival margin and the tooth. This change in the environment permits subgingival bacteria to colonize into bacterial plaque on the root or before or in the sulcus. Next, aerobic bacteria become organized subgingivally in attached and unattached plaque. Toxins, enzymes, and metabolic by-products then injure the periodontium and cause an immune response that results in indirect toxicity. As the host responds to the irritant, periodontal destruction occurs by immunopathologic reaction; that is, periodontal tissues are altered as a result of immune or allergic reactions to the irritant.

In conclusion, elimination of supragingival plaque is critical in preventing periodontal diseases. In addition, control of supragingival and subgingival plaque biofilm is critical to successful periodontal therapy. Patients are continually challenged to remove plaque biofilm. It is difficult for a patient to be 100% effective in controlling plaque, especially when it is located subgingivally; therefore, self-care without professional mechanical removal, such as periodontal instrumentation, results in less healing.[33-35] Professional subgingival mechanical instrumentation is mandatory to complement patient self-care to achieve and maintain periodontal health.[36] *Nonsurgical periodontal therapy* is the professional treatment rendered and is defined as "plaque (biofilm) removal, plaque (biofilm) control, supragingival and subgingival scaling, root planing, and the adjunctive use of chemical agents."[37] Presently, the relationship between bacterial plaque and forms of periodontal diseases is complex; however, approaches to clinical care and self-care therapies for patients are improving rapidly.

CELLULAR DEFENSE IN THE PERIODONTAL DISEASE PROCESS

The body has three key functions of immunologic defense: (1) to protect it from outside invaders (antigens), (2) to destroy or neutralize the antigens that do penetrate the epithelial defenses, and (3) to repair any damage caused by the antigen–antibody reactions. To accomplish this task, the body uses cellular immunity and humoral immunity. The cells responsible for the cellular defense are the granular cells, which consist of granulocytes (basophils, eosinophils, and polymorphonuclear neutrophils [PMN, polys]), monocytes (macrophages), and those cells of lymphoid origin, and T and B lymphocytes.

DID YOU KNOW ?

A chemotactic signal initiates the cellular immune response.

During the cellular response to a periodontal infection, there is first a chemotactic (movement of a cell along a chemical concentration gradient away from the chemical stimulus) signal from an inflamed gingival site, which initiates the cellular immune response.[38,39] This signal possibly arises from the epithelial cells under bacterial attack. For example, in laboratory studies, it was demonstrated that the gingival epithelial cells can cause an increase in the secretion of potent neutrophil chemotactic interleukin-8 following an *Actinobacillus actinomycetemcomitans* challenge (currently now called *Aggregatibacter actinomycetemcomitans*).[40] The defense cells then arrive at the inflamed site in a definite sequence. Initially, during the acute phase of inflammation, large numbers of PMN enter the connective tissue underlying the sulcus. The acute phase may last from a few days to a few weeks. However, if the inflammation continues, the PMN decreases in number and is replaced by lymphocytes. This stage lasts a few weeks to a few months. Finally, if healing does not occur, the lymphocytes are replaced largely by plasma cells, macrophages, and mast cells. The inflammation is now in the chronic stage.

The immune response just described can be linked to predictable histopathologic events. Within 2 to 4 days of plaque biofilm accumulation, the microscopic picture of the connective tissue is one of early inflammation. Vasculitis (inflammation of blood vessels) is present, and large numbers of extravascular PMNs begin to appear in the connective tissue. Edema (excessive fluid in local body tissues) is present because of fluid permeation through the capillary walls. After 4 to 7 days, the vasculitis becomes clinically apparent with the four primary signs of inflammation (i.e., heat, redness, swelling, and pain). Cellular infiltrate is predominated by lymphocytes.

The heat and the change of color of the marginal gingiva from pink to red are caused by the increased blood flow to the area. The gingival swelling is caused by the edema that is caused by leakage from the dilated (enlarged) capillaries. The fluid pressure of edema on nerve endings can cause an acute soreness. When the pain and swelling of the gingiva are sufficiently painful, altered eating habits can result. At this point, if the gingivitis is treated by professional care and subsequent self-care, the gingiva can make a complete return to normal. The shallow sulcus is soon cleared of destroyed bacteria and dead cells by the GCF, and the saliva flushes and neutralizes residual oral debris.

The development of a chronic stage of gingivitis, especially with pocket formation, is accompanied by a different series of reactions. The bacteria possess enzymes that can be lethal to the defense cells,[41] and the defense cells contain enzymes to destroy the bacteria. Thus, there are cellular or humoral reactions, such as dying cells and dying bacteria in the inflamed area, while destruction of epithelial cells, fibroblasts, and bone occurs. Also, the macrophage kills agents such as oxygen and nitrogen as well as hypochlorite. Other products of an activated macrophage include numerous proteins that affect coagulation and multiplication of cells that generate new tissue and repair damaged tissue.[42] This bacteria–epithelial–defense cell exchange is continuously taking place in the small pocket area. The low oxygen tension and low circulation within the pocket aid in perpetuating the pathogenicity of the inflamed periodontal site. Table 6–1 provides an overview of the stages of inflammation in the periodontal lesion.

Because of its complexity, a detailed discussion of the humoral defense of the periodontal site is beyond the scope of this book. (See Chapter 9 for discussion of host defense mechanisms.) Growing evidence points to the immune system playing an important role in the pathogenesis of periodontitis. One genetic factor, interleukin-1, should be mentioned because it has received attention as a marker that can help predict the risk for periodontal disease.[43] Interleukin-1 is a proinflammatory cytokine that is a key regulator of host responses to microbial infection, and it is a major modulator of the catabolism (breakdown) of extracellular matrix and bone resorption.[44] Other cytokines, such as interleukin-8, interleukin-10, and interleukin-11, are involved in tissue destruction.

Because interleukin-1 is a genetic factor, it may serve as a marker for a lifetime risk factor. A great advantage of such a marker is that it would help identify higher-risk individuals early in the periodontal disease process.[44] A positive genetic marker would serve to focus immediate attention on the daily requirement for meticulous mechanical and chemical biofilm control to negate the effect of the plaque bacteria. For a clinical practice, the genetic marker would aid in developing the periodontal care plan, an appropriately planned and individualized reevaluation, and follow-up visit intervals.[45] There is one or more tests for interleukin-1 on the market; thus, this genetic marker can be used to help predict the future course of the disease.

As the chronic inflammation continues, the epithelial attachment slowly migrates apically on the cementum. Alveolar bone and soft tissue continue to be lost, and the periodontal pocket becomes deeper, making the control of disease difficult.

Eventually, this continuing loss of tooth support results in a loosening of the tooth or teeth. The destruction of hard and soft tissues can continue until little or no support remains for the tooth or teeth if professional nonsurgical and/or surgical care is not sought. Extraction might become necessary, at which time all components of the periodontium are lost. Infrequently, even with professional care, tooth loss is inevitable.

CLASSIFICATIONS OF PERIODONTAL DISEASES

The most current classification system for periodontal diseases was developed in 1998. Classification systems aid in studying the etiology, pathogenesis, and treatment of diseases and provide a way to organize patients' health care needs.[46] Classification systems also enhance communication about periodontal diseases among oral health professionals and other health care providers and serve to classify periodontal diseases for insurance-reporting purposes. The previous classification system from 1989 was changed because it had overlapping disease categories, no gingival disease category, an inappropriate emphasis on age of onset of disease and its progression rate, and inadequate or unclear classification criteria.[46]

DID YOU KNOW?

There are two major categories of gingival diseases and seven categories of periodontitis in the current Classification of Periodontal Diseases that aid in studying the etiology, pathogenesis, and treatment of diseases.

The two major categories of gingival diseases are plaque induced and nonplaque induced. Gingivitis that is initiated by plaque biofilm (i.e., *plaque induced*) can be modified by systemic factors, medications, and malnutrition. *Nonplaque-induced* gingival lesions include diseases of bacterial, viral, or fungal origin, genetic manifestations of systemic conditions, traumatic lesions, and foreign body reactions.

The seven categories of periodontitis are chronic, aggressive, and systemic periodontitis; **necrotizing disease**; abscesses; endodontic lesions; and developmental or acquired deformities and conditions.[46] Chronic periodontitis is the most commonly diagnosed disease category. Chronic periodontitis implies disease that occurs over a period of time, that is usually treatable and can be controlled, and that is usually responsive to appropriate treatment. Generally, this disease state progresses slowly; however, some patients experience short periods of rapid progression. The three stages of chronic periodontitis are slight (early), moderate, and advanced (severe). Each stage has specific therapeutic goals, clinical features, treatment options, and prognoses or outcomes.[47,48]

Aggressive periodontitis is a highly destructive form of periodontal disease that can be localized or generalized. It occurs in otherwise healthy individuals and has a familial aggregation (i.e., tends to occur in most members of a family). Characteristics of aggressive periodontitis include (1) microbial deposit accumulation that is inconsistent with the severity of the disease (i.e., not much deposit but significant destruction) and (2) advancement of loss of attachment and bone loss that can be self-arresting (stopped on its own without recent treatment). Features of the localized form include onset around puberty, destruction to permanent first molars and incisors, association with the periodontal pathogen *Aggregatibacter actinomycetemcomitans (serotype b),* and abnormalities in neutrophil function.[49]

Although exceptions exist, generalized aggressive periodontitis usually affects people under the age of 30. Generalized attachment loss is present and affects at least three permanent teeth in addition to the first molars and incisors. The loss of attachment occurs in major episodic periods of destruction, and it is associated with *Aggregatibacter actinomycetemcomitans* and *Porphyromonas gingivalis* as well as abnormalities in neutrophil function.[49]

Periodontitis as a manifestation of systemic disease includes diseases associated with hematologic disorders (e.g., leukemias), and genetic disorders, such as cyclic neutropenia, Down syndrome, Papillon-Lèfevre syndrome, Cohen syndrome, and hypophosphatasia, to name a few.[46] These diseases actually cause periodontal destruction and loss of attachment.

Necrotizing periodontal diseases encompass necrotizing ulcerative gingivitis (NUG) and necrotizing ulcerative periodontitis (NUP). NUG is a condition of sudden onset, and the patient might have a history of stress, change in living habits, inadequate rest, debilitating disease, and/or respiratory tract infection. In NUG, the lesions appear punched out and craterlike; the necrotic tissue separates from the healthy gingiva, forming a gray pseudomembrane (false membrane), and the gingiva shows pronounced linear erythema (redness). Spontaneous bleeding is another characteristic accompanied by a fetid odor and increased salivation. If left untreated, NUG might advance to the supporting structures. When bone loss occurs, the condition has become necrotizing ulcerative periodontitis.

The **periodontal abscess** category relates to gingival, periodontal, or pericoronal lesions (gingival lesions close to the crown), which require special diagnostic and treatment approaches. Also, the periodontic–endodontic lesion classification recognizes the possible connection between periodontitis and endodontic lesions.

The last category of periodontal diseases, developmental or acquired deformities and conditions, refers to modifiers of the susceptibility to periodontal diseases, not to separate diseases. These modifiers such as recession, lack of keratinized gingiva, or decreased depth of the vestibule directly influence the outcomes of nonsurgical or surgical treatment.[46]

Future classifications are inevitable as more is learned about the etiology and pathogenesis of periodontal diseases. The reader is referred to the American Academy of Periodontology Web site (www.perio.org) for scientific and position papers related to the specific categories of periodontal diseases.

RISK FACTORS

A risk factor is a behavioral, biological, or environmental factor associated with a disease.[50] Risk factors are associated with incidence, extent, and progression of periodontal diseases and are usually identified through longitudinal studies (research studies in which the subjects are followed for a long period of time to study the natural course of a disease). Risk assessment can help dental professionals assess a patient's risk of developing periodontal disease and helps to improve clinical decision making related to oral health care and prognosis. Risk assessment has the potential to reduce the need for complex periodontal therapy and to improve patient outcomes that will lead to reduced cost for oral health care.[51,52] Specific examples of risk factors for periodontal diseases are age, gender, socioeconomic status, genetics, plaque biofilm, self-care, tobacco, stress, and diabetes.[53] Some risk factors cannot be changed or modified (nonmodifiable or determinant), such as age and gender, whereas others are modifiable, such as smoking and plaque biofilm. The difference between these two types of risk factors is important in educating patients about risk factors that can be changed in the future. Through education and risk assessment in the dental practice, patients will understand the significance of their individual risk factors and be motivated to strive to change and/or control those factors that are modifiable. This model represents the medical or wellness model of patient care versus the "repair" or treatment model that was used formerly for dental care.[54]

Periodontal disease is not a disease of aging; however, greater periodontal destruction is found in the elderly population as a result of lifetime disease accumulation rather than an age-specific condition.[53] By the time 90% of persons are 55 years of age, they have at least one site of 2 mm or more clinical attachment loss, and 53.6% have 4 mm or more loss of attachment at one or more sites.[54] Clinical attachment loss does increase with age; however, extensive loss of tooth function in the affected teeth is not prevalent. Pocket depth also relates somewhat to age.[53] Periodontitis seen in youth and early adulthood could be diagnosed as aggressive periodontitis, as previously discussed, depending on clinical conditions and other findings. The most rapid disease progression with periodontitis is seen in the small number of patients who manifest disease at an early age. Genetic predisposition probably contributes to this aggressive periodontitis.[49]

In reference to gender, clinical attachment loss is more prevalent in males than females.[50] This finding has been consistent in national surveys conducted over the years.[54] Genetic factors are not thought to be responsible for this gender difference in clinical attachment loss. Rather, it is thought that males are less compliant with self-care and routine oral health care visits and have a less positive attitude toward oral health.

Socioeconomic status is another risk factor for periodontal diseases that is complex and multifactorial and includes a variety of cultural factors.[53] It is accepted that patients who are well educated, relatively wealthy, and live in advantageous circumstances have better health status than those who are less educated, not wealthy, and live in poorer conditions.

Gingivitis and poor oral hygiene are clearly related to socio-economic status; however, the relationship of periodontitis to socioeconomic status is less established.[53] Even though racial and ethnic differences are evident in periodontal status, these differences are not due to true genetic differences. Instead, these differences are due to enhanced self-care among those who are better educated, have positive health attitudes, have a higher frequency of health care visits, and are aware of the need and have insurance.[53] This risk factor points to the need for culturally relevant education related to self-care practices and biofilm bacteria.[55]

Genomics is the study of structure and function of organisms in terms of their DNA sequences.[56] Genomics provides the means to discover hereditary factors in disease. Genes, by themselves, do not always determine disease; however, genetic factors alter how patients interrelate with environmental agents such as smoking. The key to a patient's development of periodontitis appears to be controlled by the response to microflora.[56] The first reported genetic components in periodontitis were discovered in 1997.[57] A specific genotype of a polymorphic interleukin-1 gene cluster, which is a key regulator of the host response to microbial infection, is associated with only severe periodontitis only in nonsmokers. This finding means that the genetic factor was not as strong a risk factor as smoking.

DID YOU KNOW ?

An individual's genetic component is a factor in periodontitis to some degree.

There is little doubt that the genetic component is a factor in periodontitis; however, the strength of the component is currently being studied. Most research is based on clinical and laboratory procedures versus epidemiologic surveys (i.e., incidence, distribution, and control of disease in a population); therefore, future studies of patients with and without disease are necessary to determine the genetic contribution to the initiation and progression of periodontitis.[53] Genetic studies have been conducted in relation to aggressive and chronic forms of periodontitis. Aggressive periodontitis appears to have several forms, and it currently is not clear how many genes may be responsible for this disease.[58] The difficulty of studying the gene identification for this disease is its rarity.[56] The genetic component for chronic periodontitis comes from studying twins in whom 50% of the susceptibility may be due to genetic factors.[59] Hopefully, the future will reveal how genetic information will help in identifying, managing, and treating those with periodontitis.

Plaque biofilm and self-care (oral hygiene) are two very significant risk factors for periodontal disease; dental professionals routinely educate patients about these factors. Plaque biofilm or, more specifically, the microbiota was previously discussed in this chapter. It is thought that the current culprits of disease are the gram-negative anaerobes found at many disease sites including *Aggregatibacter actinomycetemcomitans, Tannerella forsythia, Porphyromonas gingivalis, Prevotella intermedia, Fusobacterium nucleatum, Campylobacter rectus,* and *Treponema denticola.* It is not known whether all gram-negative anaerobes are pathogenic; however, they are found most often in the broad gram-negative groupings of bacteria from disease sites.[53] It is important for patients to realize that not all types of bacteria are equally detrimental to their periodontal health and that this variation is why the amount of plaque biofilm deposit is not as important to health as the quality or type of bacteria. Unfortunately, without efficient and cost-effective chairside tests, practitioners usually teach patients that the less plaque biofilm one has, the less chance there will be of developing periodontal disease or perpetuating an existing disease. This information is somewhat of a problem because patients often leave the education session believing quantity or amount is more important than quality of plaque biofilm.

DID YOU KNOW ?

Oral hygiene positively affects the subgingival microflora in shallow and moderate pocket depths; however, self-care has little effect on the microflora in deep pockets.

It is clear there is a relationship between poor oral hygiene and manifestation of gingivitis.[53] In fact, the better the self-care, the less gingivitis one seems to develop. On the other hand, oral hygiene positively affects the subgingival microflora in shallow and moderate pocket depths; however, self-care has little effect on the microflora in deep pockets. Some of the detrimental gram-negative pathogens identified earlier can be established in young children; these pathogens are found in supragingival plaque. Supragingival plaque microflora can migrate subgingivally when the host response is overwhelmed in the individual. Therefore, frequent supragingival prophylaxis and good self-care together can have a beneficial effect on subgingival microflora in shallow to moderately deep pockets. In conclusion, it is important to educate the patient about the importance of removing supragingival plaque to prevent and arrest progression of periodontitis.

Tobacco use is a health behavior that, as a major environmental factor, causes or contributes to various oral diseases and adverse conditions including periodontal disease. There is no doubt that tobacco users are at more risk for periodontal diseases than nonusers. Smokers make up 90% of individuals with refractory periodontal disease (periodontal disease that continues to progress or recur despite professional care and self-care).[60] In fact, smoking is one of the most significant risk factors for periodontal disease.[60] Smoking produces heat that may enhance attachment loss, reduces collagen synthesis and protein secretion, and inhibits bone formation. It also inhibits immunologic function and negatively affects immunoglobulin levels, which may increase susceptibility to microbial pathogens.[61] Also, most research concludes that healing is slower in smokers, possibly because of the suppressed growth and attachment of fibroblasts in the periodontal ligament of smokers and the slower reduction of white blood cells and neutrophils after therapy.[53] It is thought that smokers display a favorable environment for the detrimental periodontal pathogens to grow; therefore, they may have a higher prevalence of subgingival pathogenic species.[53] Some studies show more calculus and plaque accumulates in smokers, and other studies show the opposite.

It seems that further study on how smoking affects gingival bleeding is needed. Some studies show that smoking masks the signs of inflammation; therefore, smokers have less bleeding than nonsmokers. In contrast, other studies show that bleeding increases in smokers because of increased vascularity. Still other studies show that bleeding is equal among smokers and nonsmokers.[53] Smoking also seems to inhibit granulocyte function, and interactions between smoking and the interleukin-1 gene cluster have also been identified, as mentioned previously. Dentists and dental hygienists are responsible for educating patients about tobacco use as a risk factor for periodontitis and prevention strategies and cessation programs. *The Healthy People 2020* objectives call for increasing the proportion of adults who receive information from a dentist or dental hygienist focusing on reducing tobacco use or ceasing smoking in the past year as well as increasing tobacco screening and tobacco cessation counseling in dental care settings.[62] The dental office is a credible source of information about smoking and tobacco use intervention.

DID YOU KNOW?

Did you know that oral health practitioners assess the patient's current level of glycemic control because of its relationship to periodontal disease?

It is also known that stress is a risk factor for many different diseases. Likewise, stress seems to be associated with the progression of periodontitis, lending credibility to the theory that periodontitis is related to systemic diseases.[50,53]

There is strong evidence suggesting that diabetes, an abnormal elevation in blood glucose levels, is a risk factor for both gingivitis and periodontitis and that the level of glycemic control appears to be important in this relationship.[63] Diabetes is a very prevalent disease, affecting 21 million Americans, 6 million of whom are unaware they have the disease because it is undiagnosed.[63] Older individuals, Hispanics, Native Americans, and non-Hispanic blacks have more diabetes compared with younger people and non-Hispanic whites.[63] Multiple studies indicate that the presence of diabetes is usually associated with increased gingival inflammation and that the level of glycemic control may be a factor in how the gingiva responds to plaque biofilm. Not only does diabetes increase the risk of periodontitis, but it does so at any age. Also, poorly controlled diabetes increases the extent and severity of periodontitis as well as the progression of periodontal destruction. The oral health professional should always be mindful of this relationship when

reviewing health histories, educating patients, and assessing and treating periodontal diseases.

Risk calculator is available to assess a patient's risk of periodontal disease. It is a computer-based risk assessment tool called the Periodontal Risk Calculator (Dental Medicine International, Inc., Philadelphia, Pennsylvania). Use of a computer-based risk assessment tool showed valid and accurate prediction of risk of periodontal deterioration as measured by change in alveolar bone status and tooth loss with the use of the calculator.[51] The findings show a strong association between the assigned risk score and the actual periodontal deterioration observed during a 15-year period.[51,52] Risk assessment factors, tools, and models of the future will aid clinicians in the ability to help patients prevent and control disease as well as aid practitioners in selecting and delivering appropriate individualized periodontal therapy.

PRIMARY PREVENTION OF PERIODONTAL DISEASES

The most important strategy for preventing periodontal disease is to exercise prevention from the earliest age. Prevention requires daily mechanical plaque control (toothbrushing and interdental cleaning) often supplemented with chemical control measures for plaque biofilm (e.g., chlorhexidine, triclosan, or essential-oil mouthrinses) as an additional component (adjunct) of the primary treatment. Fluoride mouthrinses can be used to aid in preventing root and coronal caries.

DID YOU KNOW?

An oral prophylaxis and more diligent self-care are indicated for the treatment of gingivitis.

Bleeding gingiva is a first sign of periodontal disease; patients who report "bleeding gums" should be treated by a dentist and dental hygienist. A thorough prophylaxis, including removal of plaque-retention factors (e.g., calculus and overhanging restorations) plus more diligent self-care are indicated for gingivitis. For patients with early to moderate periodontitis, nonsurgical periodontal therapy is indicated with treatment focused on removal of plaque biofilm and calcified deposits from the cementum and disruption of subgingival microbial flora. Thorough debridement (scaling and root planing) of tooth surfaces is performed by manual (hand) or ultrasonic instrumentation. Flushing out toxins from the epithelial-related plaque biofilm can be achieved with some irrigation units with special tips that permit patients to irrigate shallow pockets (4 to 5 mm).[64]

Some patients have advanced periodontitis with vast tissue destruction, deep pockets (more than 5 mm), and furcation involvement, which indicate a need for periodontal surgery. Even if complex surgical procedures or intensive therapy is used to treat patients, primary preventive measures play a critical role in helping to maintain disease control after periodontal health has been reestablished.

A major challenge in primary preventive dentistry is to increase public awareness that patient self-care usually can maintain excellent oral health. Effective removal of supragingival plaque biofilm coupled with regular professional examination and appropriate oral health care established early in life will minimize periodontal disease. It was long believed that, once the subgingival plaque biofilm was permanently organized, supragingival plaque control (self-care) activities had no effect on the subgingival plaque. However, more recent evidence has demonstrated that meticulous supragingival plaque control measures can delay the initiation and organization of the subgingival plaque.

SUMMARY

Periodontitis is a disease involving pathology of one or more of the four components of the periodontium: the epithelial attachment, alveolar bone, cementum, and periodontal ligament. The term *periodontal disease* is an umbrella term for several clinically similar types of diseases attributable to different bacteria and different modifying factors. Gingivitis, by definition, becomes periodontitis when the epithelial attachment migrates apically, causing a loss of the level of clinical attachment and alveolar bone. Periodontitis is caused by a combination of bacterial species. These variables can be estimated by studying clinical signs of inflammation and past disease behavior. The bacteria associated with healthy gingiva are usually composed of aerobic, nonmotile, gram-positive cocci. In contrast, the microorganisms for the subgingival plaque that are associated with disease usually are anaerobic, gram-negative motile rods and treponema. The most common form of gingivitis is plaque induced, and the most common form of periodontitis is chronic periodontitis.

The supragingival plaque biofilm is on the enamel, and the tooth-associated subgingival plaque biofilm is on the cementum. In the area separating the supragingival from the subgingival plaque, a melding of bacteria of the two biofilms occurs. To combat the bacterial challenge when there is a site of inflammation, the body recognizes chemotactic signals that bring both cellular and humoral immune responses to the inflamed areas.

Predicting risk of periodontitis is a complex issue. It is difficult to study the effects of one risk factor in a population for many reasons. Multiple risk factors enhance the ability of an individual to acquire periodontal disease and for it to progress. It is evident, however, that tobacco use is clearly a single indicator that affects one's risk of disease development and progression.

In patients with periodontal disease, it currently is not possible to predict the speed of development and severity of the disease with complete accuracy. Research is being conducted in genetics to identify etiologic bacteria, aid in diagnosis, and enhance treatment. The Human Genome Project, a worldwide effort that decoded the DNA molecule, is expected to enhance these efforts in the future. Studies of interleukin-1, a cytokine, have indicated that laboratory evaluation of this cytokine can help identify those individuals at higher risk for developing severe periodontal diseases. Interleukin-1 is also related to bleeding on dental probing. Because interleukin-1 is a lifetime genetic factor, one test for this factor can suffice to assign risk for a lifetime. This test also can be used in developing treatment plans for individual patients. Because bacteria are essential for periodontitis, a positive marker (high blood level) of interleukin-1 should alert the dental professional and the patient to the importance of complying with daily mechanical and chemical plaque control therapies.

PRACTICAL CONSIDERATIONS

Most patients who present to dental offices have varying levels of periodontal disease. The dental provider should understand gingival and periodontal disease anatomy, physiology and disease etiology to aid in choosing the correct treatment and adjuncts and to educate patients on oral health.

SELF-STUDY QUESTIONS

1. Which of the following is the primary clinical and diagnostic difference between gingivitis and periodontitis?

   a. Sulcus depth

   b. Pocket depth

   c. Loss of attachment

   d. Evidence of gingival inflammation

Rationale: Loss of attachment is the detachment of collagen fibers from the cementum and subsequent movement of the zone of soft tissue attached to the teeth (i.e., the junctional epithelium) toward the apex of the root. The presence of gingival inflammation without loss of attachment is gingivitis. Gingival inflammation accompanied by a pathological loss of attachment is classified as periodontitis.[2]

2. Which of the following is the most apical portion of the marginal gingiva?

   a. Attached gingiva

   b. Free gingival groove

   c. Interdental papilla

   d. Free gingival margin

   Rationale: The gingiva consists of the free (or marginal) gingiva, interdental papillae, and attached gingiva (Figure 6–3). The marginal gingiva surrounds each tooth in a cuff-like fashion and is not attached to the tooth. The most coronal portion of the marginal gingiva is the edge of the gingiva that touches the tooth (free margin). Its most apical portion is the free marginal groove, which defines the boundary between the attached and marginal gingiva.

3. What is the primary location and function of the interradicular fibers of the periodontal ligament?

   a. They are found in the furcation area of a multirooted tooth and connect the cementum and tooth.

   b. They are found at the apex of the tooth and help cushion the tooth from occlusal forces.

   c. They extend obliquely from the cementum to the alveolar crest and prevent lateral movement and extrusion of the tooth.

   d. They are located at the cervical area and resist lateral forces.

   Rationale: The periodontal ligament is a network of collagen fibers. This structure surrounds the tooth root and connects it with the alveolar bone (Figure 6–8B). Its collagen fibers embed into the cementum of the root on one side and into the alveolar bone on the other side. The five principal fibers of the periodontal ligament have different orientations and functions at various levels on the tooth root. They are arranged in bundles called *alveolar crest, horizontal, oblique, apical,* and *interradicular fiber groups* (Figure 6–5). The alveolar crest fibers extend obliquely from the cementum to the alveolar crest. They prevent lateral movement and extrusion of the tooth. The horizontal fibers are located at the cervical area and resist lateral forces. The oblique fibers extend in an oblique fashion from the alveolar bone to the cementum and bear the stress of chewing. The apical fibers form at the tooth apex and are generally parallel to the long axis of the tooth to help cushion the tooth from occlusal forces. The interradicular fibers are found in the furcation area of a multirooted tooth and connect the cementum and tooth. In addition, a network of blood vessels within the periodontal ligament protects the bone and periodontal fibers from excessive occlusal forces.

4. A characteristic clinical sign of the *early lesion* of periodontal disease is which of the following?

   a. Increased flow of gingival crevicular fluid

   b. Bleeding on probing

   c. A bluish hue in the gingiva

   d. Loss of attachment

   Rationale: The early lesion is Stage II of inflammation in the periodontal lesion, which correlates with the clinical changes of erythema, bleeding on probing, and loss of tissue tone. An increase in gingival crevicular fluid is part of the initial lesion, which is Stage I and is subclinical. An underlying bluish hue in the gingiva is part of the chronic gingivitis or Stage III of the periodontal lesion. Loss of attachment and true pocketing are characteristics of Stage IV or the advanced lesion (periodontitis). Refer to Table 6–1.

5. Which of the following is the *classification* of disease that is rapid and highly destructive to the attachment apparatus, can be localized or generalized, occurs in otherwise healthy individuals, and has a familial aggregation?

   a. Plaque-induced gingivitis

   b. Nonplaque-induced gingivitis

   c. Chronic periodontitis

   d. Aggressive periodontitis

   Rationale: The two major categories of gingival diseases are plaque induced and nonplaque induced. Gingivitis that is initiated by plaque biofilm (i.e., plaque induced) can be modified by systemic factors, medications, and malnutrition. Nonplaque-induced gingival lesions include diseases of bacterial, viral, or fungal origin, genetic manifestations of systemic conditions, traumatic lesions, or foreign body reactions. Gingival diseases as a diagnosis do not have accompanying attachment loss.

   Chronic periodontitis, which is the most commonly diagnosed disease category, implies disease that occurs over a period of time, that is usually treatable and can be controlled, and that is usually responsive to appropriate treatment. This disease state progresses slowly; however, some patients experience short periods of rapid progression. The three stages of chronic periodontitis are slight (early), moderate, and advanced (severe). Each stage has specific therapeutic goals, clinical features, treatment options, and prognoses or outcomes.[47,48]

   Aggressive periodontitis is a highly destructive form of periodontal disease that can be localized or generalized. It occurs in otherwise healthy individuals and has a familial aggregation (i.e., tends to occur in most members of a family). Characteristics of aggressive periodontitis include (1) microbial deposit accumulation that is inconsistent with the severity of the disease (i.e., not much deposit but significant destruction) and (2) advancement of loss of attachment and bone loss that can be self-arresting (stopped on its own without recent treatment). Features of the localized form include onset around puberty, destruction to permanent first molars and incisors, association with the periodontal pathogen *Aggregatibacter actinomycetemcomitans,* and abnormalities in neutrophil function.[49]

REFERENCES

1. Lovegrove, J. M. (2004). Dental plaque revisited: Bacteria associated with periodontal disease. *J N Z Soc Periodontol*, 87:7–21.

2. The American Academy of Periodontology. (2003). Diagnosis of periodontal diseases. (Position paper). *J Periodontol*, 74:1237–47.

3. Bascones-Martinez, A., Matesanz-Perez, P., Escribano-Bermejo, M., González-Moles, M. A., Bascones-Ilundain, J., & Meurman, J. H. (2011 January 3 [Epub ahead of print]). Periodontal disease and diabetes—Review of the literature. *Med Oral Patol Oral Cir Bucal*.

4. Mealey, B. L., Oates, T. W. (2006). Diabetes mellitus and periodontal diseases. *J Periodontology*, 77:1289–1303.

5. Shchipkova, A.Y., Nagaraja, H. N., & Kumar, P. S. (2010). Subgingival microbial profiles of smokers with periodontitis. *J Dental Research*, 89:1247–1253.

6. Filoche, S. K., Cornford, E., Gaudie, W., Wong, M., Heasman, P., & Thomson, W. M. (2010). Smoking, chronic periodontitis and smoking cessation support: Reviewing the role of dental professionals. *N Z Dent J*, 106(2):74–77.

7. Johnson, G. K., & Hill, M. (2004). Cigarette smoking and the periodontal patient. *J Periodontology*, 75:196–209.

8. Arbes, S. J., Jr., Agerstsdottier, H., & Slade, G. D. (2001). Environmental tobacco smoke and periodontal disease in the United States. *Am J Public Health*, 91:253–57.

9. Research, Science and Therapy Committee of the American Academy of Periodontology. (2005). Implications of genetic technology for the management of periodontal diseases. *J Periodontology*, 76:850–857.

10. The American Academy of Periodontology. (2003). Periodontal diseases of children and adolescents (Position paper). *J Periodontol*, 74:1696–1704.

11. The American Academy of Periodontology. (2005). Epidemiology of periodontal diseases (Position paper). *J Periodontol*, 76:1406–19.

12. The American Academy of Periodontology. (2000). Parameter on periodontitis associated with systemic conditions. *J Periodontol*, 71 (Suppl):876–79.

13. Friedewald, V. E., Kornman, K. S., Beck, J. D., Genco, R., Goldfine, A., Libby, P., Offenbacher, S., Ridker, P. M., Van Dyke, T. E., & Roberts, W. C. (2009). Editors' consensus: Periodontitis and atherosclerotic cardiovascular disease. *American Journal of Cardiology* and *J Periodontol*, 80:1021–32.

14. Dumitrescu, A. L. (2005). Influence of periodontal disease on cardiovascular diseases. *Rom J Intern Med*, 43:9–21.

15. Kim, J., & Amar, S. (2006). Periodontal disease and systemic conditions: A bidirectional relationship. *Odontology*, 94:10–21.

16. Pizzo, G., Guiglia, R., Lo Russo, L., & Campisi, G. (2010, December) Dentistry and internal medicine: From the focal infection theory to the periodontal medicine concept. (Review). *Euro J Intern Med*, 21:496–502.

17. Slayton, R. L., & Slavkin, H. C. (2009). Scientific investments continue to fuel improvements in oral health (May 2000–Present). *Academic Pediatrics*, 9:383–85

18. Hacker, B. M., & Roberts. F. A. (2005). Periodontal disease pathogenesis: Genetic risk factors and paradigm shift. *Pract Proced Aesthet Dent*, 17:97–102.

19. Hormia, M., Owaribe, K., & Virt, I. (2001). The dento-epithelial junction cell adhesion by Type I hemidesmosomes in the absence of true basal lamina. *J Periodontol*, 72:788–97.

20. Weidlich, P., Lopez de Souza, M. A., & Opperman, R. V. (2001). Evaluation of the dentogingival area during early plaque formation. *J Periodontol*, 72:901–10.

21. Löe, H., Theilade, E., & Jensen, S. B. (1965). Experimental gingivitis in man. *J Periodontol*, 36:177–83.

22. Moore, W., Holdeman L., Smibert, R., Cato, E. P., Burmeister, J. A., Palcanis, K. G., & Ranney, R. R. (1984). Bacteriology of experimental gingivitis in children. *Infect Immun*, 46:1–6.

23. Slots, J., Möenbo, D., Langebaek, J., & Frandsen, A. (1978). Microbiota of gingivitis in man. *Scand J Dent*, 86:174–81.

24. Friedman, M. T., Barber, P. M., Mardan, N. J., & Newman, H. N. (1992). The "plaque-free zone" in health and disease: A scanning electron microscope study. *J Periodontol*, 63:890–96.

25. *Periodontal literature review.* (1996). Chicago: The American Academy of Periodontology, 68–72.

26. Fiorellini, J. P., Kim, D. M., & Uzel, N. G. (2012). Gingival inflammation. In Newman, M. G., Takei, H., Carranza, F. A., & Klokkevold, P. R., Eds. *Carranza's clinical periodontology* (11th ed.), St. Louis, MO: Elsevier Saunders, 71–76.

27. American Academy of Periodontology Academy Report. (2004). Informational paper: Drug-associated gingival enlargement. *Journal of Periodontology*, 75:1424.

28. Ronderas, M., Pihlstrom, B. L., & Hodges, J. S. (2001). Periodontal disease among indigenous people in the Amazon rain forest. *J Clin Periodontol*, 28:995–1003.

29. American Academy of Periodontology. (2001). *Glossary of periodontal terms* (4th ed.). Chicago, IL: Author.

30. Teughels W., Quirynen M., Jakubovics N. (2012). Periodontal microbiology. In Newman, M. G., Takei, H., Carranza F. A., & Klokkevold, P. R., Eds. *Carranza's clinical periodontology* (11th ed.), 232–270. St. Louis, MO: Elsevier Saunders.

31. Fine, D. H., Tabak, L., Oshrain, H., Salkind, A., & Siegel, K. (1978). Studies in plaque pathogenicity. Plaque collection limulus lysate screening of adherent and loosely adherent plaque. *J Periodontol Res*, 13:17–22.

32. Fine, D. H., Tabak, L., Oshrain, H., Salkind, A., & Siegel, K. (1978). Studies in plaque pathogenicity. II. A technique for the specific detection of endotoxin in plaque samples using the limulus lysate assay. *J Periodontol Res*, 13:127–133.

33. Caton, J., Bouwsma, O., Polson, A., & Epseland, M. (1989). Effect of personal oral hygiene and subgingival scaling on bleeding interdental gingiva. *J Periodontol*, 60: 84–90.

34. Cercek, J. F., Kiger, R. D., Garrett, S., & Egelberg, J. (1983). Relative effects of plaque control and instrumentation on the clinical parameters of human periodontal disease. *J Periodontol*, 10:46–56.

35. Kho, P., Smales, F., & Hardie, J. (1985). The effect of supragingival plaque control on subgingival microflora. *J Clin Periodontol*, 12:676–86.

36. Greenstein, G. (2000). Non-surgical periodontal therapy in 2000: A periodontal response to mechanical non-surgical therapy: A literature review. *J Amer Dent Assoc*, 131:1580–92.

37. Ciancio, S. G. (1989). Non-surgical periodontal treatment. In *Proceedings of the world workshop in clinical periodontics* (Section II). Chicago: American Academy of Periodontology.

38. Boch, J. A., Wara-aswapati, N., & Auron, P. E. (2000). Interleukin 1. Signal transduction—Current concepts and relevance to periodontitis. *J Dent Res*, 80:400–407.

39. Flood, P. M., Washington, O., Stevens, D. P., & Ptak, W. (1992). Immunological signals which control T cell responses. *J Endod,* 18:435–39.

40. Huang, G. T., Haake, S. K., & Park, N. H. (1998). Gingival epithelial cells increase interleukin-8 secretion in response to Actinobacillus actinomycetemcomitans challenge. *J Periodontol,* 69:1105–10.

41. Guthmiller, J. M., Lally, E. T., & Korostoff, J. (2001). Beyond the specific plaque hypothesis: Are highly leukotoxic strains of Actinobacillus actinomycetemcomitans a paradigm of periodontal pathogenesis? *Crit Rev Oral Biol Med,*12:116–24.

42. Gustafasson, A., Asman, B., & Bergstrom, K. (2001). Increased release of IL-B from monocytes for patients with chronic periodontitis. *J Dent Res,* 80(Spec Iss).

43. McGuire, M. K., & Nunn, M. E. (1999). Prognosis versus actual outcome. IV. The effectiveness of clinical parameters and IL-1 genotype in accurately predicting prognoses and tooth survival. *J Periodontol,* 70:49–56.

44. Deo, V. & Bhongade, M. L. Pathogenesis of periodontitis: Role of cytokines in host response. *Dent Today,* 9:60–62, 64–66, 68–69.

45. McDevitt, M. J., & Wang, H.-Y. (2000). Interleukin-1 genetic association with periodontitis in clinical practice. *J Periodontol,* 71:156–62.

46. Armitage, G. C. (1999). Development of a classification system for periodontal diseases and conditions. *Ann Periodontol,* 4:1–6.

47. American Academy of Periodontology. (2000). Parameter on chronic periodontitis with slight to moderate loss of periodontal support. *J Periodontol,* 71 (Suppl):853–55.

48. American Academy of Periodontology. (2000). Parameter on chronic periodontitis with advanced loss of periodontal support. *J Periodontol,* 71 (Suppl):856–58.

49. American Academy of Periodontology. (2000). Parameter on aggressive periodontitis. *J Periodontol,* 71 (Suppl):867–69.

50. Novak, K., Novak, J. (2012). Clinical risk assessment. In Newman, M. G., Takei, H., Carranza, F. A., & Klokkevold, P. R., Eds. *Carranza's clinical periodontolog* (11th ed.).

51. Page, R. C., Krall, E. A., Martin J., Mancl, L., & Garcia, R. I. (2002). Validity and accuracy of a risk calculator in predicting periodontal disease. *J Am Dent Assoc,* 133:569–76. St. Louis, MO: Elsevier.

52. Persson, G. R., Mancl, L. A., Martin, J., & Page, R. C. (2003). Assessing periodontal disease risk. *J Am Dent Assoc,* 134:575–82.

53. American Academy of Periodontology. (2005). Epidemiology of periodontal diseases. (Position Paper). *J Periodontol,* 76: 1406–19.

54. U.S. Public Health Service, National Institute of Dental Research. (1987). *Oral health of United States adults: National findings* (NIH Publication 87-2868). Bethesda, MD: National Institute of Dental Research.

55. Douglass, C. W. (2006). Risk assessment and management of periodontal disease. *J Am Dent Assoc,* 137 (Suppl 3):27–32.

56. Kornman, K. S., Crane, A., Wang, H.-Y., diGiovine, F. S., Newman, M. G., Pink, F. W., Wilson, T. G., Jr., Higginbottom, F. L., & Duff, G. W. (1997). The interleukin-1 genotype as a severity factor in adult periodontal disease. *J Clin Periodontol,* 24:72–77.

57. American Academy of Periodontology. (2005). Informational paper: Implications of genetic technology for the management of periodontal diseases. *J Periodontol,* 76:850–57.

58. Li, Y., Xu, L., Hasturk, H., Kantarci, A., DePalma, S. R., & van Dyke, T. E. (2004). Localized aggressive periodontitis is linked to human chromosome 1q25. *Hum Genet,* 114:291–97.

59. Michalowicz, B. S., Diehl, S. R., Gunsolley, J. C., Sparks, B. S., Brooks, C. N., Koertge, T. E., Califano, J. V., Burmeister, J. A., & Schenkein, H. A. (2000). Evidence of a substantial genetic basis for risk of adult periodontitis. *J Periodontol,* 71:1699–1701.

60. Johnson, G. K., & Slach, N. A. (2001). Impact of tobacco use on periodontal status. *J Dent Educ,* 65:313–21.

61. American Academy of Periodontology. (1999). Tobacco use and the periodontal patient. (Position Paper). *J Peridontol,* 70:1419–27.

62. healthypeople.gov/2020/topicsobjetives2020/excel/HealthyPeople2020—All objectives. xisx

63. American Academy of Periodontology. (2006). Diabetes mellitus and periodontal diseases. *J Periodontol,* 77:1289–303.

64. Cutler, C. W., Stanford, T. W., Abraham, C., Cederberg, R. A., Boardman, T. J., & Ross, C. (2000). Clinical benefits of oral irrigation for periodontitis are related to reduction of proinflammatory cytokine levels and plaque. *J Clin Periodontol,* 27:134–43.

Oral Cancer

Sandra J. Maurizio

OBJECTIVES

After studying this chapter, the student should be able to:

1. Describe the epidemiology of oral cancer.
2. Identify risk factors that contribute to oral cancer.
3. Identify signs and symptoms of oral cancer.
4. Identify factors to prevent oral cancer.
5. Describe the common locations for oropharyngeal cancers.
6. Describe the various screening and diagnostic tools used to detect oral cancer.
7. Describe the steps in a complete oral cancer examination.
8. Identify the staging system used for oral cancer.
9. Identify appropriate referral sites.
10. Describe treatment options.
11. Identify resources available to health care providers and patients.
12. Identify practical considerations for health care providers.

KEY TERMS

Actinic cheilitis, 92
Angiogenesis, 88
Apoptosis, 88
Brachytherapy, 100
Carcinogenesis, 92
Carcinoma in situ, 92
Differentiation, 88
Epithelial dysplasia, 88
Grading system, 100
Growth regulation, 88
Neoplasm, 88
Proliferation, 88
Stage, 90
Staging system, 100

INTRODUCTION

Cancer refers to a variety of malignant neoplasms that occur throughout the body. The term **neoplasm** means "new growth" and describes a rapid growth of the number of cells (**proliferation**) that exceeds normal growth.[1] This overgrowth can be caused by cells that continue proliferation after cessation of the stimuli that initiated the new growth or by cells that fail to undergo **apoptosis** (programmed cell death).[1] Neoplasms can be either benign or cancerous, depending on whether they invade surrounding or distant tissues. Carcinomas are malignant neoplasms derived from epithelial tissue.[1]

Oral cancers are defined in various ways. In this chapter, they are defined according to the primary anatomic structures. Oral cancers affect the oral cavity and the oropharynx, which is the part of the pharynx located at the back of the mouth. As discussed in this chapter, the oral cavity extends from the vermilion (red) border of the lips through the mouth to and including the pharyngeal arches. The arches are formed by the palatoglossus and the palatopharyngeus muscles. Both muscles arise from the soft palate, which is the muscular portion of the roof of the mouth located posterior to the root of the tongue. The palatoglossus muscle forms the anterior arch on each side of the throat, whereas the palatopharyngeus muscle forms the posterior arch.[1] Subdivisions of the oral cavity include the lips, floor of the mouth, buccal mucosa, palate, and alveolar processes. The oropharynx includes the entire area from the base of the tongue, the pharyngeal wall, the tonsillar fossae (the depressions between the pharyngeal arches in which the palatine tonsils are located), and the soft palate.[1] Generally, in this chapter, the term *oral cancer* includes both oral cavity and oropharyngeal cancers unless otherwise specified.

Squamous cell carcinomas represent more than 90% of cancers of the oropharynx and oral cavity. The etiology of squamous cell carcinomas of the oral cavity and oropharyngeal regions is multifactorial. Salivary gland cancers, including adenoid cystic carcinoma, mucoepidermoid carcinoma, and polymorphous low-grade adenocarcinoma, are present in the oral cavity among other sites.[2] The following brief explanation of the biologic basis for cancer formation will be helpful in discussions of preventive modalities.

Cancers are formed when normal cells undergo a sequential, multistep process from normality to eventual metastatic cancer (that has spread from its site of origin). **Epithelial dysplasia** is a premalignant condition during which cells undergo a combination of cellular and architectural changes. Cell alterations include changes in the size, shape, and number of nuclei and increased mitosis (cell division; Figure 7–1 ■). Altered architectural integrity includes formation of rete pegs (elongated ridges of epidermis that point downward), hyperplasia (abnormal increase in the number of cells) of the basilar membrane, and altered maturation.[3] Cell functions that must be disrupted for cancer to occur include (1) growth regulation, (2) apoptosis, (3) differentiation, (4) replicative senescence, (5) angiogenesis, (6) DNA repair, (7) tissue remodeling and

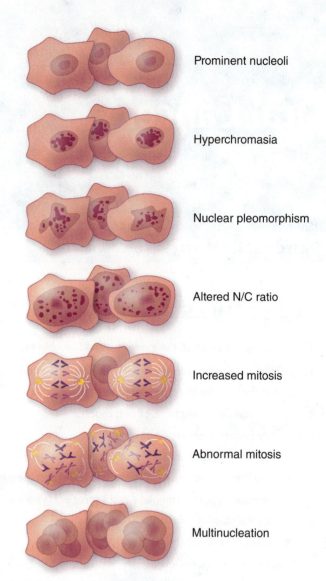

Prominent nucleoli

Hyperchromasia

Nuclear pleomorphism

Altered N/C ratio

Increased mitosis

Abnormal mitosis

Multinucleation

FIGURE ■ 7–1 Cell alterations in epithelial dysplasia. The degree of severity of an epithelial dysplasia is determined, in part, by the frequency and combination of these alterations.

migration, and (8) immune evasion. **Growth regulation** refers to proliferation beyond the number of cells expected in normal cell division. *Apoptosis* is programmed cell death, which is the process of removing aging cells or cells with damaged DNA from the body. In cancerous growths, apoptosis is "turned off" so that damaged cells are allowed to replicate (duplicate their genetic material). **Differentiation** involves the degree of alteration of cells from their normal morphology (form) and function. Poorly differentiated neoplasms no longer resemble the cells they derived from originally. Well-differentiated neoplasms retain the original cells' morphology and function (Figure 7–2 ■). *Replicative senescence* is the irreversible loss of the cell's ability to stop dividing after a finite number of divisions, which results in faulty cells. **Angiogenesis** is the buildup of vascular tissue needed to sustain cancerous growth.

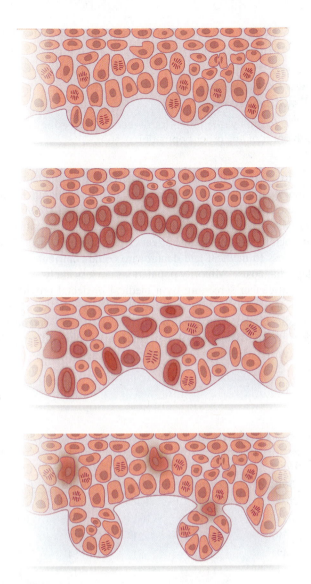

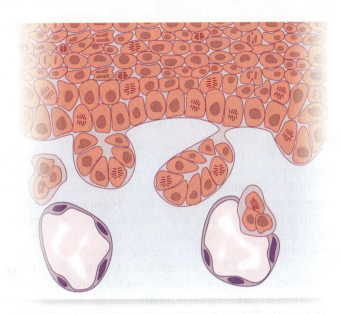

FIGURE ■ 7–3 Transition of epithelial dysplasia to invasive squamous cell carcinoma. Malignant cells have penetrated through the basement membrane into the underlying connective tissue where they are capable of eroding into lymphatic vessels.

FIGURE ■ 7–2 Architectural alterations of the epithelium found in epithelial dysplasia. The degree of severity of the epithelial dysplasia is determined by the extent of severity of these alterations combined with the individual cell abnormalities.

DNA repair is the process by which a cell monitors and repairs DNA disruptions before replication to avoid passing faulty DNA material to new cells. Mutation of the p53 gene is observed in head and neck cancers. *Tissue remodeling and migration* refers to the ability to travel beyond the normal borders of the tissue associated with a particular cell (Figure 7–3 ■). *Immune evasion* is a breakdown in the ability to monitor tissues for evidence of cancer.[3]

Some mild forms of epithelial dysplasia can be reversed if preventive measures are taken, such as dietary changes or tobacco and alcohol cessation. The role of the dental professional is critical in the process of recognizing early lesions and perhaps preventing the transformation to malignancy. Educating patients and assisting them in termination of harmful habits can accomplish these goals. Because squamous cell carcinomas represent nearly all oral cancers, the remainder of the chapter will refer to this type of cancer.

EPIDEMIOLOGY OF ORAL CANCER

The American Cancer Society estimated 36,540 new cases of oral cavity and pharynx cancers will occur in 2010, with an estimated 7,880 deaths.

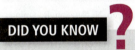

DID YOU KNOW

Incidence rates refer to the number of new cases of a disease in a specified population during 1 year per 100,000 individuals.

Incidence rates for oral cavity and pharyngeal cancers in men are roughly twice as high as those in women.[4] Estimated incidence rates by gender for 2010 reflected a 2-to-1 ratio of men to women, with 25,420 new cases expected for men and 11,120 for women.[4] Five-year survival rates for all cancers have demonstrated an increase from 53% in the mid–1970s to 63% in 2005.[4] For all stages of oral cavity and pharynx cancer patients, about 83% will survive 1 year; 5-year and 10-year survival rates are 61% and 50%, respectively.[4] The 1999–2006 Surveillance, Epidemiology, and End Results Program (SEER) data indicate that 5-year survival rates are 60.9% for all stages, 82.5% for localized lesions, 54.7% for regional cancers, 32.2% for distant cancers, and 53.2% for unstaged cancers of the oral cavity and pharynx.[5] Estimated deaths by gender for 2010 indicate a 2-to-1 ratio of men to women with 5,430 deaths expected for men versus 2,450 for women.[4] As the survival rates indicate, **stage** (extent of a cancer in the body[2]) at diagnosis is a critical factor in the expected mortality rate for oral cancer.

Oral cancer mortality is disproportionately distributed among ethnic and minority groups (see Tables 7–1 ■ and 7–2 ■). *Mortality rate* refers to the number of deaths in a specified population during 1 year per 100,000 individuals. SEER 2003–2007 data indicate oral cavity and pharynx mortality rates of 3.7 and 1.4 per 100,000 for white men and women, respectively. The mortality rate for African Americans is 6.3 for men and 1.5 for women. Rates for white and African American women are comparable, but the mortality rates for men show a much higher rate for African American males than white males. The gender breakdown in other races ranges from 3.1 and 1.2 for Asian/Pacific Islander men and women, respectively, to 3.5 and 1.6 for American Indian/Alaskan Native men

and women, and 2.5 and 0.8 for Hispanic men and women (Tables 7–1 and 7–2).[5]

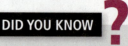

DID YOU KNOW

The mortality rate for African American men is the highest of any other population group.

Reasons for the disproportionate burden of oral cancer on minority populations are complex, and confounding factors make causes difficult to assess. In simplistic terms, *confounding factors* are two or more factors that can affect a situation, but each factor's individual effect cannot be determined.[5] Lack of access to medical and dental care could contribute to later stage diagnosis.[5] Minority populations are less likely to receive an oral cancer screening by a medical or dental provider. In addition, high-risk individuals are more likely to seek care from a medical rather than a dental provider. A lack of awareness of the signs and symptoms of oral cancer and the need for regular oral cancer screenings contribute to late diagnosis.[6]

TABLE ■ 7–1 Stage Distribution (Percentage) of Oral Cavity and Pharynx Cancer by Race and Sex, 1999–2006

	All Races			Whites			Blacks		
	Total	*Male*	*Female*	*Total*	*Male*	*Female*	*Total*	*Male*	*Female*
Number of cases	46,149	31,829	14,320	37,512	26,062	11,450	4,464	3,126	1,338
Percent	100%	100%	100%	100%	100%	100%	100%	100%	100%
Localized	33	30	42	35	31	44	21	17	31
Regional	46	49	38	45	49	37	51	54	44
Distant	14	15	13	13	13	11	21	22	18
Unstaged	7	7	7	7	6	7	7	6	7

(*Source:* S. F. Altekruse, C. I. Kosary, M. Krapcho, N. Neyman, R. Aminou, W. Waldron, J. Ruhl, N. Howlader, Z. Tatalovich, H. Cho, A. Mariotto, M. P. Eisner, D. R. Lewis, K. Cronin, H. S. Chen, E. J. Feuer, D. G. Stinchcomb, & B. K. Edward, Eds. (2010). SEER Cancer Statistics Review, 1975–2007. Bethesda, MD: National Cancer Institute. Retrieved March 4, 2012 from http://seer.cancer.gov/csr/1975_2007/, based on November 2009 SEER data submission, posted to the SEER Web site.)

TABLE ■ 7–2 Oral Cavity and Pharynx Cancer 5-Year Survival (Percent), 1999–2006, by Stage at Diagnosis, Race, and Sex

	All Races			Whites			Blacks		
	Total	*Male*	*Female*	*Total*	*Male*	*Female*	*Total*	*Male*	*Female*
All stages	60.9	59.8	63.6	62.8	62.2	64.1	42.2	37.5	53.2
Localized	82.5	81.7	83.8	83.0	82.6	83.7	74.0	66.4	83.6
Regional	54.7	55.8	51.7	56.8	58.6	51.3	36.7	34.7	42.4
Distant	32.2	31.3	34.7	32.2	31.5	34.0	24.0	22.6	27.8
Unstaged	53.2	51.9	55.8	53.7	52.5	55.7	37.2	32.7	46.6

(*Source:* Based on SEER Cancer Statistics Review, 1975–2007, National Cancer Institute. Bethesda, MD, based on November 2009 SEER data submission, posted to the SEER web site, 2010.)

RISK FACTORS

The oncology field has started to shift from a treatment-oriented philosophy toward a prevention-oriented philosophy. A similar shift occurred in cardiology when suspected risk factors were studied sufficiently to determine causal relationships. Educational campaigns directed toward health professionals and the public resulted in well-understood prevention modalities to help overcome cardiac diseases. The important shift toward identifying factors to prevent cancer as further research evolves is a critical one for dental professionals to pursue.[7]

The oral cavity is exposed to a variety of ingested and inhaled agents that may increase the risk of cancer. The multitude of possible contributors to the development of oral carcinoma confounds the difficulty in identifying causative agents. Host susceptibility, environmental factors, and exposure to protective factors all play a role in the development of oral cancer.

Primary risk factors for oral cancer include tobacco use and excessive alcohol intake. Tobacco use is the major cause of oral cancer in the United States. Other risk factors include human papillomavirus infection, increasing age, low intake of fruits and vegetables, and excessive sun exposure (lip cancers). The majority of oral cancers occur in individuals older than 40 to 45 years.[8] However, a recent upswing of cases has been identified in young people with no apparent risk factors.[8] Human papillomavirus infection is a possible contributor to this phenomenon.[8,9]

Tobacco

Tobacco contributes to an estimated 30% of cancers in the United States. Cigarette smoking has been firmly established as a direct causal link of cancer of the oral cavity and pharynx.[4] Eight of ten people with oral cancer are smokers.[4] Smokers have a 5-fold to 25-fold higher risk for developing head and neck cancers than nonsmokers.[10] In addition, 1 in 3 oral cancer patients who continue to smoke after their cancer is gone will develop second oral cancers whereas recurrent cancer will occur in only 1 in 10 former oral cancer patients who quit.[4] In other countries, particularly India, chewing betel or areca nut in a quid called *paan* is associated with a higher risk of oral cancer.[11] Recently, tobacco products appearing on the market include dissolvable orbs, sticks, and strips. Their level of risk for contributing to oral cancer is currently unknown.[12]

Alcohol

DID YOU KNOW

The combination of tobacco use and excessive alcohol use is synergistic, and individuals who use both are more likely to develop oral cancer.

Heavy alcohol consumers who do not use tobacco products have a higher risk for developing oral cancer, regardless of the type of alcohol consumed. The risk for oral cancer development is dose related with individuals consuming more than four drinks per day at greatest risk. The type of alcohol does not seem to have an effect on the incidence of oral cancer. The American Cancer Society suggests about 70% of oral cancer patients drink alcohol.[4] Individuals who consume more than 100 g (4 drinks) per day have a 30-fold higher risk of developing oral cancer than those who consume less than 15 g of alcohol per day.[13] The combination of smoking and alcohol is particularly deadly. Heavy drinkers and smokers have 100 times the risk of developing oral cancer compared with abstainers.[13] Alcohol may enhance cell permeability, contributing to the carcinogenic nature of tobacco, thus providing the mechanism of action that results in the synergistic effect.[14,15] In addition, heavy drinkers typically have nutritional deficiencies that lower the body's ability to prevent cancer.[15] When ethanol is metabolized, toxic compounds, including acetaldehyde, a recognized carcinogen, are released. The increased risk associated with the use of tobacco and alcohol products will fade after 10 years of abstinence, lessening the risk to approximately that of any nondrinker and nonsmoker.[15]

Human Papillomavirus

DID YOU KNOW

Human papillomavirus is the primary cause of tonsillar cancer in North America.

Human papillomavirus (HPV) is the most common sexually transmitted infection in the United States.[16] More than 100 types of HPV have been identified. HPV has been implicated as a causative factor in oral cavity and oropharyngeal squamous cell carcinoma and is present in 47% to 63% of these cancers. HPV–16 is most frequently associated with oropharyngeal cancer. The tongue and tonsils are primarily affected. HPV is the primary cause of tonsillar cancer in North America and Europe.[8] A recent retrospective analysis of SEER data from 1975–2006 demonstrates significant trends in oral cavity and oropharyngeal carcinoma. Tongue and tonsillar cancer have been increasing although cancer in other oral sites have decreased in cancer development.[17] Patients with HPV-associated oral cancer have different characteristics from the classic oral cancer patient. They are an average of 5 years younger (40–60 years old).[17,18] Risk factors have identified in HPV-associated cancers include beginning sexual practices at an early age, a high number of sexual partners, and a history of oral sex.[19] Nonsmokers with head and neck squamous cell carcinoma are 15 times more likely to have an HPV-positive cancer than smokers. Alcohol has a similar profile. HPV-associated tumors tend to be poorly differentiated, higher-grade tumors with frequent metastasis to cervical lymph nodes, resulting in a later stage at diagnosis.[18]

Generally, poorly differentiated tumors are associated with higher mortality rates. However, cancers associated with HPV have a better prognosis and an 80% increase in 5-year survival rate than those that are HPV-negative. Reasons for the improved prognosis may include increased sensitivity to radiation and chemotherapy for HPV-positive cancers.[18] As a result, HPV status is assessed to assist in determining treatment and prognosis of oropharyngeal carcinomas.[18] HPV causes nearly all cases of cervical cancer. Currently, vaccines are available to prevent HPV infection in girls and boys to reduce the incidence of cervical cancer and genital warts.[16] The vaccination protocol may protect against HPV-associated oropharyngeal cancers as well.[8,18,19]

Age

The 2003–2007 SEER data indicate the median age at diagnosis for cancer of the oral cavity and pharynx for all races and both sexes is 62 years with 91% of the cases occurring in adults aged 45 years and older.[5] The aging demographical profile of the U.S. population suggests an increase in oral cancer incidence in coming years. Aging may cause the immune system to become less effective and cause biophysical or biochemical processes that contribute to **carcinogenesis** (production or development of cancer).[15] Although cancer is typically a disease of older populations, several reports in the literature suggest an upturn of cases among young individuals with no apparent risk factors.[6–8] The cause for the increase is under investigation.

DID YOU KNOW?

Although oral cancer was once a disease primarily limited to older individuals, it is increasingly affecting younger individuals.

Race and Ethnicity

The influence of race and ethnicity on incidence of oral cancer is difficult to quantify. There are definite differences in the incidence and mortality rates of various racial groups, but the reason for the differences is unclear. Are they actually related to genetic alterations of races, or are they associated with lifestyle issues? The genetic code is becoming better understood, and eventual changes in the genetic code that lead to various cancers may become clear. Until then, most researchers attribute the differences to lifestyle and environmental factors.[20,21] Unraveling the confounding effects of lifestyle variations between racial and ethnic groups is extremely difficult. Brown and others attribute the vast majority of the higher level of esophageal cancer in African American men to alcohol and smoking but also express concerns that the rate is higher than that expected for alcohol and tobacco alone. They suggest there may be qualitative differences in alcohol consumption, environmental exposure differences, and differences in susceptibility to alcohol and tobacco.[20,21] Nutritional differences and lower socioeconomic status appear to play a role in increased incidence and mortality rates among minority groups. Lack of access to care and cultural issues may contribute to later detection.[20,21] Few studies

have been done on Latino or Hispanic populations; however, variations in oral and pharyngeal cancer rates occur in Hispanic groups located in different regions of the United States, which suggests behavioral, cultural, genetic, and familial risk factors may be involved. Hispanic populations have lower rates of oral cancer than other racial and ethnic groups. However, in one study, New York City Hispanic men, primarily of Puerto Rican descent, showed much higher incidence and mortality rates than those of Hispanic men and white, non-Hispanic men in other areas of the country.[21] Further research into the genetic as well as environmental factors associated with racial and ethnic groups is necessary to clarify the differences in oral cancer incidence and mortality.

Actinic Radiation (Ultraviolet Light) Exposure

Solar radiation or sun exposure is a known risk factor for cancer of the lip. Typically, the chronic overexposure of ultraviolet radiation from sunlight initially causes **actinic cheilitis**, a demonstrated precancerous lesion, usually occurring on the lower lip.[2] Actinic cheilitis frequently progresses to squamous cell carcinoma. Lip cancer is more prevalent in fair-skinned individuals, particularly men. Reasons for higher incidence in males may be that more men work in outdoor occupations and the use of cosmetic lipstick may provide some protection for women. Lip cancer is rare in dark-skinned individuals. The rates of lip cancer are decreasing,[5] presumably because of an increased awareness of the damage done to skin by exposure to sunlight and increased use of lip balms containing sunscreen.

Potentially Malignant Oral Epithelial Lesions

Leukoplakia, Erythroplakia, and Erythroleukoplakia (Speckled Leukoplakia)

Leukoplakia (white), erythroplakia (red), and erythroleukoplakia (red and white, or "speckled") lesions are considered premalignant. *Leukoplakia* refers to a white patch on oral mucosa that cannot be wiped or scraped off or classified as any other diagnosis. This term describes a clinical diagnosis only, not a histologic one.[13] The risk for malignant transformation is multifaceted. The type of leukoplakia, site, presence of dysplasia, habits, gender, age/duration of lesion, size of lesion, and other factors contribute to the possible transformation to malignancy[22] (Figure 7–4 ▪). Erythroleukoplakia and erythroplakia demonstrate a greater threat for malignant transformation[23] (Figures 7–5A, B, and C ▪, 7–6 ▪, and 7–7 ▪). More than 90% of erythroplakia lesions exhibit dysplasia, **carcinoma in situ**, or invasive carcinomas.[23] However, a recent retrospective study of 173 cases of oral epithelial dysplasia found that 89 (56.8%) lesions were white in color, 27 (17%) were red, and 20 (12.6%) exhibited both colors. The mixed white and red lesions were associated with severe oral epithelial dysplasia (30.8%).[23] Risk of malignancy cited in studies worldwide varies widely by site within the mouth and population, among other factors. Lesions on the floor of the mouth (Figure 7–8 ▪), tongue, and

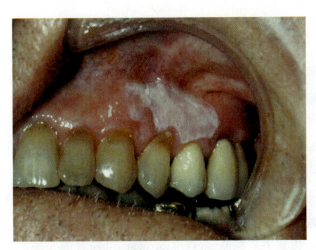

FIGURE ■ 7–4 Leukoplakia.
(*Source:* Courtesy Dr. Sol Silverman, Jr.)

retromolar/soft palate are twice as likely to develop oral squamous cell carcinoma than lesions on the buccal mucosa, gingiva, or palate.[22] Lesions with epithelial dysplasia are usually surgically excised; however, recurrence is common. Discontinuance of any contributing habits such as smokeless tobacco should be encouraged. Heavy smokers have seven times the risk of developing leukoplakias. Following cessation, many lesions regress and/or disappear.

Oral Lichen Planus

Lichen planus is a chronic inflammatory dermatologic disease that frequently manifests as lesions of the oral mucosa.[4,24] Whether oral lichen planus can transform into malignant disease has long been a controversial subject. The potential for malignant transformation appears to be small and limited to severe cases.[4] Clinicians should regularly evaluate lichen planus cases and refer for further follow-up, such as biopsy, when indicated.

Immune System Suppression

Individuals who take drugs that suppress the immune system to prevent rejection of transplanted organs may be at increased risk of developing cancers of the oral cavity and oropharynx. In addition, drugs to treat some immune system diseases may increase the risk for cancers of the oropharynx or oral cavity.[4]

SIGNS AND SYMPTOMS OF ORAL CAVITY OR OROPHARYNGEAL CANCER

A *symptom* is a change from the normal in a body structure, function, or sensation, whereas a *sign* is any abnormality that is discoverable on examination of the patient. A patient experiences a symptom; therefore, it is a subjective indication of disease. Because a sign is observable, it is an objective indication of disease.[1] See Table 7–3 ■ for a list of the most common signs and symptoms of oral cancer.

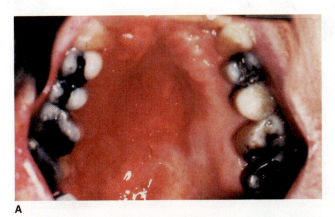

A

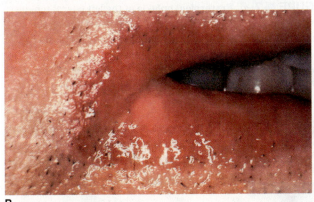

B

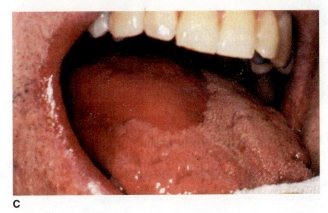

C

FIGURE ■ 7–5 Erythroplakia in a 73-year-old man. Biopsy revealed carcinoma in situ of the palate and well-differentiated squamous cell carcinoma of the tongue and labial commissure. **A. Palate. B. Labial commissure (corner of the lip). C. Tongue dorsum.**

(*Source:* R. A. Ord, & R. H. Blanchaert, Jr., eds. (2000). *Oral cancer: The dentist's role in diagnosis, management, rehabilitation, and prevention.* Carol Stream, IL: Quintessence Publishing Co., Inc. © Quintessence Publishing Co., Inc.)

DETECTION AND DIAGNOSIS OF ORAL CANCER

Health History

A thorough assessment of the patient's present and past habits must be a part of the initial and subsequent patient encounters. Tobacco assessment must include type, amount, frequency,

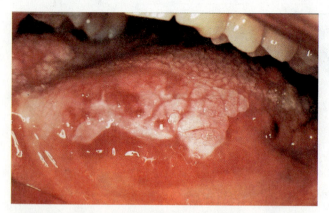

FIGURE ■ 7–6 Erythroleukoplakia of the left lateral tongue border. Note the velvety red appearance admixed among the leukoplakic plaques. Biopsy confirmed moderate dysplasia.

(*Source:* R. A. Ord, & R. H. Blanchaert, Jr., eds. (2000). *Oral cancer: The dentist's role in diagnosis, management, rehabilitation, and prevention.* Carol Stream, IL: Quintessence Publishing Co., Inc. © Quintessence Publishing Co., Inc.)

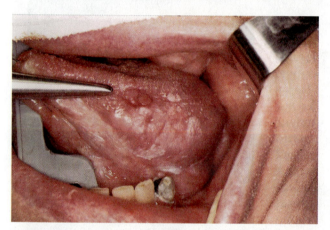

FIGURE ■ 7–7 Extensive leukoplakia of the tongue and floor of the mouth in an elderly woman. Pointer shows site of previous tongue biopsy with early focus of carcinoma.

(*Source:* R. A. Ord, & R. H. Blanchaert, Jr., eds. (2000). *Oral cancer: The dentist's role in diagnosis, management, rehabilitation, and prevention.* Carol Stream, IL: Quintessence Publishing Co., Inc. © Quintessence Publishing Co., Inc.)

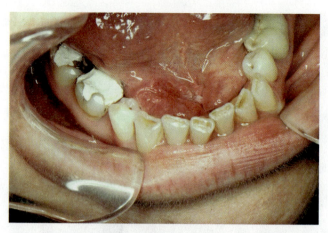

FIGURE ■ 7–8 Squamous cell carcinoma, floor of the mouth.

(*Source:* Courtesy Dr. Sol Silverman, Jr.)

duration (years of smoking), quit attempts including methods used, and current stage of change. (A detailed cessation program is included in Chapter 21.)

DID YOU KNOW?

Dental providers and other healthcare providers should assess alcohol consumption and talk to the patient about its connection to oral cancer.

Alcohol assessment should be included on the health history form and discussed with the patient. Questions similar to the tobacco assessment should be asked, including type of alcohol, amount, frequency, duration of use, and quit attempts. A study of dental school health history forms demonstrated only one-third of the forms contained questions about tobacco or alcohol use.[25] Several alcohol screening tools are available, including the Alcohol Use Disorders Identification Test

TABLE ■ 7–3   Possible Signs and Symptoms of Oral Cancer

- Presence of mucosal ulcerations that do not resolve within 2 weeks
- Red or white patchy lesions that do not resolve within 2 weeks
- Persistent pain in the mouth
- Persistent lump or thickening in the soft tissues
- Persistent sore throat or a feeling that something is caught in the throat
- Difficult or painful chewing or swallowing
- Difficulty moving the jaw or tongue
- Numbness of the tongue or other area of the mouth
- Swelling of the jaw that causes dentures to fit poorly or become uncomfortable
- Loosening of the teeth or pain around the teeth or jaw
- Hoarseness or change in voice quality
- Ear pain in one ear without hearing loss
- Trismus (difficulty opening the mouth)
- Presence of a neck mass that does not resolve after antibiotic therapy

(AUDIT), and single-question tools, among many others. Use of a screening tool may assist the dental professional in determining when to refer patients to their family physician for further evaluation.

A study of 408 patients who visited a walk-in emergency dental clinic used the AUDIT-C screening tool, a 3-question adaptation of the World Health Organization's original 10-question AUDIT questionnaire.[26] Findings indicated one-quarter of the patients had positive results for heavy alcohol use. Because of concerns that dental patients may be offended by questions about their alcohol use, they were asked how they felt about answering the questions. More than 80% of the patients indicated the dentist should feel free to ask about alcohol use; more than 90% felt the dentist should advise them to cut down if drinking were affecting their oral health; and more than 90% indicated they would provide an honest answer if asked how much alcohol they consumed. Even heavy alcohol-consuming patients did not object to answering questions about alcohol use and receiving counseling. In light of this study, dental professionals should be comfortable asking their patients about alcohol use and advising them to quit or cut down.

Oral Cancer Screening/Examination

The topic of oral cancer is seldom mentioned in the popular media, and the general public's knowledge of the risk factors, symptoms, and need for an oral cancer screening is low.[28] Health care providers, including dental professionals, have a professional responsibility to provide thorough oral cancer screenings.[29]

The American Dental Education Association includes oral cancer screenings in its list of competencies for the new dentist; this list was recently published in the *Journal of Dental Education*.[30] The competencies encompass 39 skills divided into several domains, including critical thinking, professionalism, communication and interpersonal skills, health promotion, practice management and informatics, and patient care. The list specifically includes "Obtain and interpret patient/medical data, including a thorough intra/extra oral examination" and "recognize and manage substance abuse" (p. 868).[30] The inclusion of these competencies as well as others dealing with integration of multidisciplinary treatment planning stress the expectation that dentists will perform these skills in their dental practices.

DID YOU KNOW ?

Many health care professionals do not regularly perform thorough oral cancer examinations despite their simplicity and importance.

Unfortunately, the reality is that too few practitioners perform thorough visual and tactile examinations (examinations performed by touch).[31,32] Although the amount of time an oral cancer examination takes varies among providers, it should take only a few minutes regardless of the provider's expertise level.

Performing oral cancer screenings annually on all adult patients is the standard of care for dental professionals and should not be relegated to "as time permits." It is important to remember that the screening involves more than simply a cursory glance at soft tissues. Rather, palpation of lymph nodes in the head and neck region is part of the examination. During palpation, the palms and fingers are pressed against the tissues and lymph nodes to detect evidence of disease.[1] Some dentists express concerns that patients may consider palpation as inappropriate touching, particularly of the superficial and deep cervical nodes in the sternocleidomastoid muscle area. (This muscle arises from the sternum (breastbone) and the clavicle on each side, runs up the neck and attaches to the skull at the mastoid process and occipital bone.) Patient responses express a different story. In a small study of 61 participants in Utah,[33] 97% (58 participants) reported they had never had an extraoral examination. Eighty-five percent (51 participants) indicated they felt the examination was worthwhile, a positive experience, and a valuable addition to future dental visits. Forty-seven participants (77%) felt more confident about their care, and 40 participants (66%) felt more relaxed. Carefully explaining the reason for the examination and the procedure of palpating lymph nodes should alleviate patient concerns. Because of the simplicity of the screening and the possibility that it could easily save a patient's life, it should be considered malpractice if not performed on all patients regularly!

Holmes, Dierks, Homer, and Potter found that patients with lesions detected by dental health care providers were diagnosed at an earlier stage of oral cancer than patients whose lesions were detected by primary health care providers. In addition, patients were more likely to start appropriate treatment sooner.[34] This study suggests the importance of the oral cancer screening in a dental setting as well as the need for additional education of primary health care providers in performing oral cancer screenings.

The steps involved in the examination are included in Table 7–4 ■. Identification of lesions or lumps is critical. If a lesion is found, the patient should be scheduled to return in 14 days for reevaluation. If the lesion is still present, further follow-up is needed.

The American Cancer Society does not recommend the specific frequency of the examination or the populations who should be assessed but does state that cancer-related checkups associated with periodic health examinations for individuals age 20 and older should include oral cancer screenings. The checkups should also include counseling about risk factors, such as tobacco, alcohol, sun exposure, diet, occupational and environmental exposure, and sexual practices.[35]

Oral cancer screenings should be included in periodic examinations by all health care providers, rather than just by dental professionals. Groups at particularly high risk for oral cancer, including heavy smokers and alcohol abusers, may seek medical care for an unrelated problem. If the medical provider performed an oral cancer screening as part of a medical examination, more oral lesions could be detected. Results from several studies indicate that dental professionals and physicians fail to provide oral cancer examinations for their patients on a

TABLE ■ 7–4   Steps in Performing an Oral Cancer Screening

1. Visually assess the patient's head, face, neck, ears, and eyes for absence of symmetry, enlargements, swellings, dry or crusty areas, lesions, and color changes.

2. Palpate lymph nodes to detect changes in size, consistency, and mobility.

3. Observe the lips closed and open. Note the color, texture, and presence of lesions on the upper and lower vermilion borders (area where the skin of the face and lips meet). Palpate the lips for changes in consistency and growths.

4. Assess labial mucosa by pulling the lower lip away from the teeth to observe the labial mucosa and frena. Look for changes in color, texture, or swelling.

5. Examine and palpate the buccal mucosa.

6. Examine and palpate the gingiva.

7. Observe the dorsum (upper side) of the tongue for any swelling, ulceration, coating, changes in the pattern of the papillae (small, raised projections), or variation in size, color, or texture. Grasp the tip of the tongue with a piece of gauze and gently pull the tongue out and to the side to allow complete observation of the lateral surface of the right side and then the left. Palpate the tongue to feel for any growths.

8. With the tongue raised, inspect the floor of the mouth for changes in color, texture, swellings, or ulcerations. Bimanually palpate the sublingual area using the index finger of one hand inside the mouth and the fingertips of the other hand extraorally under the chin.

9. With the patient's head tilted back, observe the hard and soft palate. Use a mouth mirror to intensify the light source. Ask the patient to move the tongue forward and/or down to help to visually assess the oropharynx, including the anterior and posterior tonsillar pillars. Look for changes in color, texture, swellings, or ulcerations. Palpate the hard palate, taking care not to stimulate the patient's gag reflex.

consistent basis.[31,32] Figure 7–9 ■ indicates the most common intraoral areas for squamous cell carcinoma.

LeHew and others surveyed dental practitioners and determined that few dentists thought they were very well trained in oral cancer examination skills. One-fifth of the dentists rarely or never palpate the cervical lymph nodes, and more than half never palpate the dorsal borders of the tongue. Because most oral cancers arise in the floor of the mouth or on the lateral borders of the tongue, it is critical that these structures be palpated for a thorough examination. Early oral cancers may not present visually but could be detected with palpation; therefore, the researchers' findings that their sample dentists did not regularly palpate these areas is disturbing.[31] Clearly, statistics on morbidity and mortality from comparisons of oral carcinomas diagnosed in early and late stages indicate that medical and dental professionals must increase their diligence in performing regular, thorough examinations.

Oral cancer can manifest as a variety of appearances. Malignant lesions often mimic other innocuous (harmless) lesions, and misdiagnosis can occur easily in the absence of appropriate follow-up. Readers should consult oral pathology texts and journal articles for further information regarding clinical manifestations of oral cancer.

Screening and Diagnostic Aids

Surgical biopsy (removal of a tissue sample) is the only definitive method available to diagnose oral carcinomas. However, in recent years, adjunctive screening aids have become available to assist clinicians in determining which lesions should be biopsied. Because many cases of dysplastic tissue and carcinomas appear innocuous, adjunctive aids that can assist the dental or medical provider in identifying possible dysplastic or cancerous lesions and to assist in the decision to subject a patient to a surgical biopsy are a welcome addition. Devices meant to assist

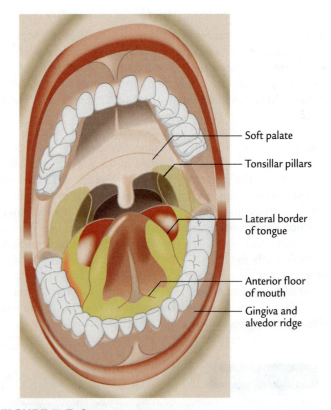

Soft palate

Tonsillar pillars

Lateral border of tongue

Anterior floor of mouth

Gingiva and alvedor ridge

FIGURE ■ 7–9   Oral Anatomy.

in visually detecting lesions include those based on the principles of tissue reflectance and tissue autofluorescence. Devices based upon tissue reflectance include MicroLux/DL (AdDent, Danbury, CT), Orascoptic DK (Orascoptic, Kerr Company, Middleton, WI), and ViziLite Plus (Zila Pharmaceuticals, a division of Tolmar, Phoenix, AZ). The VELscope (LED Dental, Burnaby, BC, Canada) is a device based on autofluorescence. The Identafi 3000 (Trimira, Houston, TX), combines both autofluorescence and tissue reflectance.[36]

Exfoliative cytology and brush biopsy   Exfoliative cytology involves the microscopic examination of cells obtained from tissue; the cells are spread on a slide, fixed in place, and then stained. Because more than 90% of oral cancers arise from epithelial tissue, exfoliative cytology is an effective screening aid to determine whether to biopsy a lesion.[37]

Exfoliative cytology is useful for lesions that appear to be innocuous and otherwise would not undergo biopsy. It can often be used when a patient will not agree to a surgical biopsy or if the patient has multiple lesions.

The OralCDx Brush Test (OralCDx Laboratories, Suffern, NY) is a device that uses transeptitheal cytology to evaluate innocuous lesions. It is not a replacement for scalpel biopsy but is used instead to identify potentially precancerous lesions. The test is similar to a cervical PAP smear. The clinician rotates a small brush through all three levels of the stratified squamous epithelium to ensure that cells from all three levels are included in the specimen, transfers the specimen to a glass slide, applies a fixative, and sends the specimen to the company laboratory for analysis. The specimen is analyzed by a computer and a pathologist and assigned one of four levels: incomplete (too few cells from all epithelial layers), negative (no evidence of pathology), atypical (abnormal cells present), or positive (contains dysplastic or cancerous cells). A surgical biopsy is recommended for atypical or positive findings to provide a final diagnosis.[36,37] The technique is helpful for patients who refuse surgical biopsy or have several lesions, which would require multiple surgical biopsies.[38]

Toluidine blue (tolonium chloride)   Tolonium chloride has been used for 40 years to aid in early recognition of abnormal mucosa in the cervix and oral cavity. The metachromatic dye acts as a nuclear stain by binding to DNA. Touidine blue appears to stain cells undergoing rapid cell division (including inflammatory, regenerative and neoplastic cells), allowing easier examination of tissue samples[38]; see Figures 7–10 and 7–11 ∎.

In spite of numerous research studies, questions remain about the use of toluidine blue as an adjunct for detection of dysplastic or neoplastic lesions. Because the dye stains inflammatory cells as well as dysplastic cells and because inflammatory cells are often present on the surface of lesions, interpretation can be problematic, resulting in concern for too many false-positive results. Controversy exists regarding the degree of staining (dark royal blue versus pale blue) necessary for a positive result. Some researchers contend that any color change is positive; others believe only dark royal blue lesions indicate a positive result.[38,39] The test is primarily useful to assist experienced clinicians in defining the margins of lesions. Its use as a screening tool in general practice settings among low-risk populations is not indicated.[36]

Light-based adjuncts. Various types of chemiluminescent devices are available for dental use, including the ViziLite Plus (Zila Pharmaceuticals), MicoLux/DL and Orascoptic DK.

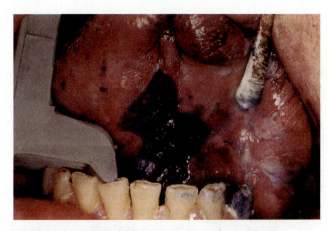

FIGURE ∎ 7–10 Intraoral area most likely to develop squamous cell carcinoma. Excluding the lip, in order of most likely area for intraoral squamous cell carcinoma to occur, are the lateral borders of the tongue (50%), anterior floor of the mouth (20%), soft palate and tonsillar pillars (15%), and gingiva and alveolar ridge (5%).

(*Source:* R. A. Ord, & R. H. Blanchaert, Jr., eds. (2000). Oral cancer: The dentist's role in diagnosis, management, rehabilitation, and prevention. Carol Stream, IL: Quintessence Publishing Co., Inc. © Quintessence Publishing Co., Inc.)

ViziLite Plus uses a disposable device and added toluidine blue whereas the MicroLux/DL and Orascoptic DK systems use a reusable insert or probe. The ViziLite Plus system consists of a chemiluminescent device, a 1% acetic acid solution, and swabs containing TBlue[630], a toluidine blue solution.

When a tissue is exposed to a light source with a specific wavelength, it gives off light with a longer wavelength (i.e., fluoresces). This property aids in the detection of cancerous tissues because the fluorescence of normal healthy tissue differs from that of precancerous or cancerous tissues. The change in appearance occurs because cellular composition causes them to reflect light at different rates. Using a simple handheld device, providers can visually assess oral tissues for abnormalities. Chemiluminescent systems provide an adjunct to direct observation with incandescent light. The utility of chemiluminescent systems has yet to be conclusively verified beyond that of a comprehensive oral examination; however, additional rigorous research studies are needed.[38]

Lesions that should be further evaluated appear distinctly bright white (acetowhite) instead of the blue color of normal tissues. The white color is caused by the increased density of nuclear content and mitochondrial matrix found in abnormal cells, which results in the reflection of light. In contrast, when the light is applied to normal epithelium, it absorbs the light and the tissue appears dark.[40]

Studies have not demonstrated that ViziLite Plus can help the clinician differentiate between dysplasia/carcinoma and benign lesions. In addition, results from studies as to the device's ability to increase the visibility of lesions beyond that of incandescent lighting are contradictory.[36,39] Other studies have demonstrated that ViziLite Plus enhanced visualization of about 60% of the lesions and identified all the lesions previously identified with standard light. No additional lesions were identified.[41] Zila Pharmaceutical representatives are quick to point out that the device is not a *diagnostic* tool but is instead a *screening* device that may help the clinician more easily visualize suspicious lesions.

Autofluorescence The VELscope (Visually Enhanced Lesion Scope) is a handheld device the clinician uses to observe changes in the appearance of oral tissues (Figure 7–11 ■). Abnormal tissue typically appears as an irregular, dark area that stands out against the otherwise normal, green fluorescence pattern of surrounding healthy tissue (Figure 7–12 ■). The VELscope system does not require the patient to rinse with a solution prior to use. A study by Lane and others demonstrated a sensitivity of 98% and specificity of 100% in distinguishing normal tissue from severe dysplasia, carcinoma in situ, and invasive carcinoma.[42] The device shows promise as an oral cancer screening aid, biopsy guide, and tool for distinguishing margins of cancerous tissue[36] (Figure 7–13 ■).

Autofluorescence and tissue reflectance The Identafi 3000 (Trimira, Houston, TX) combines both tissue reflectance and autofluorescence. There are insufficient studies to make a determination on its effectiveness at this time.

A panel convened by the American Dental Association Council on Scientific Affairs to address the benefits and limitations of oral cancer screening and adjunctive screening aids determined that there is insufficient evidence that devices based upon autofluorescence, tissue reflectance or both, enhance visual detection beyond conventional visual and tactile examination. In addition, they concluded there is insufficient evidence to assess the brush test's validity of innocuous lesions. They reported that in lesions with high malignant potential, the brush test has validity in identifying dysplastic cells. The panel clarified that "insufficient evidence" simply means that more research is needed to provide enough evidence to support a recommendation.[36]

Nevertheless, the use of imaging tools may assist dental providers during large public health screening events as well as in the more traditional in-office setting. The enhanced ability to visually assess lesions is a step forward for early detection of lesions, and rigorous studies will ultimately determine their effectiveness in the hands of primary providers as well as specialists.

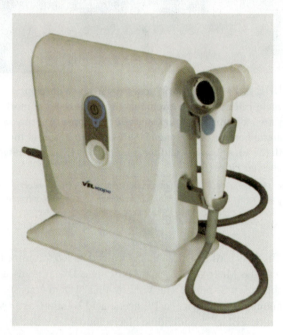

FIGURE ■ 7–11 VELscope device.
(*Source:* Courtesy of VELscope LED Dental, Inc.)

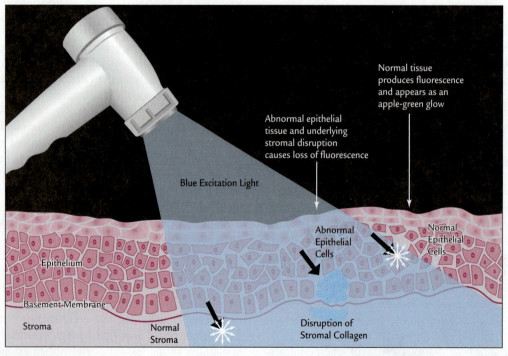

FIGURE ■ 7–12 Blue excitation light's effect on normal and abnormal tissues.
(*Source:* Cancer Staging Manual. (2010) (7th ed.). New York, NY: Springer. www.springer.com.)

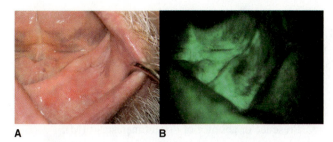

A   **B**

FIGURE ■ 7–13 A. Area appears to be chronic denture trauma (observed with naked eye). B. Intense dark area (observed through VELscope) on the ridge persisted after relief of denture irritation. Biopsy confirmed as severe dysplasia.

(*Source:* VELscope LED Dental, Inc.)

Many new techniques to assist in oral cancer diagnosis are in use and in development, including many present in saliva, biomarkers, DNA ploidy, loss of heterozygozity, and others.[36,43]

DID YOU KNOW ?

Researchers are investigating the use of saliva to provide cellular and gene markers to identify individuals who are prone to have, or have, oral cancer.

Biopsy Types

As previously stressed, the *only* way to definitely diagnose oral malignancies is with a surgical biopsy. The type of biopsy performed depends upon the size and location of the lesion. Types of biopsies encountered in oral cancer include fine-needle aspiration, punch, and scalpel biopsy.[44] Many other diagnostic tests are currently under study, including molecular tests that analyze DNA and genetic alterations that identify cells as cancerous or normal.[45]

Fine-Needle Aspiration Biopsy

Fine-needle aspiration biopsy is typically performed to differentiate benign and malignant lesions that involve the lymph nodes or salivary glands. Biopsies of this type are preferred in those areas because the biopsy does not spread the tumor or disrupt the field for surgical dissection later[4] (Figure 7–14 ■).

Punch Biopsy

Punch biopsy instruments remove a cylindrical sample of tissue for analysis. They are commercially available as disposable devices of various sizes (Figure 7–15 ■).

DID YOU KNOW ?

A scalpel biopsy is the gold standard for diagnosing oral cancer.

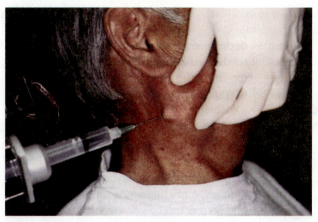

FIGURE ■ 7–14 Fine-needle aspiration biopsy. Aspiration with a syringe holder, which allows the mass to be stabilized with one hand and aspirated with the other hand.

(*Source:* R. A. Ord, & R. H. Blanchaert, Jr., eds. (2000). *Oral cancer: The dentist's role in diagnosis, management, rehabilitation, and prevention.* Carol Stream, IL: Quintessence Publishing Co., Inc. © Quintessence Publishing Co., Inc.)

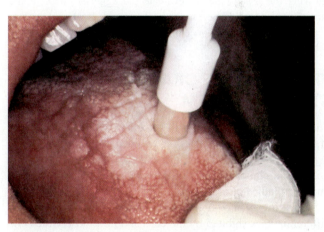

FIGURE ■ 7–15 Punch biopsy instrument.

(*Source:* R. A. Ord, & R. H. Blanchaert, Jr., eds. (2000). *Oral cancer: The dentist's role in diagnosis, management, rehabilitation, and prevention.* Carol Stream, IL: Quintessence Publishing Co., Inc. © Quintessence Publishing Co., Inc.)

Scalpel Biopsy

Scalpel biopsy types include incisional and excisional. An incisional biopsy removes a portion of the lesion; an excisional biopsy removes the lesion in its entirety. Excisional biopsies are limited to small lesions. Biopsy specimens should be representative samples of the lesion. Care must be taken when determining the type of biopsy to perform or whether the patient should be referred to a specialist for biopsy. Incisional biopsy of a small lesion could distort the appearance and consistency of the tissue, interfering with the ability to assess the tissue. A lesion that would be altered by performing a biopsy should be referred to the clinician who will ultimately treat the lesion to determine the extent of resection or irradiation.[44]

Scar tissue from a previous incisional or excisional biopsy could hamper attempts to identify subsequent cancer in the same area. In addition, cancer cells can be plunged deep into underlying tissues during the biopsy procedure.

Regardless of the biopsy method used to diagnose oral cancer, the patient should be referred for follow-up and treatment to a cancer center that specializes in head and neck cancers, an otolaryngologist (physician who treats head and neck disorders), or maxillofacial surgeon (dental specialist who treats disorders of the mouth, teeth, jaws, and face).

Imaging

Oral cancer is usually detected by clinical examination and confirmed by surgical or fine-needle biopsy. Imaging techniques are generally used to provide evidence of the extent of the disease. Imaging may also be used to detect recurrent disease after therapy. Computed tomography (CT) and magnetic resonance imaging (MRI) are the methods currently available for providing structural information nodal size but do not identify active disease well.[46] Recently, positron emission tomography (PET) and the combination of PET-CT are being utilized. PET using the tracer F-fluoro-deoxyglucose (FDG) provides information on tumor metabolism, allowing the practitioner to evaluate the aggressiveness of the tumor, stage nodal disease in the neck, provide treatment evaluation, and provide surveillance of recurrent disease.[46]

PROGNOSIS OF ORAL CANCER: STAGING SYSTEM

The prognosis, or forecast of the probable course or outcome,[1] of squamous cell carcinoma is determined by a system of grading (determining the histologic subtype) and staging (determining the clinical extent) of the tumor. Staging is the more important indicator of the two.

Grading is accomplished by determining the degree of differentiation exhibited by the cells and how closely the cells resemble normal tissue structure (Table 7–5 ■). Well-differentiated (grade 1, low-grade) tumors produce keratin, closely resemble the tissue of origin, grow less aggressively, and metastasize later. Tumors that produce little or no keratin but are still recognizable as stratified squamous epithelium are called *moderately differentiated,* or *grade 2.* Poorly differentiated (high-grade, grade 3) tumors produce no keratin, bear little resemblance to stratified squamous epithelium, lack normal architectural structure, and often grow aggressively and metastasize early in their course.[47]

TABLE ■ 7–5   Grading System for Squamous Cell Carcinoma

	Histologic Grade
GX	Grade cannot be assessed
G1	Well differentiated
G2	Moderately differentiated
G3	Poorly differentiated

Staging is based on the size and extent of metastatic spread of the lesion.[47,48] The tumor-node-metastasis (TNM) system is used to determine the stage of most cancers (Table 7–6 ■). Three clinical features specify the stage:

- Size of the tumor (T) in centimeters.
- Involvement of local lymph nodes (N).
- Presence or absence of distant metastasis (M).

TREATMENT OPTIONS FOR ORAL CANCER

Treatment modalities for oral cancer vary, primarily depending on the tumor stage, size, location, relation to the mandible, nodal involvement, and histologic type.[49] Early stage cancer (stages I and II) can be treated with surgery or radiation, although surgery is often preferred to minimize possible side effects. The treatment protocol for late stage cancer (stages III and IV) usually includes a combination of surgery, postoperative radiation, and chemotherapy. Photodynamic (laser) therapy has recently been added as a possible option for treating oral cavity cancers.[49] Its advantage is that the area heals without fibrosis (formation of fibrous tissue).[3]

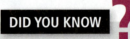

DID YOU KNOW

Oncology specialists use the stage of the oral cancer to plan the type of treatment for the patient.

Chemotherapeutic agents are generally not successful in treating oral carcinomas when used as a single modality and are used as an adjunctive procedure in combination with surgery and radiation. Smaller intraoral lesions are treated with a single modality whereas larger lesions or cases that involve lymph nodes require a combination of modalities. Oropharyngeal lesions usually receive radiation therapy. Lip lesions are typically surgically excised with excellent results. Tongue lesions are often treated surgically, which may include partial or total hemiglossectomy (removal of half or more than half of the tongue[1]) followed by radiation therapy. Segmental resection is usually necessary for alveolar ridge cancers. Selective neck dissection is performed when metastasis to local lymph nodes has occurred.[4,49]

Radiotherapy may consist of external-beam irradiation, interstitial irradiation or *brachytherapy*, and intensity modulated radiotherapy and image-guided radiation therapy.

Considerations Regarding Treatment Options

The oral cavity is a complex structure composed of muscles, nerves, jaws, tongue, and salivary glands. Nutritional intake depends on all of those factors. Losing the ability to speak drastically affects a patient's quality of life and ability to socialize.

TABLE ■ 7–6   TNM Staging System for Squamous Cell Carcinoma

PRIMARY TUMOR (T)

TX	Primary tumor cannot be assessed
T0	No evidence of primary tumor
T1S	Carcinoma in situ
T1	Tumor 2 cm or less in greatest dimension
T2	Tumor more than 2 cm but not more than 4 cm in greatest dimension
T3	Tumor more than 4 cm in greatest dimension
T4a	Moderately advanced local disease (lip) Tumor invades through cortical bone, inferior alveolar nerve, floor of mouth, or skin of face, i.e., chin or nose (oral cavity) Tumor invades adjacent structures only (e.g., through cortical bone, [mandible or maxilla] into deep [extrinsic] muscle of tongue [genioglossus, hyoglossus, palatoglossus, and styloglossus], maxillary sinus, skin of face)
T4b	Very advanced local disease. Tumor invades masticator space, pterygoid plates, or skull base and/or encases internal carotid artery

REGIONAL LYMPH NODES (N)

NX	Regional lymph nodes cannot be assessed
N0	No regional lymph node metastasis
N1	Metastasis in a single ipsilateral lymph node, 3 cm or less in greatest dimension
N2	Metastasis in a single ipsilateral lymph node, more than 3 cm but not more than 6 cm in greatest dimension; or in multiple ipsilateral lymph nodes, none more than 6 cm in greatest dimension; or in bilateral or contralateral lymph nodes, none more than 6 cm in greatest dimension
N2a	Metastasis in single ipsilateral lymph node more than 3 cm but not more than 6 cm in greatest dimension
N2b	Metastasis in multiple ipsilateral lymph nodes, none more than 6 cm in greatest dimension
N2c	Metastasis in bilateral or contralateral lymph nodes, none more than 6 cm in greatest dimension
N3	Metastasis in a lymph node more than 6 cm in greatest dimension

DISTANT METASTASIS (M)

M0	No distant metastasis
M1	Distant metastasis

ANATOMIC STAGE/PROGNOSTIC GROUPS

Group	T	N	M
Stage 0	Tis	N0	M0
Stage I	T1	N0	M0
Stage II	T2	N0	M0
Stage III	T3	N0	M0
	T1	N1	M0
	T2	N1	M0
	T3	N1	M0
Stage IVA	T4a	N0	M0
	T4a	N1	M0
	T1	N2	M0
	T2	N2	M0
	T3	N2	M0
	T4a	N2	M0
Stage IVB	Any T	N3	M0
	T4b	Any N	M0
Stage IVC	Any T	Any N	M1

HISTOLOGIC GRADE (G)

GX	Grade cannot be assessed
G1	Well differentiated
G2	Moderately differentiated
G3	Poorly differentiated
G4	Undifferentiated

(*Source:* Based on AJCC Cancer Staging Manual, 7th Edition (2010).)

Treatment planning must consider all of the functions performed by the mouth and associated structures, as well as the psychosocial issues involved with disfigurement. Rehabilitation should be considered before surgical or radiation therapy intervention, and quality of life issues must be carefully assessed.

Surgery

Surgical management of malignancies of the oral cavity may involve several approaches, depending on the extent and location of the disease. Wide local excision involves the removal of the tumor in soft tissue while leaving a 1-cm to 1.5-cm margin of clinically normal tissue at the periphery (Figure 7–16A, B ■).

Resection involves removing carcinoma that has invaded bone, leaving a 2-cm margin of radiographically normal bone tissue at the periphery.

Marginal resections involve removal of bone that leaves the inferior border of the mandible intact. Segmental resection involves removal of the full height of the mandible. Composite resection involves removal of hard and soft tissue, typically the neck nodes, mandible, and soft tissues associated with the primary tumor, as in the tongue or floor of the mouth.

Surgery to remove tongue lesions includes partial glossectomy (removing less than half of the tongue) or total glossectomy (removing more than half of the tongue).

Neck dissections are comprehensive or selective. Comprehensive neck dissections include radical neck dissection and modified radical neck dissection. Radical neck dissection removes lymph nodes of the neck, the sternocleidomastoid muscle, the internal jugular vein, and the spinal accessory nerve. Modified radical neck dissection preserves the sternocleidomastoid muscle, the internal jugular vein, or the spinal accessory nerve. Selective neck dissections preserve one or more of the groups of lymph nodes that are removed during radical neck dissection. In addition, the sternocleidomastoid muscle, internal jugular vein, and spinal accessory nerve are preserved. Weakness in raising the arm above the head and weakness of the lower lip may follow neck dissection. *Elective neck dissection* refers to the precautionary removal of lymph nodes despite negative nodal involvement. Sentinel lymph node biopsy (SLNB) is a relatively recent possible replacement for elective neck dissection. The procedure has been used for melanoma and breast cancer and is currently in clinical trials to determine its effectiveness for use in oral cancer. The technique involves a preoperative injection of a colloid around a tumor in an awake patient. During surgery, the neck is scanned with a gamma probe to determine the most radioactive area. The lymph nodes in that area are removed and immediately evaluated by a pathologist. If the nodes show evidence of metastasis, a neck dissection is performed. If metastasis is not evident, the neck is closed.[49] Reconstruction after invasive surgical procedures results in varying degrees of successful restoration of function and appearance, depending on the area involved.

Radiation therapy is indicated after surgery if the soft tissue margin is positive, one or more lymph nodes exhibit extracapsular invasion (extension of the tumor outside the lymph node capsule), bone invasion is present, more than one lymph node is positive in the absence of extracapsular invasion, comorbid (existing simultaneously) immunosuppressive disease is present, or perineural invasion (invasion of the sheath surrounding a bundle of nerve fibers[1]) is present.

Radiation Therapy

Computed tomography (CT) and/or magnetic resonance imaging (MRI), and positron emission tomography (PET) scanning or a combination of PET and CT scans (PET-CT) are used to identify the lesion and involved structures. Dental panoramic film is used to assess dental status and mandibular involvement. A dental consultation is necessary before any radiotherapy in dentulous or edentulous patients. Teeth that are periodontally involved, mobile teeth, teeth with large carious lesions and periapical pathology, and impacted teeth should be extracted before beginning radiation therapy.

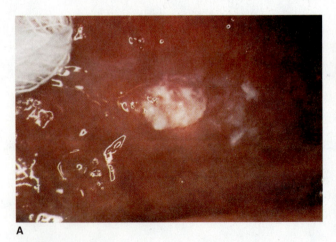

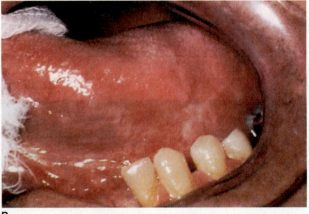

A

B

FIGURE ■ 7–16 A. Leukoplakia of the left lateral tongue border that was confirmed as squamous cell carcinoma. B. Appearance of tongue border 9 months after surgical resection.

(*Source:* R. A. Ord, & R. H. Blanchaert, Jr., eds. (2000). *Oral cancer: The dentist's role in diagnosis, management, rehabilitation, and prevention.* Carol Stream, IL: Quintessence Publishing Co., Inc. © Quintessence Publishing Co., Inc.)

Types of Radiation Therapy

Types of radiation therapy used in oral cancer include primary external-beam radiotherapy, intensity-modulated radiotherapy, brachytherapy or interstitial radiotherapy, and intraoral cone or electron-beam therapy. Conventional radiation therapy usually consists of one daily treatment per week for 7 weeks. Dosage is generally 60–70 Gy. *Hypofractionation* and *hyperfractionation* refer to treatments given less than or more than once per day, respectively. In external-beam radiotherapy, radiation is applied to a tumor from outside the body; immobilization devices are used to minimize damage to areas other than the tumor. Preserving salivary function is an important component. Intensity-modulated radiotherapy follows the contours of the tumor and spares more of the normal tissues. Brachytherapy delivers high-dose, localized radiation by implanting radioactive sources directly into the tumor.[50] Intraoral cone, or electron-beam therapy, can be used for small, superficial lesions in edentulous patients and involves the placement of the cone in contact with the oral mucosa during treatment. It is often followed by external-beam radiotherapy.[51]

Radiotherapy may also be palliative to alleviate symptoms of pain or obstruction in patients that cannot undergo curative therapies.

Chemotherapy

Chemotherapy is not typically used as a single modality in oral cancer but is frequently used as an adjunct to radiation therapy and/or surgery in late-stage cancers. Chemotherapy involves cytotoxic drugs that affect cancer cells' life cycle, normally disrupting the DNA so the cells can no longer reproduce. Various chemotherapeutic agents act on different stages of the life cycle of the cells; therefore, more than one agent may be administered simultaneously. Commonly used chemotherapy drugs include platins (cisplatin and carboplatin), taxanes, paclitaxel, docetaxel, 5 fluorouracil, methotrexate, vinblastine, and vincristine. Cisplatin and 5 fluorouracil have been used extensively. Chemotherapy may be administered as neoadjuvant (before irradiation), concurrent (during irradiation), or adjuvant (after irradiation).[52]

Early detection of lesions is critical to allow conservative treatment and to protect the patient's quality of life. Many avenues are available to treat oral cancers, and improved methods are constantly being investigated. A multidisciplinary team can help oral cancer patients adjust to the aftermath of treatment. Recurrence or development of new primary cancer requires close follow-up for all patients. Examinations typically occur every 2–3 months the first year, 3–4 months the second year, 4 months the third year, 5 months for the fourth and fifth years, and annually after five years.

MANAGEMENT OF SIDE EFFECTS FROM TREATMENT OF ORAL CANCER

The side effects of cancer therapy are numerous and can be quite debilitating (Table 7–7 ■). Radiation therapy and chemotherapy side effects may be transient (lasting a short time) or lessen with the passage of time, but many are permanent and may be severe. The dental professional must be prepared to assist patients in improving their quality of life during and after treatment.

TABLE ■ 7–7   Side Effects of Cancer Therapy

Radiation Therapy

Alterations in pigmentation of skin including white patches (vitiligo) or "tanning"

Loss of hair

Subcutaneous changes

   Telangiectasia (spider veins)

   Fibrosis

   Edema (swelling)

Acute mucositis

Xerostomia (hyposalivation or dry mouth) and changes in quality of saliva

Candidiasis (fungal overgrowth)

Hypogeusia, dysgeusia, or ageusia (partial loss, changes in perception, or complete loss of taste, respectively)

Dental caries

Osteoradionecrosis

Soft tissue necrosis (mucosal ulcer)

Trismus

Chemotherapy

Acute mucositis

Xerostomia and changes in quality of saliva

Hemorrhage

Candidiasis

Myelosuppression

Consultation with other members of the multidisciplinary team is critical. Depending on the type of treatment, side effects vary.

Surgical Reconstruction

Surgical removal of cancerous tumors may be extremely debilitating in terms of function and disfigurement. Reconstruction following surgical intervention aims to restore functioning and appearance. Patients often have difficulty dealing with body image changes, and the dental team must be prepared to assist them. Free flaps from the radial forearm, fibula, iliac crest, and scapula are frequently used in surgical reconstruction.[53] The radial forearm free flap may be used to repair soft tissue defects in the oral cavity. The fibula, iliac crest, and scapular-free flaps are typically used to reconstruct the mandible following resection.[54] (See Figures 7–17 ■ to 7–21 ■).

Deltopectoral flaps and pectoralis major mucocutaneous flaps are used to replace tissues and protect the carotid artery after removal of the sternocleidomastoid muscle. Bone and soft tissue grafts provide good cosmetic appearance and function. Osseointegrated implants (implants anchored in the bone) and dentures can be used to replace lost teeth. Obturator prostheses can be utilized to separate the oral and nasal cavities. Extraoral prosthetics provide replacement of part of the face using a lifelike silicone material. Clasps or hooks, eyeglass frames, retentive undercuts, and osseointegrated craniofacial implants may be used to retain prostheses.[55]

Toxicity and Side Effects of Radiation Therapy

The type of radiation, site of tumor, radiation dose, and length of treatment determine the side effects of radiation therapy. Complications from irradiation include pain, mucositis, xerostomia

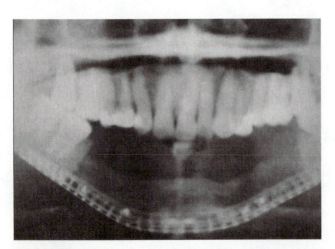

FIGURE ■ 7–17 Reconstruction of the mandible immediately after resection for large ameloblastoma. A Timesh titanium basket filled with particulate bone marrow harvested from the ilium (the largest of the three principal bones composing either half of the pelvis).

(*Source:* R. A. Ord, & R. H. Blanchaert, Jr., eds. (2000). *Oral cancer: The dentist's role in diagnosis, management, rehabilitation, and prevention.* Carol Stream, IL: Quintessence Publishing Co., Inc. © Quintessence Publishing Co., Inc.)

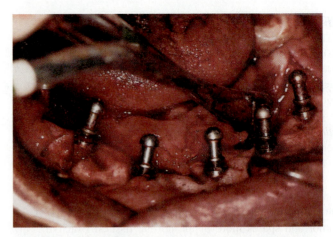

FIGURE ■ 7–18 Implant guide pins in place after all holes have been drilled. Alignment is directed slightly lingual because of the relatively larger size of the mandible compared with the maxilla.

(*Source:* R. A. Ord, & R. H. Blanchaert, Jr., eds. (2000). *Oral cancer: The dentist's role in diagnosis, management, rehabilitation, and prevention.* Carol Stream, IL: Quintessence Publishing Co., Inc. © Quintessence Publishing Co., Inc.)

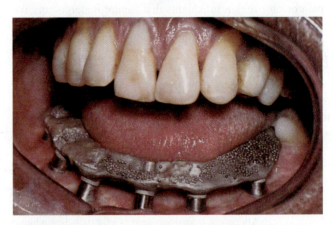

FIGURE ■ 7–19 Frame try-on to test fit.

(*Source:* R. A. Ord, & R. H. Blanchaert, Jr., eds. (2000). *Oral cancer: The dentist's role in diagnosis, management, rehabilitation, and prevention.* Carol Stream, IL: Quintessence Publishing Co., Inc. © Quintessence Publishing Co., Inc.)

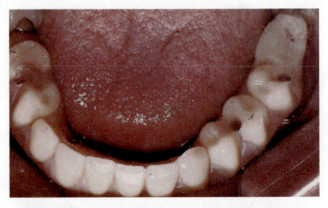

FIGURE ■ 7–20 Final prosthesis at the time of delivery.

(*Source:* R. A. Ord, & R. H. Blanchaert, Jr., eds. (2000). *Oral cancer: The dentist's role in diagnosis, management, rehabilitation, and prevention.* Carol Stream, IL: Quintessence Publishing Co., Inc. © Quintessence Publishing Co., Inc.)

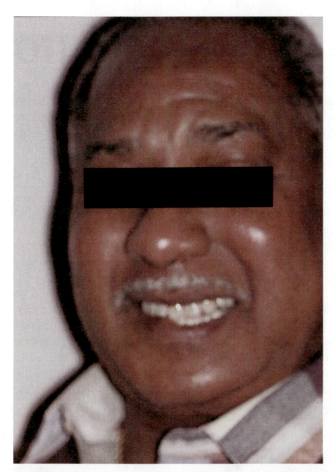

FIGURE ■ 7–21 Facial view of patient after placement of the final restoration.

(*Source:* R. A. Ord, & R. H. Blanchaert, Jr., eds. (2000). *Oral cancer: The dentist's role in diagnosis, management, rehabilitation, and prevention.* Carol Stream, IL: Quintessence Publishing Co., Inc. © Quintessence Publishing Co., Inc.)

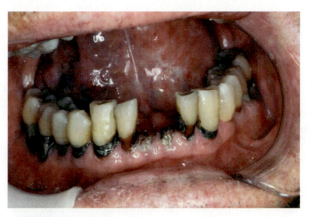

FIGURE ■ 7–22 Radiation-induced caries.

(*Source:* Dr. Sol Silverman, Jr.)

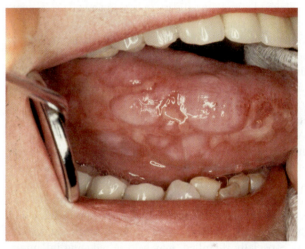

FIGURE ■ 7–23 Mucositis.

(*Source:* Dr. Sol Silverman, Jr.)

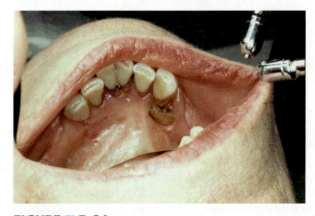

FIGURE ■ 7–24 Osteoradionecrosis.

(*Source:* Dr. Sol Silverman, Jr.)

(hyposalivation or dry mouth), dysgeusia (altered taste perception), cervical caries, epithelial atrophy, focal alopecia (hair loss), focal hyperpigmentation, telangiectasias (small enlarged blood vessels near the surface of the skin), oral candidiasis, and osteoradionecrosis (death of bone tissue)[56] (Figures 7–22 ■ to 7–25 ■).

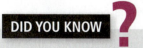

DID YOU KNOW?

Radiation therapy and chemotherapy cause numerous serious side effects.

Depending on the targeted area, radiation therapy may destroy the salivary glands, resulting in xerostomia, which can range from relatively mild to severe. It can seriously affect the patient's quality of life because it may make eating or talking difficult and dramatically increase the risk of caries. Radioprotective agents such as amifostine to prevent the severity of xerostomia have demonstrated mixed results. Various products are available that provide some lubrication, but they are temporary fixes to what can be a major source of discomfort. The dental professional can provide saliva substitutes and encourage the patient to carry water with them at all times. Saliva substitutes come in several forms, including sprays, gels, liquids, toothpastes, mouthrinses, chewing gum, and lozenges. Sugarless gum or candy may provide some relief. Sialogogues (agents that promote flow of saliva, such as pilocarpine and cevimeline) may help stimulate salivary flow in some patients, depending on the amount of salivary gland damage.[57–59] Avoidance of mouthrinses containing alcohol should be stressed due to the drying nature of alcohol. Because of the extremely high caries risk, patients should avoid foods and beverages with high sugar content. The use of custom-fitted fluoride trays with a mildly flavored 1.1% neutral sodium fluoride gel can significantly reduce cervical caries and will be a necessity for the remainder of the patient's life.[60] A casein phosphopetides-amorphous calcium phosphate product such as MI-paste may be prescribed to brush on at least once per day. These products saturate the tooth surface to assist in remineralization.[61] Acupuncture has been shown to stimulate salivary secretion and alleviate zerostomia in some studies.[58]

Cutaneous changes typically manifest as darkened (hyperpigmented) or lightened (vitiligo or hypopigmented) skin. Localized hair loss (focal alopecia) may occur if the hair follicles are in the treatment beam area. Subcutaneous changes may occur, including telangiectasia, fibrosis, and edema (retained fluids, swelling).

Acute mucositis (inflammation of mucous membranes) is a common reaction to cancer therapy and can become so severe that intake of nutrition is impossible until the condition subsides. Oral and gastrointestinal mucosa are affected. Because no curative treatment is available for mucositis, palliative care is provided. Topical solutions such as a mixture of lidocaine, cough syrup, and a coating agent (milk of magnesia, kaolin-pectin), especially if chilled, may help in reducing inflammation and discomfort. Cryotherapy such as chewing on ice chips may be helpful. Bland rinses of sodium bicarbonate or salt (1 teaspoon of sodium bicarbonate or salt per pint of water; swish one tablespoon for at least 30 seconds) can help alleviate symptoms.[62] Systemic prednisone may also help reduce these side effects. Systemic narcotics such as morphine may be required. Patients should maintain oral care as much as possible by gently debriding the oral cavity with an ultrasoft toothbrush or wet gauze. Toothbrush bristles may be further softened with warm water if necessary.[63] Chlorhexidine, sucralfate, and antimicrobial lozenges are not recommended for prevention of oral mucositis.[64] A feeding tube (gastrostomy tube) may be temporarily inserted prior to the start of radiation therapy so hydration and nutritional needs can be maintained in the event the patient cannot take fluid or foods by mouth.[65] A brief interruption in radiation and/or chemotherapy is necessary when mucositis is severe.

Dietary changes to assist in managing xerostomia and mucositis may be necessary. Sucking on ice chips or popsicles may help temporarily alleviate pain. Patients should be counseled to avoid hot, spicy, acidic, and rough-textured foods. The use of straws for liquid intake may be suggested. Mild, high moisture–content foods such as applesauce, puddings, custards, gelatins, milk shakes, scrambled eggs, mashed potatoes,

and pureed vegetables should be encouraged. Nutritional supplements including Ensure or Boost provide additional nutrition.[65]

Taste buds are sensitive to radiation and may be destroyed if they are in the path of the external beam. A partial (hypogeusia) or complete (ageusia) loss of taste may occur during treatment. Dysgeusia (altered taste perceptions) may also occur. Taste buds will usually regenerate several months after treatment terminates, but some patients may suffer permanent loss of taste. Zinc supplements may help restore or enhance the ability to taste in some patients.[66]

Fungal overgrowth of *Candida albicans* may occur, particularly in patients with xerostomia. The condition is managed with systemic antifungal drugs such as ketoconazole or fluconazole or with topical administration of nystatin or clotrimazole. In severe cases, topical or systemic pain medication may be necessary.

Trismus, severely restricted mouth opening, can be a major problem for some patients following radiation therapy. It has a detrimental effect on eating, chewing and swallowing, quality of life, and maintenance of oral health and oral rehabilitation.[67] Various interventions have been utilized to maintain or increase mouth opening, including tongue blades, spatulas, dynamic bite openers, rubber plugs, and a Therabite device.[67]

DID YOU KNOW ?

Osteoradionecrosis is a serious risk for the remainder of an oral cancer patients' life.

Osteoradionecrosis is a serious complication of head and neck irradiation and remains a major concern for the remainder of the patient's life (see Figures 7–24 ■ and 7–25 ■). As the radiation dose increases, the occurrence of osteoradionecrosis becomes more likely. Bone cells and the accompanying vascular system may be irreversibly damaged, causing sequestrated bone fragments (bone fragments separated from the bone[1]). Jaw resection may become necessary to treat the condition. Hyperbaric oxygen can be effective, but studies regarding its effect are inconclusive.[68]

Meticulous oral hygiene is critical postradiation to minimize the effects of xerostomia and osteoradionecrosis. Nutrition is also extremely important, and tooth extraction or other invasive procedures must be avoided if at all possible.

Toxicity and Side Effects of Chemotherapy

Chemotherapy may result in some of the side effects commonly observed in radiation therapy, such as acute mucositis and accompanying dysphagia, xerostomia, changes in the quality of saliva, and candidiasis. In addition, neurotoxicity is a side

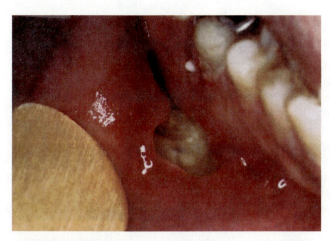

FIGURE ■ 7–25 Area of necrotic bone.

(*Source:* R. A. Ord, & R. H. Blanchaert, Jr., eds. (2000). *Oral cancer: The dentist's role in diagnosis, management, rehabilitation, and prevention.* Carol Stream, IL: Quintessence Publishing Co., Inc. © Quintessence Publishing Co., Inc.)

effect of some chemotherapeutic agents. It manifests as altered sensation, partial paresthesia (abnormal sensations such as burning, tingling, etc.) of the perioral and intraoral areas affiliated with the trigeminal nerve, or as severe, throbbing pain, particularly in the mandibular molar region. Systemic analgesics, usually narcotics, are required. Residual neuropathy may remain after chemotherapy is completed.[69]

Myelosuppression resulting from chemotherapy includes neutropenia, anemia, and thrombocytopenia, contributing to mucositis, infection, bleeding, and delayed healing of oral mucosa. Platelet levels below $30,000/mm^3$ may result in spontaneous bleeding. Oral care should continue despite the low platelet counts to help prevent or control infections and bleeding.[70]

The dental professional must closely follow the cancer therapy of the head and neck cancer patient to ensure that caries do not develop and side effects are treated quickly. Treatment coordination with the oncologist and other members of the multidisciplinary team will be required.

ROLE OF THE DENTAL TEAM

The dental team must work with other health care professionals in planning, implementing, and evaluating treatment for all patients with oral cancer. The network of health care professionals is extensive, as evidenced by the following list of potential team members:

- Otolaryngologist
- Plastic and reconstructive surgeon
- Oral and maxillofacial surgeon
- Radiation oncologist
- Radiologist
- Dietitian
- Speech language pathologist

- Social worker
- Psychologist
- Physical therapist
- Occupational therapist
- Dentist/maxillofacial prosthodontist
- Dental hygienist
- Facial prosthetics clinician
- Head and neck nurse coordinator/clinical nurse specialist

See Table 7–8 ■ for a summary of what dental professionals can do to increase the prevention and early detection of oral cancer. Public awareness is critical. The newly released *Healthy People 2020* objectives once again include objectives to increase the proportion of oral and pharyngeal cancers detected at the earliest stage (from 32.5% in 2007 to 35.8%) (OH-6) and increase the proportion of adults who received an oral and pharyngeal cancer screening from a dentist or dental hygienist in the past year (OH-14-2).[71] Through mass media, community efforts, increased vigilance, and advocacy, health care providers can work to increase awareness and meet the new objectives. Health care professionals must become proactive in ensuring that they routinely provide thorough oral cancer screenings to all patients at initial and recall appointments.[31] Oral cancer screenings must be offered at sites that are accessible and comfortable for minority populations.[72] Educational programs for health care professionals should train students to perform oral cancer screenings and use diagnostic tools, as well as provide tobacco and alcohol cessation counseling.[32,37]

TABLE ■ 7–8 Actions the Dental Team Can Take to Increase Awareness

- Provide oral cancer materials to health agencies and community centers.
- Initiate an oral cancer consortium composed of health and social service agencies, educational partners, and community groups.
- Volunteer at health fairs to provide screenings and dispense pamphlets and other information.
- Talk to clients/patients about oral cancer risk factors, prevention, and early detection.
- Perform oral cancer screenings on every patient and explain that you are doing an oral cancer examination.
- Provide continuing education programs on oral cancer for other health professionals. Assess clients'/patients' tobacco and alcohol use.
- Initiate tobacco and alcohol cessation programs in practice settings.
- Provide nutritional assessments and nutritional oral cancer prevention strategies.
- Include health promotion strategies in client/patient education.

Education

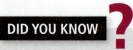

DID YOU KNOW

The public is usually unaware of the risks associated with oral cancer.

The public is woefully uninformed about oral and pharyngeal cancers.[73] This lack of knowledge is not surprising considering the paucity of oral cancer educational materials available to them through mass media and print materials.[28,74]

Health care professionals must increase their dissemination of oral cancer information among the general public and individuals in their communities and dental practices. They should obtain and distribute materials to local health departments[74] and other venues including private practices, senior centers, long-term care facilities, drug abuse treatment centers, and schools for nurses, physicians, and physician assistants. Dental professionals should ensure that dental providers are included on health boards and local health consortia.

A variety of materials is available for the education of patients and health care providers through the American Cancer Society, National Oral Health Information Clearinghouse, Oral Cancer Foundation, American Dental Association, American Academy of Otolaryngology, American Association of Oral and Maxillofacial Surgeons, and Support for People with Oral and Head and Neck Cancer, among others. Many of the materials are available free or at minimal cost.

Public Health Screening for Oral and Pharyngeal Cancers

Oral cancer screenings can be offered as a free public health service for community groups at long-term care facilities, health fairs, senior centers, and other venues. Disposable mouth mirrors and portable headlamps or flashlights make the screenings easy to do in virtually any setting. Including an educational aspect will dispense much needed information to the public. Location is especially important to reach the most at-risk populations, particularly African American males.[73] Enlisting the assistance of prominent members in African American communities, such as training barbers and members of the faith community, as health ambassadors can help reach those in underserved areas. Using local dental/dental hygiene societies and educational programs can provide expertise in performing screenings and training ambassadors.

Cultural Sensitivity

Paying attention to various cultures is crucial in health promotion activities. Many subcultures in U.S. society have unique views of health and disease. Factors affecting vulnerable populations must be assessed when designing programs. Characteristics such as religious differences, ethnicity, primary language spoken, education, and literacy level affect access to care, response to illness, health-seeking behavior, and trust of Western health providers, among others. Social customs and norms, such as touching, intimate space requirements, acceptable behaviors for gender and age groups, and eye contact, may serve as potential barriers. These concerns must be addressed before initiating health promotion programs.[75]

SUMMARY

Oral cavity and oropharyngeal cancers are life-threatening diseases that can often be prevented through the avoidance of causative agents. Tobacco remains the primary cause of oral cancers; it acts synergistically with alcohol, so tobacco users who consume excessive amounts of alcohol are particularly at risk. Squamous cell carcinoma makes up more than 90% of oral cancers. Early detection and treatment are critical to prevent morbidity and mortality. Oral cancer strikes a disproportionate number of minority populations and is especially deadly for African American men who are typically diagnosed at later stages.

Treatment is based on the disease stage at diagnosis and usually entails surgery and/or radiation, sometimes with the addition of chemotherapy. Side effects can affect quality of life. Surgical interventions may result in disfigurement, and the individual's social, psychological, and physical states are impacted.

Every medical and dental provider has the responsibility to perform annual examinations on patients to screen for lesions. In addition, volunteering at screening events takes little time and provides an excellent public health service, particularly for underserved populations with little access to dental care. Various screening tools are available, including the brush test and chemiluminescent devices. Educating the public and patients about the risk factors as well as signs and symptoms of oral cancer is critical. The public receives little information through mass media and is unaware of the disease as well as the availability and importance of an oral cancer screening. It is up to health care providers to ensure they regularly receive the information and screenings they deserve.

PRACTICAL CONSIDERATIONS

What does the information in this chapter mean for a student in a dental professional program? What should you do as a result of what you have learned? How does this fit into your daily

practice? The answers to these questions are clear. First, dental professionals and students should carefully perform thorough oral cancer examinations, including palpations, on every patient. Do not assume that young adults will not develop oral cancer. In particular, assess the tongue and tonsillar area. Every member of the dental team should be alert to changes in the oral cavity and oropharngeal region. If you are a dental hygienist, do not assume the dentist will see or feel suspicious areas. It is your responsibility to thoroughly assess and notify the dentist of any suspicious areas.

Second, educating patients and family members about oral cancer is critical. Because it receives very little media attention, patients are unaware of the disease and the need to immediately bring anything unusual to the attention of the dentist or physician. Tobacco and alcohol cessation should be stressed and provided when appropriate.

Third, get involved with community events. Arrange oral cancer screenings and education at fairs, churches, senior centers, factories, and other opportunities. Work with other health professionals to ensure that they are knowledgeable about oral cancer. Ask if you can join other health topic community events, such as diabetes or prostate screening events. Provide blood pressure checks and nutrition information as well as oral cancer screening.

Stay alert and take advantage of every opportunity to share information on oral cancer. Together we can save lives and help limit the morbidity that accompanies oral cancer.

SELF-STUDY QUESTIONS

1. How long is the oral cancer patient at risk for developing osteoradionecrosis?

   a. 1 year

   b. 5 years

   c. 10 years

   d. Lifetime

   Rationale: The patient remains at risk for osteonecrosis for the remainder of his or her life.

2. Mucositis is a concern for patients who have which treatment types?

   a. Radiation therapy

   b. Chemotherapy

   c. Surgery

   d. a & b

   Rationale: Oral cancer patients are at risk for developing mucositis if they undergo radiation therapy or chemotherapy.

3. The population group most likely to die from oral cancer is

   a. Caucasian males

   b. African American males

   c. Caucasian females

   d. African American females

   Rationale: African American males are much more likely to die from oral cancer than the other groups.

4. The most common area for intraoral squamous cell carcinoma to occur is the

   a. Tongue

   b. Alveolar ridge

   c. Soft palate

   d. Floor of the mouth

   Rationale: About half of the intraoral squamous cell carcinoma occurs on the lateral borders of the tongue.

5. Squamous cell carcinoma accounts for what percentage of oral and oropharyngeal cancers?

   a. 10%

   b. 35%

   c. 50%

   d. 90%

   Rationale: About 90% of oral and oropharyngeal cancers are squamous cell carcinomas.

REFERENCES

1. *Stedman's medical dictionary for the dental professions* (2nd ed.) (2012). Philadelphia: Wolters Kluwer Health/Lippincott Williams and Wilkins.

2. Jones, A., Freedman, P., & Phelan, J. (2009). Neoplasia. In Ibsen, O., & Phelan, J., Eds. *Oral pathology for the dental hygienist* (5th ed.). St. Louis: Saunders Elsevier, 232–75.

3. Saunders, N. A., Coman, W. B., & Guminski, A. D. (2007). Cancer of the head and neck. In E. C. Ward, & C. J. van As-Brooks (Eds.), *Head and neck cancer: Treatment, rehabilitation, and outcomes.* San Diego, CA: Plural Publishing, 1–26.

4. American Cancer Society Cancer Facts and Figures 2010. (2010). Atlanta: American Cancer Society. Retrieved September 26, 2012 fromhttp://www.cancer.org/acs/groups/cid/documents/webcontent/003128-pdf.pdf.

5. Altekruse, S. F., Kosary, C. L., Krapcho, M., Neyman, N., Aminou, R. Waldron, W., et al., Eds. *SEER cancer statistics review, 1975–2007.* Bethesda, MD: National Cancer Institute. http://seer.cancer.gov/csr/1975_2007/results_merged/sect_20_oral_cavity_pharynx.pdf

6. Edwards, J. (2011). A strong foundation for battling oral cancer. *Access,* 25(3):18–19.

7. American Cancer Society. *Cancer facts & figures 2009.* (2009). Atlanta: American Cancer Society.

8. Marur, S., D'Souza, G., Westra, W., & Forastiere, A. (2010). HPV-associated head and neck cancer: A virus-related cancer epidemic. *Lancet Oncology,* 11:781–89.

9. Peres, J. (2010). HPV-Positive oropharyngeal cancer: Data may justify new approach. *Journal of the National Cancer Institute,*

112(19), 1456–59. Retrieved January 19, 2011 from http://www.jnci.oxfordjournals.org.

10. Marur, S., & Forashiere, A. (2008). Head and neck cancer: Changing epidemiology, diagnosis, and treatment. *Mayo Clin Proc,* 83:489–501.

11. Hashmani, K. (2011). The effects of paan, gutkha and betel nut in the oral cavity. *Access,* 25:16–17.

12. Snyder, J. (2011). Emerging tobacco products. *Access,* 25:12–14.

13. Kademani, D. (2007). Oral cancer. *Mayo Clin Proc,* 82:878–887.

14. Lubin, J., Purdue, M., Kelsey, K., Zhang, Z., Winn, D., Wei, Q., . . . & Hayes, R. (2009). Total exposure and exposure rate effects for alcohol and smoking and risk for head and neck cancers: A pooled analysis of case-control studies. *American Journal of Epidemiology,* 170:937–47.

15. Oral Cancer Foundation. (2011). Alcohol and tobacco. Retrieved July 11, 2011 from http://oralcancerfoundation.org/facts/alcohol_tobacco.htm.

16. Centers for Disease Control and Prevention. (2011). Genital HPV infection fact sheet. Retrieved April 6, 2011 from http://www.cdc.gov/std/hpv/stdfact-hpv.htm.

17. Mehta, V., Yu, G., & Schantz, S. (2010). Population-based analysis of oral and oropharyngeal carcinoma: Changing trends of histopathologic differentiation, survival and patient demographics. *Laryngoscope,* 120:2203–12.

18. Westra, W. (2009). The changing face of head and neck cancer in the 21st century: The impact of HPV on the epidemiology and pathology of oral cancer. *Head and Neck Pathol,* 3:78–81.

19. Ramqvist, T., & Dalianis, T. (2010). Oropharyngeal cancer epidemic and human papillomavirus. *Emerging Infectious Diseases,* 16. Retrieved March 16, 2011 from http://www.cdc.gov/EID/content/16/11/1671.htm.

20. Warnakulasuriya, S. (2009). Risk factors for oral cancer. *British Journal of Healthcare Management,* 15:557–61.

21. Cruz, G., Salazar, C., & Morse, D. (2006). Oral and pharyngeal cancer incidence and mortality among Hispanics, 1996–2002: The need for ethnoregional studies in cancer research. *American Journal of Public Health,* 96:2194–2200.

22. Napier, S., & Speight, P. (2008). Natural history of potentially malignant oral lesions and conditions: An overview of the literature. *J Oral Pathol Med,* 37:1–10.

23. Pereira, J., Carvalho, M., Henriques, A., Camara, T., Miguel, M., & Freitas, R. (2011). Epidemiology and correlation of the clinicopathological features in oral epithelial dysplasia: Analysis of 173 cases. *Annals of Diagnostic Pathology,* 15:98–102.

24. Oral Cancer Foundation. (2011). Oral cancer facts. Retrieved July 11, 2011 from http://oralcancerfoundation.org/facts/index.htm

25. Yellowitz, J. A., Goodman, H. S., Horowitz, A. M., & al-Tannir, M. A. (1995). Assessment of alcohol and tobacco use in dental schools' health history forms. *J Dent Educ,* 59:1091–96.

26. Miller, P., Ravenel, M., Shealy, A., & Thomas, S. (2006). Alcohol screening in dental patients: The prevalence of hazardous drinking and patients' attitudes about screening and advice. *J Am Dent Assoc,* 137:1692–98.

27. Vinson, D., Galliher, J., Reidinger, C., & Kappus, J. (2004). Comfortably engaging: Which approach to alcohol screening should we use? *Annals of Family Medicine,* 2:398–404.

28. Graham, J., Horowitz, A., & Canto, M. (2004). Coverage and quality of oral cancer information in selected popular press: May 1998 to July 2003. *Journal of Public Health Dent,* 64:231–36.

29. Patton, L., Ashe, T., Elter, J., Southerland, J., & Strauss, R. (2006). Adequacy of training in oral cancer prevention and screening as self-assessed by physicians, nurse practitioners, and dental health professionals. *Oral Surg Oral Med Oral Pathol Oral Radiol Endod,* 102:758–64.

30. ADEA competencies for the new general dentist. (2009). *J Dent Educ,* 73:866–69.

31. LeHew, C., Epstein, J., Kaste, L., & Choi, Y. (2010). Assessing oral cancer early detection: Clarifying dentists' practices. *Journal of Public Health Dentistry,* 70:93–100.

32. LeHew, C., Epstein, J., Koerber, A., & Kaste, L. (2009). Training in the primary prevention and early detection of oral cancer: Pilot study of its impact on clinicians' perceptions and intentions. *Ear, Nose & Throat Journal,* 88:748–53.

33. Johns, S. G. (2001). The extraoral examination from the perspective of the patient. *J Dent Hyg,* 75:282–89.

34. Holmes, J. D., Dierks, E. J., Homer, L. D., & Potter, B. E. (2003). Is detection of oral and oropharyngeal squamous cancer by a dental health care provider associated with a lower stage at diagnosis? *Journal of Oral and Maxillofacial Surgery,* 61:285–91.

35. Smith, R., Cokkinides, V., Brooks, D., Saslow, D., Shah, M., & Brawley, O. (2011). Cancer screening in the United States, 2011: A review of current American Cancer Society guidelines and issues in cancer screening. *CA Cancer Journal for Clinicians,* 61:8–30.

36. Rethman, M., Carpenter, W., Cohen, E., Epstein, J., Evans, C., Flaitz, C., . . . & Meyer, D. (2010). Evidence-based clinical recommendations regarding screening for oral squamous cell carcinomas. *J Am Dent Assoc,* 141:509–20.

37. Epstein, J., Gorsky, M., Fischer, D., Gupta, A., Epstein, M., & Elad, S. (2007). A survey of the current approaches to diagnosis and management of oral premalignant lesions. *J Am Dent Assoc,* 138:1555–62.

38. Lingen, M., Kalmar, J., Karrison, T., & Speight, P. (2008). Critical evaluation of diagnostic aids for the detection of oral cancer. *Oral Oncology,* 44:10–22.

39. Fedele, S. (2009). Diagnostic aids in the screening of oral cancer. *Head and Neck Oncology,* 1:5–10.

40. Patton, L., Epstein, J., & Kerr, A. (2008). Adjunctive techniques for oral cancer examination and lesion diagnosis: A systematic review of the literature. *Journal of the American Dental Association,* 139:896–905.

41. Epstein, J.B., Silverman, S., Jr., Epstein, J.D., Lonky, S.A., & Bride, M.A. (2008). Analysis of oral lesion biopsies identified and evaluated by visual examination, chemiluminescence and toluidine blue. *Oral Oncology,* 44:538–44.

42. Lane, P., Gilhuly, T., Whitehead, P., Zeng, H., Poh, C., Ng, . . . & MacAulay, C. (2006). Simple device for the direct visualization of oral-cavity tissue fluorescence. *Journal of Biomedical Optics,* 11:024006–7.

43. Nagler, R. (2009). Saliva as a tool for oral cancer diagnosis and prognosis. *Oral Oncology,* 45:1006-10.

44. Oliver, R., Sloan, P., & Pemberton, M. (2004). Oral biopsies: Methods and applications. *Br Dent J,* 196:329–33.

45. Haddad, R., & Shin, D. (2008). Recent advances in head and neck cancer. *New Engl J Med,* 359:1143–54.

46. Koppula, B., & Rajendran, J. (2010, April). PET-CT in head and neck cancer. *Applied Radiology.* Retrieved October 6, 2011 from www.appliedradiology.com.

47. American Society of Clinical Oncology. (2011). *Oral and oropharyngeal cancer: Staging with illustrations.* Retrieved July 12, 2011 from http://www.cancer.net/patient/Cancer+Types/Oral+and+Oropharyngeal+Cancer/ci. Oral+and+Oropharyngeal+Cancer?sectionTitle=Staging With Illustrations.

48. National Cancer Institute, National Institutes of Health. (2011). *Lip and oral cavity cancer treatment (PDQ®): Health professional version.* Retrieved July 12, 2011 from www.cancer.gov/cancertopics/Pdq/treatment/lip-and-oralcavity/HealthProfessional/page3.

49. Genden, E., Ferlito, A., Silver, C., Takes, R., Suarez, C., Owen, R., . . . & Rinaldo, A. (2010). Contemporary management of cancer of the oral cavity. *European Archives of Otorhinolaryngology,* 267:1001–17.

50. Oral Cancer Foundation. (2011). CDC oral cancer background papers, Chapter VI: Treatment. Retrieved July 11, 2011 from http://oralcancerfoundation.org/cdc/cdc_chapter6.htm.

51. Mendenhall, W., Amdur, R., & Palta, J. (2008). Head and neck cancer. In S. Levitt, J. Purdy, C. Perez, & S. Vijayakumar, Eds. *Technical basis of radiation therapy: Practical clinical applications* (4th ed.). Berlin, Germany: Springer. 453–84.

52. Furness, S., Glenny H. A., Worthington, J., Pavitt, S., Oliver, R., . . . & Conway, D. (2011). Interventions for the treatment of oral cavity and oropharyngeal cancer: Chemotherapy (Review). *The Cochrane Library,* 4. Retrieved July 12, 2011 from http://www.thecochranelibrary.com.

53. Bak, M., Jacobson, A., Buchbinder, D., & Urken, M. (2010). Contemporary reconstruction of the mandible. *Oral Oncology,* 46:71–76.

54. Shah, J., & Gil, Z. (2009). Current concepts in management of oral cancer—Surgery. *Oral Oncology,* 45:394–401.

55. Guttal, K., Naikmasur, V., Rao, C., Nadiger, R., & Guttal, S. (2010) Orofacial rehabilitation of patients with post-cancer treatment: An overview and report of three cases. *Indian Journal of Cancer,* 47:59–64.

56. Ko, C., & Citrin, D. (2009). Radiotherapy for the management of locally advanced squamous cell carcinoma. *Oral Diseases,* 15:121–32.

57. Chambers, M., Rosenthal, D., & Weber, R. (2007). Radiation-induced xerostomia. *Head and Neck,* 29:58–63.

58. Jensen, S., Pedersen, A., Vissink, A., Anderson, E., Brown, C., . . . & Brennan, M. (2010). A systematic review of salivary gland hypofunction and xerostomia induced by cancer therapies: Management strategies and economic impact. *Support Care Cancer,* 18:1061–79.

59. Brosky, M. (2007). The role of saliva in oral health: Strategies or prevention and management of xerostomia. *Journal of Supportive Oncology,* 5:215–25.

60. Chambers, M., Mellberg, J., Keene, H., Bouwsma, O., Garden, A., Sipos, T., & Fleming, T. (2006). Clinical evaluation of the intraoral fluoride releasing system in radiation-included xerostomic subjects—Part 1: Fluorides. *Oral Oncology,* 42:934–45.

61. Reynolds, E. (2009). Casein phosphopeptide-amorphous calcium phosphate: The scientific evidence. *Adv Dent Res,* 21:25–29.

62. Harris, D., Eilers, J., Harriman, A., Cashavelly, B., & Maxwell, C. (2008). Putting evidence into practice: Evidence-based interventions for the management of oral mucositis. *Clinical Journal of Oncology Nursing,* 12:141–52.

63. Manne, D. S. (2006). Oral mucositis and xerostomia: Challenging oral health conditions. Part I: Oral mucositis. *Access,* 20:34–37.

64. Peterson, D., Bensadoun, R., & Roila, F. (2008). Management of oral and gastrointestinal mucositis: ESMO clinical recommendations. *Annals of Oncology,* 19(Suppl 2), ii122–25.

65. Hayward, M., & Shea, A. (2009). Nutritional needs of patients with malignancies of the head and neck. *Seminars in Oncology Nursing,* 25:203–11.

66. Kamprad, F., Ranft, D., Weber, A., & Hildebrandt, G. (2008). Functional changes of the gustatory organ caused by local radiation exposure during radiotherapy of the head-and-neck region. *Strahlenther Onkol,* 184:157–62.

67. Scott, B., Butterworth, C., Lowe, D., & Rogers, S. (2008). Factors associated with restricted mouth opening and its relationship to health-related quality of life in patients attending a maxillofacial oncology clinic. *Oral Oncology,* 44:430–38.

68. Lyons, A., & Ghazali, N. (2008). Osteoradionecrosis of the jaws: Current understanding of its pathophysiology and treatment. *British Journal of Oral and Maxillofacial Surgery,* 46:653–60.

69. Williams, J., Yen, J., Parker, G., Chapman, S., Kandikattu, S., & Barbachano, Y. (2010). Prevalence of pain in head and neck cancer out-patients. *Journal of Larngology & Oncology,* 124:767–73.

70. McClure, D., Essary, D., & Gurenlian, J. (2007). A collaborative team approach for symptom management for head and neck cancer patients. *Grand Rounds Oral-Sys Med,* 2:43-51.

71. United States Department of Health and Human Services. *Healthy People 2020 Topics and Objectives.* Retrieved from http://www.healthypeople.gov/2020/topicsobjectives2020/.

72. Gourin, C., Kaboli, K., Blume, E., Nance, M., & Koch, W. (2009). Characteristics of participants in a free oral, head and neck cancer screening program. *Laryngoscope,* 119:679–82.

73. Choi, Y., Dodd, V., Watson, J., Tomar, S., Logan, H., & Edwards, H. (2008). Perspectives of African Americans and dentists concerning dentist-patient communication on oral cancer screening. *Patient Education and Counseling,* 71:41–51.

74. Maurizio, S., Lukes, S., & DeMattei, R. (2005). An assessment of printed oral cancer materials from local health departments in Illinois. *J Dent Hyg,* 79:10.

75. Pender, N., Murdaugh, C., & Parsons, M. (2006). *Health promotion in nursing practice* (5th ed.). Upper Saddle River, NJ: Pearson Prentice Hall.

Dental Trauma

Gary Cuttrell

OBJECTIVES

After studying this chapter, the student will be able to:

1. Define *dental trauma*.
2. Describe the etiology of dental trauma.
3. Describe the assessment of trauma.
4. List and describe the categories of dental trauma.

INTRODUCTION

Dental trauma of some form happens to almost everyone. The outcomes are as variable as the injuries themselves. The overwhelming majority involves anterior teeth, so injury to these teeth is the primary focus of this chapter. Research throughout the world has been making steady progress in defining how to increase the successes of preventive measures and therapies rendered to patients with dental trauma. The continued effort in clinical research holds great promise that the outcomes for dental trauma will continue to improve.

Damage to soft tissues, alveolar ridge, and dentition require the dental provider to have diagnostic and clinical skills that will minimize permanent damage. This chapter is intended to aid providers in delivering appropriate emergency and follow-up care.

The periodontium is made up of the gingival unit as well as the attachment apparatus and alveolar bone. The attachment apparatus consists of the cementum, periodontal ligament, and the alveolar process. These attachment components are involved in traumatic teeth injuries. The periodontal ligament attaches the tooth root to the bony socket (i.e., alveolar process). In addition, the periodontal ligament's specialized cells replace the cementum, periodontal ligament, and alveolar bone. Maintaining the blood supply and health of the periodontal ligament is one of the most important considerations in enabling repair of dentition injuries.[1] Trauma to the attachment apparatus requires proper diagnosis and assessment to maximize healing. Periodontal ligament healing depends on several factors. These include the type of stabilization, the extent of damage, contamination of tissues with toxins from necrotic dental pulp, amount of time the tooth was out of the socket (**extra-alveolar time**), and the storage method used to preserve the tooth (i.e., wet versus dry).[2] **Dry storage** means the tooth is not placed in a fluid or solution to keep its structures moist. The length of time the tooth is stored under dry conditions (dry storage time) affects the ability to save the tooth.

Regardless of the patient's age, dental trauma can be emotional and painful. Cost of the repairs can also be a substantial economic burden. Psychologically, children can be especially troubled because of unsightly fractures.[3,4] This embarrassment is not limited to children; it affects all ages when the front teeth are adversely affected. Another burden is the amount of time involved in the healing process and in receiving treatment. The effects of dental trauma include tooth death, root resorption (disintegration of the root), tooth loss, and altered potential to develop permanent teeth.[5] **Root resorption** is the breakdown or destruction and subsequent loss of the root structure of a tooth. This is caused by living body cells attacking part of the tooth. When the damage extends to the whole tooth, it is called tooth resorption. Severe root resorption is very difficult to treat and often requires the extraction of teeth.

DID YOU KNOW ?

Root resorption sometimes occurs during or after orthodontic work because of dental trauma caused by moving teeth.

The term **avulsion** refers to the traumatic removal of a tooth, usually through accidents or sports injuries. (See Figure 8–1 ■.) An avulsed tooth can be reinserted into the alveolus (tooth socket); this procedure is called **reimplantation.** If avulsed teeth are reimplanted more than 15 minutes after avulsion, healing will vary according to the factors listed earlier that affect healing of the periodontal ligament. Even if patients or parents are informed of a poor prognosis, the choice often is to reimplant the avulsed tooth even when there are better long-term treatment options.[6] Often the strong desire to restore the tooth overrules the costs of treatments and the final outcome. Therefore, clinicians need to understand the outcomes of different types of treatments of dental trauma to guide patients in their decisions.

ETIOLOGY

Many researchers worldwide have studied traumatic dental injuries, and dental providers have developed parameters for treating them. It is reported that about 33% of 5-year-old children have suffered tooth **luxation** (dislocation) of primary teeth. Uncomplicated fracture of a permanent tooth's crown is highly reported among 12-year-old children. Primary dentition trauma peaks at ages 2 to 3 years and corresponds to young children's development of walking skills. Trauma to permanent dentition in boys peaks at 9 to 10 years; active play and sports injuries with falls are the leading causes.[7]

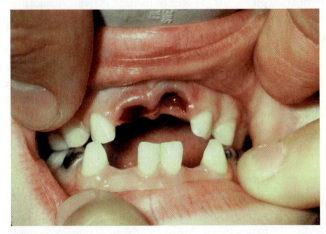

FIGURE ■ 8–1 Avulsion.

(*Source:* Courtesy of Gary Cuttrell.)

DID YOU KNOW ?

Various types of mouth guards are available for protection of such injuries. Besides custom mouth guards available from dentists, sporting goods stores carry a variety of inexpensive "boil and bite" athletic mouth guards that are easy for parents to help protect teeth during all sorts of sporting events.

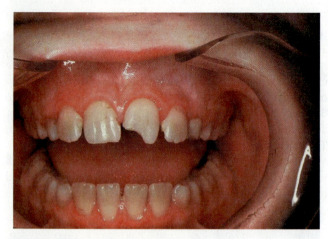

FIGURE ■ 8–2 Incisor fracture.

(*Source:* Courtesy of Gary Cuttrell.)

Other epidemiologic studies have found that 50% of boys have a dental injury between the ages of 8 and 12 years.[8] The upper central incisors in both primary and permanent teeth are most affected because of their position (Figure 8–2 ■) followed by the remaining anterior teeth, the upper and lower lateral incisors, and the upper canines.[9]

The acute stage of trauma begins when teeth and supporting structures are subjected to traumatic forces sufficient for injury. Dental injuries include tooth fracture, luxation, intrusive crushing injury, and separation from the attachment apparatus (i.e., avulsion) of the tooth. Two types of tooth displacement are intruded teeth, which are pushed inward into the tooth socket, and extruded teeth, which are pushed outward from but not out of, the tooth socket. Intrusive crushing injury involves a much greater inward force.

DID YOU KNOW ?

In medicine, ischemia (from Greek ισχαιμία, *ischaimía*; *isch:* root denoting a restriction or thinning or to make or grow thin/lean; *haema:* blood) is a restriction in blood supply generally due to factors in the blood vessels with resultant damage or disfunction of tissue.

The more severe injuries compromise the vascularization (blood flow) of pulpal and periodontal ligament tissues through obstruction of the blood supply to the tissues. This process is called *ischemia,* and it results in an interrupted blood supply.

Wound healing is delayed and complicated by bacteria at the injury site. Bacterial contamination of pulpal tissue occurs through direct exposure to bacteria from the object that caused the injury, from blood clots in the periodontal ligament, or from bacteria introduced to the affected area through the blood stream or through the dentinal tubules (tubules that extend throughout the surface of dentin).

With appropriate treatment, the periodontal ligament will begin significant healing within 1 to 2 weeks. Pulp tissue may heal within 4 days, but such quick healing usually occurs only

for teeth with open apices.[7] Limited periodontal ligament damage leads to limited inflammation, which leads, in turn, to healing with new replacement cementum. More severe periodontal ligament damage leads to a severe inflammatory response over a diffuse (wide) area of the root.

Resorption

Resorption refers to the removal of enamel and other tooth components that are composed of calcium salts (calcific), such as dentin and cementum. This process may occur naturally during the shedding of deciduous (primary) teeth; this type of resorption is called *surface resorption.* In dental trauma, the tooth root undergoes resorption. Root resorption is classified as either replacement resorption or inflammatory resorption.[10] Replacement resorption is much more common than inflammatory resorption.

The greatest prevalence of resorption is seen in teeth reimplanted after a delay of more than 1½ hours. Teeth with dry storage of less than 5 minutes may still have a resorption rate of 36%. Teeth stored dry longer than 30 minutes suffer root resorption at a rate of 90%. The best predictor of overall resorption was total time of dryness prior to storage or reimplantation. The total time the tooth was outside the mouth (extra-alveolar time) was the only significant factor in predictors of replacement resorption. After 30 minutes of dry time, root resorption occurs at a high rate. The onset of resorption varies from 102 to 997 days.[10]

Replacement Resorption Cementoblasts are responsible for depositing cementum on dentin that covers the root. Osteoblasts are responsible for producing the alveolar bone that lies under the periodontal ligament. Damage to the periodontal ligament cells and cementum leads to resorption of the root surface through a series of processes. Osteoblasts respond to traumatic injury by producing new bone to repair the alveolar bone. This process is called remodeling. The damage to the slow-growing cementoblasts allows osteoblasts to attach areas of bone directly to the root before the cementoblasts can cover the root with cementum. The direct attachment of bone leads to **recontouring** of the physiologic bone, with the entire root being replaced by bone. This process is called **replacement resorption.**[11] If the area of damage is large, replacement resorption is irreversible. Replacement resorption is better in younger patients because remodeling occurs faster.[10]

Replacement resorption is characterized by the loss of root surface (cementum) accompanied by loss of periodontal ligament space and loss of lamina dura (the hard layer lining the tooth alveoli). Consequently, bone is seen to be in direct contact with the root surface. This phenomenon is often referred to as **ankylosis** and may occur in the absence of inflammation.[10]

DID YOU KNOW ?

Ankylosis is common in other body joints. Diseases (i.e., chronic rheumatoid arthritis) and dental trauma can destroy the membrane that lines joints.

Cementum, or root, resorption is defined radiographically as the evidence of loss of root substance accompanied by its replacement with bone, such that periodontal ligament space has been lost, but radiolucency is not evident. One clinical test for root resorption is the percussion test, which involves tapping the tooth with a tool and listening for the sound produced. A high percussion note indicates resorption. Teeth with no physiologic mobility are another clinical sign of resorption. If there is no radiographic evidence of root resorption but the tooth is clinically ankylosed, replacement resorption has occurred. Resorption of the root may not be visible in x-rays of labial or palatal tooth surfaces (i.e., surfaces located adjacent to the lips or palate, respectively). Resorption is more commonly visible on the mesial or distal tooth surfaces.[10]

Inflammatory Resorption

Death of the pulp tissue (pulpal necrosis) always occurs after an avulsion injury. Necrotic tissue becomes infected and releases toxins. The wider dentin tubules provide a physiologic path for these inflammatory products to reach the root surface. Inflammatory resorption occurs when surface or replacement resorption involves dentin and the inflammatory toxins of a necrotic, infected pulp. The inflammatory products cause a loss of root surface (cementum) accompanied by the loss of adjacent bone and the formation of an area of radiolucency. In luxation trauma, if revascularization (restoration of blood flow) or endodontic procedures on dental pulp and periapical tissues are not successful, necrosis will lead to external inflammatory resorption and rapid loss of the tooth.[11]

Revascularization is possible if the apex of the injured tooth is open, but not if it is closed. Limiting inflammation around the root (periradicular inflammation) tips the balance toward favorable (cemental resorption) rather than unfavorable (inflammatory resorption) healing.[11]

INITIAL EXAMINATION

Obtaining a complete history of the injury will guide the treatment plan for repair. The soft tissue examination often helps in diagnosing areas of trauma and planning where to place necessary sutures to promote healing. The hard tissue examination involves looking for loosened teeth, fractured teeth, fractured alveolar process, displaced teeth, and missing teeth.[5] Radiographs are always necessary to evaluate the extent of injury to the root and alveolus. If there is extensive soft tissue damage, radiographs may be needed to determine whether embedded teeth or tooth fragments are present. Movement of the alveolar process and several teeth together is diagnostic of an alveolar fracture.[10] Detection of horizontal root fracture often requires multiple x-rays from different angles to diagnose the fracture.[12] The two main factors of the prognosis include extra-alveolar time and dry storage time. Prolonged drying causes loss of the periodontal ligament and dehydration of the pulp. Prolonged dry storage time is directly related to root resorption. The total extraoral time is the strongest single predictor of which type of resorption will occur.

DID YOU KNOW

In any kind of trauma, the "golden hour" is often spoken of in getting a patient treated and having the best chance of healing from one's injury. This has been shown to be very important in car injuries and war injuries, and it illustrates that teeth are living tissue that respond best to treatment in the first golden hour.

It appears that contamination, endodontic treatment or the initial stage of root development appears not to affect the prognosis significantly.[10] Diagnosis will determine the treatment plan and improve prognosis of the involved teeth. It may be helpful to use a standard checklist during the examination to provide good documentation for treatment planning and potential legal questions. It is also a good practice to have pictures as a permanent part of the patient's chart.

It is important at the initial visit to obtain a good history including medical history, prior dental trauma, timing of current trauma, clinical examination of injuries, radiographs, and discussion of treatment options and prognosis of outcomes. The dental provider needs to be aware that a neurologic injury is possible. Closed head or cervical spinal injury should at least be considered if the force was strong enough to fracture, intrude, or avulse a tooth.[13] The patient should be referred to a physician for neurologic evaluation (Table 8–1 ■). Of course, if any doubt exists, emergency transport is appropriate.

Pain control is necessary for the patient's well-being and often to permit controlled evaluation. The character of the pain will help with assessment of the injury. Pain as a result of temperature change is consistent with pulpal inflammation. Pain related to occlusion may mean that a tooth has been displaced or that swelling of periodontal or supporting tissues has occurred. If teeth are mobile, the vascular blood supply may have been disrupted. Extreme tooth mobility leaves little chance that the blood supply has not been damaged, and pulpal necrosis will likely develop.

Electric vitality testing involves placing an electrode on the injured tooth and then passing an electric current through the tooth. The current is increased until the patient feels a sensation in the tooth.

TABLE ■ 8–1 Neurologic Evaluation of Patient

A neurologic examination may include the following:
- The history: questions concerning symptoms and condition
- An evaluation of neurologic function
- Diagnostic tests
- Electrodiagnostic tests
- Blood tests
- Other common tests

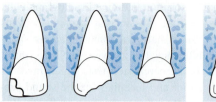

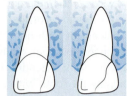

FIGURE ■ 8–3 Crown fractures.

This test, however, is of limited use during the acute injury phase because the normal anatomy is disrupted. Thermal testing can be more useful in the acute phase, but it also can be misleading. A nontraumatized tooth in another area of the mouth should be tested first. This tooth is referred to as a *baseline control* because it establishes the level of heat to which a normal tooth responds. A quick response to heat indicates inflammation, which is expected at this stage. No response to heat indicates that pulpal necrosis is highly likely. Cold testing is another form of thermal testing; it involves application of ice, cold air, or a vapocoolant (a substance that produces a cooling effect when it evaporates). If the pain stops when the cold is removed, the tooth is normal. A prolonged reaction of pain to cold is diagnostic of pulpal damage that will need further assessment. A follow-up evaluation after a healing period of 7 to 10 days will provide a better assessment. Laser Doppler flowmetry provides a real-time measurement of the flow of red blood cells in minute vessels (venules or capillaries) of the circulatory system. This microvascular blood flow is referred to as **perfusion**. Researchers have used this technique to provide an objective measurement of pulpal damage, but the cost is currently prohibitive unless the dental office deals with frequent cases of dental trauma.[14]

SOFT TISSUE INJURIES

Soft tissue injuries often are associated with facial trauma. Tears of the gingival tissue and displacement of teeth often are present. Lips commonly have puncture wounds caused by bite injuries when the open mouth is forcibly closed during the accident. Wounds should be rinsed with saline and, if necessary, gently debrided with gauze wetted with mild soapy water to remove foreign material and dead or damaged tissue. This cleaning is often needed to adequately perform the initial examination. Appropriate suturing of tissue is needed for tissue repair and healing. It may be necessary to refer patients to a plastic or oral surgeon if facial or complex suturing is required. It is important to refer patients to their physician to determine if tetanus immunization or booster injections are needed.

CATEGORIES OF TRAUMATIC DENTAL INJURIES

Crown fractures have been classified from class I through IV. Class I involves just the enamel, class II includes enamel and dentin, and class III involves enamel, dentin, and pulpal tissues. Class IV is the complete loss of the clinical crown[15] (Figure 8–3 ■).

INJURY TO PRIMARY TEETH

Treatment of pediatric patients may involve behavioral issues, especially with a painful injury. Fortunately, primary teeth allow conservative treatment in most situations (see Figure 8–4 ■). Definitive treatment for pulpal exposures, soft tissue injuries, painful fractures, and necessary extractions are not easily accomplished in the uncooperative patient. Because children's alveolar bone is softer than that of adults due to less mineralization and their inability to provide feedback, the extent of the injury may be difficult to diagnose. If injury is suspected, young children may need referral for examination under general anesthesia.

Mobile, nondisplaced primary teeth generally heal without treatment (self-heal) and require only reassurances to the child and parents. Displaced primary teeth require assessment of occlusal interferences and pain to decide the appropriate

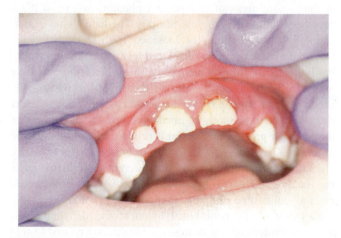

FIGURE ■ 8–4 Primary teeth trauma.

(*Source:* Courtesy of Gary Cuttrell.)

care. Generally, if the primary tooth interferes with the child's bite or endangers the permanent tooth development, the tooth is extracted. If neither condition exists, the tooth is left and allowed to heal. Intruded teeth are assessed for potential endangerment to the permanent tooth, which would require extraction of the primary teeth.

Intruded Primary Teeth

Intrusions of primary central incisors typically do not require treatment. Natural re-eruption of intruded teeth permits a conservative approach to reduce damage to the developing permanent teeth.[16] Fortunately, the structures from which permanent teeth are formed (tooth germs, or buds) are lingual to primary root tips. Intrusions and avulsions of great force would be required to injure the tooth buds; these injuries are more associated with secondary damage to the developing permanent teeth.[9] Children younger than 3 years are more likely to suffer damage to successor permanent teeth because bone mineralization is incomplete at this age and dental germs are still developing.[9] In rare cases, if the primary teeth are obviously intruded lingually, it may be necessary to extract the primary tooth in an attempt to avoid developmental problems with the permanent teeth. Radiographic confirmation should be completed before deciding to extract the teeth.

Avulsed Primary Teeth

Many cases of avulsed primary teeth may not be well documented, but studies list these injuries as 7% to 13% of primary tooth trauma.[17] The most frequently avulsed primary teeth are the maxillary incisors at 89%.[18] Avulsed primary teeth are seldom reimplanted. Many recommend that primary teeth never be replaced[19,20] because of concern that permanent teeth may be damaged. Damage to the permanent tooth germ occurs 30% of the time after avulsion of primary teeth. Discoloration is the most common damage and occurs more often in children younger than 2 years.[18] Always of concern is the need to use traditional space maintenance appliances to prevent potential loss of arch space. This procedure will require follow-up evaluations by the dentist.

Parents often are concerned about the discoloration of traumatized primary teeth. These teeth often will naturally exfoliate without treatment and need only conservative monitoring. It is important to use other clinical symptoms such as infection to determine whether pulpal therapy is necessary.[16,21] Treatment is indicated if any symptoms develop that could affect the development of permanent teeth.

INJURY TO PERMANENT TEETH

Trauma to young permanent teeth may lead to devitalization of the pulp with arrest in root development, resulting in open apices,[22] which are difficult to seal and require apexification procedures. **Apexification** involves placing a root canal dressing, traditionally calcium hydroxide, at the apex, which may induce closure of the root apex.[23] This time-honored treatment requires several months and requires follow-up appointments. A wide range of researchers has reported successes in healing rates in the 70% to 100% range.[24]

Avulsed Secondary Teeth

Recommendations for reimplanting avulsed teeth with open apices are quite varied. The International Association of Dental Trauma does not recommend reimplanting such teeth. However, the debate as to the proper treatment is still ongoing. Without doubt, the emotional element alone is the reason that most teeth are reimplanted. If possible, performing endodontic therapy before reimplantation provides a good seal for the open apices and avoids the apexification procedure. This treatment should be completed as aseptically as possible and with minimal trauma to the periodontal ligament on the root surface to yield the best prognosis.[11]

Preservation of Avulsed Teeth

Proper storage of avulsed teeth is essential to the viability of reimplantation if immediate reimplantation is not practical. Although it is known that air drying rapidly reduces the chance of successful reimplantation, proper transport and storage will help maintain the periodontal ligament, thus buying precious time. Matching the osmolality of the storage medium to the tissue fluid will help preserve the periodontal ligament. Research has identified several valid storage media. Hanks balanced salt solution (HBSS), milk, saline, and the patient's own saliva have proved beneficial.[25] Viaspan, a storage medium used for transport of transplant organs, has also been effective for avulsed teeth.[26] Viaspan is expensive and not readily available, however, and HBSS provides similar results. Milk has proved very effective in preserving the periodontal ligament but may not be available in many emergency settings because of its need for refrigeration. Milk substitutes do not need refrigeration and offer an advantage over natural whole milk. Of the different milk substitutes studied, whole milk and the reconstituted baby formulation Enfamil were within the physiologic pH range (6.6–7.8) for periodontal ligament cells and within the physiologic osmolarity range (230–400).[25] Although other milk substitutes were within the physiologic osmolarity range, they were not as effective as storage media, probably because their pH values were outside the physiologic range.[25] Tap water often is used for storage because of its ready availability, but it is a very poor storage media. In fact, water's low osmolality results in cell death of the periodontal ligament.[25,27] Storage of avulsed teeth on ice is a low alternative if none of the approved storage media is available. Although time of reimplantation of avulsed teeth is critical, allied health and laypeople would do well to learn proper storage to increase survival in the hands of dental professionals. Some commercial products offer proper storage media and containers for avulsed teeth.[28,29] It seems that, unless immediate reimplantation or storage in an acceptable media is available, avulsed teeth have poor survival rates.

Preservation of Periodontal Ligament

Preserving the periodontal ligament is a race to minimize the inflammation that occurs when avulsion damages the ligament and to minimize the pulpal infection that follows damage of the vascular bed.[11] Inflammatory resorption follows in subluxated (partially dislocated) and luxated teeth when pulp necrosis develops but is controlled with timely endodontic treatment.[30] Although it is well known that reimplantation in less than 15 minutes provides the greatest chance of survival, proper storage and handling of avulsed teeth increase the survival rate after they are implanted.[31] Splinting materials and fixation with slight mobility will aid reorientation of the periodontal membrane fibers and help preserve the periodontal ligament.[32]

Case reports of reimplanted teeth after prolonged air drying (18 hours) indicate that their appearance can be improved and their functionality restored; nevertheless, long-term root resorption leads to a poor prognosis.[33]

Clinical Steps for Reimplantation

Final clinical steps involve the removal of any obstructions in the socket. Obstructions may include collapsed alveolar bone or the coagulum of the clot (i.e., the soft, insoluble mass of the clot). Coagulum may be gently rinsed out with saline. A blunt instrument can be used to reposition the socket bone to allow replacement of the avulsed tooth.[11]

Splinting

Semirigid or flexible splints show less root resorption and improved periodontal ligament healing compared with rigid fixation.[34] Rigid fixation time of less than 2 weeks reduces the chance of ankylosis.[35,36] A semirigid (physiologic) splint to reposition the teeth is placed for 7 to 10 days. The splint should not impinge on the gingiva and cannot interfere with occlusion. (See Figure 8–5 ■.) If the injury involved fractures of the alveolar ridge, splint placement is necessarily increased up to 8 weeks even though the chances of tooth ankylosis are increased. Radiographs are needed to verify splint placement and the course of healing.[11]

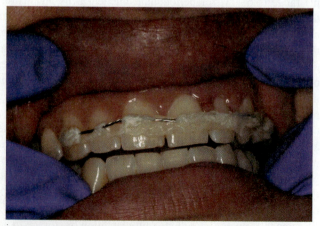

FIGURE ■ 8–5 Splinting.
(*Source:* Courtesy of Gary Cuttrell.)

Healing of the Pulp

Pulp healing in permanent teeth varies with the degree of trauma to the crown and periodontal ligament. Crown fractures with no luxation heal in 99% of cases with no apparent long-term effects.[37] Crown fractures with luxation result in pulpal necrosis in 25% of cases, and 70% heal with no apparent long-term effects. The pulpal necrosis is associated with periodontal ligament damage, emphasizing that the primary factor in pulp healing is related to compromised circulation that occurs with luxation.[38]

Fractured Secondary Teeth

Fractured anterior coronal fragments are often saved and presented to the dentist after injury. If there is a good fit of the fragment, it is possible to use a reattachment process that involves an acid-etch bonding treatment. (See Chapter 16 for discussion of etching processes.) Fragment retention provides an alternative to conventional resin composite restorations, but weakness of the bonding junction may lead to poor long-term results.[39]

Displaced Secondary Teeth

Displaced teeth incur injury to the periodontal ligament, the pulp, and the bone in the alveolar sockets. Dental professionals must decide which treatments give the teeth the best chance to heal. The act of repositioning in itself often requires force that can lead to more injury. In cases of young teeth still in formation, the pulp has the ability to heal and complete tooth development. The edges of significantly displaced alveolar bone will need to be approximated to encourage bony healing and to provide a better foundation for gingival repair. Repositioning the periodontal ligament portions of the bony socket and root from avulsed and severely displaced teeth provides a good chance for healing. Repositioning the ligament in some categories of injury is still under investigation; therefore, discretion should be taken in selecting a clinical treatment. Displacement of teeth to the side of the socket (lateral luxation) may be better treated with spontaneous repositioning for young patients and orthodontic repositioning for patients older than 12 years.[40] An extra-alveolar time of 60 minutes makes survival of the periodontal ligament cells unlikely.[10]

Intruded Secondary Teeth

Intrusion injury accounts for 3% of permanent teeth injuries; its prognosis for healing is directly related to the stage of root development. Apical diameters less than 0.7 mm have a higher probability of developing necrosis than apical diameters larger than 1.2 mm.[40] Treatment of intruded secondary teeth follow three general recommendations: (1) spontaneous re-eruption, (2) immediate surgical repositioning and fixation, and (3) orthodontic repositioning.[40] An intruded tooth with mature root formation and closed apices has the best prognosis if repositioning occurs within 90 minutes of the injury, followed by timely pulpal therapy to prevent a necrotic pulp.[41] Necrotic pulps trigger inflammatory root resorption, which leads to tooth loss.[42]

PUBLIC EDUCATION ON DENTAL TRAUMA

More than 60% of avulsion injuries occur at home or school.[43] Availability of emergency kits on-site and to emergency personnel would help prevent dry storage or use of inappropriate storage media and would help to ensure better healing results. Provision of regular and frequent information for educators and health care providers is necessary to ensure the best treatment. The correct protocols to increase the survivability and viability of traumatized teeth are simple, but they often are not followed because often the information about their use has been forgotten. Proper medical and dental treatments, such as evaluation for tetanus injections, neurologic examinations, and proper storage and stabilization of injured tooth structures, provide safe and effective treatment for this common emergency.[27] It is important to let the public know that dry storage of avulsed teeth results in irreversible injury to the periodontal membrane and usually leads to loss of the tooth, making it a temporary solution.[27] Surveys of schoolchildren have shown them to be better versed in emergency treatments for other body parts. Lack of basic knowledge for emergency treatment of avulsed teeth reduces the chance of a favorable prognosis.[44] Education of teachers, parents, and students in the basic management of dental trauma should be encouraged to improve outcomes.[45] Educational programs need reinforcement so that the public retains the knowledge needed to properly handle dental traumas.[46]

RESEARCH ON DENTAL TRAUMA

Carl E. Misch has looked at life expectancies of both fixed prosthodontic (cemented) bridge work and removable prosthodontic (noncemented) bridge work appliances; he found that, since 1993, dental implants have had the highest survival rate for single-tooth implants than for any other method of tooth replacement.[47] Misch acknowledges that the longevity of implant crowns needs a longer history before such a blanket statement can be made. Use of implants requires, as stated, a clinical judgment of **abutment teeth** (teeth used to support fixed or removable prosthodontic appliances) and the risks associated with their potential loss. Implants with a high success rate (i.e., above the 90th percentile) should be strongly considered in some categories of traumatic dental injury replacement. Further research and evaluation of success rates in traumatic dental injuries and treatments need to consider the best initial treatment options. This investigation should look at total costs and final outcomes for patient function and aesthetics. Of course, implants are an option only for patients of an age that allows implants to be a valid choice.

The Cochrane Collaboration, an international organization that prepares, maintains, and disseminates systematic reviews of health care interventions, offers an electronic resource for locating high-quality information. The Cochrane Library focuses primarily on systematic reviews of controlled trials of therapeutic interventions. Two Cochrane protocols provide guidance in the research of dental trauma. The first deals with "Interventions for treating traumatized permanent front teeth: Root fracture."[48] The second protocol deals with "Interventions for treating traumatized permanent front teeth: Luxated (dislodged) teeth."[49] Continued research in all categories is providing guidelines for more defined and appropriate treatment for dental trauma.

SUMMARY

Maintaining a viable, functioning tooth is the desirable outcome after traumatic dental injuries. When this outcome is not possible, timing and restorative options need to be addressed. If the tooth is lost immediately or has a poor prognosis, the patient needs to be aware of options to restore function and aesthetics. These options range from removable and fixed prosthodontics to dental implants.

All of these procedures are acceptable restorative options. The newest option for dental implants has shown very good results, has become a reliable choice, and has inherent benefits. As evidenced by worldwide articles dealing with dental trauma, this subject will continue to be studied because dental trauma is one of the common accidents that occur in everyday life.

PRACTICE CONSIDERATIONS

Many times patients present with dental trauma to dental offices and need information. However, an important role may be to provide education on types of dental emergencies and how to respond when asked to speak to teachers, parent's groups, and other target populations because this can be valuable information in helping save teeth and to prevent further destruction.

The Internet provides a ready reference for parents to find information on their child's trauma. When educating the public, remind them of this valuable resource. School nurses can go to the Internet and print out readily available dental trauma management sheets to have on hand in the office.

SELF-STUDY QUESTIONS

1. Primary dentition trauma peaks at age
   a. 2–3 years old
   b. 4–5 years old
   c. 9–10 years old
   d. 11–12 years old

   Rationale: The age when children begin to walk make children very susceptible to injuring their front teeth.

2. Movement of teeth and alveolar process together indicate
   a. Minimal trauma
   b. Advanced periodontal disease
   c. Alveolar ridge fracture
   d. Age of patient

   Rationale: Recognizing that the alveolar ridge is possibly fractured is important and may require referral to a specialist such as an oral surgeon to promote proper healing

3. The initial exam of dental trauma includes
   a. Soft tissue exam
   b. Hard tissue exam
   c. X-rays
   d. Neurologic evaluation
   e. All the above

   Rationale: The initial exam needs to focus on all the possible injuries that a patient may have obtained including brain trauma from head injuries.

4. A class III crown fracture involves
   a. Enamel
   b. Enamel and dentin
   c. Enamel, dentin, and pulpal tissue
   d. Alveolar ridge fracture

   Rationale: Crown fractures involving the pulpal tissue need evaluation and immediate treatment by a dentist for restoration.

5. Of the following, which is the best storage media for avulsed teeth
   a. Tap water
   b. Bottled water
   c. Carbonated beverage
   d. Milk

   Rationale: Although not the perfect storage media, milk is commonly available.

REFERENCES

1. Roberson, T. M., Heymann, H. O., & Swift E. J., Jr., (2006). *Sturdevant's art and science of operative dentistry* (5th ed.) St. Louis, MO: Mosby Elsevier. 38–39.
2. Von Arx, T., Filippi, A., & Lussi, A. (2001). Comparison of a new dental trauma splint device (TTS) with three commonly used splinting techniques. *Dent Traumatol,* 17:272.
3. Slack G. L., & Jones, J. M. (1955). Psychological effect of fractured incisors, *Br Dent J,* 99:386–88.
4. Cortes, M. I., Marcenes, W., & Shelham, A. (2002). Impact of traumatic injuries to the permanent teeth on the oral health-related quality of life in 12- to 14-year old children. *Community Dent Oral Epidemiol,* 30:193–98.
5. Douglass, A. B., & Douglass, J. M. (2003). Common dental emergencies. *Am Fam Phys,* 67:515.
6. Nguyen, P.-M. T., Kenny, D. J., & Barrett, E. J. (2004). Socioeconomic burden of permanent incisor replantation on children and parents. *Dent Traumatol,* 20:124–29.
7. Andreasen, J. O., Andreasen, F. M., Bakland, L. K., & Flores, M. T. (2003). *Traumatic dental injuries: A manual* (2nd ed.). Ames, IA: Blackwell Munksgaard, Blackwell Publishing, 8–11.
8. Flores, M. T., Andreasen, J. O., & Bakland, L. K. (2001). Guidelines for the evaluation and management of traumatic dental injuries. *Dent Traumatol,* 17:193–96.
9. Sennhenn-Kirchner, S., & Jacobs, H.-G. (2006). Traumatic injuries to the primary dentition and effect of the permanent successors—A clinical follow-up study. (Abstract). *Dent Traumatol,* 22:1.
10. Boyd, D. J., Kinirons, M. J., & Gregg, T. A. (2000). A prospective study of factors affecting survival of replanted permanent incisors in children. *Int J Paediatr Dent,* 10:200–4.
11. Trope, M. (2002). Clinical management of the avulsed tooth: Present strategies and future directions. *Dent Traumatol,* 18:1–11
12. Bramante, C. M., Menezes, R., Moraes, I. G., Bernardinelli, N., Garcia, R. B., & Letra, A. (2006). Use of MTA and intracanal post reinforcement in a horizontally fractured tooth: A case report. *Dent Traumatol,* 10:277.
13. Davis, J. J., & Vogel L. (1995). Neurological assessment of the child with head trauma. *J Dent Child,* 62:93–96.
14. Mesaros, S. V., & Trope, M. (1997). Revascularization of traumatized teeth assessed by laser Doppler flowmetry. *Endod Dent Traumatol,* 13:24–30.
15. Ellis, R. G., & Davey, L. W. (1970). *The classification and treatment of injuries to the teeth of children* (5th ed.). St. Louis, MO: Mosby.
16. Spinas, E., Melis, A., & Savasta, A. (2006). Therapeutic approach to intrusive luxation injuries in primary dentition. A clinical follow-up study. (Abstract). *Eur J Paediatr Dent,* 7:179–86.
17. Andreasen, J. O., & Andreasen, F. M. (1994). *Textbook and color atlas of traumatic injuries to the teeth* (3rd ed.). Copenhagen, Denmark: Blackwell Munksgaard, 19–425,750.
18. Christophersen, P., Freund, M., & Harild, L. (2005). Avulsion of primary teeth and sequelae on permanent successors. *Dent Traumatol,* 21:321–23.

19. McTigue, D. J. (2000). Diagnosis and management of dental injuries in children. *Pediatr Clin North Am,* 47:1067–84

20. Flores, M. T., Andreasen, J. O., & Bakland, L. K. (2001). Guidelines for the evaluation and management of traumatic dental injuries. *Dent Traumatol,* 17:49–52.

21. Holan, G., & Fuks, A. B. (1996). The diagnostic value of coronal dark-gray discoloration in primary teeth following traumatic injuries. *Pediatr Dent,* 18:224–27

22. Andreasen, J. O. (1970). Etiology and pathogenesis of traumatic dental injuries. A clinical study of 1,298 cases. *J Dent Res,* 78:339–42.

23. Ghose, L. J., Baghdady, V. S., & Hikmat, B. Y. M. (1987). Apexification of immature apices of pulpless permanent anterior teeth with calcium hydroxide. *J Endod,* 13:285–90.

24. Pradhan, D. P., Chawla, H. S., Gauba, K., & Goyal, A. (2006). Comparative evaluation of endodontic management of teeth with unformed apices with mineral trioxide aggregate and calcium hydroxide. *J Dent Child,* 73:79–84.

25. Pearson, R. M., Liewehr, F. R., West, L. A., Patton, W. R., McPherson, J. C., & Runner, R. R. (2003). Human periodontal ligament cell viability in milk and milk substitutes. *Am Assoc Endod,* 29:184–86.

26. Trope, M., & Friedman, S. (1992). Periodontal healing of replanted dog teeth stored in Viaspan, milk and Hanks' balanced salt solution. *Endo Dent Traumatol,* 8:183–88.

27. Andersson, L., Al-Asfour, A., & Al-Jame, Q. (2006). Knowledge of first-aid measure of avulsion and replantation of teeth: An interview of 221 Kuwaiti schoolchildren. *Dent Traumatol,* 22:57, 60, 558.

28. Emergency Medical Treatment Toothsaver (EMT Toothsaver). Phoenix, AZ: SmartPractice.

29. Emmanouil, S., Regan, J. D., Kramer, P. R., Witherspoon, D. E., & Opperman, L. A. (2004). Survival of human periodontal ligaments for transport of avulsed teeth. *Dent Traumatol,* 20:21–28.

30. Qin, J., Ge, L., & Bai, R. (2002). Use of a removable splint in the treatment of subluxated, luxated and root fractured anterior permanent teeth in children. *Dent Traumatol,* 18:81–85.

31. Krasner, P., & Person, P. (1992). Preserving avulsed teeth for replantation. *J Am Dent Assoc,* 123:80–88.

32. Oikarinen, K. (1990). Tooth splinting: A review of the literature and consideration of the versatility of a wire-composite splint. *Endod Dent Traumatol,* 6:237–50.

33. Cho, S. Y., & Cheng, A. C. (2002). Replantation of an avulsed incisor after prolonged dry storage: A case report. *J Can Dent Assoc,* 68:297–300.

34. Berude, J. A., Hicks, M. L., Sauber, J. J., & Li, S. J. (1988). Resorption after physiological and rigid splinting of replanted permanent incisors in monkeys. *J. Endod,* 14:592–600.

35. Nasjleti, C. E., Castelli, W. A., & Caffesse, R. G. (1982). The effect of different splinting times on replantation of teeth in monkeys. *Oral Surg,* 53:557–66.

36. Von Arx, T., Filippi, A., & Lussi, A. (2001). Comparison of a new dental trauma splint device (TTS) with three commonly used splinting techniques. *Dent Traumatol,* 17:267.

37. Robertson, A., Andreasen, F. M., Andreasen, J. O., & Noren, J. G. (2000). Long-term prognosis of crown-fractured permanent incisors. The effect of stage of root development and associated luxation injury. *Int J Paediatr Dent,* 123(3):191.

38. Andreasen, F. M., Noren, J. G., & Andreasen, J. O., Engelhardtsen, S., & Lindh-Strombert, U. (2006). Long-term survival fragment bonding in the treatment of fractured crowns: A multicenter clinical study. The Cochrane Library, Issue 4. Retrieved from The Cochrane Central Register of Controlled Trials (Central) database.

39. Andreasen, J. O., Andreasen, F. M., Bakland, L. K., & Flores, M. T. (2003). *Traumatic dental injuries: A manual* (2nd ed.). Ames, IA: Blackwell Munksgaard, Blackwell Publishing Professional, 14.

40. Gungor, H. C., Cengiz, S. B., & Altay, N. (2006). Immediate surgical repositioning following intrusive luxation: A case report and review of the literature. *Dent Traumatol,* 10:340–43.

41. Kenny, D. J., Barrett, E. J., & Casas, M. J. (2003). Avulsions and intrusions: The controversial displacement injuries. *J Can Dent Assoc,* 69:308–13.

42. Hedegard, B., & Stalhone, I. (1973). A study of traumatized permanent teeth in children aged 7–15 years. Part I. *Swed Dent J,* 66:431–38

43. Loh, T., Sae-Lim, V., Yian, T. B., & Liang, S. (2006). Dental therapists' experience in the immediate management of traumatized teeth. *Dent Traumatol,* 22:66–70.

44. Kinoshita, S., Kojima, R., Taguchi, Y., & Noda, T. (2002). Tooth replantation after traumatic avulsion: A report of 10 cases. *Dent Traumatol,* 18:153–56.

45. Kahabuka, F. K., Willemsen, W., Wan't Hof, M., & Burgerskijk, R. (2006). The effect of a single educational input given to school teachers on patient's correct handling after dental trauma. The Cochrane Library, Issue 3. Retrieved September 12, 2012 from Cochrane Central Register of Controlled Trials database.

46. Misch, C. E. (2005). *Dental implant prosthetics.* St. Louis, MO: Mosby, 2–3.

47. Guyatt, G., & Rennie, D. (Eds). (2005). *Users' guide to the medical literature* (5th ed.). Chicago: American Medical Association Press, 32.

48. Al-Hennawi., D., Day, P. F., & Duggal, M. S. (2005). Interventions for treating traumatized permanent front teeth: Root fracture. (Protocol). *Cochrane Database Syst Rev,* Issue 3. Art. No.: CD005408. DOI: 10.1002/14651858.CD005408.

49. Belmonte, F. M., Abrao, C. V., Day, P. F., Macedo, C. R., Saconato, H., & Trevisani, V. F. M. (2006). Interventions for treating traumatized permanent front teeth: luxated (dislodged) teeth. Flávia Monari Belmonte—São Paulo, 2006.

Host Defense Mechanisms in the Oral Cavity

Beth E. McKinney

OBJECTIVES

After reading this chapter, the student should be able to:

1. List the four host defense mechanisms operational in the oral cavity.
2. Describe how the epithelium functions as a microbial barrier in the mouth.
3. Describe how an ideal dentition functions as a defense mechanism.
4. Describe the cycle of enamel demineralization and remineralization and assess its presence in patients.
5. Evaluate caries treatment plans to include a medical model of disease prevention and non-surgical treatment.
6. Identify early and late colonizers in bacterial plaque, and discuss their roles in the disease process.
7. Incorporate systemic assessments of host defense mechanisms into periodontal therapy.
8. Explain the significance of plaque pH.
9. Differentiate between cellular and humoral immunity.
10. Describe the role of granulocytes in host defense.
11. List the major salivary glands and functions of saliva.
12. Prescribe appropriate therapies for a patient with compromised salivary function.
13. Discuss the functions of the immunoglobulins.
14. Integrate concepts of host defense mechanisms into patient treatment plans.

Humans share this planet with billions of microorganisms. The human body is home to millions of tiny microbes whose eradication is neither possible nor desirable. Typically, human beings and microbes coexist peacefully and in many cases have forged mutually beneficial (**symbiotic**) relationships. Infection is the state in which disease is caused when pathogenic microbes are able to proliferate and the host's protective mechanisms fail or are inadequate. Environmental factors play a significant role in determining whether or not the host's defensive mechanisms are sufficient to prevent disease. Both dental caries and periodontal disease are infectious disease processes.

This chapter provides an overview of host defense mechanisms in the oral cavity and is not a substitute for a course in immunology. The reader who finds this subject intriguing is referred to the medical literature that teaches pathophysiology and the study of clinical disease processes. This topic is the focus of new research in the dental field as advances are made in the study of stem cells, gene therapy, and priiobotics.

The mouth is the gateway for food and drink destined for the gastrointestinal tract. It is also the structure with which we communicate most frequently (i.e., it handles speech). As such, the mouth is constantly exposed to the outside environment and potential invasion by microbial pathogens. To ensure the safety of the body from infection, a number of defensive systems exist: (1) anatomic barriers, (2) normal oral flora, (3) the immune system, and (4) saliva.

Anatomic barriers include the **epithelium** and an ideal dentition. Normal oral flora includes bacteria that discourage colonization by pathogenic microbes. The immune system includes cellular and **humoral** components, which refer to antibody production and its accompanying processes, which are found in body fluids. The saliva is a mucosal secretion and contains **immunoglobulins** (antibodies).

ANATOMIC BARRIERS: THE ORAL EPITHELIUM

The skin is the largest organ in the human body. Epithelium is a formidable barrier to microbial invasion. Microbes cannot cause infection without first getting past this anatomic barrier. Until breached, no infection can occur. As long as the epithelium is intact, most microbes find this barrier exceedingly difficult to penetrate. Like personal protective equipment worn for patient care, an intact epithelium is an excellent protective mechanism for the oral cavity. Like a torn latex glove, cuts, scrapes, and abrasions all provide possible routes of entry for a pathogen. Minute insults to the oral epithelium occur with disturbing regularity; a patient with a floss cut, pizza burn, or tortilla chip scrape is a good example.

The epithelium in the oral cavity does not differ appreciably from the rest of the body except for the fact that it is always wet. The majority of oral epithelium is keratinized. **Keratin** is a fibrous, sulfur-containing protein, which cannot be penetrated, even by gastric acid. (Pills that must be absorbed intact in the intestines are often coated with keratin so that they will not dissolve in the stomach.) The junctional epithelium at the bottom of the gingival sulcus/crevice lacks any keratin at all and is perhaps the oral site most susceptible to invasion by microorganisms.

Mucosal epithelium in the mouth is more highly vascularized than the skin on the hand. Because of the increased blood perfusion, any injury to the barrier is immediately met with the blood's defensive components. Healing time in the oral cavity can then occur more rapidly. Conversely, activities such as smoking cause a decrease in the diameter of capillaries (vasoconstriction) in the oral tissues, leading to exacerbation of periodontal disease where it exists.

The epithelial barrier is such a good defense mechanism that the body will often go to great lengths to recreate one when it is lost. For example, pulpal polyps (Figure 9–1 ■) are made of granulomatous tissue, which occasionally forms in large carious lesions that have invaded the pulp.[1] **Granulomas** are inflammatory responses to foreign substances that have invaded a body tissue. A large number of different types of immune cells and fibroblasts form the granuloma as they surround the foreign substance.[2] Typically granulomas are not painful. Pyogenic granulomas are another exacerbated attempt of the body to respond to a foreign substance (Figure 9–2 ■). They occur most often following an injury in an exuberant attempt by the body to heal itself. They are highly vascularized and bleed easily. Oral pyogenic granulomas are often seen during

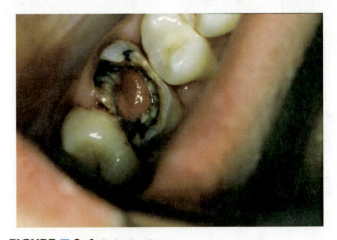

FIGURE ■ 9–1 Pulpal polyps.
(*Source:* Courtesy of Beth E. McKinney.)

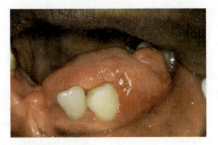

FIGURE ■ 9–2 Pyogenic granuloma.
(*Source:* Courtesy of Beth E. McKinney.)

pregnancy; however, they can occur in any patient and at any site in the body. The usual treatment is complete excision of the lesion because they can recur.

During infancy, the oral environment is relatively uncolonized by microbes. At the presence of the first tooth, the microbial tenants of the oral cavity undergo a vast change. This change can be significant, not to mention pathologic, if the baby's caregivers happen to have active dental caries, untreated periodontal disease, or an active oral herpetic lesion, all of which are easily transmissible to the baby. As humans age, achievement and maintenance of an ideal anatomic dentition afford maximum protection against microbial dental infection. In other words, esthetically pleasing teeth are not just the goal of models and actors. Possession of twenty-eight teeth in class 1 occlusion and with healthy interdental papillae is the oral anatomic condition most naturally resistant to microbial onslaught.

DID YOU KNOW

Restorations with overhangs, lack of interdental papillae, periodontal pockets, or drifting or crowded teeth are all examples of anatomic situations that give microbial pathogens an advantage in colonization of the tooth structure, thereby contributing to dental disease.

An ideal dentition also includes the anatomic barrier of tooth enamel. Tooth **enamel** is the hardest substance in the human body, harder even than cortical bone. Enamel is more mineralized than bone or dentin. It is estimated that enamel is composed of approximately 96% mineral by weight and is therefore highly inorganic. The inorganic phase of enamel is based on the mineral hydroxyapatite, which is made up mainly of calcium, phosphate, and hydroxyl ions. After teeth are fully erupted, the hydroxyl group is often substituted by fluoride, giving additional protection against caries. When the substitution occurs, the enamel is composed of **fluorapatite**.

Tooth enamel is constantly undergoing a process of demineralization and remineralization. Demineralization occurs with exposure to the acids found in foods, beverages, and the stomach and to acids produced by bacteria in plaque. **Remineralization** is the repair of the enamel rods after prolonged exposure to an acidic environment. When teeth erupt, they are anatomically complete but histologically incomplete and immature. After eruption, the missing ions are supplied from the saliva, a process termed *posteruptive maturation*. For this reason, partially erupted first permanent molars are particularly susceptible to developing occlusal caries. In addition, newly improved glass ionomer products have been developed to seal such teeth when a dry environment cannot be achieved. Without specific knowledge of the caries process, the development of a caries lesion is likely to be seen as a continuous process resulting in the ever-increasing loss of tooth mineral until a clinically discernible hole in the tooth structure is present. This conception is incorrect. The process of demineralization is not irreversible or inevitably progressive. If damage has not progressed beyond a still yet to be defined point, lost mineral can be replaced. As dentistry moves more from a surgical model toward a medical model, emphasis is on enamel repair during the early stages of the caries process. Although dentistry has typically focused on the surgical treatment of caries, the practice of dental hygiene with its more preventive approach is ideal for adopting a medical model that focuses on the reversal of the caries process by alternative interventions.

In a long-term study, Backer-Dirks noted that more than 50% of the proximal lesions seen at the initial examination did not progress, indicating an arrestment phenomenon resulting from remineralization.[3] Additional support for remineralization is derived from the frequent observations of teeth that are acid-etched prior to placement of pit-and-fissure sealants. For those etched areas not covered with the resin, the chalky white appearance disappears over a period of a few days, and the enamel regains its initial translucent, glossy appearance.

Remineralizing conditions in the mouth are usually fairly constant. For example, the local pH can be lowered to the point at which enamel demineralization occurs from ingestion of acidic foods or from the production of acid by bacteria after ingestion of carbohydrates, particularly refined foods. If the insults are brief and widely separated in time, remineralizing conditions can be restored in the intervening periods and the slight damage repaired. On the other hand, frequent or protracted periods of acid exposure with insufficient time intervals for remineralization ultimately lead to the development of overt caries. Recent developments in oral hygiene products have remineralization as a goal. Toothpastes and chewing gums are being formulated with bioavailable calcium and phosphate ions in a milk-derived protein called *Recaldent.*™

Saliva, which will be discussed in more detail later in the chapter, is an important factor in remineralization. Individual capacity for salivary remineralization varies depending on both the quantity and quality of saliva. Throughout life, minerals from the saliva are used to repair acid-damaged tooth structure. This repair process can range from an almost immediate replacement of daily ion losses from the enamel surface to a slow repair (under proper conditions) of more extensive subsurface (white spot) lesions.

Fluoride has a major influence on both demineralization and remineralization.[4] Only small concentrations of fluoride are needed to inhibit demineralization or to enhance remineralization. As little as 0.1 ppm fluoride can reduce the amount of enamel dissolution in vitro (i.e., under artificial conditions in a laboratory). The presence of fluoride at the remineralizing site can accelerate rehardening by a factor of up to 5-fold. Fluoride enhances tooth mineralization both through systemic routes and topical applications. In the mouth, fluoride can come from a variety of sources:

- Short-term contact with fluoridated drinking water.
- The continual low fluoride output of the salivary glands.
- The bound fluoride in the plaque, which is released when the pH drops to around 5.5.
- The fluoride contained in the mature enamel layer after demineralization.

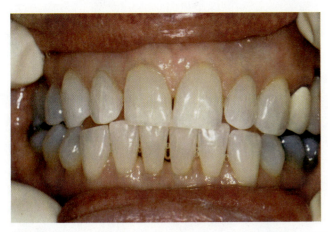

FIGURE ■ 9–3 Healthy dentition, healthy periodontium, and excellent occlusion.

(*Source:* Courtesy of Beth E. McKinney.)

- Dental restorations such as glass ionomers, which release fluoride.
- Topical fluoride applications in forms ranging from toothpaste to varnishes.

The reader is referred to Chapter 15 for a more complete discussion of the uses, types, and benefits of fluoride.

See Figure 9–3 ■, which is a photograph of a 76-year-old woman who has healthy dentition, healthy periodontium, and excellent occlusion. People with normal immune function and regular preventive dental care can maintain healthy, aesthetically pleasing teeth for a lifetime. Dentures are neither a natural, nor inevitable, part of the aging process. Caries and periodontitis are disease states, not naturally occurring conditions.

NORMAL ORAL FLORA

The formation of supragingival dental plaque begins with the acquired (salivary) pellicle, which is an acellular protein layer of saliva components adsorbed onto the surface of the enamel. The bacteria colonize on this pellicle. The pellicle plus the bacteria and the gel they create constitute a biofilm (dental plaque).[5] For several hours after a prophylaxis or toothbrushing has removed the biofilm, there is a steady change in the quantity and composition of the pellicle because new proteins are added from the saliva. The more the plaque matures, the denser it becomes and the more it retains acid against the tooth. In subgingival plaque, a sample of only a cubic millimeter can contain as many as a hundred million organisms. In a healthy sulcus, loose gram-positive cocci such as *Streptococcus gordonii* and *Streptococcus oralis* predominate. In periodontal pockets, the bacterial population becomes predominately colonized by gram-negative anaerobes.[6] Later colonizers responsible for the disease process include *Porphyromonas gingivalis* and *Actinobacillus actinomycetemcomitans.* In the periodontal pocket, bacteria are shielded from salivary flow. Bacteria with limited attachment ability are contained within the walls of the gingival pocket.

The most variable factor in the pathogenicity of plaque colonies is the makeup of the microbial population.[7] Not all bacteria are bad. Some species discourage the attachment of other more pathogenic species, whereas others serve as a bridge.[8] Early colonizers include *Streptococcus mitis* and *Streptococcus sanguis. Veillonella,* when present, metabolizes lactic acid generated by the later colonizers *Streptococcus mutans* and *Lactobacillus,* which are responsible for caries formation. This action decreases the amount of acid available to demineralize tooth structure. Several studies indicate that the presence of *Veillonella* decreases caries risk. It becomes evident that the varieties, metabolic characteristics, and interrelationships of the bacteria are important in determining whether disease will occur.

Probiotics (beneficial bacteria such as are found in live yogurt cultures) have been a field of interest in treating gastrointestinal ailments. It is thought that probiotics can also hold promise in the prevention of dental disease, and in fact some companies are already marketing bacteria for this purpose. For a more thorough discussion of probiotics, see Chapter 22.

The pH of plaque can drop to as low as 4.0 on the **Stephan curve** after use of a glucose mouth rinse.[9] Damage control from acid in the plaque is achieved by dilution and chemical buffering and by increasing the protective ions (mainly, calcium, phosphate, and fluoride) in the vicinity of the teeth.[10] The water content of the saliva and plaque aid greatly in diluting the acid and in transporting acid into the main flow of saliva where it is further diluted and swallowed. Saliva acts as a strong buffer for the acidic plaque. This higher adsorption capacity for fluoride in the plaque also increases bicarbonates, phosphates, and ammonia concentrations derived from the saliva. These neutralizing actions serve as a brake in the rapidity and extent to which the pH can drop during periods of acidogenesis.

Each individual has a different potential for modifying the drop and recovery of the pH represented by the person's individual Stephan curve. For example, if a group of individuals are given a glucose mouthrinse, each person demonstrates a different, but reproducible, pH pattern. Once the pH begins to drop, the salivary buffers help to shorten the time that the pH is at its lowest and most damaging level.

DID YOU KNOW ?

More than 400 drugs that have **xerostomia** as a possible side effect are now on the market. This can have a significant negative impact on one of the oral cavity's primary host defensive mechanisms in caries prevention and repair.

Refer to Figure 9–4 ■, which depicts the complicated arrangement of the community known as *bacterial plaque.* The early colonizers represented here are desirable organisms to have in an environment that can never be sterile. It is the later colonizers that cause disease. The goal of preventive dentistry then is not the eradication of all microorganisms but the selective encouragment of the right mix.

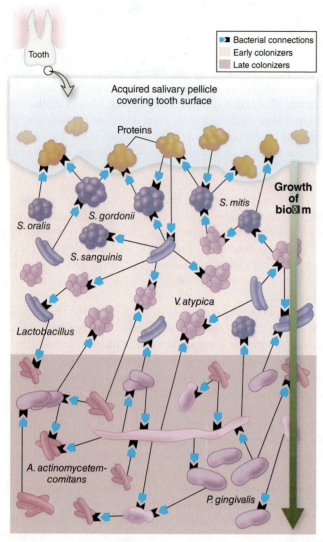

FIGURE ■ 9–4 Complicated arrangement of the community known as *bacterial plaque*.

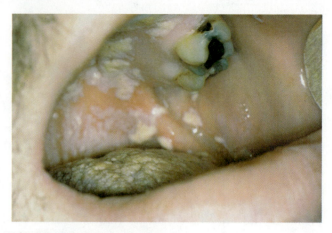

FIGURE ■ 9–5 *Candida albicans*.
(*Source:* Courtesy of Beth E. McKinney.)

THE IMMUNE SYSTEM IN THE ORAL CAVITY

The body's immune system has several components, all of which are active in the oral cavity. These components all monitor the body and distinguish it from anything that is foreign. Anything deemed not to belong is attacked. This process can be good in the case of a flu virus or a parasite; conversely, this process is bad in the case of a transplanted organ. Most significant for this discussion, in periodontal disease, the immune system causes as much or more tissue damage than the bacteria.

The lymph system is composed of two parts: cellular and humoral immunity. **Cellular immunity** is carried out by T cells from the thymus; humoral immunity is carried out by B cells from the bone marrow.[11] The cells from which T cells are formed (precursors) also originate in the bone marrow; however, the thymus is where they become fully functional. From the thymus, the T cells migrate to the lymph nodes, spleen, and

blood. Both parts of the lymph system are involved in defending the body against bacteria and viruses. The tonsils contain a large proportion of B cells. Another part of the immune system is the complement system, which is composed of about 20 proteins whose primary function is to lyse foreign cells.

Candida albicans (Figure 9–5 ■) is a yeast organism that resides in very small quantities on human mucosa. It is kept from proliferation by saliva, normal oral flora, and T lymphocytes.[12] When there is a defect in any or all of these defense mechanisms, the candida organism can proliferate and cause infection as seen here in this patient with AIDS. If candida is also present in the blood and spreads throughout the body, it can be fatal.

The blood also has a myeloid (bone marrow) system of **granulocytes** (mature granular **leukocytes**) whose function is to find and attack foreign invaders. Granulocytes include eosinophils, neutrophils, basophils, and macrophages.[13] The main access that phagocytic cells and their antibacterial products have to the oral cavity is through the gingival sulcus/crevice and the tonsils. Polymorphonuclear leukocytes (PMNs) are the first neutrophils found in the gingival sulcus/crevice in response to plaque bacteria. They are able to migrate through the junctional epithelium to the site of infection. PMNs are the body's first responders to the site of injury or infection and our most abundant type of white blood cell. They also produce pus and other infection-fighting products such as interleukin 8 (IL-8). Neutrophils and macrophages are the cells most responsible for forming the periapical lesions seen on x-rays of abscessed or traumatized teeth. About 500 leukocytes per second are estimated to emigrate from the tissues through the gingival sulcus/crevice into the oral cavity. Because lymphocytes secrete a number of toxic substances, they destroy not only foreign cells but also the body's own cells over a period of time. Some of these secretions include interleukins, cytokines, collagenase, C-reactive protein, and tumor necrosis factor. As this army of components indicates, the development of periodontal disease is a complicated process that starts only with the colonization of pathogenic microflora. The presence of pathogenic bacteria alone, however, is insufficient to cause disease.

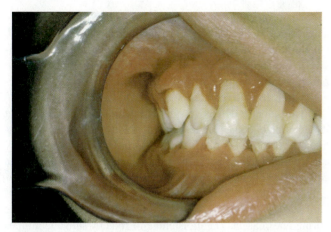

FIGURE ■ 9–6 Child, aged 5 years, with LAD with severe bone loss around all of her primary teeth.

(*Source:* Courtesy of Beth E. McKinney.)

Genetic and metabolic disorders which alter the host defense response can increase the susceptibility of a person to periodontal pathogens.[14] Leukocyte adhesion disorder (LAD) is a rare genetic disease of the white blood cells. Leukocyte is another term for white blood cells and includes neutrophils, basophils, eosinophils, monocytes, lymphocytes, and macrophages. In LAD, the leukocytes cannot migrate to sites of infection. One of the first signs of this disorder is severe periodontal disease in a child. Figure 9–6 ■ is a 5-year-old child with LAD with severe bone loss around all of her primary teeth. It is untreatable by current methodologies. Typically, people with LAD die from infection by early adulthood. New gene therapies can hold some promise in treating this disorder.

A new area of research is human beta-defensin **peptides**; to date, three (hBD-1, 2, and 3) have been identified.[10,15–18] These peptides have been found in the mucosa, the salivary glands, and the gingiva. They have a broad spectrum of antimicrobial activity and offer little opportunity for bacteria to develop resistance. Another antimicrobial peptide, designated LL-37, has been found in human neutrophils, skin, gingiva, and junctional epithelium. Peptides are believed to play important roles in the immune defense mechanism. Another category of PLUNC (palate, lung, and nasal epithelium clone) proteins, only recently identified, seem to act as sensors for gram-negative bacteria in the oral cavity.[19] These three categories of newly found proteins appear to play more of a role in periodontal disease than in the caries process. Immunoglobulins are also part of the body's immune system and will be discussed further in the section on saliva.

Periodontal Disease and Host Defense Mechanisms

The body's immune system plays a bigger role in periodontal disease than it does in the caries process. Like tooth fissures, the gingival sulcus is home to millions of bacteria, some of which are not harmful. In some acute forms of periodontal disease such as necrotizing ulcerative gingivitis, bacteria can cause destruction in host tissue by direct invasion. The two bacteria most often implicated in routine periodontal disease are *Porphymonous gingivalis* and *Actinobacillus actinomycetecomitans*. These organisms cause destruction by the way in which they activate the host's immune system.

Analysis of gingival crevicular fluid in people with advanced periodontal disease show high levels of many components of the host immune system, including white blood cells (primarily neutrophils), more than 30 proteins, immunoglobulins (primarily IgG and IgA), tumor necrosis factor (TNF), cytokines, peroxidases, interleukins. and prostoglandins.[21–23] The bacteria produce surface proteins that trigger this inflammatory response. At least some are also able to produce proteases and other molecules, which help them to evade the host's immune system. As these products and by-products are absorbed into the circulatory system for disposal, they travel to other areas of the body (e.g., the heart) where it is postulated they can be factors in other disease processes. Scaling and root planing are procedures that induce a transient bacterimia in the patient, and serve to increase the activity of their immune system. The link between oral and system disease is currently under intense investigation. Although recent research has shown associations between, for example, heart disease and periodontal disease, well-controlled prospective studies have not yet been able to establish causal relationships (e.g., periodontal disease and preterm/low-birth-weight infants). The strongest evidence so far between periodontal disease and systemic disease is in diabetes. Although current methodologies might be sufficient to arrest the periodontal disease process, at least under favorable circumstances, the regeneration of periodontal tissue has been heretofore impossible. Gene therapy and stem cell therapy offer exciting promise as future techniques to regrow periodontal structures as well as repair damaged salivary glands. For a more detailed discussion of the potential use of gene therapy in dental practice see Chapter 22.

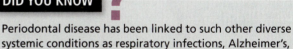

DID YOU KNOW ?

Periodontal disease has been linked to such other diverse systemic conditions as respiratory infections, Alzheimer's, kidney disease, and rheumatoid arthritis.

SALIVA AND ITS ROLE IN PROMOTING ORAL HOMEOSTASIS

The importance of saliva as a host defense mechanism cannot be understated. The same watery fluid that used to make placement of the perfect sealant on a second molar so difficult is actually filled with a wide variety of antimicrobial properties. The defense functions of the saliva are part of the body's ability to maintain **homeostasis**, that is, the ability to remain in balance and successfully resistant to challenges by chemical and bacterial agents.[24] Disease ensues only when the bacterial challenge exceeds the body's defense capabilities and/or a person lacks commitment to self-care. Saliva helps modulate and augment the previously described major body defense systems in the protection of oral tissues.

Salivary Glands

The salivary glands are exocrine glands, meaning that their secretion (saliva) leaves the glands to bathe the oral cavity. Saliva is derived mainly from the major salivary glands—the parotid, submandibular, and sublingual glands. Of these, the parotid gland secretes a serous watery fluid that contains electrolytes but is relatively low in organic substances. The parotid gland secretes the majority of the sodium bicarbonate that is essential in neutralizing acids produced by cariogenic bacteria in the dental plaque and the majority of the enzyme amylase, which initiates intraoral digestion of carbohydrates.[25] The submandibular gland secretes a mixed serous and mucous fluid whereas the sublingual gland has a higher proportion of mucous output than the other major glands. The minor glands (Figure 9–7 ■), which include palatal, lingual, buccal, and labial salivary glands, empty onto the mucous membrane in many locations on the palate, under the tongue, and on the inner sides of the cheeks and lips. These minor glands are mainly mucus-secreting glands that lubricate these surfaces and allow for improved mastication and passage of food into the esophagus.[26] The minor salivary glands also contribute fluoride that bathes the teeth and enhances caries resistance.[27–29]

Pure saliva produced by the oral glands is sterile until it is discharged into the mouth. When the fluids from all major and minor glands mix with each other, this secretion becomes known as *whole saliva*. It is further altered by the presence of particles of food, tissue fluid, sloughed epithelial cells, and lysed bacteria (whose cellular components have disintegrated from the action of enzymes, antibodies, or complement). It becomes even more complex with the inclusion of living cells and their metabolic products such as bacteria and leucocytes; the latter are derived from the gingival sulci/crevices and tonsils.

> **DID YOU KNOW ?**
>
> The average person produces about 700 mL of saliva per day, which is slightly less than a quart.

The protective functions of saliva can be divided into five categories (1) lubrication, (2) flushing/rinsing, (3) chemical, (4) antimicrobial (including antibacterial, antifungal, and antiviral), and (5) maintenance of supersaturation of calcium and phosphate ions bathing the enamel, and helping to buffer demineralization and aid remineralization of tooth structures.[30,31]

The salivary defensive system functions continuously, but its secretion becomes highest and most active during food ingestion. The lowest flow rate is during sleep. This is one reason why early childhood caries caused by a baby sleeping with a bottle containing milk or other sugary substances occurs so rapidly.

A very thin microscopic layer of mucus protects the oral hard and soft tissues from the often harsh and abrasive foods during mastication. The moistening of food by saliva facilitates chewing and swallowing. Speech is enhanced by the reduced friction between the dry tongue and soft tissues. In addition, less saliva results in a greatly increased risk of caries because of the decreased buffering ability, which results in the salivary pH becoming more acidic and the prolonged bacterial plaque adherence to tooth surface.

> **DID YOU KNOW ?**
>
> A normal child will show a stimulated salivary flow rate of more than 1.0 mL/min, somewhat higher than the value for an adult (0.7 mL/min). Dry mouth occurs when the resting salivary flow rate is less than the rate of fluid loss from the mouth either by evaporation or by absorption of water through the oral mucosa.

Chewing, swallowing, and speaking are all adversely affected by xerostomia. In addition to changes in taste, a chronic burning often occurs. When this condition persists, it is termed *burning mouth syndrome*. In someone who has xerostomia, mild candidiasis, tooth erosion, and caries are often found even in the presence of good oral hygiene and dietary habits. Good oral hygiene cannot completely overcome deficits in the host's defense mechanisms.

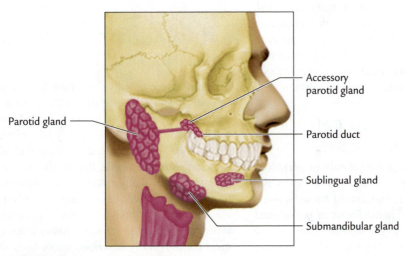

Accessory parotid gland

Parotid duct

Sublingual gland

Submandibular gland

Parotid gland

FIGURE ■ 9–7 Salivary gland.

Providing continuous lubrication is probably the most important defensive function of the salivary glands. It is the fluid that transports the buffering agents, the antimicrobials, and the demineralization and remineralization properties of saliva. In addition, the fluid output of the glands is essential for (1) diluting acids, (2) flushing food particles embedded around the teeth, (3) clearing refined carbohydrates, and (4) physically removing any free-floating bacteria.[31]

The composition of saliva varies, depending on whether it is stimulated or unstimulated. During the day, submandibular glands secrete the highest proportion of unstimulated saliva. The flow rate of resting saliva for all three glands is very low and is about one-tenth of that during stimulated flow. Approximately two-thirds of the resting saliva is derived from the submandibular glands; one-quarter is from the parotids; and approximately one-twentieth is from the sublingual glands. The minor salivary glands secrete almost one-tenth of the total amount of saliva. The customary unstimulated flow rate of the salivary glands is subject to a circadian rhythm with the highest flow in mid-afternoon and the lowest around 4:00 A.M.

DID YOU KNOW ?

No one really knows why radiation therapy to treat oral cancer destroys salivary glands. Salivary gland cell turnover is slow, and theoretically salivary glands should not be so susceptible to the effects of radiation.

Upon moderate stimulation, the submandibular and parotid glands secrete approximately equal amounts of saliva whereas at full stimulation, the parotid has the greatest output. When salivary flow is stimulated by chewing gum, 1 to 2 mL of whole saliva per minute can be expected. The minimum level of stimulated salivary flow necessary to maintain oral health is unknown, but when the flow is below 1 mL per minute, occurrence of xerostomia is a cause for concern. Once the flow rate is below 0.7 mL per minute, a diagnosis of xerostomia can be rendered. In the course of a single day, up to 1 liter of saliva is secreted into the oral cavity.

The total amount of saliva secreted varies considerably between and within individuals, depending on the environmental factors. Seasonal variations occur; flow is lower in warm weather and higher in cold. Salivary flow is higher during standing than sitting and when one is lying down. These postural changes parallel changes in systemic blood pressure. Recent product developments in dental health have led to the creation of kits designed to assess salivary quantity and quality. These materials are currently available and can assess the saliva's viscosity (ability to flow), pH, flow rate, and buffering capacity. Currently, private general dental practitioners do not commonly use these tests. In addition, the test data are rarely routinely collected as part of an oral examination and recorded in a patient record. Although the importance of the presence of adequate saliva is known, very few treatments are available once a salivary problem is diagnosed. Even the treatments that currently exist, such as saliva substitutes and drugs such as cevimeline, are poor substitutes for the real thing.

Stimulated saliva flow results from physiologic, psychologic, pharmacologic, and disease effects.[32,33] Examples of physical stimulation are the simple acts of chewing food and gum. Psychologic stimulation can be evoked by the same anticipation experienced by Pavlov's now famous dogs. Saliva can also be stimulated by the use of cholinergic drugs that increase exocrine gland secretions, such as pilocarpine or cevimeline. Under certain conditions, saliva flow can be abnormally high—a condition termed **sialorrhea** (or *ptyalism*), which is manifested by drooling. Ptyalism can occur with forms of mental impairment and some neurologic conditions and occasionally during pregnancy.

The suppression of salivary flow is more serious. This condition also can result from physiologic, pharmacologic, and/or disease effects. The dry mouth sensation that accompanies panic is an example of a physiologic response. Disease states of the glands include sialoliths (stones) within the gland ducts, resulting in obstruction of saliva flow, Sjögrens syndrome, or postradiation exposure of the glands during cancer therapy.[34,35]

Sjögrens syndrome is an autoimmune disease that typically affects older women. Its primary oral symptom is xerostomia (Figure 9–8 ■). People with xerostomia are at high risk for the development of caries, including caries in unusual places, such as the incisal edges of teeth. Treatment includes the use of drugs such as cevimeline, saliva substitutes, and lots of fluoride. Even with treatment, individuals with compromised salivary glands are usually affected for life.

Organic Components of Saliva

In addition to the secretion of different proportions of electrolytes, salivary glands secrete organic molecules that can be categorized into five major groups: amylase, mucins, phosphoproteins, glycoproteins, and immunoglobulins. Two of the families of small salivary proteins—histidine and statherin—deserve specific mention because they help control the status of calcium and phosphate in the saliva. These proteins prevent fallout

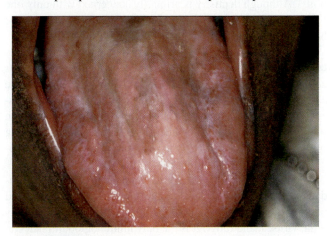

FIGURE ■ 9–8 Xerostomia as seen in a patient with Sjögren's syndrome.

(*Source:* Courtesy of Beth E. McKinney.)

of the calcium and phosphate that maintain supersaturation in relation to hydroxyapatite. They prevent a rapid drop in saliva pH and aid in its faster recovery. In addition, both of these proteins are antifungal and bacteriostatic (i.e., capable of inhibiting bacterial growth without destroying the bacteria).

> **DID YOU KNOW ?**
>
> Saliva can be used to easily and painlessly test for such things as HIV, drugs, DNA, and hormone levels.

The salivary glands also produce various enzymes. Salivary peroxidase reacts with saliva to form the antimicrobial compound hypothiocyanate, which inhibits the capability of the bacteria to fully use glucose. Lactoperoxidase strongly adheres to hydroxyapatite as a component of the acquired pellicle and can influence the qualitative and quantitative characteristics of the microbial population of dental plaque.

Salivary Mucins

The salivary glands secrete **salivary mucins**.[36] The **pellicle** that covers enamel is rich in mucins, which help clear carbohydrates from the mouth and protect against caries. Mucins also help modulate calcium channel activity in the mouth, thereby assisting in the maintenance of tissue integrity. The passage of calcium into and out of cells helps regulate enzymes, such as zinc, that are responsible for tissue repair. It is believed that the presence of salivary mucins and their ability to modulate this activity enhance the repair process in oral soft tissues.

Immunoglobulins

The human body has five categories of immunoglobulins: immunoglobulin M (IgM), immunoglobulin G (IgG), immunoglobulin A (IgA), immunoglobulin D (IgD), and immunoglobulin E (IgE). Immunoglobulins are antibodies made of protein. They, too, defend the body against all types of infection and, sometimes, even when there is no infection (i.e., allergic reactions). Although dentistry is primarily concerned with only one of the immunoglobulins, a brief review of all of them can be helpful in obtaining a basic understanding of their functions.

Immunoglobulin M is located on B cells and is found circulating in the blood. It is the largest of the immunoglobulins and, as such, cannot easily exit the circulatory system. It is the earliest of the group to appear at the site of infection. Its presence in a blood test indicates recent infection. It is also the main immunoglobulin that reacts when someone is given the wrong type of blood during a transfusion. IgM is the first immunoglobulin to be found in a fetus.

Immunoglobulin G has four subtypes. It is the most abundant of the immunoglobulins and is found in both blood and other tissue liquids. Immunoglobulin G is effective against bacteria, viruses, and fungi. It is the only immunoglobulin that can pass through the placenta. This immunoglobulin is also responsible for food allergies and is found in egg yolks (in birds it is called IgY).

> **DID YOU KNOW ?**
>
> Lucy was both right and wrong in her fear of dog germs from Snoopy's licking. Dog bacteria and salivary enzymes are peculiar to dogs and cannot cause either disease or increased healing time in humans. However, dog saliva can possibly transmit diseases such as rabies, roundworms, leptospirosis, salmonella, and *E. coli* to humans.

Immunoglobulin A has two subtypes: serum IgA and secretory IgA (Figure 9–9 ■). Dentistry is most concerned with secretory IgA. All exocrine gland secretions are rich in IgA, and it can be found not only in tears and saliva but also in vaginal fluid and colostrum. Secretory IgA initiates the inflammatory process. It prevents both bacteria and viruses from adhering to mucous membranes. IgA deficiency is the most common type of immunoglobulin deficiency and is seen in autoimmune diseases such as rheumatoid arthritis and lupus.

Immunoglobulin D occurs in the smallest concentrations. Little is known about it, but it is closely linked to IgM and is found on B cells. Its function largely remains a mystery.

Immunoglobulin E is found only in mammals and is widespread throughout the body. It can be found in blood, tissue fluid, and exocrine gland secretions as well as attached to leukocytes, basophils, eosinophils, macrophages, and platelets. It is the major defense against parasitic infections and can also play a role in the defense against cancer cells. This immunoglobulin is responsible for most allergic reactions and for anaphylaxis (a systemic allergic reaction that can be fatal). New allergy therapies that specifically target IgE are being developed.

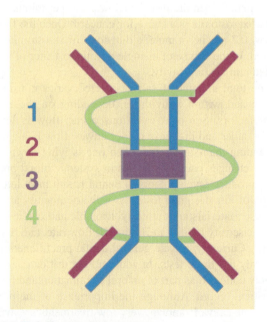

FIGURE ■ **9–9** Immunoglobulin A.

Job's syndrome is also known as "hyper-IgE syndrome"; this rare disorder is characterized by an overabundant production of IgE. Its symptoms are recurrent staphylococcal infections of the skin, lung infections, and some changes in the bone (e.g., scoliosis, or lateral curvature of the spine). The disorder was named for the skin infections that were thought to resemble those suffered by the biblical character Job. This syndrome also has an interesting dental component. The primary dentition does not exfoliate, which can result in two very crowded sets of teeth being present at the same time. Treatment includes chronic antibiotic use for the skin infections and very carefully timed extraction of the primary dentition.

SUMMARY

The oral cavity is intricately connected to the rest of the body. It serves as the entrance to the digestive system and, as such, is never a sterile environment. The oral cavity has a number of host defense mechanisms that operate to prevent infection. Some, such as saliva, are unique to the oral environment. Others, such as cellular and humoral immunity, operate throughout the entire body. Oral disease, as with any other disease, occurs when the challenge posed by pathogens exceeds the body's capability for defense and repair. In the case of dental caries, the defense and self-repair mechanisms of the body operate continuously in the saliva, the plaque, and the enamel. In the case of periodontal disease, the immune system also plays a large part, providing protection as well as causing its own damage. In the case of soft tissue infections (e.g., candidiasis), the epithelial barrier, normal oral flora, and saliva play the biggest roles in preventing infection.

As is readily apparent to even the most inexperienced dentist or dental hygiene clinician, the maintenance of a healthy mouth is not an easy task. All the host protective mechanisms available in the oral cavity are often inadequate for the job. Personal self-care, such as toothbrushing and flossing, is a necessity. The level of self-care needed to achieve and maintain health differs for every individual, depending, in part, on how strong or compromised that person's host defenses are. Regular professional dental care is also usually required to maintain a healthy mouth. This care can include everything from appropriately timed professional prophylaxes to orthodontics to correct malocclusion. The host defense mechanisms in the oral cavity, together with delivery of modern dental care, make dental disease both a preventable and highly treatable disorder.

PRACTICE CONSIDERATIONS

Dental professionals in practice can use information on host defense mechanisms to supplement questions in the health history that can impact a patient's oral condition. Knowledge of the effects of a compromised immune system can allow the practitioner to focus the patient on other helpful therapies in addition to mechanical removal of plaque. An understanding that disease processes might not always be within a patient's direct control and increasing the options offered to patients to improve their oral health beyond just a toothbrush and floss will not only improve patient compliance but also reduce stress and frustration in the practitioner. Finally, an appreciation of the role that the host's body plays in its own response to pathogens and the healing process can help the practitioner to better address cases that do not respond to conventional treatment in a predictable manner. Dentists and hygienists can be more attuned to recognize case "failures" as a potential signal that further investigation into systemic issues is warranted.

SELF-STUDY QUESTIONS

1. Which of the following components is *not* a part of a person's natural oral defenses against infection?

   a. Intact oral epithelium

   b. Saliva

   c. Enamel containing fluorapatite

   d. Class 2 occlusion

   Rationale: Malocclusion in which the teeth are not in proper anatomical relationship is a condition that exacerbates the potential for disease occurrence. Malocclusion should be corrected not only for appearance but also for the promotion of long-term oral health.

2. In which of the following oral disease states is the host's defense response more responsible for tissue destruction than the pathogens themselves?

   a. Dental caries

   b. *Candida albicans*

   c. Periodontal disease

   d. Squamous cell carcinoma

Rationale: Periodontal disease stimulates the immune system to produce a persistent and complicated response that produces more destruction than the bacteria themselves. In fact, the presence of bacteria by themselves is not sufficient to cause periodontal disease.

3. Which of the following is not a function of saliva?

   a. Lubrication

   b. pH buffering

   c. Production of tumor necrosis factor (TNF alpha)

   d. Initial carbohydrate digestion

Rationale: Saliva has many functions including some not listed here, but it does not produce TNF alpha.

4. Which of the following immunoglobulins is of most concern in the practice of dentistry?

   a. IgA

   b. IgG

   c. IgE

   d. IgM

Rationale: IgA is the immunoglobulin present in saliva. It helps to prevent bacteria from adhering to oral tissues but it also stimulates the immune response.

5. If a dental practitioner wanted to incorporate the concept of strengthening the patient's own defense processes in the treatment of dental disease, which of the following components might the practitioner employ in her or his practice?

   a. Sealant placement on the primary dentition

   b. Salivary testing and fortification

   c. Use of antibiotics early in periodontal disease treatment

   d. Placement of dental implants rather than other types of prosthetics

Rationale: Although salivary testing is still in its beginning stages and options to augment poor saliva or replace lost saliva are currently inadequate, this field holds a great deal of promise in helping people maintain oral health.

REFERENCES

1. Jontell, M., Okiji, T., Dahlgren, U., & Bergenholtz, G. (1998). Immune defense mechanisms of the dental pulp. *Crit Rev Oral Biol Med,* 9:179–200.
2. *Stedman's medical dictionary.* (2006). Baltimore, MD: Lippincott Williams & Wilkins.
3. Backer-Dirks, O. (1970). Posteruptive changes in dental enamel. *J Dent Res,* 4:131–48.
4. Tenouvo, J. (1997). Salivary parameters of relevance for assessing caries activity in individuals and populations. *Community Dent Oral Epidemiol,* 25:82–86.
5. Kolenbrander, P., & Palmer, R. (2004). Human oral bacterial biofilms. In Ghannoum, M., & O'Toole, G. A., Eds. *Microbial biofilms.* Washington, DC: ASM Press, 85–117.
6. Laforce, F., Hopkins, J., Trow, R., & Wang, W. (1976). Human oral defenses against gram-negative rods. *Am Rev Respir Dis,* 114:929–35.
7. Kolenbrander, P., Palmer, R., Rickard, A., Jakubovics, N., Chalmers, N., & Diaz, P. (2006). Bacterial interactions and successions during plaque development. *Periodontology 2000,* 42:47–79.
8. Kolenbrander, P., Andersen, R., Blehert, D., Egland, P., Foster, J., & Palmer, R. (2002). Communication among oral bacteria. *Microbiol Molec Biol Rev,* 66:486–505.
9. Edgar, W. M., Higham, S. M., & Manning, R. H. (1994). Saliva stimulation and caries prevention. *Adv Dent Res,* 8:239–45.
10. Dale, B., Kimball, J., Krisanaprakornkit, S., Roberts, F., Robinovitch, M., O'Neal, R., Valore, E., Ganz, T., Anderson, G., & Weinberg, A. (2001). Localized antimicrobial peptide expression in human gingiva. *J Periodontal Res,* 36:285–94.
11. Lehner, T. (1972). Cell-mediated immune responses in oral disease: A review. *J Oral Pathol,* 1:39–58.
12. Lilly, E., Shetty, K., Leigh, J., Cheeks, C., & Fidel, P. (2005). Oral epithelial cell antifungal activity: Approaches to evaluate a broad range of clinical conditions. *Med Mycol,* 43:517–23.
13. Merrell, W., Cripps, A., & Clancy, R. (1980). An overview of immunology with special reference to oral disease. *Aust Dent J,* 25:84–92.
14. Pizzo, G., Lo Re, D., Piscopo, M. R., Pizzo I., & Guiliana G. (2009). Genetic disorders and periodontal health: A literature review. *Med Sci Monit,* 15:167–78.
15. Dale, B., & Fredericks, L. (2005). Antimicrobial peptides in the oral environment: Expression and function in health and disease. *Curr Issues Mol Biol,* 7:119–33.
16. Dunsche, A., Acil, Y., Dommisch, H., Siebert, R., Schroder, J., & Jepsen, S. (2002). The novel human beta-defensin-3 is widely expressed in oral tissues. *Eur J Oral Sci,* 110:121–24.
17. Dunsche, A., Acil, Y., Siebert, R., Harder, J., Schroder, J., & Jepsen, S. (2001). Expression profile of human defensins and antimicrobial proteins in oral tissues. *J Oral Pathol Med,* 30:154–58.
18. Komatsuzawa, H., Ouhara, K., Kawai, T., Yamada, S., Fujiwara, T., Shiba, H., Kurihara, H., Taubman, M.A., & Sugai, M. (2007) Susceptibility of periodontopathogenic and cariogenic bacteria to defensins and potential therapeutic use of defensins in oral diseases. *Curr Pharm Des,* 13:3084–95.
19. Bingle, C., & Gorr, S. (2004). Host defense in oral and airway epithelia: Chromosome 20 contributes a new protein family. *Int J Biochem Cell Biol,* 36:2144–52.
20. Bissell, J., Joly, S., Johnson, G., Organ, C., Dawson, D., McCray, P., & Guthmiller, J. (2004). Expression of beta-defensins in gingival health and in periodontal disease. *J Oral Pathol Med,* 33:278–85.
21. Deo, V., & Bhongade, M.L. Pathogenesis of periodontitis: Role of cytokines in host response. (2010) *Dent Today,* 29:60–66.
22. Ashby, V.T. Inorganic chemistry of defensive peroxidases in the human oral cavity. (2008). *J Dent Res,* 87:900–1014.
23. Bascones-Martinez, A., Munoz-corcuera, M., Noronha, S., Nota, P., Bascones-Ilundain, C., & Campo-Trapero, J. (2009).

Host defense mechanisms against bacterial aggression in periodontal disease: Basic mechanisms. *Med Oral Patol Oral Cir Bucal*, 14:680–85.

24. Tandler, B., Gresick, E. W., Nagoto, T., & Philliss, C. J. (2001). Secretion by striated ducts of mammalian major glands: A review of ultrastructural, functional and evolutionary perspective. *Anat Rec*, 264:125–45.

25. Bardow, A., Madson, J., & Nautofte, B. (2000). The bicarbonate concentration in human saliva does not exceed the plasma level under normal physiological conditions. *Clin Investig*, 42:45–53.

26. Pedersen, A. M., Bardow, A., Jensen, S. B., & Nauntofte, B. (2002). Saliva and gastrointestinal functions of taste, mastication, swallowing and digestion. *Oral Dis*, 8:117–29.

27. Boros, I., Kesler, P., & Zelles, T. (1999). Study of saliva secretion and the salivary fluoride concentration of the human minor labial glands by a new method. *Arch Oral Biol*, 44 (Suppl. 1):511–14.

28. Feruson, D. B. (1999). The flow rate and composition of human labial gland saliva. *Arch Oral Biol*, 44 (Suppl.):1511–14.

29. Lagerof, F., & Oliveby A. (1994). Caries-protective factors in saliva. *Adv Dent Res*, 8:229–38.

30. Dowd, F. J. (1995). Saliva and dental caries. *Dent Clin North Am*, 43:579–97.

31. Lageroff, F. (1998). Saliva: Natural protection against caries. *Rev Belge Med Dent*, 337–481.

32. Chausau, S., Becker, A., Chausau, G., & Sharpiro, J. (2002). Stimulated parotid saliva flow rates in patients with Down syndrome. *Spec Care Dentist*, 103:378–83.

33. Sommers, M. (2003). Response of the body to immunologic challenge. In Price, S., & Wilson, L., Eds. *Pathophysiology: Clinical concepts of disease process* (6th ed.). St. Louis: C.V. Mosby.

34. Salerno, S., Cannizzaro, F., Lo Castro, A., Loinbardo, F., Barress, B., Speciale, R., & Lagalla, R. (2002). Interventional treatment of sialoliths in main salivary glands. *Radiol Med* (Torino), 13:378–83.

35. Stern, Y., Feinmesser, R., Collins, M., Shotts, S. R., & Cotton, R. T. (2002). Bilateral submandibular gland excision and parotid duct ligation for treatment of sialorrhea in children: Long term results. *Arch Otolaryngol Head Neck Surg*, 128:801–803.

36. Slomianyk, B., Murty, V., Piotrowski, J., & Slomiany, A. (1996). Salivary mucins in oral mucosal defense. *Gen Pharmacl*, 27:761–71.

PEARSON myhealthprofessionskit™

Visit www.myhealthprofessionskit.com to access the interactive Companion Website for this textbook. Simply select "Dental Hygiene" from the choice of disciplines. Find this book and log in by using your user name and password to access additional learning tools.

Toothbrushes and Toothbrushing Methods

Christine N. Nathe

KEY TERMS

OBJECTIVES

After studying this chapter, the student will be able to:

1. Describe the history of the toothbrush.
2. Describe manual toothbrush designs including size, shape, and texture.
3. Demonstrate toothbrushing methods and techniques.
4. Describe the rationale for each toothbrushing method.
5. Describe design, methods, and uses of powered toothbrushes.
6. Describe toothbrush efficiency and safety evaluations.
7. Recommend appropriate toothbrushing time and frequency.
8. Determine appropriate time for toothbrush replacement.
9. Demonstrate brush care for dentures, orthodontic appliances, and tongues.

INTRODUCTION

Microbial dental plaque biofilm continually forms on the tooth surfaces and is the primary agent in the development of dental caries and periodontal diseases. If plaque biofilm is completely removed with self-care procedures, dental caries and periodontal diseases can be prevented. Unfortunately, the majority of the population is unable, uninstructed, or unwilling to spend the time to adequately remove plaque from all tooth surfaces. Plaque deposits can be removed either mechanically or chemically. The focus of this chapter is the mechanical removal of plaque by using toothbrushes and toothbrushing techniques.

THE HISTORY OF THE TOOTHBRUSH

The exact origin of mechanical devices for cleaning teeth is unknown. However, since ancient times, individuals have chewed twigs from plants with high aromatic properties. Chewing these twigs freshened breath and spread out fibers at the tips of the twig, which were then used for cleaning the teeth. Toothbrushing twigs actually date back to 3500–3000 B.C. when the Babylonians and the Egyptians made these brushes by fraying the end of a twig. Tombs of the ancient Egyptians containing toothsticks alongside their owners have been found.[1]

In Arabic countries, individuals used a piece of the root of the arak tree because the root fibers stood out like bristles; this device was called a *siwak*. These chew sticks not only helped to physically clean teeth but also helped to prevent plaque development because the fibers contained antibacterial oils and tannins.[2] To this day, the siwak and other chew twigs are used throughout the world to remove plaque. In the seventh century, Mohammed developed rules about oral hygiene and promoted the use of siwak.

During the Tang dynasty (618–907 A.D.), the Chinese invented a toothbrush with a handle and bristles. They used hog bristles similar to those in some contemporary brushes. The premise exists that the Chinese version of the toothbrush spread to Europe when travelers brought it back from China.[3]

In 1780 in England, William Addis manufactured "the first modern toothbrush."[4,5] This brush had a bone handle and holes for placement of natural hog bristles. In the early 1900s, celluloid began replacing the bone handle. This change came about during World War I when bone and hog bristles were in short supply. As a result of this supply issue, nylon bristles were introduced. Initially, nylon bristles were copies of natural bristles in length and thickness; however, they were stiffer than the natural bristles. They did not have the hollow stem of natural bristles; therefore, they did not allow water absorption. Other advantages of nylon bristles, or **filaments**, were the ability to form the bristles in various diameters and shapes and to round the bristle ends to be gentler on gingival tissues. For various reasons, toothbrushing spread throughout the world.

In 1916, Dr. Alfred C. Fones, founder of dental hygiene, wrote a textbook, *Mouth Hygiene,* which specifically directed dental hygienists to teach defined toothbrushing methods to schoolchildren (Figure 10–1 ■). In 1919, the American Academy of Periodontology developed guidelines for both toothbrush design and brushing techniques.[6]

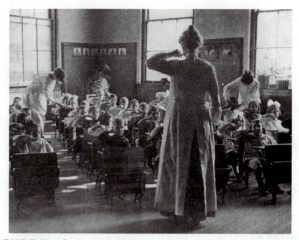

FIGURE ■ 10–1 Fones School of Dental Hygiene instructors and students during a toothbrush drill, circa early 1900s.
(*Source:* Courtesy of Fones School of Dental Hygiene, University of Bridgeport, CT)

DID YOU KNOW ?

The first dental hygienists used to conduct "toothbrush drills" in the schools where they practiced. Students would be supervised to ensure proper brushing techniques.

In 1939, the first power toothbrush was developed in Switzerland. This brush had a power cord and was introduced in the United States in the 1960s by Squibb under the name Broxodent.[7] This product was a great success. Soon afterward, battery-powered brushes were developed and marketed. Unfortunately, problems with these battery-powered products, including short "working times" and mechanical breakdowns, were encountered. The enthusiasm for the powered toothbrush declined and was recommended mainly for those with dexterity problems and developmental disabilities.[7]

In the 1980s, powered toothbrushes were revitalized with the introduction of the InterPlak. Compared with manual toothbrushes, powered toothbrushes have shown an increased **efficacy** (ability to produce a desired effect); this result was consistent in published studies.[5,8–12] Since then, sonic-powered toothbrushes have been developed, and studies continue to report that they remove plaque adequately compared with manual toothbrushes. Most recently, battery-powered, disposable toothbrushes have been introduced.

MANUAL TOOTHBRUSH DESIGNS

Manual toothbrushes vary in size, shape, texture, and design (Figure 10–2 ■).[13] A manual toothbrush consists of a head with bristles and a handle. When the bristles are bunched together, they form **tufts**. The head is arbitrarily divided into the toe, which is at the extreme end of the head, and the heel, which is closest to the handle (Figure 10–3 ■). The shank is a constriction that usually occurs between the handle and the head. The handle

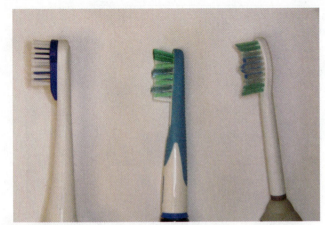

FIGURE ■ 10–2 Lateral profiles of selected toothbrushes.
(*Source:* Courtesy of Christine N. Nathe.)

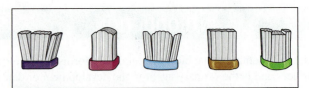

FIGURE ■ 10–4 Cross-sectional profile of five toothbrushes.

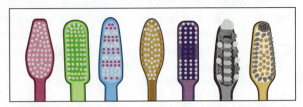

FIGURE ■ 10–5 Overhead appearance of selected toothbrushes.

the head could be most useful for increased cleaning of facial tooth surfaces. Convex shapes with longer bristles in the middle of the head appear more useful for improved cleaning of lingual surfaces.[13] In laboratory and clinical studies, toothbrushes with **multilevel profiles** were consistently more effective, especially when interproximal efficacy was evaluated, than flat profiles in which the bristles are the same length.[8,15–18]

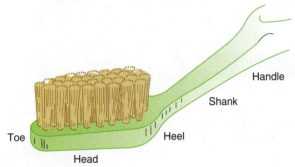
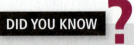

FIGURE ■ 10–3 Parts of a toothbrush.

is the area held by the hand during brushing. Toothbrushes are manufactured in different sizes—large, medium, and small—to adapt better to the oral anatomy of different individuals.[13,14]

DID YOU KNOW ?

The toothbrush is the most commonly used instrument in plaque removal.

Toothbrushes also differ in their defined hardness or texture and are classified as hard, medium, soft, or extra soft. Extra soft and soft toothbrush bristles are preferred because hard bristles damage teeth by causing abrasion of the tooth surface. More recently, toothbrush heads have been altered to vary bristle lengths and placement in attempts to better reach interproximal areas (Figures 10–4 ■ and 10–5 ■). Handles have also been ergonomically designed to accommodate multiple dexterity levels to work efficiently and safely without causing stress to hand muscles or damage to the gingiva.

TOOTHBRUSH PROFILES

When viewed from the side, toothbrushes have four basic lateral profiles: concave, convex, flat, and multileveled rippled or scalloped. The concave shape with shorter bristles in the middle of

NYLON VERSUS NATURAL BRISTLES

The nylon bristle is superior to the natural hog bristle in several aspects. Nylon bristles flex as many as 10 times more often than natural bristles before breaking; they do not split or abrade and are easier to clean. The shape and stiffness of nylon bristles can be standardized. Natural bristle diameters vary greatly in each filament. This can lead to wide variations in the resulting texture.

DID YOU KNOW ?

Mass production of toothbrushes began in the United States around 1885.

BRISTLE SHAPE AND TEXTURE

Nylon bristles can be manufactured in various dimensions that influence their shape and texture. *Texture* is defined as bristle resistance to pressure and is referred to as firmness, stiffness, or hardness. A thinner diameter filament allows the bristle to be softer and more resilient. The usual range of diameters for adult toothbrush bristles is 0.007 to 0.015 inches. The shorter a filament, the stiffer and less flexible it will be. In addition, an increase in the number of bristles within a tuft will make it feel stiffer. Angled filaments may remove direct pressure from the tooth and gingiva and appear to be more flexible. Factors such as temperature, uptake of water, and frequency of use also influence the bristle texture.

End rounding is a term used to describe the heat treatment in which each filament end is sealed and rounded (Figure 10–6 ■). Originally, individual toothbrush bristles were

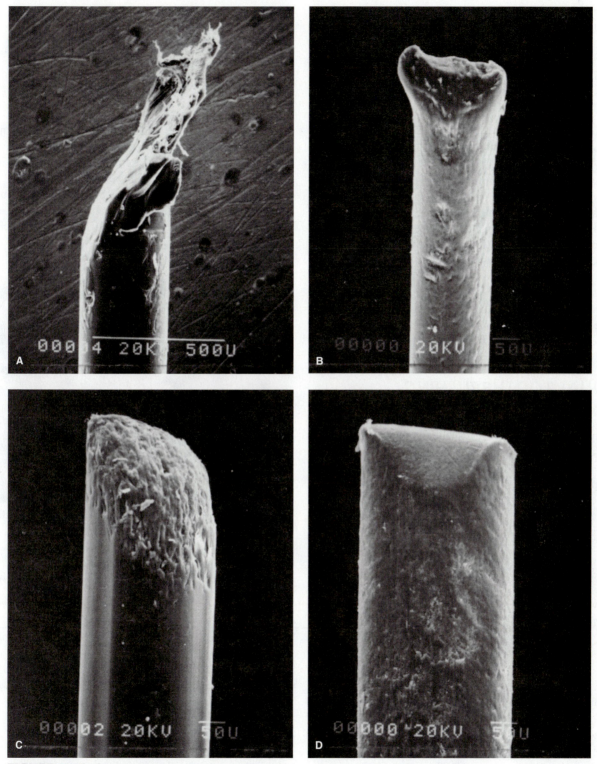

FIGURE ■ 10–6 End rounding of toothbrush bristle.

A: A coarse-cut toothbrush bristle end, probably the result of an incomplete single-blade cut during the manufacturing process. These sharp projections can reduce the bristles' overall cleaning efficiency and damage oral tissues.

B. A slightly enlarged, bulbous nylon bristle end, resulting from a double-blade or scissor cut during the manufacturing process.

C. A tapered or round-end nylon bristle produced by heat or a mechanical polishing process.

D. The scrubbing, mechanical action of a toothbrush wear machine has nicely rounded off this bristle removed from a brush that was originally coarse cut.

(*Source:* Courtesy of K. K. Park, B. A. Matis, A. G. Christen, Indiana University Dental School.)

cut bluntly and often had sharp ends. In 1948, Bass reported that these bristle tips could damage the soft tissues and that rounded, tapered, or smooth bristle tips were less abrasive.[19] Although Bass's research was not performed according to strict research protocol, his findings have remained undisputed for more than 60 years. To this day, end-rounded tips are recommended for the safety of hard and soft oral tissues.[20]

HANDLE DESIGNS

Most toothbrushes have some type of plastic handle. The plastic allows the handle to be durable and resistant to water. Plastic is also inexpensive and easily manipulated for an attractive design. Handle design and length can provide comfort and compliance during toothbrushing (Figure 10–7 ■). These factors have been documented to improve the quality of toothbrushing, particularly in children whose dexterity is not highly developed.[8,9] The most important aspects of a toothbrush handle are that it is easy to hold and does not slip or rotate during use and that it does not have sharp corners or projections. Angled shanks may help to adapt the brush into hard-to-reach areas of the mouth.

MANUAL TOOTHBRUSHING METHODS

The purposes of toothbrushing include (1) removal of plaque biofilm and disturbance of plaque re-formation, (2) removal of food, debris, and stain from the oral cavity, (3) stimulation of the gingival tissues, and (4) application of a toothpaste containing specific ingredients to prevent demineralization of tooth structure, periodontal diseases, and tooth sensitivity or to attain remineralization of demineralized tooth structures.

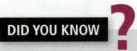

DID YOU KNOW

More people use blue toothbrushes than red toothbrushes.

During the last 50 years, many toothbrushing methods have been introduced, and most are identified by an individual's name, such as Bass, Stillman, or Fones, or by a term indicating a primary action to be followed, such as "roll" or "scrub" (Table 10–1 ■). The most natural brushing methods used by patients are a reciprocating horizontal scrub technique, a rotary motion such as the Fones technique, or the Leonard technique,

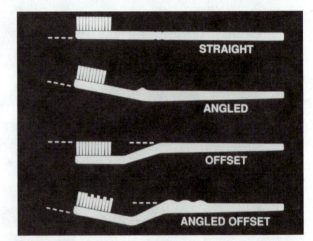

FIGURE ■ 10–7 Four basic shapes of toothbrush handles.

(*Source:* Courtesy of *Journal of Clinical Dentistry.*)

TABLE ■ 10–1 Manual Toothbrushing Methods

Technique	Bristle Position	Brushing Motion	Effect Claimed
Bass	At 45 degrees with tips in sulcus	Vibratory, horizontal jiggle	Subgingival cleansing, gingival stimulation
Rolling	Apically against attached gingiva	Swept in arc toward occlusal surface	Supragingival cleansing, gingival stimulation
Stillman	Against apical part of gingiva and cervical part of tooth	Vibratory, pulsing strokes	Gingival stimulation
Charters	With tips toward occlusal plane	Circular, vibratory strokes	Gingival stimulation, interproximal cleansing
Fones	At 90 degrees to tooth	Large circles over teeth and gingiva	Supragingival cleansing, gingival stimulation
Leonard	At 90 degrees to tooth	Vertical strokes	Supragingival cleansing, gingival stimulation
Horizontal	At 90 degrees to tooth	Horizontal strokes	Supragingival cleansing, gingival stimulation
Smith	At occlusal surface	Sweep toward gingiva	Supragingival cleansing
Modified (in combination with a previously mentioned method)		Sweep toward occlusal surface	Supragingival cleansing

(*Source:* Toothbrush Focus. *Dimensions of Dental Hygiene.* 2007; 5(5):24–25.)

a simple up-and-down motion over the maxillary and mandibular teeth.[21–23] All of these techniques are able to adequately clean the facial, lingual, and to some extent, the occlusal surfaces of the teeth; all, however, are relatively ineffective in cleaning interproximal areas. Only the Bass technique is effective in cleaning the sulcus.

Bass Method

The **Bass method** is acceptable for all patients, specifically for those with periodontal involvement. This method is effective at removing plaque at the gingival margin and directly below it. The toothbrush bristles are angled apically at a 45-degree angle to the long axis of the tooth. The filaments are then gently placed subgingivally into the sulcus. With very light pressure, the brush is vibrated with very short horizontal strokes while keeping the bristles in the sulcus. After several vibrations, the bristles are removed from the sulcus, and the brush is repositioned on the next two or three teeth (Figure 10–8 ■).

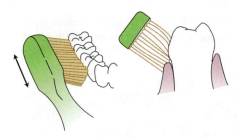

FIGURE ■ 10–8 Bass technique.

Rolling Method

The **rolling technique** is most appropriate for children whose dexterity is not sufficient to master the Bass technique. The bristles are positioned apically along the long axis of the tooth. The edge of the brush head should be touching the facial or lingual aspect of the tooth. Then with light pressure, the bristles are rolled against the tooth from the apical position toward the occlusal plane. This motion is repeated several times; then the brush is repositioned on the next teeth with bristles overlapping a portion of the teeth previously cleaned. The heel or toe of the brush is used on the lingual aspect of the anterior teeth (Figure 10–9 ■).

Stillman Method

The **Stillman method** was originated to massage and stimulate the gingiva while cleansing the cervical areas. The bristles are positioned apically along the long axis of the tooth. The edge of the brush head should be touching the facial or lingual aspect of the tooth. A slight blanching effect should be seen; then the brush is slightly rotated at a 45-degree angle and vibrated over the crown (Figure 10–10 ■).

Charters Technique

The **Charters technique** is effective for cleaning around devices used to correct improper contact of opposing teeth (orthodontic appliances) and plaque under abutment teeth of a fixed bridge. The bristles are placed at a 45-degree angle toward the occlusal or incisal surface of the tooth. The bristles should touch at the junction of the free gingival margin and tooth. A circular vibratory motion is then activated (Figure 10–11 ■).

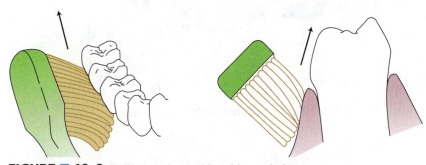

FIGURE ■ 10–9 Rolling stroke toothbrushing technique.

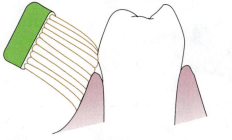

FIGURE ■ 10–10 Stillman toothbrushing technique seen diagrammatically.

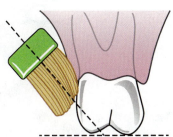

FIGURE ■ 10–11 Charters toothbrushing technique.

Fones Method

The **Fones method** is not to be used by adults but can be an easy technique for young children to learn. The teeth are clenched, and the brush is placed inside the cheeks. The brush is moved in a circular motion over both maxillary and manibular teeth. In the anterior region, the teeth are placed in an edge-to-edge position and the circular motion is continued. On the lingual aspect, an in-and-out stroke is used against all surfaces. This technique can be damaging if done too vigorously (Figure 10–12 ■).

Leonard Technique

In the **Leonard technique**, the toothbrush is placed at a 90-degree angle to the long axis of the tooth. The teeth are held in an edge-to-edge position. Next the toothbrush is moved in a vertical, vigorous motion up and down the teeth. The maxillary and mandibular teeth are brushed separately (Figure 10–13 ■).

Horizontal Technique

In the **horizontal technique**, the teeth are placed edge to edge while the brush maintains a 90-degree angle to the long axis of the tooth. The brush is then moved in a horizontal stroke. This technique is known to cause excessive toothbrush abrasion (Figure 10–14 ■).

Smith Method

The **Smith method** is a physiologic technique that follows the pattern that food follows when it is in the mouth during mastication. The bristles are positioned directly onto the occlusal surface. The brush is then moved back and forth with the bristles reaching from the occlusal surface to the gingiva. Smith

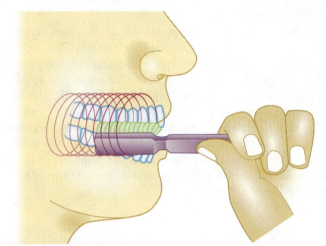

FIGURE ■ 10–12 Fones toothbrushing technique: Circulatory motion extending from maxillary to mandibular teeth.

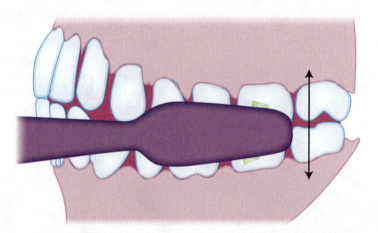

FIGURE ■ 10–13 Leonard toothbrushing technique.

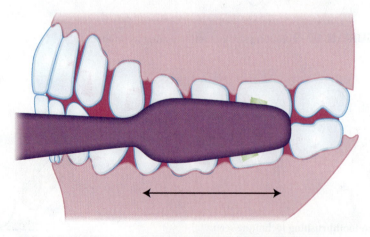

FIGURE ■ 10–14 Horizontal toothbrushing technique.

also recommends a few gentle horizontal strokes to clean the sulcus areas near furcations (Figure 10–15 ■).

Scrub Toothbrushing Technique

The **scrub toothbrushing technique** is a combination of horizontal, vertical, and circular strokes. It also incorporates vibration movements in certain areas. This is not an appropriate method to choose, and care should be taken with this technique to avoid excessive pressure (Figure 10–16 ■).

Modified Brushing Technique

In attempts to enhance brushing of the entire facial and lingual tooth surfaces, the original techniques have been modified. The **modified brushing technique** integrates a rolling stroke after use of the vibratory motion to any type of brushing method. The position of the brush is maintained after the completion of the original method's stroke. The bristles are then rolled coronally over the gingiva and teeth. During this rolling motion, care should be taken that some of the filaments reach the interdental areas.

POWERED TOOTHBRUSHES

Design

Powered toothbrushes were first advertised in *Harper's Weekly* in February 1886[10] but did not become a factor in the U.S. marketplace until Broxadent was introduced in the 1960s.

Since then, the design of the powered toothbrush has changed significantly (Figure 10–17 ■). Today powered toothbrushes can be categorized as mechanical, sonic, or ionic. A **mechanical brush** literally uses the motion of the bristles to remove the plaque and debris. The sonic toothbrush emits sound waves in addition to the movement of the filaments. The vibration is said to help loosen the plaque and food particles for removal. Lastly, the ionic toothbrushes are believed to temporarily reverse the negative ionic charge of a tooth to a positive charge. A portion of the toothbrush that is also positively charged is thought to attract the plaque and food particles away from the tooth, allowing bristles to brush the loosened particles away.

The main patterns of movements in the modern powered toothbrushes are oscillation, reciprocation, and rotational. The **oscillation movement** takes the bristles in a consistent back-and-forth movement. Next reciprocation moves the bristles up and down or back and forth. Lastly, rotational movements are circular. The category of sonic powered toothbrushes refers to the speed at which the bristles move (Figure 10–18 ■).

Powered toothbrushes also have varied power sources. A direct source brush has a cord that can be plugged into an electrical outlet. Although this type of brush will never slow because of a lack of power, the cord could interfere with the toothbrushing technique. Battery-powered brushes, as well as rechargeable battery-powered brushes, are also available. The battery-powered brushes' initial cost is low, but the cost of battery replacement could add up. In addition,

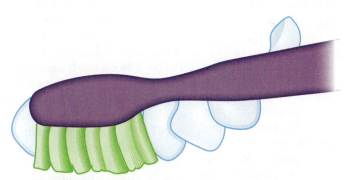

FIGURE ■ **10–15** Smith toothbrushing technique.

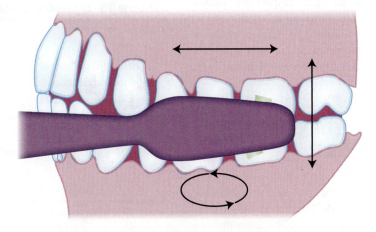

FIGURE ■ **10–16** Scrub toothbrushing technique.

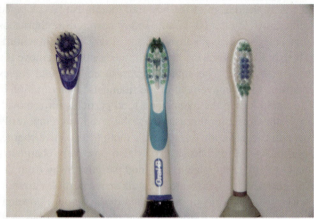

FIGURE ■ 10–17 Selected power toothbrushes, from left to right: Crest SpinBrush; Oral-B Sonic Complete; Sonicare Elite.

(*Source:* Courtesy of Christine N. Nathe.)

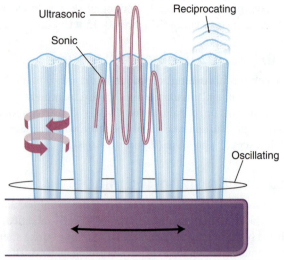

FIGURE ■ 10–18 Movements of power-assisted toothbrushes.

the batteries can corrode if they come in contact with water. With the rechargeable style, the charger may be bulky and must accompany the toothbrush. Some brushes come with a switch that the patient must hold down while the toothbrush is in operation. This brush could cause difficulty for patients who have dexterity problems.

The speed of a powered toothbrush varies widely. The movements of the typical reciprocating brushes can range from 3,800 to 7,600 pluses per minute. In comparison, the action of a pulsation-type head can produce approximately 40,000 pulses per minute.

Powered Toothbrush Methods and Uses

Most powered toothbrush manufacturers do not recommend a specific brushing method. However, some guidelines for using a powered brush are available. It is recommended that the brush be positioned slightly differently for each surface of the tooth. Each tooth and corresponding gingival areas should be brushed separately, always with light, steady pressure. Pressure should never be exerted on the bristles of a powered toothbrush because this could damage the tissues.

Powered toothbrushes can be beneficial for a variety of reasons. Their brushes have been found helpful for parents who brush their children's teeth. Powered toothbrushes are especially helpful for people who have disabilities or dexterity issues. These brushes are also highly recommended for patients who require a larger handle because powered models are easier to grasp.

TOOTHBRUSH EFFICIENCY AND SAFETY EVALUATIONS

Published testing methods are now available to evaluate both safety and efficacy of manual and powered toothbrushes. Differences between products can be determined and, in several areas, are predictive of clinical results. The areas that are

evaluated are listed in Table 10–2 ■. These tests can be predictive of the products' ability to remove clinical plaque and can report clinical differences between toothbrush designs.[8,9,18] As far as safety is concerned in powered toothbrushes, a large body of published research in the preceding two decades has consistently shown oscillating-rotating toothbrushes to be safe compared to manual toothbrushes, demonstrating that these powered toothbrushes do not pose a clinically relevant concern to hard or soft tissues.[24]

Even with these evaluation methods, clinical advantages of various toothbrush-head configurations for removing dental plaque and debris (i.e., cleaning efficacy) have been difficult to substantiate. This problem is attributed to the wide variations in how patients brush their teeth, such as the amount of toothbrushing time, type of motion, and amount of applied pressure. The shape and number of teeth also vary among patients. Published studies on the clinical superiority of newly designed manual or powered toothbrush have been inconsistent.

One study revealed that a powered toothbrush was significantly more effective than a manual toothbrush in the reduction of plaque after two and four weeks of product use and

TABLE ■ 10–2   Toothbrush laboratory testing procedures

Toothbrush evaluation

- Abrasion
- Depth of deposit removal
- Distal surface cleaning
- Gingival margin cleaning
- Efficacy of interproximal access
- Polishing
- Removal of smooth surface (area) deposit
- Stain removal
- Efficacy of subgingival ACCESS

(*Source:* Toothbrush Focus. *Dimensions of Dental Hygiene.* 2007; 5(5):24–25.)

significantly more effective in the reduction of gingivitis and bleeding sites than a manual toothbrush after four weeks.[25] However, a systematic review reported that in general there was no evidence of a statistically significant difference between powered and manual brushes. However, rotation oscillation powered brushes significantly reduce plaque and gingivitis in both the short and long-term. The clinical significance of this reduction is not known.[26]

TOOTHBRUSHING TIME AND FREQUENCY

For many years, dental providers advised patients to brush their teeth after every meal. Research has indicated that, if plaque is completely removed every other day, no harmful effects will occur in the oral cavity.[27] On the other hand, very few individuals completely remove plaque; therefore, frequent brushing is still extremely important and recommended. These repeated brushings will maximize sulcular cleaning as a measure to control periodontal diseases and introduce more frequent use of fluoride toothpastes to control caries. In areas with periodontal pockets, even more frequent oral hygiene procedures are indicated to decrease infection.

Thorough toothbrushing requires a different amount of time for each individual, depending on such factors as the tendency to accumulate plaque and debris; the individual's psychomotor skills; and the adequacy of clearance of foods, bacteria, and debris by the saliva. Often a compromise is made by suggesting 5 to 10 strokes in each area or by advocating the use of a timer. A patient should be encouraged to brush for up to 2 minutes and, if necessary, to use a timing device. In addition, many powered toothbrushes are designed with built-in timers that signal the patient when to move to another area of the mouth; the timers shut off when the designated number of minutes has passed.

A routine brushing pattern should also be established to avoid exclusion of any area. One systematic pattern is to begin with the distal surface of the most posterior tooth and to continue brushing the surfaces around the maxillary arch until the last molar on the other side of the arch has been reached. The mandibular arch is then brushed in a similar manner. Explaining to the patient that the bristles should always overlap previously cleaned teeth is important.

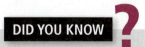

DID YOU KNOW ?

The average American spends an average of 38.5 total days brushing teeth over her or his lifetime.

Patients tend to apportion more time and effort on the facial areas of the anterior teeth.[28] Often, right-handed people do not brush the right side of the arch as well as the left side; left-handed people similarly neglect the left side of the arch.

Patients should be instructed on specific brushing tips on an individualized manner to their brushing needs.

CLINICAL ASSESSMENTS OF TOOTHBRUSHING

Whatever techniques are recommended, the main purpose of toothbrushing is to remove dental plaque biofilm from the teeth and the gingival crevice without damaging the teeth and surrounding structures. Disclosing agents provide a means of evaluating the thoroughness of cleaning the teeth.[29]

Disclosing agents, or disclosants, can be in either a liquid or tablet form. They allow the patient to see plaque in the mouth before or after brushing. These agents can give patients a literal road map to remove the plaque. The chewable tablet or the liquid disclosant should be swished around in the mouth for 15 to 30 seconds and then expectorated. Home use of disclosants by the patient can be encouraged to permit self-evaluation of the effectiveness of plaque-control programs.

Toothbrush abrasion, or the wearing away of oral tissues as a result of toothbrushing, can occur from the use of highly abrasive toothpastes, brush bristles that are too firm, incorrect brushing methods, or excessive pressure during brushing. Common abrasion locations are on the facial surfaces of the teeth and on the cervical areas of exposed root surfaces. Measures to reduce progression of the abrasion include the use of soft-bristled brushes, changes in brush angulation, the use of less-abrasive toothpastes, and application of less pressure during brushing.

One study reported that when brushing with water, the harder toothbrush caused more abrasion, but when adding the toothpaste, the softer toothbrush caused more abrasion. This study also suggested that a softer toothbrush can cause as much and in some cases more abrasion than harder ones. When researchers conduct abrasivity studies, it is important to look at both the quantitative and qualitative aspect of abrasivity.[30]

Toothbrush abrasion should not be confused with dental erosion, which is the irreversible loss of tooth structure due to chemical dissolution by acids not of bacterial origin. Possible casues of dental erosion include the ingestion of acidic foods and beverages such as citrus fruits, soft drinks, and wine. Other possible sources of erosion could be regurgitation of gastic acids as seen in patients with gastroesophageal reflux disease (GERD) and from exposure to chlorinated swimming pool water.

Loss of tooth substance in the cervical region usually has been attributed to toothbrush abrasion or dental erosion or a combination of both factors. Recently the role of occlusal loading, termed *abfractions,* has become increasingly prominent.[31] The abfraction theory focuses on the potential role of occlusal loading in the loss of cervical tooth tissue so that management of the occlusion can be incorporated into a treatment plan for patients with wearing away of the cervical tooth structure.[31]

TOOTHBRUSH REPLACEMENT

Toothbrush wear (e.g., splayed, bent, or broken bristles) is influenced more by the brushing method than by the length of time or number of toothbrushings per day. The average life of a manual toothbrush is 2 to 3 months. This estimate can vary greatly depending on brushing habits. It is also sound advice for patients to have several toothbrushes and to rotate the use of them to ensure use of a dry brush. Toothbrushes can become contaminated. Drying the toothbrush gives a less favorable environment for the contaminants to survive. In addition to regular replacement, replacement after contagious illness is imperative.

TONGUE BRUSHING

The tongue is anatomically perfect for harboring bacteria. The fungiform (mushroom-shaped) papillae create elevations and depressions in the tongue, which can house debris and microorganisms. A patient with a fissured tongue (deep grooves on the tongue surface) is more prone to accumulate bacterial plaque and debris. The tongue can transmit organisms during toothbrushing and infection or reinfection of a periodontal pocket. Interestingly, halitosis (oral malodor, or bad breath) most often originates on the tongue. For these reasons, the tongue, especially those with fissuring or prominent papilla, should be regularly cleaned.

The brushing of the tongue helps reduce the debris, plaque, and number of oral microorganisms. Appropriate technique involves placing the head of the toothbrush near the middle of the tongue, with the bristles pointed toward the throat. Then the tongue is extruded, and the brush is swept forward. This motion is repeated six to eight times across the entire tongue. Using a toothpaste on the brush helps the cleansing action.[32]

Commercial tongue cleaners, made of plastic or a flexible metal, are also available. They are curved so they can be placed over the tongue without touching the teeth. These instruments are swept over the dorsum of the tongue to remove bacterial plaque and debris.

THE AMERICAN DENTAL ASSOCIATION ACCEPTANCE PROGRAM

The American Dental Association (ADA) acceptance program is a voluntary program for evaluation of toothbrushes.[33] Companies may submit their toothbrushes and, if the brushes meet the ADA criteria, the companies may use the ADA Seal of Acceptance as a marketing tool on their toothbrush package and in advertisements. As always, dental providers should recommend products that they have thoroughly evaluated.

SUMMARY

A toothbrush is the primary instrument used for oral hygiene care. There are many different types of toothbrushes manual and powered toothbrushes with each having various designs of the handle, head, and bristles. These variations all have unique benefits.

The several different toothbrushing methods remove plaque most efficiently, depending on the patient and the anatomy of the oral cavity. Any method that is taught should be effective and used routinely and should not damage hard or soft tissues or cause excessive tooth wear. In initiating effective toothbrushing, it is necessary to (1) select the appropriate toothbrush(es) for the patient, (2) create individual goals for toothbrushing and explain the need for good oral hygiene, (3) teach a technique or combination of brushing methods necessary to meet established goals, and (4) assess and refine toothbrushing techniques as a part of the total oral hygiene program.

PRACTICAL CONSIDERATIONS

The most common questions that patients ask dental providers pertain to toothbrush effectiveness and proper toothbrushing techniques. Individually, toothbrush types and methods are important parts of a dental prevention regimen. Toothbrushing remains one of the constants in preventive modalities for the removal of dental plaque.

SELF-STUDY QUESTIONS

1. A patient with a fissured tongue (deep grooves on the tongue surface) is more prone to accumulate bacterial plaque and debris. The tongue can transmit organisms during toothbrushing and infection or reinfection of a periodontal pocket.

   a. The first statement is true; the second statement is false.

   b. The first statement is false; the second statement is true.

   c. Both statements are true.

   d. Both statements are false.

Rationale: A patient with a fissured tongue (deep grooves on the tongue surface) is more prone to accumulate bacterial plaque and debris. The tongue can transmit organisms during toothbrushing as well as infection or reinfection of a periodontal pocket.

2. A mechanical brush literally uses which of the following to remove the plaque and debris?

   a. Oscillation of the brush

   b. Reciprocation of the brush

   c. Motion of the bristles

   d. Tuft spins of the bristles

   Rationale: A mechanical brush literally uses the motion of the bristles to remove the plaque and debris.

3. The American Dental Association (ADA) acceptance program is a mandatory program for evaluation of toothbrushes. Companies may submit their toothbrushes and, if the brushes meet the ADA criteria, the company may use the ADA Seal of Acceptance as a marketing tool on its toothbrush package and in advertisements.

   a. The first statement is true; the second statement is false.

   b. The first statement is false; the second statement is true.

   c. Both statements are true.

   d. Both statements are false.

   Rationale: The American Dental Association (ADA) acceptance program is a voluntary program for evaluation of toothbrushes. Companies may submit their toothbrushes and, if they meet the ADA criteria, the company may use the ADA Seal of Acceptance as a marketing tool on its toothbrush package and in advertisements.

4. If plaque biofilm is completely removed with self-care procedures, which of the following diseases can be prevented?

   a. Dental caries

   b. Oral cancer

   c. Asthma

   d. No disease can be prevented

   Rationale: If plaque biofilm is completely removed with self-care procedures, dental caries and periodontal diseases can be prevented.

5. Which is the term that describes the heat treatment in which each filament end is sealed and rounded?

   a. Tuft bristling

   b. End rounding

   c. Tuft rounding

   d. End bristling

   Rationale: *End rounding* is a term used to describe the heat treatment in which each filament end is sealed and rounded. Originally, individual toothbrush bristles were cut bluntly and often had sharp ends. In 1948, Bass reported that these bristle tips could damage the soft tissues and that rounded, tapered, or smooth bristle tips were less abrasive.

REFERENCES

1. History of Toothbrushes and Toothpastes. Retrieved November 18, 2011, from http://www.colgate.com/app/CP/US/EN/OC/Information/Articles/Oral-and-Dental-Health-Basics/Oral-Hygiene/Brushing-and-Flossing/article/History-of-Toothbrushes-and-Toothpastes.cvsp.

2. Hattab, F. N. (1997). Meswak: The natural toothbrush. *J Clin Dent,* 8:125–29.

3. "Who invented the toothbrush and when was it invented?" The Library of Congress. 2007-04-04. Retrieved April 12, 2008 from http://www.loc.gov/rr/scitech/mysteries/tooth.html.

4. Golding, P. S. (1982). The development of the toothbrush. A short history of tooth cleansing. *Dent Health* (London), 21:25–27.

5. Smith, C. (2000). Toothbrush technology—Even the Pharaohs brushed their teeth. *J Dent Technol,* 17:26, 27.

6. American Academy of Periodontology. (1920, March). Committee report: The tooth brush and methods of cleaning the teeth. *Dent Items Interest,* 42, 193.

7. Penick, C. (2004). Power toothbrushes: A critical review. *Int J Dent Hygiene,* 2:40–44.

8. Saxer, U. P., & Yankell, S. L. (1997). Impact of improved toothbrushes on dental diseases. I. *Quintessence Int,* 28:513–25.

9. Saxer, U. P., & Yankell, S. L. (1997). Impact of improved toothbrushes on dental diseases. II. *Quintessence Int,* 28:573–93.

10. Ring, M. E. (1985). *Dentistry: An illustrated history.* St. Louis: C.V. Mosby, 1–319.

11. Boyd, R. L. (1997). Clinical and laboratory evaluation of powered electric toothbrushes: Review of the literature. *J Clin Dent,* 8:67–71.

12. Warren, P. R., Smith, R. T., Cugini, M., & Chater, B. V. (2000). A practice-based study of a power toothbrush: Assessment of effectiveness and acceptance. *JADA,* 131:389–94.

13. Yankell, S. L., & Emling, R. C. (1978). Understanding dental products: What you should know and what your patient should know. *Univ Pa Cont Dent Educ,* 1:1–43.

14. Mintel, T. E., & Crawford, J. (1992). The search for a superior toothbrush design technology. *J Clin Dent,* 3:C1–C4.

15. Volpe, A. R., Emling, R. C., & Yankell, S. L. (1992). The toothbrush—A new dimension in design, engineering and clinical evaluation. *J Clin Dent,* 3:S29–S32.

16. Volpenhein, D. W., Handel, S. E., Hughes, T. J., & Wild, J. (1996). A comparative evaluation of the in vitro penetration performance of the improved Crest Complete toothbrush versus the current

Crest Complete toothbrush, the Colgate Precision toothbrush and the Oral-B P40 toothbrush. *J Clin Dent,* 7:21–25.

17. Saxer, U. P., & Yankell, S. L. (1997). A review of laboratory methods to determine toothbrush safety and efficacy. *J Clin Dent,* 8:114–19.

18. Beals, D., Ngo, T., Feng, Y., Cook, D., Grau, D. J., & Weber, D. A. (2000). Development and laboratory evaluation of a new toothbrush with a novel brush head design. *Am J Dent,* 13:5A–14A.

19. Bass, C. C. (1948). The optimum characteristics of toothbrushes for personal oral hygiene. *Dent Items Int,* 70:697–718.

20. Drisko, C., Henderson, R., & Yancy, J. (1995, July). A review of current toothbrush bristle endo-rounding studies. *Compend Contin Educ Dent,*16:694, 696–98.

21. Tsamtsouris, A., White, C. E., & Clark, E. R. (1979). The effect of instruction and supervised tooth brushing on the reduction of dental plaque in kindergarten children. *J Dent Child,* 465:204–209.

22. Home care of the mouth. (1934). In Fones, A. C., Ed. *Mouth hygiene* (4th ed.). Philadelphia, PA: Lea & Febiger, 294–315.

23. Leonard, H. J. (1939). Conservative treatment of periodontoclasia. *JADA,* 26:1308–18.

24. Van der Weijden, F. A., Campbell, S. L., Dörfer, C. E., González-Cabezas, C., & Slot, D. E. (2011, January). Safety of oscillating-rotating powered brushes compared to manual toothbrushes: A systematic review. (Epub 2010). *J Periodontal,* 82:5–24.

25. Moritis, K., Jenkins, W., Hefti, A., Schmitt, P., & McGrady, M. (2008). A randomized, parallel design study to evaluate the effects of a Sonicare and a manual toothbrush on plaque and gingivitis. *J Clin Dent,* 19:64-68.

26. Deery, C., Heanue, M., Deacon, S., Robinson, P. G., Walmsley, A. D., Worthington, H., Shaw, W., & Glenny, A. M. (2004, March). The effectiveness of manual versus powered toothbrushes for dental health: A systematic review. *J Dent,* 32: 197–211.

27. Lang, K. P., Cumming, B. R., & Löe, H. (1973). Tooth brushing frequency as it relates to plaque development and gingival health. *J Periodontol,* 44:396–405.

28. Tsamtsouris, A. (1978). Effectiveness of tooth brushing. *J Pedod,* 2:296–303.

29. Carranza, F. A., & Newman, M. G., Eds. (1996). *Clinical periodontology* (8th ed.) Philadelphia, PA: W.B. Saunders, 1–1033.

30. Tellefsen, G., Lilioborg, A., Johannsen, A., & Johannsen, G. (2011, November). The role of the toothbrush in the abrasion process. *Int Jour Dent Hyg,* 9:284–290.

31. Rees, J. S., & Jagger, D. C. (2003). J Abfraction lesions: Myth or reality? *Esthet Restor Dent,* 15:263–71.

32. Christen, A. G., & Swanson, B. Z., Jr. (1978). Oral hygiene: A history of tongue scraping and brushing. *J Am Dent Assoc,* 96:215–19.

33. ADA Seal: Frequently asked questions. Chicago: American Dental Association. Retrieved on September 6, 2012 from http://www.ada.org/adasealfaq.aspx.

Dentifrices, Mouthrinses, and Chewing Gums

Meg Horst Zayan

OBJECTIVES

After studying this chapter, the student should be able to:

1. Differentiate between a cosmetic and a therapeutic dentifrice, mouthrinse, and chewing gum.

2. Explain the three phases of research necessary when applying to investigate a new drug.

3. Discuss how approval or nonapproval of a new product by the Food and Drug Administration (FDA) differs from acceptance or rejection by the American Dental Association (ADA).

4. List and define the purpose of each dentifrice ingredient including percentage quantities.

5. Explain the various reasons that the same abrasive material in toothpaste can cause different levels of abrasion on tooth structure.

6. Define the three types and amounts of fluoride compounds commonly used in dentifrices.

7. Identify the agents used in dentifrices to produce anticaries, anticalculus, whitening, and antihypersensitivity effects.

8. Explain the active ingredients in antiplaque and antigingivitis mouthrinses sold over the counter and as a prescription item.

9. Describe the advantages and disadvantages of mouthrinses containing alcohol.

10. Describe the benefits of chewing gum and the ingredients used to help reduce oral disease.

KEY TERMS

INTRODUCTION

Dentifrices and mouthrinses are major products for routinely administering effective cosmetic and therapeutic agents in the mouth. **Dentifrices** (toothpastes) are substances used to clean the teeth. **Mouthrinses** are used to flush food debris from the oral cavity, freshen breath, or if fluoridated, to deposit fluoride on the teeth. These products are the most widely used by consumers, generating the largest sales of all dental products. **Chewing gums** are a newer category of products with cosmetic claims and the ability to deliver therapeutic compounds.

Dentifrices and mouthrinses differ considerably. Dentifrices are complex and difficult to formulate. Tremendous innovations have occurred in the past 25 years in the appearance and packaging of dentifrices. The contemporary consumer faces many alternatives in appearance (pastes, gels, stripes) and packaging (conventional tubes, stand-up tubes, pumps) as well as products marketed specifically for children and adults. In addition, numerous claims are made for dentifrices including the prevention or reduction of calculus formation, dental caries, plaque, gingivitis, **hypersensitivity**, and the ability to whiten teeth. Because the public routinely uses dentifrices one to three times per day, they could be the most beneficial dental products. Some of this benefit can be lost when patients rinse immediately after brushing because rinsing decreases the concentration or reservoir of the active agent in the oral cavity.

Mouthrinses are available in liquid form, the traditional method for stabilizing and delivering many pharmaceutically active agents. Mouthrinses are considered by consumers to have primarily cosmetic benefits (i.e., breath freshening); therefore, mouthrinses are not used as frequently or routinely as dentifrices in the daily oral-hygiene regimen. The Food and Drug Administration (FDA) has approved products that contain **chlorhexidine**, a therapeutic agent in mouthrinses as prescription-only products.

Chewing gums have the potential to be used by the consumer for periods of 5 to 20 minutes several times a day or until the flavor of the product dissipates. This product form enables delivery of a cosmetic or therapeutic agent for a longer time than do dentifrices or mouthrinses. In addition to prolonged delivery of an agent, chewing gums stimulate salivary flow, which can provide a buffer effect and ensure removal of debris from occlusal and interproximal sites. To ensure safety and avoid harmful gastrointestinal effects, active agents delivered by chewing gums must be safe for swallowing at the dose delivered in one use or contained in the entire product sold in one package.

SAFETY AND EFFICACY

Caution is needed before introducing a new therapeutic product to the market. Some of the concerns surrounding new products are: Will the active agent disrupt the "normal" bacterial balance of the mouth? Should the search for an ideal agent focus on depressing or eliminating specific disease-related organisms or a broad spectrum of organisms? Should a product be used to preserve a disease-free state while risking possible development of drug resistance? Regardless of the apparent effectiveness of any new product in the laboratory or in controlled clinical studies, the public safety of the product is paramount because it will have widespread availability and will be used unsupervised by consumers.

Various processes exist by which oral-care agents are evaluated and regulated in the United States to ensure standards for safety and efficacy standards. These standards apply not only to prescription medications but also to over-the-counter (OTC) drugs. There are two government levels of regulation of oral chemotherapeutic agents (chemical substances or drugs). These levels include the Food and Drug Administration (FDA) and the Federal Trade Commission (FTC). The FDA regulates the safety, efficacy, and security of OTC and prescription drugs, and the FTC regulates advertising of OTC and prescription drugs to protect consumers against false claims as to the uses, effectiveness, and safety of these drugs. Safety refers to the potential to create no harm or discomfort to patients whereas efficacy is the ability to create a positive outcome.

DID YOU KNOW ?

Efficacy means that a product is likely to be at least as good as other available interventions to which it will have been compared.

The United States Pharmacopoeia (USP) is an independent public health organization. It establishes public standards for prescription and OTC drugs available in the United States. Federal law requires that these drugs meet the USP public standards. Other groups that review these agents include consumer advocacy organizations and review panels for advertising standards. One voluntary reviewer is the Council on Scientific Affairs (CSA) of the American Dental Association (ADA). Interestingly, each of the major television networks also has an in-house review committee.

The FDA conducts an ongoing review of all OTC products. One aim of regulation is to protect the patient–consumer from useless or harmful products. All approval or disapproval decisions by the FDA have the force of law. The stages of FDA approval include (1) the manufacturer's preclinical research and development (animal testing, laboratory testing, and toxicity evaluation), (2) FDA review of manufacturing information on the drug product, which is submitted as part of an investigational new drug (IND) application, and (3) clinical research conducted by the manufacturer after approval of the IND application. The investigative process usually includes three phases: In phase 1, the study is limited in scope and uses 30 to 80 healthy volunteer subjects to determine the safe dose for humans.[1] For dental products, this phase usually involves taking agents into the body through the mouth (ingestion) or using exaggerated (three or four times per day) topical applications to the surface of oral mucosa or teeth, or both. Phase 2 usually involves several hundred subjects with the disease or condition to demonstrate the initial clinical efficacy of the drug and to define a dose range that is safe and efficacious. Phase 3 generally includes expanded controlled and uncontrolled trials with "final" formulas to demonstrate long-term safety and efficacy. These trials range from 3 to 6 months for plaque and gingivitis studies, to 2 or 3 years for caries studies. Generally, phase 3 studies involve several hundred to several thousand people. After the investigation process is completed, the company submits a new drug application (NDA), which contains data on the results from the trials. After the FDA reviews and approves the NDA, marketing can begin, but postmarketing surveillance of the product is mandatory.

Over the years, the FDA has requested that manufacturers of OTC products submit a listing of the active (i.e., therapeutic) and inactive ingredients in their products as a basis for helping to codify regulations governing OTC sales. The requirement that all inactive ingredients be listed alphabetically on the product label is among the many FDA recommendations to provide better control of OTC oral therapeutic products.[2] Active ingredients, as well as inactive agents, should be in no higher concentrations than necessary for the intended purpose. In addition, the indicated objective of the active agent(s) must be on the label. Furthermore, the FDA would consider the inclusion of the name of an active agent(s) without stating the proposed benefits as misleading. Proof must exist to substantiate any claim for a specific therapeutic benefit. For example, if a dentifrice has not been subjected to laboratory or clinical trials but its label lists "decay-fighting fluorides" without listing the proposed benefits of the fluorides, the product manufacturer cannot claim that the dentifrice is anticariogenic. The manufacturer can claim only that the product contains fluoride. It is possible that the fluoride in the untested dentifrice might not be compatible with other dentifrice ingredients or that the fluoride cannot be released in an active ionic form and therefore be totally ineffective.

Recommendations also apply to packaging and labeling guidelines, which help to regulate advertising. For example, the recommendations suggest that all containers for OTC therapeutic dentifrices, rinses, and gels containing fluoride have the following information on the label:

- Identification of the product, such as "anticaries dentifrice."
- The product's use, such as "aids in the prevention of dental caries."
- A warning, such as, "Do not swallow. Developing teeth of children under 6 years of age can become permanently discolored if excessive amounts of fluoride are repeatedly swallowed."
- Directions for product use, such as "Adults and children 6 years of age or older should brush teeth thoroughly at least twice daily, or as directed by a dentist or physician."

In April 1997, the FDA issued a labeling requirement for fluoride toothpaste: "Keep out of reach of children under 6 years of age. If you accidentally swallow more than used for brushing, seek professional help or contact a poison control center immediately." This recommendation may be an exaggerated response

because most experts believe that neither an adult nor a child could absorb enough fluoride to cause a serious problem.

For products bearing antiplaque and antiplaque related claims, such as "for the reduction or prevention of plaque, tartar, calculus, film, sticky deposits, bacterial buildup and gingivitis," the FDA reviews submitted data to determine whether these products are generally regarded as safe and effective and not misbranded for the label uses. The U.S. Attorney General also enforces policy governing the marketing of OTC drug products bearing antiplaque and antiplaque-related claims during the pendency of this review. This is part of the ongoing review of OTC drug products conducted by the FDA.

In 2003, the FDA published its call for rulemaking, stating,

> The Food and Drug Administration issued an advanced notice of proposed [sic] that would establish conditions under which OTC drug products for the reduction or prevention of dental plaque and gingivitis are generally recognized as safe and effective and not misbranded. This notice is based on the recommendations of the Dental Plaque Subcommittee of the Non Prescription Drugs Advisory Committee (NDAC) and is part of the FDA's on going review of OTC drug products.[3]

In addition to the FDA's regulation of OTC products, the American Dental Association's CSA reviews dental products on a *voluntary* basis. A product does not need to undergo review by ADA; in fact, the major reason products go under the review process is to carry the ADA Seal of Acceptance, which helps advertise the product to the public. The CSA is directed to study, evaluate, and disseminate information with regard to dental therapeutic agents, their adjuncts, and dental cosmetic agents that are offered to the public or to the profession. The most important activity of the CSA in meeting this charge is its acceptance program. Unlike the FDA review process, the primary review responsibilities for the acceptance program are conducted by consulting dental professionals who are appointed by the CSA but are not the ADA's employee. If the product is considered safe and effective after extensive clinical and laboratory research, the Seal of Acceptance is granted and can be used by the manufacturer in marketing the product. Studies have shown that 7 of 10 consumers recognize this seal.[4] It is important to realize that the ADA is a professional, private organization that does not have mandatory regulations comparable to those of the FDA.

DENTIFRICES

According to the dictionary, the term dentifrice is derived from *dens* (tooth) and *fricare* (to rub). A simple, contemporary definition of a dentifrice is a mixture used on the tooth in conjunction with a toothbrush.

Dentifrices are marketed as toothpastes and gels, and to a lesser extent, toothpowders. Some dentifrices are sold as liquid gels, liquid pastes, and stripes and with breath strips. All are sold as either therapeutic or cosmetic products. A *therapeutic dentifrice* must reduce some disease-related process in the mouth. Usually the actual or alleged therapeutic effect is to reduce caries incidence, gingivitis, plaque, or tooth sensitivity. The purpose of a *cosmetic toothpaste* is to clean and polish the teeth. The sales appeal of either product, however, is strongly linked to its flavor and foaming action.

Packaging

The development of the toothbrush provided the stimulus to market commercial dentifrices. Toothpowders were popular because boxes and cans from which they could be dispensed already existed. The formulas consisted of little more than water, soap, and flavor.

Toothpastes began to appear on the market following the development of lead tubes for packaging. The change to plastic packaging during World War II simultaneously caused the following effects:

• Eliminated the possibility of the user ingesting lead.
• Reduced the possibility of incompatibility of the tube and paste components.
• Aided the expelling of the paste by squeezing.
• Permitted an easier and more economic production of tubes.
• Provided a good surface for the printing of decorative designs and information.

The initial plastic tubes were permeable, which allowed the liquids in the dentifrices to seep through pores in the plastic and through the packaging. As a result, the flavors were lost. This problem has been resolved with the use of new plastic materials and of laminated or layered packaging materials.

In 1984, Colgate introduced the plastic pump dispenser to the market. Separate color compartments used to dispense "striped" products were introduced in Stripe dentifrice by Lever Brothers and are now used in Aquafresh (GlaxoSmithKline Consumer Healthcare, L.P.) and Colgate Total Stripe (Colgate-Palmolive Co.). Chesebrough-Pond introduced a dual-chamber pump dispenser to keep the peroxide and baking soda components of their dentifrice, Mentadent, separate until immediately before use; then they are delivered together on the toothbrush.

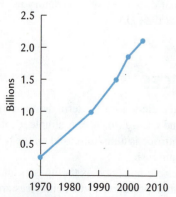

FIGURE ■ 11–1 Rapid seven-fold increase in toothpaste sales over the past 30 years, including 2005.

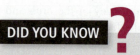

Of the variety of packaging, plastic tubes dominate the market with consumers having the option of a gel or a paste dentifrice. GlaxoSmithKline introduced Sensodyne Fresh Impact, which provides a combination of paste and gel. And Church & Dwight Co., Inc., recently marketed Arm & Hammer Advance White dentifrice in a new liquid gel.

Dentifrice Ingredients

Dentifrices were originally developed to provide a cosmetic effect and deliver a pleasant taste. They are effective in removing extrinsic stains, which occur on the surface of the tooth. These stains, which are often the end products of bacterial metabolism, range in color from green to yellow to black. Stains can also result from smoking; eating foods; and drinking coffee, tea, cola-containing beverages, and red wines. OTC dentifrices do not remove intrinsic stains, which are a result of altered formation or maturation of dental enamel (amelogenesis). Examples are the white-to-brown color changes seen in fluorosis (mottling on teeth caused by ingestion of excessive amounts of fluoride) or the grayish-blue appearance of enamel after ingestion of tetracycline. Dentifrices and other OTC products are also ineffective in altering the yellowing color of teeth seen with physiologic aging and in altering the hues of tooth color produced by differing shades of dentin. Therefore, they can only claim to "make your teeth their whitest or brightest"; they cannot state, "Makes your teeth whiter or tooth color lighter."

Toothpastes contain several or all of the ingredients listed in Table 11–1 ■. Gel dentifrices contain the same components as toothpastes except that gels have a higher proportion of the thickening agents. Both tooth gels and toothpastes are equally effective in plaque removal and in delivering active ingredients.

Abrasives

The degree of dentifrice abrasiveness depends on the inherent hardness of the abrasive, size of the abrasive particle, and the shape of the particle. Several other variables can affect the abrasive potential of the dentifrice: the brushing technique, the pressure on the brush, the hardness of the bristles, the direction of the strokes, and the number of strokes. Results for an abrasive tested alone can differ from those for the same abrasive tested as part of a dentifrice formula. The salivary characteristics of individuals can also affect dentifrice abrasiveness.

The most common types of abrasives used are carbonates, phosphates, and silicas. Carbonates include calcium carbonate (chalk) and sodium carbonate (baking soda). **Calcium carbonate** is an economical and highly effective abrasive, although the calcium ion limits the amount of soluble fluoride in toothpaste

TABLE ■ 11–1   Toothpaste Constituents

Ingredient	Percentage
Abrasives	20–40
Water	20–40
Humectants	20–40
Foaming agent (soap or detergent)	1–2
Binding agent	Up to 2
Flavoring agent	Up to 2
Sweetening agent	Up to 2
Therapeutic agent	Up to 5
Coloring or preservative	<1

up to 7 ppm. When the combination of fluoride and calcium carbonate is desired, it is recommended that **sodium monofluorophosphate** be used. Sodium fluoride, which provides soluble fluoride, is compatible with sodium bicarbonate. Phosphate abrasives include calcium pyrophosphate and dicalcium phosphate dihydrate. These phosphates are effective in having the teeth feel clean and white. **Silicas**, such as silicon oxides, mechanically cleanse the tooth, are chemically inert, and do not react with other dentifrice ingredients. They are currently the most commonly used abrasive found in dentifrices. Aluminum oxides and perlites have also been introduced into dentifrice formulas with additional efficacy claims.

Abrasiveness Testing

Standard laboratory testing for abrasiveness uses a machine with several brushes.[5] The length of the reciprocating stroke, number of strokes, and pressure of the brush can be adjusted. According to the experimental objectives, enamel, dentin, or cementum is brushed, and the amount of calcium or phosphorus in the resultant slurry is analyzed. Another method of testing abrasiveness in dentifrices is to measure surface roughness using a tester equipped with a diamond tip stylus and applying the dentifrice slurry of abrasives to mounted teeth at 2500 rpm for 5 seconds under a load of 145 g.[6]

Abrasives usually do not damage enamel, but they can dull the tooth luster. To compensate for this, polishing agents are added to the dentifrice formulation. These **polishing agents** are usually small-sized particles of aluminum, calcium, tin, magnesium, or zirconium compounds. Typically, the manufacturer blends the abrasives and the polishing agents to form an abrasive system. Agents, such as chalk or silica, can have both polishing and abrasive effects. Smaller particles (1 mm) have a polishing action, and larger particles (20 mm) have an abrasive action.

In selecting a dentifrice, the abrasiveness and polishing characteristics should meet individual needs. The majority of the population do not accumulate visible stain when engaged in their own style of personal oral hygiene. For these individuals, a dentifrice with high polishing and low abrasion should be recommended. For other individuals, an additional amount of abrasive is needed to control accumulating stain. As the abrasive level increases, greater care must be taken to perfect brushing techniques to avoid self-inflicted injury to the teeth or soft tissues. Such injuries can result from excessive pressure, hard bristles, and prolonged brushing.

When toothbrush abrasion damage does occur, it usually appears as a V-shaped notch in the cementum apical to the cementoenamel junction (Figure 11–2 ■). This area is vulnerable because enamel is about 20 times harder than dentin or cementum. More serious defects usually occur in older individuals who maintain a very high level of oral hygiene.

Humectants

Toothpaste consisting of only a toothpowder and water results in a product with several undesirable properties. Over time, the solids in the paste tend to settle out of solution and the water evaporates. This process can result in caking of the remaining dentifrice. Until the 1930s, most toothpaste had a short shelf life because of this problem. When the tube was opened, it first expelled paste that was liquid, but the last paste in the tube was either impossible to expel or too hard to use. To solve this problem, **humectants** were added to maintain the moisture and prevent hardening. Commonly used humectants are sorbitol, mannitol, glycerol, and propylene glycol. These humectants are nontoxic, but mold or bacterial growth can occur in their presence. For this reason, **preservatives** such as sodium benzoate, dichlorinated phenols, and alcohols are added to prevent their growth.

Humectants help maintain the consistency of toothpaste, but despite their presence, the solids tend to settle out of the paste. To counteract this, thickening or **binding agents** are added to the formula. Gums, such as gum tragacanth, were first used. These were followed by colloids derived from seaweed, such as carrageenan. These, in turn, were replaced by synthetic celluloses. In low concentrations, these celluloses are also often used as humectants; in higher concentrations, they function as gelling agents in the formulation of gel dentifrices. At high concentrations (>40%), humectants also act as preservatives.

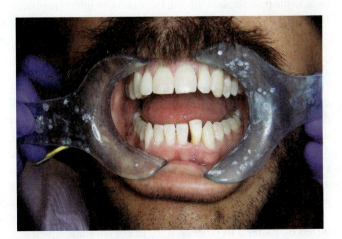

FIGURE ■ 11–2 V-shaped notches in maxillary lateral incisors resulting from use of a dentifrice with a harsh abrasive system.
(*Source:* Courtesy of Vicki Gianopoulos.)

Soaps and Detergents

Because toothpastes were originally manufactured to keep the teeth clean, soap was the logical cleansing agent. As the toothbrush bristles dislodge food debris and plaque biofilm, the foaming or sudsing action of the soap aids in the removal of the loosened material. However, soaps have several disadvantages: They can be irritating to the mucous membrane, their flavor is difficult to mask and often causes nausea, and many times soaps are incompatible with other ingredients, such as calcium.

When detergents appeared on the market, soaps largely disappeared from dentifrices. Today, **sodium lauryl sulfate** (SLS) is the most widely used detergent. It is stable, possesses some antibacterial properties, and has a low surface tension, which facilitates the flow of the dentifrice over the teeth. Sodium lauryl sulfate is active at a neutral pH, has a flavor that is easy to mask, and is compatible with the current dentifrice ingredients. Rantanen and others have suggested that some dentifrices containing SLS can cause mucosal irritation in humans.[7] Low-SLS dentifrices that claim a lower incidence of oral ulcers have been marketed, or it can be suggested to use a dentifrice containing cocamidopropyl betaine that is found in Colgate Luminous®, Sensodyne®, or Pronamel®.

Flavoring

Flavor, along with smell, color, and consistency of a product, are important characteristics that lead to public acceptance of a dentifrice. If dentifrices did not possess these characteristics, they would probably be poorly accepted. For taste acceptance, the flavor must be pleasant, provide an immediate taste sensation, and be relatively long lasting. Usually synthetic flavors are blended to provide the desired taste. Spearmint, peppermint, wintergreen, cinnamon, and the most recently introduced flavor, vanilla give toothpaste a pleasant taste, aroma, and refreshing aftertaste. It is difficult to formulate a flavor that is universally acceptable because people have different color and taste preferences. Some manufacturers use essential oils such as thymol, menthol, and so forth, which can provide a "medicinal" taste to the product. In addition, these oils can impart antibacterial effects, as will be discussed later in this chapter.

Sweetening Agents

In early toothpaste formulations, sugar, honey, and other sweeteners were used. Because these materials can be broken down in the mouth to produce acids and lower plaque pH, they can increase caries. They have been replaced with saccharin, cyclamate, sorbitol, and mannitol as primary noncariogenic sweetening agents. Sorbitol and mannitol serve a dual role as sweetening agents and humectants. Glycerin, which also serves as a humectant, adds to the sweet taste. A new sweetener in some dentifrices is xylitol. In laboratory studies, it is not metabolized by bacteria to produce acid. In human studies, where it was placed in chewing gums and food, xylitol was noncariogenic and demonstrated an anticaries capability by facilitating the remineralization of incipient carious lesions.

Baking-Soda Dentifrices

Baking soda (sodium bicarbonate) has had a long history of use as an oral-hygiene aid. Church and Dwight, a manufacturer of baking soda and the manufacturer of the original baking-soda toothpaste, suggests that dentists and hygienists recommend brushing with baking soda for healthier teeth and gums. Sodium bicarbonate dentifrices are known to reduce plaque and gingivitis, remove extrinsic stain, and reduce malodor.[8,9]

Some dental providers also have suggested the mixture of baking soda with peroxide as an alternative to the use of commercial dentifrices. Many patients attribute benefit to the routine use of these products. It was inevitable that these products would be incorporated into toothpastes. All contain hydrated silica, which is compatible with fluoride. Baking-soda dentifrices actually contain only a small amount of baking soda in addition to the standard fluoride-compatible abrasives.

Methods of Controlling Plaque and Gingivitis

The most intriguing method of controlling plaque and gingivitis is the concept of chemical plaque control by which chemical compounds are used to supplement the usual brushing, flossing, and use of auxiliary aids employed in mechanical plaque control. Antiplaque agents can act directly on the plaque bacteria or can disrupt different components of plaque to permit easier and more complete removal during toothbrushing and flossing. This opportunity to use chemistry to enhance oral-hygiene procedures is important because manual plaque-control methods can be difficult to teach and monitor, tedious to perform, time-consuming, and impossible to accomplish by some persons who have disabilities. In addition, nonmotivated individuals may not use manual methods.

The present chemical plaque-control agents should not be considered a panacea, or cure for all plaque problems because these agents have not been proven to be a total substitute for routine oral-hygiene measures. Excessive emphasis on chemical control can encourage some patients to de-emphasize proven oral-hygiene methods. The properties of an ideal form of such an agent are listed in Table 11–2 ■. Colgate Total® brands contain triclosan, and Colgate Pro-Health® uses a combination of sodium hexametophosphate, a whitening and anticalculus agent, and stabilized stannous fluoride. Triclosan will be discussed later in this chapter.

Therapeutic Dentifrices

The most commonly used therapeutic agent added to dentifrices is fluoride, which aids in the control of caries. In 1960, the Council on Dental Therapeutics of the American Dental Association classified Crest toothpaste with stannous fluoride as a caries prophylactic dentifrice on the basis of several studies that indicated its effectiveness. For the first time, a therapeutic dentifrice was awarded the Seal of Provisional Acceptance.

TABLE ■ 11–2   Properties of an Ideal Agent to Control Gingivitis

- High, immediate antimicrobial activity
- Broad-spectrum efficacy against bacteria and yeasts
- Chemical stability in formulations and in the oral cavity
- Substantivity (ability to stick) to oral tissues and to be released over time in an active form
- Toxicologic and ecologic safety
- No topical adverse reactions (staining, burning)
- No taste or aftertaste problems
- No inhibition of taste perception
- No systemic toxicity
- No change in oral or gastrointestinal flora
- Neither carcinogenic nor teratogenic
- No adverse reactions
- Compatibility with dentifrice or mouthwash formulations

In 1964, on the basis of additional new and favorable data, the classification was upgraded to full acceptance.

The original level of fluoride in OTC dentifrices and gels was restricted to 1,000 to 1,100 ppm fluoride and a total of no more than 120 mg of fluoride in the tube with a requirement that the package include a safety closure. Most dentifrices today still contain 1,000 ppm. Therapeutic toothpastes, dispensed on prescription, could contain up to 260 mg or 4,950 ppm of fluoride in a tube. Other therapeutic dentifrices include active ingredients for calculus control, hypersensitivity, biofilm formation reduction, and remineralization.

Anticaries Agents

Fluoride is the most commonly used anticaries agent added to dentifrices. The following fluorides are generally recognized as effective and safe for OTC sales: 0.22% sodium fluoride (NaF) at a level of 1,100 ppm, 0.76% sodium monofluorophosphate (MFP) at a level of 1,000 ppm, and 0.4% stannous fluoride (SnF_2) at a level of 1,000 ppm. Fluoride levels were increased to 1,500 ppm sodium monofluorophosphate in OTC Aim Cavity Protection toothpastes. A prescription dentifrice, Colgate PreviDent 5,000, contains 5,000 ppm of fluoride.

One baking soda–peroxide–fluoride dentifrice (Mentadent) contains a combination of 0.75% stable peroxide gel in conjunction with baking soda and 1,100 ppm of sodium fluoride. The materials are packaged in a two-chamber pump to permit the baking soda and peroxide components to be mixed with the fluoride at the time of delivery.

Multiple clinical studies of fluoride dentifrices containing NaF, MFP, or SnF_2 in the presence of compatible abrasives and stable formulations have been submitted to and accepted by the ADA. The ADA, therefore, awards the Seal of Acceptance to fluoride dentifrices solely on the basis of laboratory data—that is, if the experimental design protocol is identical or similar to that of previous ADA-accepted products.[10] Not all fluoride-containing dentifrices have demonstrated anticaries activity. The level of active fluoride must be adequate and must be maintained over the shelf life of the dentifrice.

A combination of calcium-phosphate in dentifrices with fluoride has also gained momentum in today's market. Dentifrices containing calcium phosphate help prevent the formation of dental caries and rapidly remineralize demineralized tooth structure. Calcium phosphate encourages the remineralization of enamel by rapidly hydrolyzing to form apatite. The addition of calcium and phosphate ions to a fluoride dentifrice can improve the ability of enamel to resist caries initiation and subsequent progression of a lesion.

Stannous fluoride (SnF_2), specifically the stannous ion, has reported activity against caries, plaque, and gingivitis. Although SnF_2 has a long record as an anticaries agent, long-term stability in dentifrices and mouthrinses has been questioned. The development and subsequent laboratory and clinical efficacy of a stabilized SnF_2 dentifrice were marketed in the United States by Procter & Gamble as Crest Pro-Health. This product combines a stabilized stannous fluoride (0.454%) and sodium hexametophosphate. Superior efficacy has been shown for Crest Pro-Health in antimicrobial, plaque acidogenicity, gingivitis or gingival bleeding, and calculus control.[11] Other clinical studies compared the antigingivitis benefits of standard sodium fluoride dentifrices with the benefits of triclosan-containing dentifrices containing pyrophosphate/copolymer. Results demonstrated superior benefits for the stabilized 0.454% stannous fluoride/sodium hexametophosphate dentifrice in reducing gingivitis compared with the triclosan/copolymer dentifrice.[12] These studies support the strong retention and lasting antimicrobial efficacy of highly stabilized stannous fluoride/sodium hexametophosphate dentifrices.

Antibacterial Agents

Triclosan is a broad-spectrum antibacterial agent effective against a wide variety of bacteria and is widely used as an antibacterial agent in OTC consumer products in the United States, including deodorant soaps and antibacterial skin scrubs. Triclosan, a bisphenol, has also been shown to be a useful antibacterial agent in oral products such as dentifrices and mouthrinse products; however, concern regarding its use is on the rise.

Many dentifrices and mouthrinses containing triclosan are marketed in Europe. In the United States, Colgate Total and Colgate Total Advanced® developed by Colgate-Palmolive contains triclosan, a patented copolymer, "Gantrez," and fluoride. When added with a copolymer, substantivity is increased up to 12 hours. Colgate Total has undergone extensive safety and clinical efficacy testing and was approved in 1997 by the FDA as the first dentifrice *to help prevent gingivitis, plaque, and caries* [emphasis added].[13] Additional research supports the fact that a triclosan dentifrice inhibits plaque regrowth and provides anticalculus activity, thereby reducing gingival inflammation and caries.[14]

Dentifrice products containing a **zinc citrate** and triclosan combination have also received attention. Clinical evaluation has shown this combination to be effective in reducing acid production and plaque formationand in preventing gingivitis. Summaries of the zinc citrate–triclosan studies have been published.[15]

Anticalculus Dentifrices

Calculus-control dentifrice formulations are designed to interrupt the process of mineralization of plaque to calculus. Plaque has a bacterial matrix that mineralizes because of the supersaturation of saliva with calcium and phosphate ions. Crystal growth inhibitors can be added to dentifrices to provide a reduction in calculus formation.

In the late 1970s, anticalculus dentifrices began to appear on the market without any evidence of effectiveness. In 1985, Procter & Gamble supplemented its existing Crest anticariogenic toothpaste with a similar anticaries formula that also contained a combination of tetrasodium phosphate and disodium dihydrogen pyrophosphate. These **soluble pyrophosphates** are crystal growth inhibitors, which retard the formation of calculus.[16] This combination has been demonstrated in clinical studies to significantly reduce the amount of calculus formed. Zinc citrate and zinc chloride also reduce calculus formation. Dentifrices containing these agents are labeled as tartar control toothpastes.

Antihypersensitivity Products

Many patients experience pain when exposed areas of the tooth root, especially at the cementoenamel junction, are subjected to heat or cold. Treatment for this sensitivity includes the stimulation of secondary dentin, blocking of the pulpal neural response, obturation (closure) of dentinal tubules, and coagulation or precipitation of tubular fluids. In coagulation, the fluid in the tubules becomes thicker whereas in precipitation, the minerals in the fluid separate and form a deposit. Both mechanisms help to close the tubules. Antihypersensitivity agents include potassium oxylate strontium chloride, sodium citrate, and potassium nitrate. Most recently, the FDA approved fluoride varnish as an agent to treat hypersensitivity; this agent is a thin resin that contains fluoride and is brushed onto tooth surfaces.

Potassium nitrate is a commonly used, FDA-approved OTC **desensitization agent**; that is, it reduces the reaction of nerves in the teeth to stimuli such as heat and cold. Potassium nitrate is known to desensitize the nerve by penetrating through the length of the dentinal tubules and to depolarize sensory nerve endings located at the dentin–pulpal interface. These actions interrupt the transmission of pain signals to the brain. OTC dentifrices include Sensodyne Fresh Impact® Toothpaste, Crest Sensitivity Protection Fluoride®, Crest ProHealth® Toothpastes, Colgate Sensitive® Toothpastes, and Orajel Sensitive Pain Relieving Toothpaste® for Adults. Most dentifrices containing potassium nitrate also contain fluoride. Colgate PreviDent® with 5,000 ppm fluoride is prescribed to help treat sensitivity. Prior to the development of potassium nitrate as a desensitizing agent, the occluding (blocking) or **sclerosing** (hardening) of exposed dentinal tubules was the primary method used to control hypersensitivity. Strontium chloride, potassium oxylate, potassium nitrate, and sodium citrate are examples of OTC agents used to occlude the exposed dentinal tubules.[17]

Whiteners

Considerable controversy surrounds the use of stain removers and tooth whiteners. Products are being marketed for professional or in-home use by patients. The cosmetic benefits of these dentifrices remain important to patients, and the OTC sales of these products continue to increase. Many claims for efficacy and safety are under review by agencies and government panels.

Surveys reveal a growing U.S. market share for dentifrices claiming "whitening" or "stain control" properties. These dentifrices control stain via physical methods (abrasives) and chemical mechanisms (surface-active agents or bleaching/oxidizing agents). Although the public perceives these products as more abrasive than ordinary toothpastes, their abrasiveness is usually intermediate among the products tested.

Dentifrices marketed with tooth-whitener claims are available as a toothpaste or gel and are used in a two- or three-step treatment "process." These products usually contain hydrogen peroxide, carbamide peroxide, or papain as their bleaching or whitening ingredient. **Carbamide peroxide** breaks down to form urea and hydrogen peroxide. **Hydrogen peroxide**, in turn, forms a free radical that contains oxygen, which is the active bleaching molecule. Papain, a naturally occurring enzyme that destroys protein is rapidly diluted by saliva. Home-bleaching products can contain other chemicals to aid in the delivery of the bleaching agent. Glycerin or propylene glycol is commonly added to thicken the solution and prolong contact with the tooth surface. In the two- or three-step products, agents can be delivered to the teeth via a custom-made tray or by toothbrushing.

Remineralization Paste—Recaldent

Casein phosphopeptide—amorphous calcium phosphate (CPP-ACP), a protein found in cow's milk—is used in some pastes to promote remineralization of enamel in areas that have demineralized. Known as Recaldent, it replaces calcium and phosphate ions that were lost to demineralization. It has also been successful in reducing teeth sensitivity. Recaldent is marketed in the United States as GC Corporation MI Paste® and MI Paste Plus®.

MI Paste® is not a dentifrice; it is a paste that is dispensed through a tube. It is used after the teeth have been properly brushed with a fluoride dentifrice. The paste is generously applied by a gloved finger or cotton swab around the tooth surfaces. For three minutes the applied paste is not to be disturbed, which means the patient should not rinse, swish or otherwise move the paste. Recaldent is not currently found in toothpaste or mouthrinses but research continues to progress in these areas. It is found in Trident White gum.

CPP-ACP is an excellent source of calcium and phosphorous. Fluoride update to the tooth requires the presence of calcium and phosphorous. It is recommended that fluoride and CPP-ACP be used in conjunction to achieve the optimal benefits of tooth remineralization and prevention of dental caries.

DID YOU KNOW?

Recaldent™ (CPP-ACP) is milk derived and therefore not recommended for people with milk allergies, but it is digestible by people with lactose intolerance.

MOUTHRINSES

Freshening bad breath has been the traditional purpose of mouthrinses. However, they can be cosmetic, therapeutic, or both. Cosmetic benefits include a pleasant taste and sensation, a decrease in microorganisms, and halitosis control. Therapeutic benefits include a reduction in bacterial plaque, gingivitis, and dental caries. Therapeutic mouthrinses are available over the counter and by prescription. They are regulated by the FDA and voluntarily by the ADA. Mouthrinses are often used daily by patients; therefore, it is important that patients understand proper usage of mouthrinses to achieve successful outcomes. When antimicrobial mouthrinses are used daily along with brushing and flossing, they are most effective in reducing plaque and gingivitis.

The claimed active ingredients of mouthrinses include quaternary ammonium compounds, phenolic compounds, sanguinarine, chlorhexidine, essential oils, fluoride, and triclosan. Ammonium compound and sanguinarine mouthrinses have not shown consistent efficacy and therefore are not recommended as part of an antiplaque/antigingivitis self-care program. As with dentifrices, commercial sales of cosmetic rinses have been related to taste, color, smell, and the pleasant sensation that follows use. The pleasant sensation is often enhanced by the addition of astringents. Commonly used astringents are alum, zinc stearate, zinc citrate, and acetic or citric acids. Triclosan has been added to mouthrinses as a claimed antiplaque ingredient.

Alcohol in mouthrinses is used as a solvent, a taste enhancer, and an agent providing an aftertaste. The alcohol content of commercial rinses, ranging up to 27%, can constitute a danger for children, especially those from 2 to 3 years of age. According to the American Association of Poison Control (AAPC), 5 to 10 ounces of a mouthrinse containing alcohol can be lethal for a child weighing 26 pounds. Between 2006 and 2009, the AAPC's poison-control centers logged approximately 44,000 reports of exposures to mouthrinses containing alcohol; 14,000 cases concerned persons younger than 6 years of age, 9,000 were between the ages of 6–19 years, and 17,000 were older than 19 years of age. Of these exposures, 5 died and another 71 had major outcomes of permanent injuries.[18] The American Academy of Pediatrics recommends that OTC liquid preparations be limited to 5% ethanol, that safety closures be required, and that the packaged volume be kept to a reasonable minimum to prevent the potential for lethal ingestion.

The ADA's CSA requires child-resistant caps on all alcohol-containing mouthrinses that bear the ADA Seal of Acceptance. The council also requires manufacturers of ADA-accepted mouthrinses that contain more than 5% alcohol to include the following statement on the label: "Warning: Keep out of reach of children. Do not swallow. Contains alcohol. Use only as directed." Although some research links alcohol-containing rinses to oral cancer, numerous published studies support the safety of these mouthrinses. The ADA reports that mouthrinses containing alcohol are considered safe and effective.

Cosmetic Mouthrinses: Halitosis

Bacterial proliferation and plaque accumulation on the surface of the tongue are major factors contributing to halitosis. Ninety percent of halitosis originates from the oral cavity and 10% from systemic or nonoral causes.[19] The effects of this oral malodor can cause patients to become insecure in social situations and self-conscious during daily living. The seriousness of this condition elicits many patient requests for treatment and for validation that mouthrinses claiming to aid in malodor actually do so.

The effect of most breath-fresheners is caused by flavors and has no effect after 3 to 5 hours. These mouthrinses mask odors and provide little antibacterial function. They usually contain a flavoring agent that provides a pleasant taste, an astringent that refreshes the mouth, ethyl alcohol that acts as a solvent and a taste enhancer, water, and an active ingredient to reduce the number of microorganisms.[20] Antibacterial components such as chlorhexidine, sanguinarine, cetylpyridinium chloride, triclosan, essential oils, phenolic compounds, quaternary ammonium compounds, benzalkonium chloride hydrogen peroxide, sodium bicarbonate, zinc ions, and combinations of these components have all been considered to reduce halitosis.

A study performed by Borden and others tested the effects of four mouthrinses on halitosis. Results showed that all four mouthrinses were effective in reducing oral malodor within 4 hours after a single use.[21] Another study tested the effectiveness of mouthrinses containing an antibacterial agent to reduce malodor when used alone and in conjunction with tongue brushing and toothbrushing. Results showed that, although a reduction in halitosis was evident for mouthrinses used as a sole treatment, the reduction was significantly higher with the combination of mouthrinses and tongue brushing and toothbrushing.[22]

Zinc chloride found in some mouthrinses has gained momentum in its efficacy claims for reducing malodor in patients with good oral health. Studies report that zinc chloride is effective in neutralizing volatile sulfur compounds (VSC) and in killing the gram-negative bacteria responsible for VSC formation for longer than 3 hours. A combination of zinc chloride, thymol, and eucalyptus oil found in BreathRx products has also been reported to be effective in reducing halitosis.[23,24]

A quantitative assessment of bad breath, including the smelling of exhaled air (**organoleptic assessment**), identifying the oral cavity as the source, and measuring VSC is effective in verifying product claims for treating halitosis. In diagnosing and treating complaints of bad breath, the clinician should consider psychologic as well as physical factors.

Xerostomia Mouthrinses

Many people experience dry mouth (xerostomia) traceable to several possible causes, such as damage to the salivary glands after radiation therapy for head and neck cancer, Sjögren syndrome, and drug usage such as antihistamines, anticholinergics, antihypertensives, diuretics, narcotics, anticonvulsants, and antianxiety and tranquilizing drugs, especially the tricyclic antidepressants. In such cases, the oral mucous membrane is continually dry and uncomfortable. Artificial salivas have been developed to ameliorate the dryness (i.e., make it more tolerable); these products are used ad libitum (as desired) by the patient to moisten the mucous membrane.

Because xerostomia is correlated with an increased caries incidence, the rinses usually contain fluoride as well as chemical compounds, such as carboxymethylcellulose, calcium, and phosphorous, in concentrations that closely parallel those of saliva. The rinses that contain fluoride can, in reality, be remineralizing solutions.

Commonly used xerostomia mouthrinses include Oasis Mouthwash by Sensodyne, Biotène Mouthwash, and Orazyme Dry Mouth Mouthwash. Oasis Mouthwash claims to moisturize the mouth from its mucoadhesive formula, to lock in moisture from a xanthum gum polymer and carboxymethyl cellulose compound, and to help protect the mouth from dryness owing to a glycerin coating of the mucosal surface. A study reported in 2006 states that Oasis Mouthwash's mucoadhesion formula (i.e., its ability to adhere to mucosa) helps manage symptoms up to 2 hours. The recommended usage is to rinse with the mouthwash in the morning and at bedtime as part of a daily oral care regimen.[25] Biotène Mouthwash is a combination of natural salivary enzymes (glucose oxidase, lactoperoxidase, and lysozyme) and protein. It claims to boost and replenish the natural defenses of saliva while killing harmful bacteria and maintaining healthy bacteria. The recommended usage is to swish 1 tablespoon (15 mL) of the mouthwash for 30 seconds, two to three times per day. Orazyme Dry Mouth Mouthwash is a natural product whose enzymatic delivery system inhibits the growth of microorganisms and helps maintain moisture in the mouth.

Therapeutic Mouthrinse Agents

Chlorhexidine Gluconate

The FDA has approved prescription plaque-control rinses containing 0.12% chlorhexidine. Directions call for a twice-daily, 60-second rinse with one-half ounce of such solutions. Chlorhexidine has proved to be one of the most effective antiplaque agents to date.[26,27] Chlorhexidine is a cationic compound that binds to the hydroxyapatite of tooth enamel, the pellicle, plaque bacteria, the extracellular polysaccharide of the plaque, and especially to the mucous membrane. The chlorhexidine adsorbed to the hydroxyapatite is believed to inhibit bacterial colonization and prevent pellicle formation. After binding, the agent is slowly released in an active form over 8 to 12 hours. This ability of the oral tissues to adsorb an active agent and to permit its slow release in active form over a prolonged period is known as *substantivity*. As the substantivity of an antiplaque agent decreases, the frequency of use needs to be increased.

The use of chlorhexidine in periodontal therapy is often recommended for some patients. It has not proved beneficial as the sole method of treating periodontitis with deep pockets, but chlorhexidine irrigation following root planing (smoothing of root surfaces), prophylaxis, or periodontal surgery can be effective in helping to control inflammation and subgingival plaque.[28]

In some countries, such as the United States, chlorhexidine products are available only by prescription. In others, such as the United Kingdom, they are available over the counter. Although chlorhexidine is quite effective, it is not active against all relevant anaerobic bacteria. A high minimal concentration is necessary for efficacy.

Some side effects are associated with chlorhexidine use; staining of the teeth, tongue, and tooth-colored restorations is the most common effect. Occasionally altered taste sensation, irritation of the oral mucosa, and burning sensation are reported.[29] Chlorhexidine is inactivated by most dentifrice surfactants; therefore, it is not included in dentifrices. Also, because of this inactivation, it is critical for dental professionals to alert patients not to use chlorhexidine mouthrinses within 30 minutes before or after regular toothbrushing.

Although chlorhexidine can be more effective than any other current antiplaque agent and has a definite role in preventive and control dental procedures, it is not a "magic bullet." Its side effects and inadequate activity range somewhat limit its use.

Essential Oils

It is reported that **essential oil** mouthrinses are effective in controlling plaque and gingivitis because the oil alters the bacterial cell wall.[30,31] The active ingredients (essential oils) used in these mouthrinses include a combination of thymol, menthol, eucalyptol, and methyl salicylate in a hydroalcoholic vehicle containing 21.6% to 26.9% alcohol.[32] Although the safety of essential oils is well established, some patients can have difficulty tolerating the burning sensation associated with the alcohol content. In addition, slight extrinsic staining has been reported with the use of essential oils rinses, which is a possible transient (short-term) side effect of any antimicrobial agent. Essential oil mouthrinses are indicated for patients who need and are compliant with antiplaque/antigingivitis mouthrinses. They cannot be indicated for patients who belong to religious organizations that prohibit the use of alcohol in any form, patients in orthodontic devices (e.g., braces), or patients who have a chemical dependency, diabetes, or xerostomia.

Listerine Antiseptic was the first OTC antiplaque and antigingivitis mouthrinse to be approved by the ADA in 1988. Patients are advised to rinse twice daily with one-half ounce of Listerine for 30 seconds in addition to their usual oral-hygiene regimen. Listerine has been used as a mouthrinse for more than 110 years. The original formula contains 26.9% alcohol. Flavor variations of the original product include Cool Mint, Smart Rinse, Soft Mint, Agent Cool Blue, and Fresh Burst Listerine Antiseptics; these products, which contain 21.6% alcohol, also received the ADA seal.

Microorganisms do not develop a resistance to the antibacterial effects of essential oils, such as clove oil (eugenol) and thyme oil (thymol). As with chlorhexidine, just rinsing with an essential oil mouthrinse is unlikely to be effective in treating periodontitis because the solution does not reach the depths of the periodontal pockets. For the dental professional, these mouthrinses are recommended in patients prior to aerosol-generating procedures. Unless the dental professional uses an effective dry-field technique in a 30-second period, the bacterial aerosol generated by an ultrasonic scaler that removes calculus, an air-powered tooth polisher, or a slow-speed or high-speed hand piece can be roughly equivalent to the aerosols received from a patient directly sneezing into the dental provider's face.

Quaternary Ammonium Compounds (Cetylpyridinium Chloride)

The most common quaternary ammonium compound used in mouthrinses is **cetylpyridinium chloride (CPC)**. This compound is a clinically studied bactericidal agent that interacts with the bacterial cell membrane and, through cellular pressure, weakens and disrupts the membrane to effectively kill bacteria. It has been shown to reduce plaque and gingivitis for up to 12 hours and to reduce plaque biofilm and gingivitis by 14% to 24%.[33-35] Crest Pro-Health Rinse by Procter & Gamble uses this bactericidal agent and markets the product as an antigingivitis/antiplaque alcohol-free mouthrinse that contains CPC. Its recommended usage is to swish 20 mL of Crest Pro-Health Rinse twice daily, 30 seconds at each use, for the product to provide all the benefits indicated. Because of the absence of alcohol content, this product claims to have little-to-no burning sensation and can have some benefit in reducing halitosis. Other mouthrinses that fall under this category include Scope, Cepacol, Clear Choice, and Rembrandt.

Fluoride Rinses

Fluoride mouthrinses are effective in the reduction of the incidence of dental caries. They are intended for daily or weekly use, depending on their categorization as low-concentration/high-frequency or high-concentration/low-frequency rinses. Some low-concentration mouthrinses are available over the counter, whereas most others require a prescription. The active agents in fluoride mouthrinse products are NaF, acidulated phosphofluorides, or SnF. Their concentration for daily use is 0.05% (250 ppm); for weekly use, the concentration of each agent is 0.2% (900 ppm), 0.44% (440 ppm), and 0.63% (250 ppm), respectively. The dose directions are 5 mL (1 teaspoon) of product to be used once daily or 10 mL of product to be used once weekly. The rinse is to be swished for 60 seconds and then expectorated. For stannous fluoride, the daily rinse concentration is diluted with water to produce a 0.1% concentration. Stannous fluoride and acidulated phosphofluoride-mouthrinses are *not* recommended for weekly usage.

Published long-term clinical studies have consistently shown the anticaries effectiveness of fluoride mouthrinses to be equal or superior to fluoride dentifrices. It has been found that the fluoride in mouthrinses is retained in dental plaque and saliva to help prevent dental caries. Studies report a 30% to 40% average reduction in the incidence of dental caries for fluoride mouthrinse users. Their use is recommended for persons in fluoridated andnonfluoridated communities.

Fluoride mouthrinses are highly indicated for patients who have a history of moderate-to-rampant caries, who are undergoing orthodontia, or who wear prosthetic appliances (e.g., dentures or bridges) that aid in adherence of plaque biofilm. Moreover, patients with inadequate oral-hygiene habits, patients with dentition areas of demineralization or root exposure/sensitivity, and patients experiencing xerostomia should also use these mouthrinses. Fluoride mouthrinses are not recommended for children under 6 years of age or those who have difficulty swishing and expectorating. It is important to reduce the risk of swallowing the fluoride.[36]

Triclosan

Triclosan, found in mouthrinses and dentifrices, is known to reduce the production of biofilm and gingivitis. Mouthrinses containing triclosan are not marketed in the United States but are commonly available in Europe. Triclosan, a bisphenol, is considered an organic antimicrobial and antigingivitis agent.[37,38] Studies have shown its success in the reduction of plaque production, treatment of individuals undergoing radiation therapy, and tooth sensitivity. Commercially available mouthrinses include Colgate Total and Plax.

Including the additives polyvinyl-methoxyethylene and maleic acid (PVM/MA) copolymer (Gantrez) to triclosan allows for prolonged substantivity and efficacy. Dentifrices containing triclosan and PVM/MA are shown to be more effective in plaque and gingivitis reduction than in their mouthrinse counterparts. Triclosan is also available in cleaning supplies, soaps, deodorants, shaving cream, and cosmetics and reported to help reduce bacterial contamination.

DID YOU KNOW ?

Chewing gum is considered the world's most common habit. Approximately 100,000 tons are chewed each year.

CHEWING GUM

Because gum chewing is pleasurable, people normally chew for longer periods of time than they spend brushing their teeth. In addition, chewing gum is especially advantageous during the course of the day when toothbrushing is not possible or convenient. Likewise, gum can complement toothbrushing by reaching many of the tooth surfaces commonly missed during brushing. The average American fails to contact approximately 40% of tooth surfaces, especially the posterior teeth and lingual surfaces, during toothbrushing. Regular toothbrushing removes only about 35% to 40% of dental plaque on tooth surfaces.

Beneficial effects of gum chewing include increased saliva production, resulting in the mechanical removal of dental plaque and debris.[39,40] Studies have shown that chewing sugared or sugar-free gum is an effective means of reducing plaque accumulation and that gum chewing can also effectively reduce established plaque on many tooth surfaces.

In the United States, published research devoted solely to chewing gum and its potential oral health benefits has increased. The interest of researchers in effective gum additives coupled with the acceptance and use of chewing-gum products by the general public makes this a new and potentially important category to be considered by dental professionals. Globally, chewing gum is the fastest-growing sector of the confectionary market, ahead of both chocolate and sweets.[39] The attraction is influenced through the marketing appeal of sugar-free gums, gums that whiten or strengthen teeth, and gums that help in mental concentration or act as a snack substitute between meals. Adults are particularly interested in the product appeal.[41]

During gum chewing, salivary flow rates increase, especially in the first few minutes because of both mechanical and gustatory (taste) stimulation. Increased salivary stimulation can continue for periods of 5 to 20 minutes, usually until the flavor in the product dissipates. However, even with unflavored chewing gum, saliva flow, as evidenced by swallowing rates, increases over the baseline.[42] The beneficial effects of additional saliva in the mouth include increased plaque biofilm calcium levels and increased buffer capacity and mineral supersaturation; the latter two effects help regulate or increase plaque pH. In addition, increased saliva flow can assist in loosening and removing debris from occlusal or interproximal sites and can be beneficial to xerostomia patients.

The focus of chewing gum research to date has been on "sugar-free" products, which contain polyol sweeteners such as sorbitol or xylitol. These sweeteners are not broken down by plaque or oral microorganisms to produce acid. Plaque pH studies have documented reduction of plaque acidity and maintenance of plaque neutrality both during and after chewing gum with xylitol, for periods of 2 to 3 weeks after the gum chewing. In addition, gums containing xylitol have shown anticaries activity in several long-term studies.[43] Xylitol is considered nonacidogenic and not fermentable by bacteria responsible for caries production. It is recommended that 6 grams to 10 grams of xylitol gum be chewed daily, three to five times per day, for 5 minutes at each session.[44]

Sorbitol, although effective, is not as effective as xylitol. When compared with sugar-sweetened gum, sorbitol-sweetened gum had low carcinogenicity when it was chewed no more than three times per day, and xylitol-sweetened gum was noncariogenic in all the protocols tested.[45] It can be concluded that sorbitol is slowly fermented through anaerobic metabolism by *Streptococcus mutans,* whereas xylitol is not fermented at all.[46]

Studies have shown that a commercial chewing gum containing 5% sodium bicarbonate (Arm & Hammer Dental Care) is capable of removing significant amounts of plaque and reducing gingivitis when used as an adjunct to regular toothbrushing. Stain removal is also of interest to the consumer. Studies simulating a realistic situation (twice-daily brushing and unsupervised use of a baking soda chewing gum) demonstrated reduction in stain after 4 weeks.[47]

Consumers have relied on chewing-gum products for "fresh breath." A recent report on reducing VSC associated with oral malodor and organoleptic scores indicates that the products tested are effective primarily as masking agents (flavor) and for the mechanical role of cleaning tooth surfaces. Wrigley's Orbit and Extra sugar free chewing gums were the first chewing gums to be awarded the ADA Seal of Acceptance.

Casein phosphopeptide (CPP) has been introduced to chewing gum as a mechanism to remineralize early carious lesions. Trident Xtra Care gum, with Recaldent, makes use of this technology through the addition of CPP and amorphous calcium phosphate (ACP). Two studies compared remineralization of enamel with sugar-free gum containing CPP–ACP to equivalent gum not containing these agents.[48,49] Superior results were obtained in the gum containing CPP–ACP. See Table 11–3 ■ for an overview of selected agents added to chewing gums in the United States.

Compounds such as chlorhexidine and fluorides delivered to the oral cavity through a gum would appear to be useful. Compared with dentifrices that contain abrasives and mouthrinses that contain water and alcohol vehicles, the gum product would contain a minimum of potentially interfering agents. Gum would also provide a sustained time of release and availability in the oral cavity. In addition, the active agents would be available at occlusal sites, which are prime areas for plaque growth and pit-and-fissure decay. Neither of these agents is available in the United States and research in this area is limited. However, some studies done outside the United States show some level

TABLE ■ 11–3   Examples of Agents Added to Chewing Gums

Agent	Purpose/Claim	U.S. Example(s)
Aspirin	Pain relief	Aspergum
Caffeine	Increase alertness	Stay Alert, Jolt
Calcium carbonate	Neutralize stomach acid	Chooz
Casein phosphopeptide–amorphous calcium phosphate	Remineralize and strengthen teeth	Trident Xtra Care
Chlorhexidine	Antiplaque, antigingivitis	None
Dimenhydrinate	Motion sickness	Sea-Band Ginger
Fluoride	Anticaries	Guide
Sodium bicarbonate	Freshen breath	Arm & Hammer Dental Care
	Whiten teeth	Trident White
	Reduce plaque	
Xylitol	Anticaries	TridentXtra Care
		Omni Theragum

of significance in caries decline with the use of chlorhexidine and fluoride added to chewing gum.[50,51] One study reported increased staining on baseline-stained teeth with chlorhexidine chewing gum.[52] Because chewing-gum products are often in the mouth several times a day, the concentration of ingredients released, especially fluoride, must be safe for swallowing.

DID YOU KNOW **?**

The average woman smiles about 62 times a day and a man smiles 8 times a day. Children laugh about 400 times a days and adults 15.

SUMMARY

The self-use of dentifrices and mouthrinses is proving to be an important preventive dental health measure. Dentifrices, mouthrinses, and chewing gums can be categorized as either cosmetic or therapeutic. Cosmetic products have traditionally been used to remove debris, provide a pleasant "mouth feel," and temporarily reduce halitosis. To improve their products' marketability, manufacturers have added flavors, stripes, sprinkles, and colors to dentifrices and mouthrinses. Recently, other ingredients have also been added to temporarily depress the oral bacterial population, or to prevent or moderate some disease process in the mouth.

The widespread use of therapeutic fluoride dentifrices and mouthrinses is credited with helping to reduce the worldwide prevalence of dental decay. Other agents are now being used to target other oral-health problems.

The FDA has developed rigid guidelines for testing the safety and efficacy of products before their introduction on the market. Part of the function of the regulatory process is to differentiate between products whose potential risks are sufficiently low to allow them to be sold over the counter and those whose possible hazards justify restriction to prescription use.

Although the ADA considers antiplaque, anticalculus, and breath-freshening claims as cosmetic, it reviews data and allows manufacturers to make these statements if the claims are coupled with a disease-related activity (e.g., prevents gingivitis or caries). Toothpastes containing potassium nitrate, strontium chloride, and sodium citrate have antihypersensitivity properties; other toothpastes with tetrasodium phosphate and disodium dihydrogen pyrophosphate retard the formation of calculus. Ricaldent and triclosan are agents currently used more often in countries other than the United States. Chlorhexidine is a highly effective antiplaque and antigingivitis agent, but it has significant side effects and can be dispensed by prescription only. Listerine, which contains essential oils, has been popular for over a century and has demonstrated the same properties but not the side effects of chlorhexidine.

Chewing gum products are in a new dental category for which manufacturers are making claims for cosmetic and therapeutic effectiveness. At this time, the FDA has not approved any chewing gum products for dental therapeutic claims.

PRACTICAL CONSIDERATIONS

Dental professionals often must answer questions from patients regarding dentifrices, mouthrinses, and chewing gums. This chapter provides a practical guideline to help in answering common questions. The product market for all three types of these products is constantly changing. It is recommended that the dental office or community health center oral health practitioners share in the responsibility in keeping abreast of these changes.

A newsletter to patients or a posting of current information in the patient reception area is an effective way to disseminate information. Periodically reviewing current research, maintaining membership in professional organizations, and speaking to dental manufacturer representatives are excellent ways to remain current withthe literature.

SELF-STUDY QUESTIONS

1. What is the major reason that oral health products go under the review process in order to carry the ADA Seal of Acceptance?

   a. ADA Seal of Acceptance is needed for FDA approval.

   b. Dental product companies can charge more for the product with the ADA Seal of Acceptance.

   c. Dental offices cannot promote products without the ADA Seal of Acceptance.

   d. Products that carry the ADA Seal of Acceptance help to advertise the product to the public.

   Rationale: The ADA Seal of Acceptance lets patients know that product is safe and effective and recommended by the American Dental Association.

2. Which of the following types of fluoride is most compatible with calcium carbonate used in dentifrices?

   a. Sodium monofluorophosphate

   b. Stannous fluoride

   c. Acidulated phosphofluoride

   d. Neutral fluoride

   Rationale: Sodium monofluorophosphate. When the combination of fluoride and calcium carbonate is desired in a dentifrice, sodium fluoride is the soluble fluoride compatible with sodium bicarbonate.

3. The antibacterial agent effective in OTC dentifrices and mouthrinses and in deodorant soaps and antibacterial skin scrubs is:

   a. Potassium nitrate

   b. Triclosan

   c. Zinc sulfate

   d. Soluble pyrophosphates

   Rationale: Triclosan is a broad-spectrum antibacterial agent marketed by its manufacturer, Ciba-Geigy, for use in oral products under the trade name Irgacare. Triclosan is effective against a wide variety of bacteria and is widely used as an antibacterial agent in OTC consumer products in the United States, including deodorant soaps and antibacterial skin scrubs. It has been shown to be a useful antibacterial agent in oral products and is considered safe for use in dentifrice and mouthrinse products.

4. The ability of the oral tissues to adsorb an active agent such as chlorohexidine and to permit its slow release in active form over aprolonged period of time is referred to as

   a. Efficacy

   b. Mucoadhesion

   c. Substantivity

   d. Aerosol generation

   Rationale: This is the definition of substantivity, the ability of the oral tissues to adsorb an active agent and permit its slow release in active form over a prolonged period of time. As the substantivity of an antiplaque agent decreases, the frequency of use needs to be increased.

5. The ingredient found in chewing gum that is capable of remineralizing early carious lesions and known as Recaldent is referred to as which of the following?

   a. CPP-ACP

   b. Casein

   c. Sorbitol

   d. Xylitol

   Rationale: CPP-ACP is casein phosphopeptide–amorphous calcium phosphate has been introduced to chewing gum as a mechanism to remineralizeearly carious lesions. Recaldent uses this technology.

REFERENCES

1. United States Department of Health and Human Services, Food and Drug Administration, Center for Drug Evaluation and Research. (2008). Drug Applications—Phase 1 Clinical Studies, Phase 2 Clinical Studies, Phase 3 Clinical Studies. Retrieved June 13, 2011, from http://www.fda.gov/Drugs/DevelopmentApproval Process/SmallBusinessAssistance/ucm069898.htm#Phases of an Investigation.

2. United States Department of Health and Human Services, Food and Drug Administration, Center for Drug Evaluation and Research. (1998). Guidelines for industry, national uniformity for non prescription drugs—Ingredient listing for OTC drugs. Retrieved June 12, 2011, from http://www.fda.gov/downloads/Drugs/GuidanceComplianceRegulatoryInformation/Guidances/ucm078733.pdf.

3. U.S. Food and Drug Administration. (2003, May 29). Oral health care drug products for over-the-counter human use; Antigingivitis/antiplaque drug products. Establishment of a monograph. *Fed Reg, 68:*32232–34. Retrieved November 26, 2007, from http://www.fda.gov/OHRMS/DOCKETS/98fr/03-12783.pdf.

4. American Dental Association. (2011). Guidelines for earning the seal. Retrieved September 14, 2012 , from http://www.ada.org/participationguidelines.aspx.

5. Richmond, R., MacFarlane T. V., & McCord, J. F. (2004). An evaluation of the surface changes in PMMA biomaterial formulations as a result of toothbrush/dentifrice abrasion. *Dent Mater,* 20:124–32.

6. Avey, K. D., Debiase, C. B., Gladwin, M. A., Kao, E. C., & Bagby, M. D. (2006). Development of a standardized abrasive scale: An analysis of commercial prophylaxis paste. *JDent Hyg,* 80.1

7. Rantanen, I., Jutila, K., Nicander, I., Tenovuo, J., & Soderling, E. (2003). The effects of twosodium lauryl sulphate containing toothpastes with and without betaine on human oral mucosa in vivo. *Swed Dent J,* 27:31–34.

8. Putt, M. S., Milleman, K. R.,Ghassemi, A., Vorwerk, L. M., Hooper, W. J., Soparkar, P. M, Winston, A. E., & Proskin, H. M. (2008). Enhancement of plaque removal efficacy by toothbrushing with baking soda dentifrices: Results of five clinical studies. *J Clin Dent,* 19:111–19.

9. Ghassemi, A. V., Hooper, L. M., Putt, W. J., & Milleman, K. R. (2008). A four-week clinical study to evaluate and compare the effectiveness of a baking soda dentifrice and an antimicrobial dentifrice in reducing plaque. *J Clin Dent,* 19:120–12.

10. American Dental Association. (2005). *Council on Scientific Affairs. Acceptance program guidelines: Fluoride-containing dentifrices.* Chicago, IL: American Dental Association.

11. White, D. J., Kozak, K. M., Gibb, R., Dunavent, J., Klukowska, M., & Sagel, P. A. (2006). A 24-hour dental plaque

prevention study with stannous fluoride dentifrice containing hexametaphosphate. *J Contemp Dent Pract,* 7:1–11.

12. Archila, L., Bartizek, R. D., Winston, J. L., McClanahan, S. E., & He, T. (2004). The comparative efficacy of stabilized stannous fluoride/sodium hexametaphosphate dentifrice and sodium fluoride/triclosan/copolymer dentifrice for the control of gingivitis: A 6-month randomized clinical study. *J Periodontol,* 75:1592–99.

13. Panagakos, F. S., Volpe, A. R., Petrone, M. E., DeVizio, W., Davies, R. M., & Proskin, H. M. (2005). A review of comprehensive advanced oral antibacterial/anti-inflammatory technology of the clinical benefits of a triclosan/copolymer/fluoride dentifrice. *J Clin Dent,* 16 (Suppl 1-19).

14. McClanahan, S. F., Bollmer, B. W., Court, L. K., McClary, J. M., Majeti, S, Crisanti, MM, Beiswaner, B. B., & Mau, M. S., (2000). Plaque regrowth effects of a Triclosan/pyrophosphate dentifrice in a 4-day non-brushing model. *J Clin Dent,* 11:107-13.

15. Adams, S. E., Theobald, A. J., Jones, N. M., Brading, M. G., Cox, T. F., Mendez, A., Chesters, D. M., Gillam, D. G., Hall, C., & Holt, J. (2003). The effect of toothpaste containing 2% zinc citrate and 0.3% triclosan on bacterial viability and plaque growth in vivo compared to a toothpaste containing 0.3% triclosan and 2% copolymer. *Int Dent J,* 53:398–403.

16. Zacherl, W. A., Pfeiffer, H. J., & Swancar, J. R., (1985).The effect of soluble pyrophosphateson dental calculus in adults. *J Am Dent Assoc,* 110:737–738.

17. Haywood, V. B., Cordero, R., Wright, K., Gendreau, L., Rupp, R., Kotler, M., Littlejohn, S., Fabyanski, J., & Smith S. (2005). Brushing with a potassium nitrate dentifrice to reduce bleaching sensitivity. *J Clin Dent,* 16:17–22.

18. American Association of Poison Control. (2010). 2006–2009 Annual AAPCC Reports of the NPDS. *Clinical Toxicology, 2007–2010,* 45-48:815–917, 927–1057,911–1084, 979–1178.

19. Farrell S., Bake, R. A., Somogyi-Mann, M., Witt, J. J., & Gerlach, R. W. (2006). Oral malodor reduction by a combination of chemotherapeutic and mechanical treatments. *Clin Oral Invest,* 10:157–63.

20. Darby, M. L., & Walsh, M. M. (2010). *Dental hygiene theory and practice* (3rd ed.). Philadelphia, PA: Saunders Elsevier.

21. Borden, L. C., Chaves, E. S., Bowman, J. P., Fath, B. M., & Hollar, G. L. (2002). The effect of four mouthrinses on malodor. *Compend Contin Educ Dent,* 23:531–36.

22. Loesche, W. J. (2003). Microbiology and treatment of halitosis. *Curr Infect Dis Rep,* 5:220–25.

23. Codipilly, D. P., Kaufman, H. W., & Kleinberg, I. (2004). Use of novel group of oral malodor measurements to evaluate an anti-oral malodor mouthrinse (TriOral^TM) in humans. *J Clin Dent,* 15:98–104.

24. Pedersen, E. J. (2003). *U.S. Patent No. 660,7711.* Mouth hygienic composition in the treatment of halitosis. Washington, DC: U.S. Patent and Trademark Office. Retrieved November 26, 2007, from http://www.patentstorm.us/patents/6607711-description .html.

25. Corcoran, R. A. (2006). Evaluation of a combined polymer system for use in relieving the symptoms of xerostomia. *J Clin Dent,* 17 (Spec Iss):34–38.

26. Lorenz, K., Bruhn, G., Heumann, C., Netuschil, L., Brecx, M., & Hoffman, T. (2006). Effect of two new chlorhexidinemouthrinses on the development of dental plaque, gingivitis, and discoloration. A randomized, investigator blind, placebo-controlled, 3-week experimental gingivitis study. *J ClinPeriodontol,* 33:561–67.

27. Kolahi, J., & Soolari, A. (2006). Rinsing with chlorhexidine gluconate solution after brushing and flossing teeth: A systematic review of effectiveness. *Quintessence Int,* 37:605–12.

28. Faveri, M., Gursky, L. C., Feres, M., Shibli, J. A., Salvador, S. L., & deFiqueiredo, L. C. (2006). Scaling and root planing and chlorhexidine mouthrinses in the treatment of chronic periodontitis: A randomized, placebo controlled clinical trial. *J ClinPeriodontol,* 33:81928.

29. Gurgan, C. A., Zaim, E., Bakirsoy, I., & Soykan, E. (2006). Short term effects of 0.2% alcohol-free chlorhexidine mouthrinse used as an adjunct to non-surgical periodontal treatment: A double blind clinical study. *J Periodontol,* 77:370–84.

30. von Fraunhofer, J. A., Kelley, J. I., DePaola, L. G., & Miller, T. F. (2006). The effect of a mouthrinse containing essential oils on dental restorative materials. *Gen Dent,* 54:403–7.

31. Sekino, S., & Ramberg, P. (2005). The effect of a mouthrinse containing phenolic compounds on plaque formation and developing gingivitis. *J Clin Periodontol,* 32:1083–88.

32. U.S. Department of Health and Human Services. (2003). Oral health care drug products for over-the-counter human use; anti-gingivitis/antiplaque drug products; establishment of a monograph; proposed rules. *Fed Reg,* 68:32231–87. (Codified at 21 CFR pr 356).

33. Stookey, G. K., Beiswanger, B., Mau, M., Isaacs, R. L., Witt, J. J., & Gibb, R. (2005). A 6-month clinical study assessing the safety and efficacy of two cetylpyridinium chloride mouthrinses. *Am J Dent,* 18 (Spec Iss):24A–28A.

34. Kozak, K. M., Gibb, R., Dunavent, J., & White, D. J. (2005). Efficacy of a high bioavailable cetylpyridinium chloride mouthrinse over a 24-hour period: A plaque imaging study. *Am J Dent,* 18 (Spec No.):18A–23A.

35. Blenman, T. V., Morrison, K. L., Tsay, G. J., Medina, A. L., & Gerlach, R. W. (2005). Practice implications with an alcohol-free, 0.07% cetylpyridinium chloride mouthrinse. *Am J Dent,* 18 (Spec No.):29A–34A.

36. Ramos-Gomez, F. L., Crall, J., Gansky, S. A., Slayton, R. L., & Featherstone, J. D. (2007). Caries risk assessment appropriate for the age 1 visit (infants and toddlers). *J Calif Dent Assoc,* 35:687–702.

37. Villalpando, K. T., Casarin, R. C., Pimentel, S. P., Cirano, F. R., & Casati, M Z (2010). A randomized clinical evaluation of triclosan-containing dentifrice and mouthwash association in the control of plaque and gingivitis. *Quint Int,* 41:855–61.

38. Patel, M., Ndlovu N. N., Owen, C. P., &Veale, R. (2010). Properties of a new mouthrinse for patients receiving radiation therapy. *SADJ,* 65:410, 412–14.

39. Dawes, C., & Kubinec, K. (2004). The effects of prolonged gum chewing on salivary flow rate and composition. *Arch Oral Biol,* 49:665–69.

40. Ribelles, L. M., Guinot, J. F., Mayné, A. R., & Bellet, D. L. J. (2010). Effects of xylitol chewing gum on salivary flow rate, pH, buffering capacity and presence of Streptococcus mutans in saliva. *Eur J Paediatr Dent,* 11:9–14.

41. Cadbury Schweppes. (2006, October 30). (Press Release). Cadbury Schweppes enters UK Chewing Gum Market. Retrieved May 5, 2008, from http://www.cadburyschweppes.com/EN/ MediaCentre/PressReleases/uk_gum_launch.htm.

42. Yankell, S. L., & Emling, R. C. (1999). Clinical effects on plaque pH, pCa and swallowing rates from chewing a flavored or unflavored chewing gum. *J Clin Dent,* 10:86–88.

43. Gutkowski, S. (2005). X marks the spot. *Contemp Oral Hygiene,* 5:10–13.

44. Beebe, S. (2006). The expanding utility of xylitol. *Dimensions,* 10:34–36.

45. Burt, B. A. (2006). The use of sorbitol- and xylitol-sweetened chewing gum in caries control. *J Am Dent Assoc,* 137:190–96.

46. Duane, B. (2010). Xylitol gum, plaque pH and mutans streptococci. *Evid Based Dent,* 11:109–10.

47. Kleber. C. J., Putt, M. S., Milleman, J. L., Davidson, K. R., & Proskin, H. M. (2001, July). An evaluation of sodium bicarbonate chewing gum in reducing dental plaque and gingivitis in conjunction with regular toothbrushing. *Compend Contin Educ Dent,* 22:4–12.

48. Iijima, Y., Cai, F., Shen, P., Walker, G., Reynolds, C., & Reynolds, E. C. (2004). Acid resistance of enamel subsurface lesions remineralized by a sugar-free chewing gum containing casein phosphopeptide-amorphous calcium phosphate. *Caries Res,* 38:551–56.

49. Shen, P., Cai, F., Nowicki, A., Vincent, J., & Reynolds, E. C. (2001). Remineralization of enamel subsurface lesions by sugar-free chewing gum containing casein phosphopeptide-amorphous calcium phosphate. *J Dent Res,* 80:2066–70.

50. Thorild, I., Lindau, B., & Twetman, S. (2006). Caries in 4-year-old children after maternal chewing of gums containing combinations of xylitol, sorbitol, chlorhexidine, and fluoride. *Eur Arch Paediatr Dent,* 7:241–45.

51. Thorild, I., Lindau, B., & Twetman, S. (2004). Salivary mutan streptococci and dental caries in three-year-old children after maternal exposure to chewing gums containing combinations of xylitol, sorbitol, chlorhexidine, and fluoride. *Acta Odontol Scand,* 62:245–50.

52. Thorild, I., Lindau, B., & Twetman, S. (2003). Effect of maternal use of chewing gums containing xylitol, chlorhexidine, or fluoride on mutans streptococci colonization in the mothers' infant children. *Oral Health Prev Dent,* 1:53–57.

Self-Care Adjuncts

Christine French Beatty
Amy Teague

OBJECTIVES

After studying this chapter, the student should be able to:

1. Describe the reasons that adjuncts to toothbrushing are needed to supplement oral health self-care.
2. Identify factors in addition to oral conditions that influence selection of self-care adjunctive devices and techniques.
3. Identify the process of developing an oral health self-care plan.
4. State the purposes, indications, contraindications, techniques, advantages, and limitations of various adjunctive oral hygiene devices and procedures.

KEY TERMS

Cannula, 185
Dental floss holder, 172
Dental floss threader, 173
End-tuft brush, 177
Halitosis, 186
Interdental brush, 175
Irrigation, 183
Loop method of flossing, 169
Power flosser, 175
Rubber tip stimulator, 181
Spool method of flossing, 169
Tongue cleaner, 190
Tongue scraper, 190
Toothpick, 178
Toothpick holder, 179
Triangular wooden stick, 179
Variable-thickness floss, 167
Waxed dental tape, 167

INTRODUCTION

It has long been recognized that the plaque biofilm that forms and remains on tooth surfaces is the primary etiologic factor in the development of both dental caries and periodontal diseases.[1] Patients need to understand that prevention and management of periodontal diseases and caries depends on effective daily removal and control of this plaque biofilm.[2,3,4] Studies have documented that long-term maintenance of a high level of oral hygiene results in a greatly reduced incidence of dental caries, periodontal diseases, and tooth loss.[5] In addition because other medical conditions are affected by oral diseases,[6] failure to practice adequate oral hygiene can have adverse effects on overall health.[7]

Although toothbrushing is effective in cleaning the buccal, lingual, and occlusal surfaces, it leaves the proximal surfaces essentially untouched.[8] Limitations of the toothbrush in removing plaque biofilm from the proximal surfaces and other hard-to-reach areas indicate a need to recommend supplemental measures.[9] Regular removal of interproximal plaque biofilm should be recommended for a number of reasons (Box 12–1 ■).

The dentition or periodontal tissues can be altered as a result of disease or repair or from architectural tissue changes after therapy.[10] When alterations occur, a device and/or technique must be introduced to accommodate them. Although it has been shown that removal of supragingival plaque biofilm influences the subgingival plaque biofilm composition, plaque biofilm removal efforts should also extend as far subgingivally as possible. Identifying the most effective supplemental oral hygiene aids is accomplished by applying the process of care model,[11] conducting a thorough assessment of the patient's oral health disease risk factors,[12] reflecting the human needs conceptual model,[13] and adhering to an evidence-based approach to establish best practices.[14] See Chapter 3 for a more detailed discussion of process of care.

Consideration of lifestyle issues is especially important to ensure that the patient can realistically follow through with recommendations to use supplemental aids.[15] This promotes a personal and individualized approach to self-care recommendations. In addition, involving the patient in the decision-making process of determining appropriate supplemental aids will increase the level of long-term commitment to, and success of, behavioral changes.[15] Finally, use of supplemental aids for self-care should be introduced, monitored, reinforced, and evaluated during appointments for therapy to increase compliance.[16] Recommendations should be documented and modified as needed throughout the patient's life span based on patient outcomes and changes in modifiable risk factors.[17]

DID YOU KNOW **?**

Just as in making decisions about treatment considerations, evidence-based practice principles should be applied to the selection of supplemental aids.

Recommending oral self-care products to boost office productivity is a commonly suggested approach.[18] However, this practice does not consider the principles of evidence-based practice. According to evidence-based principles, recommendations for a self-care plan should be based on the best available scientific evidence; the patient's needs, values, and desires; and the professional judgment and clinical expertise of the oral health care practitioner.[14] Continual involvement of the patient in self-care decisions supports the practice of these evidence-based principles.

There is frequently a gap between the published evidence and the evidence practitioners use to make clinical decisions.[19] As researchers learn more about oral diseases, risk factors, and ways to prevent and control these diseases, clinicians will need to adjust their recommendations to match the new knowledge. The provider needs to continually learn to become aware of new evidence in relation to oral diseases, the efficacy and safety of self-care products, and procedures to prevent oral diseases.[20] Development of a self-care plan should follow a systematic approach that incorporates prescribed techniques based on sound evidence to enhance plaque biofilm removal and reduction of risk without causing trauma to the hard and soft oral tissues. Although the American Dental Association (ADA) seal of approval program may be used to evaluate products, it is a voluntary program, so it is not mandatory for manufacturers to submit their products for review. Therefore, a variety of peer-reviewed sources should be consulted as well.[21]

This chapter will discuss various self-care adjunctive aids for oral hygiene (Table 12–1 ■), application of these oral hygiene aids (Table 12–2 ■), and evidence of their effectiveness and potential for trauma. This information is for the practitioner's consideration in developing supplemental self-care recommendations. This discussion includes self-care adjunctive aids

---

BOX 12–1 | **Reasons to Recommend Regular Interproximal Plaque Biofilm Removal**

- Incomplete plaque biofilm removal can increase the rate and growth of new plaque bioflim.
- Plaque biofilm regrowth occurs first in the interproximal areas.
- Allowing plaque biofilm to remain on some tooth surfaces can facilitate development of a complex microflora on other clean surfaces.
- Individuals who clean interproximally on a daily basis have less plaque biofilm and calculus.
- Gingivitis, periodontitis, and caries occur more frequently in interproximal areas.
- Daily effective interproximal plaque biofilm removal can facilitate prevention of caries.
- Interproximal plaque biofilm removal is beneficial for preventing gingival and periodontal infections, as well as for reducing or eliminating diseases in these tissues.[1]
- Daily effective interproximal plaque removal can facilitate prevention of caries.[20]

TABLE ■ 12–1   Self-Care Adjunctive Aids

- Dental floss
- Dental floss holder
- Dental floss threader
- Power flosser
- Interdental (interproximal) brush
- Uni-tuft (end-tuft) brush
- Toothpick
- Toothpick holder
- Wooden or plastic triangular stick
- Rubber tip stimulator
- Yarn
- Pipe cleaner
- Gauze strip
- Oral irrigator
- Tongue cleaner

TABLE ■ 12–2   Application of Interproximal Supplemental Aids

- Proximal surfaces
- Hard-to-reach areas
- Rotated teeth
- Malaligned teeth
- Partially erupted teeth
- Irregular tooth morphology
- Embrasure spaces
- Isolated teeth[a]
- Furcations
- Orthodontic appliances
- Implants
- Fixed prosthetic appliances

[a]An isolated tooth occurs when the teeth that normally surround the tooth are missing.

for interdental cleaning, adjunctive procedures for antibacterial effects, and procedures and aids for control of halitosis.

ORAL HEALTH SELF-CARE

Self-care includes all activities and decisions made by an individual in relation to the prevention, diagnosis, and treatment of personal ill health, and the maintenance or control of chronic conditions. This concept, as applied to care of the oral cavity, is referred to as *oral self-care* or *oral health self-care*. The term is used in place of earlier terms such as *personal plaque control* and *oral physiotherapy* to emphasize the client's responsibility for his or her preventive oral health decisions and practices. One primary purpose of oral health self-care is to prevent or arrest periodontal diseases and caries by reducing plaque biofilm accumulation.[22] Less-than-optimal oral self-care is regarded as a major risk factor for

oral diseases. An appropriate oral self-care plan for each individual is based on the results of a comprehensive assessment, as discussed previously.

DID YOU KNOW ?

The term *oral health self-care* indicates the patient's responsibility for personal oral hygiene and better expresses the comprehensive approach required for maximum effectiveness.

On the basis of the assessment, an oral health self-care plan should be recommended before initiating therapy for treatment of disease. It is adjusted as needed during and after therapy according to the results of evaluation. A one-size-fits-all approach to making recommendations to patients regarding their oral self-care plan does not work. There is no universally accepted oral hygiene method, practice, device, or frequency of cleaning.[15] Critical thinking must be applied to develop an individualized, appropriate oral hygiene regimen based on the dictates of the individual's oral condition, personal preferences, abilities, dexterity, and lifestyle.

Once the oral health self-care plan has been developed, the oral health professional must provide adequate education about the need for oral health self-care as well as instruction in the use of any recommended procedure, method, or device. Selecting the right device, minimizing the number of recommended devices, simplifying the instructions, and providing effective strategies to motivate the patient will help promote successful implementation of, and increase compliance with, the oral self-care plan. Patient education should be based on solid health promotion theory[23] and should include the strategies of codiscovery, observation, explanation, demonstration, guided practice, and request for a return demonstration to assess understanding.[16] Codiscovery is the process in which the oral care professional explains diagnostic methods and results to the patient during dental examinations; this sharing of information allows the patient and professional to learn about the patient's oral condition at the same time. In addition, reasons for noncompliance should be explored so they can be addressed in an attempt to overcome them (see Chapter 19).[23]

FREQUENCY OF SELF-CARE

Although mechanical plaque biofilm removal is important to the prevention of dental caries, it appears that only a very high level of personal mechanical plaque biofilm removal impacts the dental caries rate. This level is difficult for the average person to sustain.[24] Control of dental caries involves a complex approach including the use of fluorides and other chemical therapies such as calcium, phosphates, xylitol, and chlorhexidine; management of healthy saliva; use of dental sealants; and appropriate dietary control in addition to plaque biofilm removal for optimal effect on the caries rate of proximal

TABLE ■ 12–3   Comparison of Various Types of Dental Floss

Type of Floss	Indications	Advantages	Disadvantages
Waxed dental tape (broad/flat)	Embrasure: II and III Loose contact Large surface areas Can use with dentifrice	Tear resistance More control	Difficult to use in tight contacts
Waxed dental floss	Embrasure: I Around rough tooth surfaces and restorations	Strength and durability Shred resistance Ease of insertion Prevents tissue trauma	Patient discomfort due to thickness
Unwaxed round floss	Embrasure: I Tight contacts	Slips in easily	Tears easily on contact with calculus and defective restorations Patient discouragement
Tufted super floss (stiff end) Variable-thickness	Embrasure: II and III Fixed bridge (stiff end) Exposed furcation Orthodontic appliances Implant prosthesis	Covers more surface area Stiff end Easier insertion Ease of reaching hard-to-access areas Easier to use than floss threaders	Requires coordination Catches on rough surfaces
Colored floss	Visualization of plaque biofilm and debris Use by beginner Use by those with weak eyesight	Motivational and educational Increases compliance	NA
Flavored floss	More appealing Lack of motivation	Motivational Easy to see	NA
Impregnated floss/tape, containing fluoride, baking soda, herbal extracts, abrasives, and antimicrobials	Caries control Therapeutic effect on gingiva	Ease of application to hard-to-access areas	Abrasiveness of some agents Efficacy not well documented

NA, not applicable.

surfaces.[4,25] Although thorough removal of interproximal plaque biofilm with daily professional flossing has been shown to decrease caries incidence in children,[26] increased use of fluorides and antimicrobials will provide greater protection than self-flossing in high-risk children.[25]

Research has shown that effective oral hygiene every 48 hours is the longest interval that will maintain gingival health.[24] However, with more daily attempts, it is more probable that the additive efforts will maximize the removal of plaque biofilm. Intervals that exceed 48 hours between removal of plaque biofilm will likely result in the development of gingivitis.[24] For those with existing gingival inflammation or periodontal infection, plaque biofilm removal every 48 hours is not frequent enough.[3] It has been shown that colonization and maturation of plaque biofilm occurs more rapidly in the presence of inflammation. Therefore, to control gingivitis versus preventing its onset, patients should practice the meticulous removal of plaque biofilm from all surfaces at least on a daily basis.

DID YOU KNOW ?

The frequency of and length of time required for adequate self-care varies from one patient to another, depending on her or his oral health status and needs.

Because the ideal frequency of interproximal plaque biofilm removal has not been identified, individual factors such as the amount of inflammation; susceptibility to caries, gingivitis, and periodontitis; efficiency of removing plaque biofilm; and accumulation and virulence of plaque biofilm must be considered in the recommendation of frequency.[27] Determining the risk factors that increase susceptibility to caries and periodontal diseases can help identify the frequency needed for both toothbrushing and interproximal cleaning.[24] Regardless of the disease of interest, the frequency of mechanical plaque biofilm removal for self-care must be tailored to the patient. The frequency of interproximal cleaning should generally be between 12 and 48 hours, and most patients who adhere to the traditional recommendation of brushing twice a day and flossing once a day can achieve oral cleanliness.[26]

The length of time that should be devoted to self-care is also not consistent. How much time is needed will depend on the degree of susceptibility, the extent of periodontal breakdown, the condition of the teeth and restorations, the patient's dexterity and motor skills, and the presence of obstacles to self-care.[24]

DENTAL FLOSS

Dental floss is best indicated for plaque biofilm and debris removal from a type I embrasure (Figure 12–1A ■) because the papilla fills the interproximal space, and the teeth are in contact.[28] For type II (Figure 12–1B ■) and III embrasures (Figure 12–1C ■), special devices other than floss may be more effective to remove plaque biofilm from proximal surfaces.[29] Effective use of dental floss accomplishes a number of objectives (Box 12–2 ■).[24,28–33]

Not all interproximal contact areas, whether natural or restored, have the same countour or configuration. Consequently, several types of dental floss are available to accommodate these differences.[29] See Table 12–3 ■ and Figure 12–2 ■ for various types of floss.

DID YOU KNOW?

The first dental floss was manufactured in 1882 in the United States from an unwaxed silk thread. This was replaced during the 1940s by nylon floss that was stronger and allowed for the development of waxed floss.

Dental floss varies from thin unwaxed varieties to thicker waxed tapes and includes variable-thickness floss. Unwaxed floss is frequently recommended because it is thin and slips easily through tight contact areas.[24] Thin silk floss has the advantage of "squeaking" when the proximal surface is clean.[26] However, unwaxed floss can fray or tear if used around heavy calculus deposits, defective and overhanging restorations, or rotated teeth, which may discourage continued use. In these situations, shred-resistant, lightly waxed, or waxed floss are recommended.

Some types of unwaxed floss, such as those made of polytetrafluoroethylene (PTFE, Teflonlike, also called Gore Tex), are stronger, more shred resistant, and may be preferable for tight contacts, rough proximal tooth surfaces, and rough restorations.[26] **Waxed dental tape**, unlike round dental floss, is broad and flat and is recommended for class I and class II embrasures and to clean an interproximal space that does not have tight contact points.[24] Tape can also be used with dentifrice to polish interproximal stain.

Another variety of dental floss is **variable-thickness floss**, which has increments of soft tufts alternating with standard floss. The standard floss can be passed through the contacts, and the tufts can be used to clean larger proximal surface areas of

BOX 12–2 Objectives Accomplished with Effective Use of Dental Floss

1. Removing plaque and debris that adheres to proximal surfaces of the teeth and restorations, orthodontic appliances, undersurfaces of fixed prostheses and pontics, and implant abutments
2. Helping to control bleeding even before initiation of scaling and root planing
3. Controlling the formation of calculus
4. Aiding the clinician in identifying the presence of interproximal calculus deposits, overhanging restorations, or interproximal carious lesions
5. Contributing to the arrest or prevention of interproximal carious lesions
6. Reducing gingival bleeding and inflammation
7. Reducing malodor
8. Applying polishing or chemotherapeutic agents to interproximal and subgingival areas

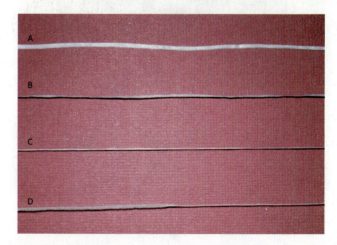

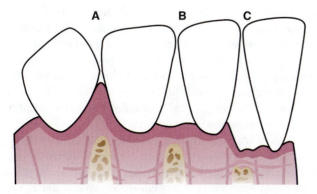

FIGURE ■ 12–1 Embrasure types. A. Type I—papilla fills interproximal space. B. Type II—slight to moderate recession of papilla. C. Type III—extensive recession or complete loss of papilla.

FIGURE ■ 12–2 A variety of types of floss. A. Waxed dental tape. B. Waxed dental floss. C. Unwaxed round floss. D. Variable-thickness floss.

(*Source:* Courtesy of Amy Teague.)

type II and III embrasures more effectively than regular floss.[24] Variable-thickness floss may be recommended for use in cleaning implant abutments, areas with open contacts, wide embrasures, or sites where recession and bone loss permit access to furcations. Another type of tufted floss is a thicker mesh that stretches for easy insertion. These thicker types of floss are also useful to remove plaque biofilm from the distal aspect of the most distal tooth in all quadrants or spaces adjacent to missing teeth. Some types of tufted floss have a stiff end to allow for threading under bridges (Figure 12–3 ■), beneath tight contact areas, under splints, under pontics, through exposed furcations, and around orthodontic wires without having to use floss threaders.

Some brands of dental floss and tape are colored and/or flavored. In addition to increased appeal, color provides a visual contrast to plaque biofilm and oral debris, thus enabling one to see what is being removed and possibly increasing the motivation to floss. Some individuals prefer waxed over unwaxed floss and flavored floss over plain waxed floss. These patient preferences can improve compliance with flossing.[24]

Various agents have been impregnated into dental floss and have the potential to help prevent and control oral diseases. Examples of these include floss treated with baking soda, fluoride, herbal extracts, antimicrobial agents, or abrasives for whitening. Although use of these agents as rinses or other means has demonstrated effectiveness, limited research has been published relative to their effectiveness when impregnated into dental floss.[26] However, chlorhexidine gel applied with dental floss has been shown to reduce caries incidence in children,[30,34] and the use of chlorhexidine-impregnated floss has reduced plaque biofilm and gingivitis.[31] A study with fluoride-impregnated dental floss demonstrated higher fluoride concentration

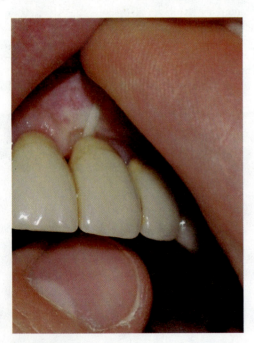

FIGURE ■ 12–3 **Variable-thickness floss with stiff end used to clean under the pontic and on the proximal surfaces of abutments of a fixed bridge.**

(*Source:* Courtesy of Amy Teague.)

of the saliva in the treated interproximal sites, which lasted up to 30 minutes.[35]

Clinical trials have shown no significant differences in the plaque biofilm removal efficacy, comfort, or ease of use of various types of floss, including the cleansing ability of unwaxed floss compared with waxed floss.[26,36] A common myth is that wax residue remains on the tooth surfaces after cleaning with waxed floss, but research has indicated that this is not accurate.[37] Study participants have expressed varying preferences in different studies, sometimes for waxed floss, sometimes for tape, and sometimes for polytetrafluoroethylene (Glide®) floss. One study found that a difference in force is required to use the thicker floss types.[38] The issues of preference and force could affect flossing frequency. Because the evidence does not identify a best type of floss, recommendations should be based on the patient's specific oral conditions, preference, and ability.

DID YOU KNOW ?

A "one-size-fits-all" approach cannot be applied to the selection of interproximal cleaning aids; the decisions must be individualized based on the patient's needs.

A limitation of flossing is its inability to conform to a concave proximal root surface such as the mesial surface of the maxillary premolar.[29] When these surfaces are exposed, other interproximal devices should be considered as supplements to clean those surfaces more effectively (Figure 12–4 ■). These aids are discussed in a later section of this chapter.

Although the occurrence is uncommon, bacterial endocarditis has been reported in susceptible individuals who have gingivitis or periodontitis and floss only sporadically.[39] Susceptible patients should be made aware of this risk and counseled to floss regularly or use some other form of interproximal plaque biofilm removal to maintain health of the gingival tissues for protection against bacteremia.[40]

Dental Flossing Methods

Two frequently used flossing methods are the spool method and the circle, or loop, method.[26] Both methods facilitate control of the floss and ease of handling. The spool method is particularly suited for teenagers and adults who have acquired the necessary neuromuscular coordination required to use floss. The loop method is suited for children as well as adults with less nimble hands or physical limitations caused by conditions such as poor muscular coordination or arthritis.

Flossing is a complex skill. Therefore, until children develop adequate dexterity, usually around the age of 10 to 12 years, their attempts at flossing will be ineffective. The American Academy of Pediatric Dentistry has recommended that an adult should perform flossing on the child.[41] To accomplish this, the adult should support the child's head in the adult's lap, against the chest, or in some other stable position, preferably flossing

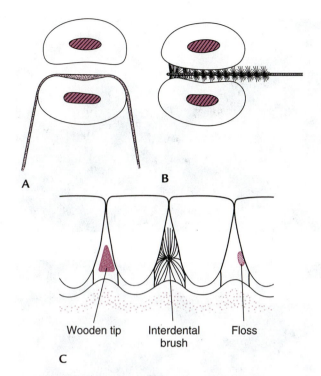

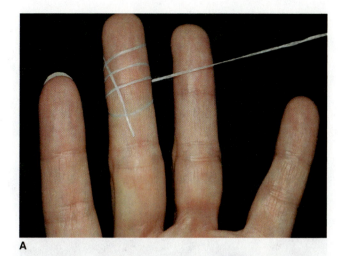

A

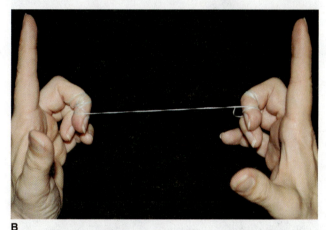

B

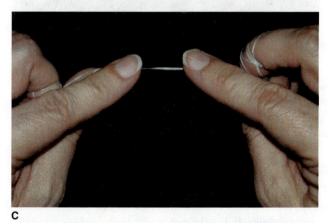

C

FIGURE ■ 12–4 Surface coverage comparison of different interdental aids. A. Floss adapted to a mesial surface of a maxillary molar shows its inability to fully cover the concave surface. B. Interproximal brush in the same area shows how it adapts into the concave surface. C. Comparable access of a wooden triangular stick, an interdental brush, and dental floss in an open embrasure.

Wooden tip   Interdental brush   Floss

FIGURE ■ 12–5 Spool method of flossing. A. Floss is lightly wound and spaced around the middle finger of each hand. B. The last three fingers are clenched, pulling the floss taut and leaving the index finger and the thumb of each hand free. C. The floss is held with the index finger and thumb of each hand by grasping a section ¾ to 1 in long between the hands.

(*Source:* Courtesy of Amy Teague.)

from behind. Younger children whose teeth still exhibit primate spaces with no interproximal contacts will not require flossing.

In the **spool method of flossing**, a piece of floss approximately 18 inches long is used. The bulk of the floss is lightly wound around the middle finger. Space should be left between wraps to avoid impairing circulation to the fingers (Figure 12–5A ■). The rest of the floss is similarly wound around the same finger of the opposite hand. This finger can wind, or take up, the floss as it becomes soiled or frayed to permit access to an unused portion. The last three fingers are clenched and the hands are moved apart, pulling the floss taut, thus leaving the thumb and index finger of each hand free (Figure 12–5B ■). The floss is then secured with the index finger and thumb of each hand by grasping a ¾- to 1-inch length section between the hands (Figure 12–5C ■).

In the **loop method of flossing**, the ends of the 18-inch piece of floss are tied in a knot to form a circle. All of the fingers, but not the thumbs, of the two hands are placed close to one another within the loop (Figure 12–6 ■). The circle of floss is rotated to advance to clean floss.

In both flossing methods, the same basic procedures are followed. The thumb and index finger of each hand are used in various combinations to floss the teeth. Index fingers are used to floss the mandibular teeth. On the maxillary arch, it is easier to use either the thumb of both hands or the thumb of one hand and the index finger of the other hand. Use of the index finger rather than the middle finger makes it easier to reach the

posterior teeth and guide the floss for correct adaptation. The fingers should be placed about an inch apart to enhance control of the floss to ensure safe insertion into the interproximal space and maintenance of correct adaptation during flossing. When

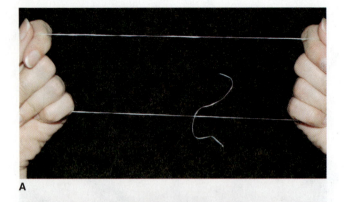

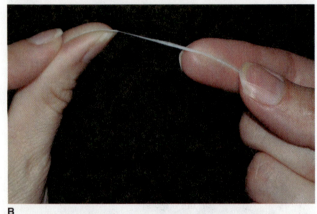

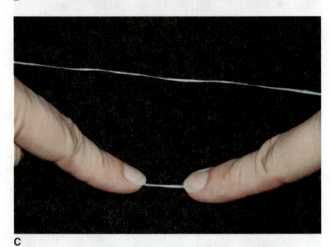

FIGURE ■ 12–6 Loop method of flossing. **A. All fingers except the thumbs are placed within the loop for easy maneuverability. B. For the mandibular teeth, the floss is guided with the two index fingers.** (*Source:* Courtesy of Amy Teague.) **C. For the maxillary teeth, the floss is guided with two thumbs or one thumb and one index finger.** (*Source:* Courtesy of Amy Teague.)

inserting the floss, it is gently eased between the teeth with a seesaw motion at the contact point. The gentle seesaw motion flattens the floss, making it possible to ease through the contact point and prevent snapping it through, thus avoiding trauma to the interdental papilla (Figure 12–7A ■). Placement of the fingers in close proximity makes it possible to ease the floss interproximally and prevent snapping of the floss.

Once past the contact point, the floss is adapted to each interproximal surface by creating a C-shape (Figure 12–7B ■).

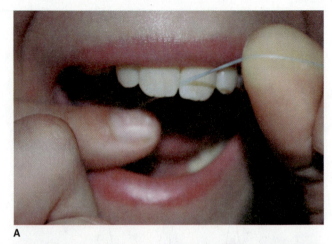

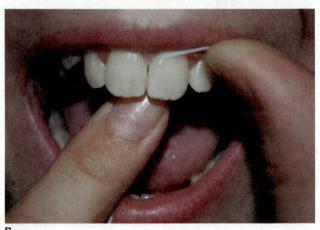

FIGURE ■ 12–7 Flossing technique. **A. The floss is gently inserted between the teeth with a back-and-forth sawing motion at the contact point. B. After this, the floss is adapted to each proximal surface by creating a C-shape, directed apically into the sulcus. Then the floss is slid down to the contact area with pressure against the proximal surface, repeating several times or until the surface is clean.**

(*Source:* Courtesy of Amy Teague.)

The floss is then directed apically into the sulcus and back to the contact area (up and down against the side of the tooth) several times or until the tooth surface is clean. This stroke must be gentle to avoid damaging the sulcular area and causing floss cuts. The number of strokes required depends on the thickness of the plaque biofilm. If floss is used daily, fewer strokes are required. Also, the use of Teflon-type floss may require more strokes to "grab" the plaque biofilm for complete removal. The procedure is repeated on the adjacent tooth in the proximal area; care is used to prevent damage to the papilla while readapting the floss to the adjacent tooth.

In general, flossing is best performed by cleaning each tooth in succession, including the distal surface of the last tooth in each quadrant. A clean, unused portion of floss should be used for each interproximal area to prevent fraying as well as for sanitary purposes. The individual should be assisted with problem areas and encouraged to use whichever method produces the best results.

Criteria for evaluation are based on the efficacy of plaque biofilm removal and safety of the flossing method.[26] Because adequate flossing will result in reduction of gingival inflammation and bleeding as well as less calculus formation, these results are cues available for evaluation. Incorrect flossing can often be detected through clinical observation of the technique (Figure 12–8 ■). Significant damage from flossing has been reported.[42] Signs that suggest incorrect use of dental floss include gingival cuts, soft tissue clefting, and cervical wear on proximal root surfaces (Figure 12–9 ■). If flossing trauma is evident, further instruction should be given until the individual becomes adept; if proficient flossing is not an achievable goal for the individual, an alternative to floss should be considered.

A variation in the method of flossing can be used to clean the lingual surfaces of lower anterior teeth when a lingual orthodontic bar (permanent retainer) is in place. The floss is inserted under the bar through both proximal surfaces, looped around the lingual surface, and crossed over on the facial. This allows a polishing action on the lingual surface under the lingual bar that is difficult to clean effectively with a toothbrush (Figure 12–10 ■).

Promoting Flossing Behavior

It is important to note that a flossing habit has traditionally been difficult for people to embrace. In reality, only a very small proportion of individuals practice daily flossing. A recent study found frequency from 8% to 19% of patients, depending on the type of dental practice.[43] Floss may be superior to other interproximal cleaning methods, but for those who have not or will not adopt a flossing behavior, another interproximal device may be more effective than no interproximal cleaning.[44] Use of a less effective device on a regular basis is superior to sporadic use of a more effective device. A frank discussion of the patient's willingness to floss or use another interdental device will aid in the discussion of alternatives. It is important that the clinician not influence patients to agree to floss just to please the practitioner when they are not willing or able to follow through with the practice.

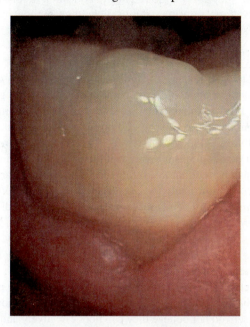

FIGURE ■ 12–9 Flossing damage. Gingival cut and cleft created by failure to adapt the floss to the interproximal surface in a C-shape.

(*Source:* Courtesy of Amy Teague.)

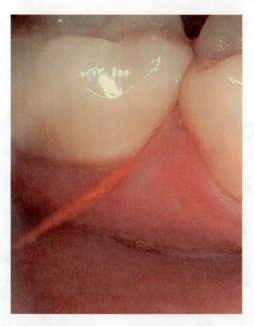

FIGURE ■ 12–8 Improper dental floss technique with potential for gingival "floss-cuts." Floss should adapt to the proximal surface in a C-shape without cutting into the gingiva.

(*Source:* Courtesy of Amy Teague.)

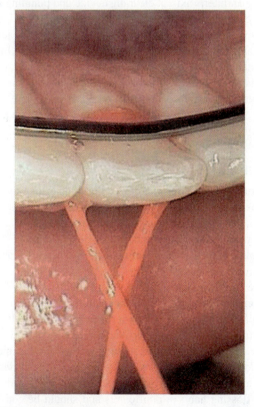

FIGURE ■ 12–10 Use of colored floss to clean the lingual surface under a lingual orthodontic retainer by "crossing over" the floss.

(*Source:* Courtesy of Amy Teague.)

Systematic reviews of studies of the effectiveness of floss in reducing plaque biofilm, clinical parameters of gingivitis, and interproximal dental caries indicate that flossing does not significantly add to the effectiveness of toothbrushing in most studies although there was a nonsignificant trend for reduced plaque biofilm scores with the addition of floss.[30,45] It is hypothesized that this failure of floss to reduce caries and gingivitis is most likely the consequence of plaque biofilm not being removed efficiently for a variety of reasons including lack of ability, dexterity, or motivation.[46]

Flossing should be encouraged although routinely recommending floss is not supported by scientific evidence. Rather, recommendations should be made in accordance with patient characteristics such as motivation and dexterity, and patients should be carefully trained in its use.[45] Research has shown that nonflossers do not believe they can floss effectively and easily. Application of sound health education theory can result in adoption of the behavior[47] (see Chapter 19). Continual reinstruction, reinforcement, and encouragement are needed to help patients maintain the flossing habit.[26] The individual's participation in selecting an interproximal cleaning device and planning a regimen is crucial to improving and/or enhancing compliance.[48] Proper instruction and practice allows most motivated adults to master either the spool or loop method of flossing.[26] In some circumstances, the use of a floss holder, floss threader, or floss picks may be indicated. In other cases, variable-thickness floss or precut floss strands with a stiff end may be more effective. Sometimes other alternatives are needed. All of these alternatives will be discussed in this chapter.

Dental Floss Holder

The **dental floss holder** is a device that holds floss and eliminates the need for placing fingers in the mouth.[28] It is recommended for specific individuals who lack the dexterity for handheld floss or who find flossing cumbersome (Box 12–3 ■).[24,49,50] The floss holder may also be helpful when one person is assisting another with flossing.[51]

The use of a floss holder is equivalent to finger flossing in reducing plaque biofilm, inflammation, and bleeding with no significant trauma found as a result of its use.[24] It is also frequently preferred over finger-manipulated flossing, especially for individuals who have not already learned the technique of finger flossing or do not have highly developed finger dexterity. Use of a floss holder may be more effective in establishing a regular flossing habit in nonflossers and should be considered when individuals experience difficulty with manual flossing.

A variety of different floss-holder designs are available (Figure 12–11 ■). They usually consist of a yokelike device with a 3/4- to 1-inch space between the yoke's two prongs. The floss is secured tightly between the two prongs, and the handle is grasped to guide the floss during use. The width and length of the handle are important features to consider when recommending the use of a floss holder to those with limited gripping abilities.[51] Most floss holders require that floss be strung around various parts of the holder before each use. This assembly mechanism allows for rethreading the floss whenever the working portion becomes soiled or begins to fray. Some devices have a floss reservoir in the handle. This improvement allows for ease of threading and advancing the floss while maintaining the proper tautness. A new device (Reach Access®) has replaceable, snap-on heads with preloaded floss to avoid having to thread the floss onto the handle (device on left in Figure 12–11).[50]

The use of a floss holder involves inserting the floss interproximally and applying the same technique used for finger-manipulated flossing. Once through the contact point, the floss and holder are pushed distally to clean the mesial surface of a tooth and pulled mesially to clean the distal surface (Figure 12–12 ■). This pulling or pushing motion makes the floss conform to the tooth convexities, thus allowing it to slide apically into the sulcus. The floss is then activated in the same manner as with finger-manipulated flossing by moving the floss in the direction of the long axis of the tooth.

The use of a floss holder requires thorough instruction to use it effectively and safely. Strict attention should be given to

BOX 12–3 **Floss Holders Recommended for These Patients**

- Physical disabilities
- Poor manual dexterity
- Large hands
- Limited mouth opening
- Strong gag reflex
- Low motivation for traditional flossing

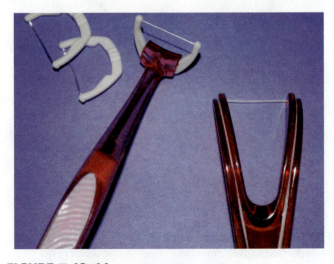

FIGURE ■ 12–11 **A variety of floss holders.**

(*Source:* Courtesy of Amy Teague.)

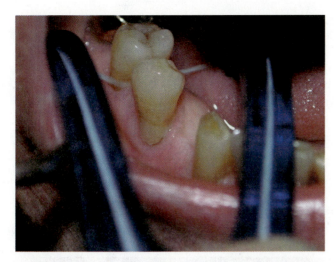

FIGURE ■ 12–12 Correct use of a floss holder on the mesial surface of a second premolar. Floss is taut, and the holder is pushed back toward the mesial surface to adapt the floss to the mesial surface in a C-shape. Then the floss is slid up and down to floss the surface in the usual manner.

(*Source:* Courtesy of Amy Teague.)

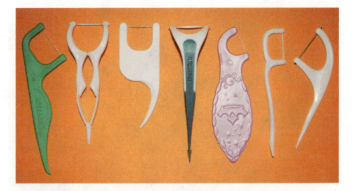

FIGURE ■ 12–13 A variety of prethreaded floss holders for one-time use.

(*Source:* Courtesy of Amy Teague.)

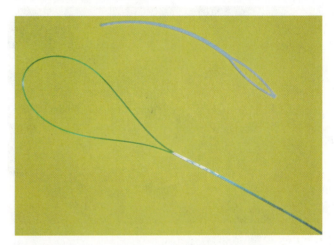

FIGURE ■ 12–14 Two examples of floss threaders.

(*Source:* Courtesy of Amy Teague.)

achieving the desired floss tension during assembly of the floss holder. To ensure tautness, the user can force the prongs together while securing the floss. The most persistent problems with the yokelike devices are the difficulties in loading and threading the floss and maintaining tension of the floss between the prongs as well as the decreased ability to adapt the floss into a C-shape around the proximal surface. Any device recommended should allow for ease of threading, maintenance of proper tautness, and easy manipulation by the user.

Several brands of prethreaded, one-time-use floss holders, referred to as *floss picks,* are also available (Figure 12–13 ■). They require minimal dexterity to control the floss tension, factors that may help improve compliance. Very limited research is available on these devices. One older study showed that the use of disposable floss aids resulted in equivalent plaque biofilm, inflammation, and bleeding reduction compared with finger flossing with no significant gingival trauma.[52] Individuals tend to prefer disposable floss aids similar to floss holders compared to using regular floss. They may be preferable to the use of a floss holder for many patients because of convenience. However, the expense of disposable floss aids may reduce compliance in some patients.

Dental Floss Threader

A **dental floss threader** is a plastic loop into which a length of floss is inserted, similar to threading a needle (Figure 12–14 ■). The floss threader is used to carry the floss under the contact point for class I embrasures[24] when the teeth are splinted or the contact is too tight for floss insertion. Floss threaders also facilitate access to clean around abutment teeth, beneath the pontic of fixed bridges, and around orthodontic appliances (Figure 12–15 ■). Care should be taken to prevent trauma to the gingival tissues when inserting the floss threader.

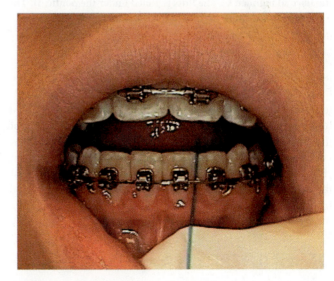

FIGURE ■ 12–15 Floss threader being used to aid in gaining access under the orthodontic arch wire.

(*Source:* Courtesy of Amy Teague.)

When cleaning under a fixed bridge, the floss threader is inserted from the facial aspect and pulled completely through to the lingual aspect until the floss is against the abutment or

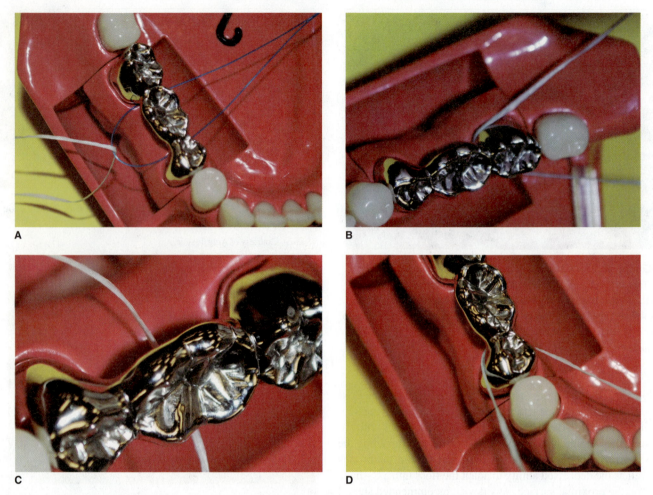

FIGURE ■ 12–16 Flossing under a fixed bridge A. The floss threader is inserted under the pontic from the facial aspect and pulled completely through to the lingual. B. The floss is adapted in a C-shape to one abutment proximal tooth surface to floss that surface in the normal manner. C. The floss is glided under the pontic. D. The floss is adapted to the opposite abutment proximal tooth surface with a C-shape to floss that surface in the usual manner.

(*Source:* Courtesy of Amy Teague.)

pontic (Figure 12–16A ■). The floss may then be disengaged from the threader to clean the proximal surface of each abutment and the under surface of the pontic. The floss is adapted to the proximal surface of one abutment tooth in the area of the embrasure (Figure 12–16B ■), used in the standard manner, then passed under the pontic to clean the underside of it (Figure 12–16C ■), and finally used on the proximal surface of the other abutment (Figure 12–16D ■). The floss is removed from between the abutment and pontic by pulling it out from the facial aspect.

OTHER INTERDENTAL AIDS

Because periodontal diseases and dental caries develop most frequently in the interdental and proximal areas, it is important to select effective devices to remove plaque biofilm from the proximal tooth surfaces.[29] Low patient compliance and limited effectiveness of floss in open embrasure spaces and exposed root concavities has led to a search for alternative interproximal aids.[53]

Clinical attachment loss as a result of disease or trauma and difficult-to-reach sites will likely require selected aids to supplement toothbrushing and flossing. Clinical attachment loss results in enlargement of embrasure spaces and exposure of root concavities, both of which limit the effectiveness of dental floss. In general, an aid that fills the interdental space is preferred for more effective cleaning.[29]

Despite the fact that effective toothbrushing leaves 30% of tooth surfaces untouched and removes only about 50% of plaque biofilm present on the teeth, patient compliance with manual flossing is low.[24] This is because it is a complex and time-consuming task that requires a great deal of coordination, manual dexterity, and motivation. People get discouraged about flossing because it is technique sensitive, is difficult to learn, can turn the fingertips blue, requires concentration, and demands the use of two hands. Others think it must be done first thing in the morning or last thing at night when they have little time and energy for it.

Although it is beneficial to help nonflossers find other ways to supplement toothbrushing, it is also important to understand that, in some cases, the use of an alternative aid instead of flossing may compromise the patient's oral hygiene and ultimately his or her future oral health.[26] Also, many aids have the potential to cause trauma to soft and hard tissues. On the other hand, in some cases other interproximal aids are superior to floss.[54] Hence, evidence-based decisions should be made concerning the selection of aids, and they should be recommended with caution and with careful instruction about their use. In addition, patients should be fully informed of any risks associated with their oral hygiene practices.

The number of supplemental aids that are recommended should be limited to one to two to avoid overwhelming the patient.[55] Thorough assessment is important to determine which aids might be most useful. In addition, careful instruction, monitoring, and reinforcement are required for successful application of supplemental aids. Although these aids may be easier to use than dental floss, the use of all aids requires dexterity, time, and motivation. Coaching patients is required to achieve compliance with interproximal aids.[56]

The selection of other interproximal aids must be based on a number of factors related to the patient's oral health status, including the periodontal condition, size and shape of the interdental embrasure space, morphology of the proximal tooth surfaces, contour and consistency of the gingiva, tooth position and alignment, and restorative work that is present. In addition, the patient's age, motivation, ability, manual dexterity and preference will affect compliance with recommendations and should be considered.[46] Numerous choices are described in this chapter to guide the oral health professional in making appropriate recommendations to patients.

Power Flosser

In response to poor compliance with flossing, **power flossers**, also called *automated flossers,* have been developed in an attempt to find a device to replace floss and provide effective interproximal plaque biofilm removal without causing trauma. These power cleaners are marketed to and for patients who are unable or unwilling to floss. Because power flossers are more convenient to use, can be used with one hand, and require less manual dexterity, they may be helpful for individuals who have physical disabilities or limited dexterity. They are also useful in difficult-to-clean areas such as around orthodontic appliances.[57] Various designs are comparable to dental floss in their ability to remove plaque biofilm and improve gingivitis and bleeding with no significant pathology resulting from their use.[36] Ease of use and patients' preference for use of a power flosser compared to dental floss may increase compliance with its use.

Various power flosser designs have been developed.[58] The Waterpik® Power Flosser (Figure 12–17 ■) is the best known

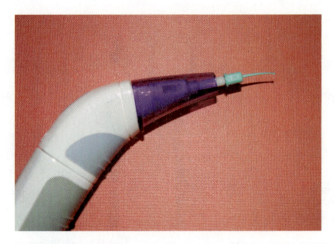

FIGURE ■ 12–17 Power flosser with a single nylon filament tip (WaterPik®).

(*Source:* Courtesy of Amy Teague.)

and has research studies to support its efficacy comparable to manual floss in reducing plaque, bleeding, and gingivitis.[58] It has a single nylon filament tip that reaches from the buccal surface to the lingual surface and electronically moves up and down at 10,000 linear strokes per minute, spinning rapidly in the interproximal space to clean the proximal surfaces.

A new power flosser, the Sonicare® AirFloss, uses new microburst technology by which microdroplets of water are accelerated by pressurized air to disrupt and remove interproxiamal plaque biofilm. In clinical trials, use of the AirFloss significantly removed interproximal plaque biofilm and reduced gingivitis. In addition, in surveys, the Sonicare AirFloss was preferred, resulted in improved compliance, and was reported to be easier to use compared to traditional dental floss or an oral irrigator.[59] Both these designs can be used when it is not possible to pass floss through the contact of adjacent teeth to reach the interdental space.

Interdental Brush

Interdental brushes, also known as *interproximal brushes,* are manufactured in different sizes and designs (Figure 12–18 ■). The brush consists of a plastic handle and a small tapered or cylindric filamentous brush tip (Figure 12–19 ■) that is either attached to the handle (nonreplaceable) or inserted into the handle (replaceable). Some long-handled designs have a straight handle, and others have an angled handle. The angled handle provides better access to difficult-to-reach areas. With other short-handled designs, it is possible to bend the tip to improve access. The available brush tips are of varied sizes to accommodate the size of the embrasure space, and the core of the brush that holds the bristles is made of plastic, wire, or nylon-coated wire.[60]

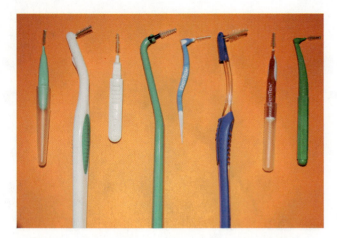

FIGURE ■ 12–18 A variety of interproximal brushes.

(*Source:* Courtesy of Amy Teague.)

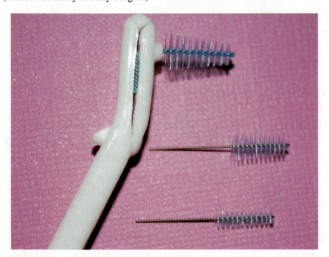

FIGURE ■ 12–19 Replaceable interproximal brush inserts in varied sizes and shapes.

(*Source:* Courtesy of Amy Teague.)

Interdental brushes are recommended for interproximal areas and other spaces that are large enough to easily receive the device.[29] Box 12–4 ■ provides a list of uses that are illustrated in Figures 12–20 ■, 12–21 ■, 12–22 ■, and 12–23 ■. Caution should be exercised when using an interdental brush to prevent damage to the tooth or soft tissues from the firm wire or plastic core of the brush. Only brushes with a plastic or nylon-coated core should be used around implant abutments to prevent scratching of the titanium surface.[44]

The brush tip should be moistened and inserted at an angle that follows the form of the gingiva. A buccolingual movement is used to remove plaque biofilm and debris from interdental spaces and furcations.[26] The type of embrasure or furcation determines the selection of the design and size of the interdental brush. The recommended brush tip should be slightly larger than the space and should provide equal coverage on both adjacent surfaces to adequately clean them. Using the interproximal brush too aggressively or too fast, or forcing the interproximal brush into an area that is too small will likely result in trauma.[44]

Interdental brushes have been shown to be effective in removing plaque biofilm and reducing bleeding. In open embrasures,

BOX 12–4   Uses of Interdental Brushes

- Type II & III embrasure spaces
- Class IV furcations
- Root concavities
- Orthodontic appliances
- Space maintainers
- Small diastemas
- Fixed prostheses
- Splints
- Dental implants

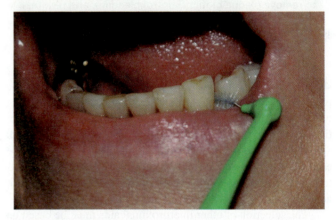

FIGURE ■ 12–20 Interproximal brush in an open embrasure space with the brush following the contour of the gingiva.

(*Source:* Courtesy of Amy Teague.)

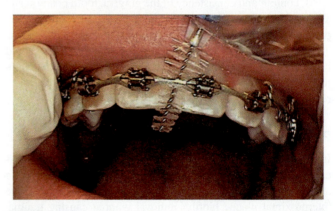

FIGURE ■ 12–21 Interproximal brush applied to orthodontic appliances.

(*Source:* Courtesy of Amy Teague.)

these brushes are superior to other interdental devices including dental floss because the bristles fill the space and reach the surfaces within the root concavities.[61] Results of a study indicated that use of the interproximal brush resulted in improved periodontal health, even before scaling and root planning.[33] Another study found them to be as effective as dental floss to remove subgingival plaque biofilm.[62] Interdental brushes have been shown to be effective also around brackets of orthodontic patients,[62] and they are preferred by patients compared to floss.[63] A special design is

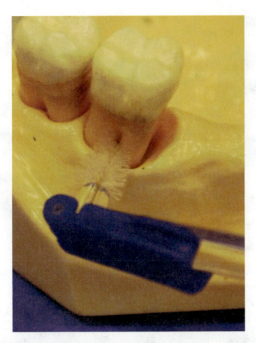

FIGURE ■ 12–22 Interproximal brush directed into an exposed furcation.

(*Source:* Courtesy of Amy Teague.)

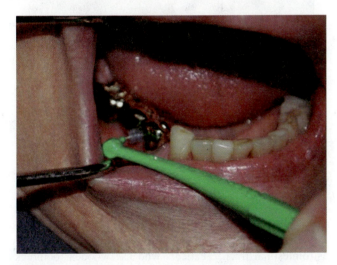

FIGURE ■ 12–23 Interproximal brush inserted between the abutment and pontic of a fixed prosthesis at an angle approximating the gingival contour. Brush can be inserted under the pontic if space allows.

(*Source:* Courtesy of Amy Teague.)

available that is intended for use with implants. (See Chapter 13.) Interproximal brushes can be used for delivery of antimicrobial, fluoride, and desensitizing agents by inserting the brush tip into the medicament and applying it into the hard-to-access areas.[26] In a study comparing various ways to apply fluoride to proximal surfaces, dipping the interproximal brush in a fluoride gel was shown to significantly increase the fluoride concentration of the proximal tooth surfaces.[64]

Some powered toothbrushes have an interproximal brush attachment, which can be used in the same way as manual interproximal brushes.[28] Limited studies have been done with powered interproximal brushes. One study demonstrated that its use was safe and effective in reducing gingivitis and removing plaque biofilm from accessible proximal surfaces.[65] Another study indicated that it removed more plaque biofilm than dental floss.[66] However, some patients may have trouble controlling the device once it is turned on.

End-Tuft Brush

The **end-tuft brush**, also called *uni-tuft brush* or *single-tuft brush,* consists of a small group of tufted bristles that are flat or tapered and are attached to a straight or angled handle[60] (Figure 12–24 ■). The handles of some uni-tuft brushes can be bent by softening them in very hot or boiling water. An angled handle will allow easier access to hard-to-reach areas. Uni-tuft brushes can be used as an alternative to floss for removal of plaque biofilm from type III embrasures, the distal surface of the most posterior teeth (Figure 12–25 ■), and proximal surfaces of teeth adjacent to edentulous spaces. Other areas where it is useful include the lingual surface of mandibular teeth, crowded or misaligned teeth, and around orthodontic appliances. This device can be adapted to clean under and around

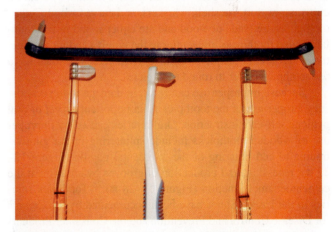

FIGURE ■ 12–24 A variety of uni-tuft brushes.

(*Source:* Courtesy of Amy Teague.)

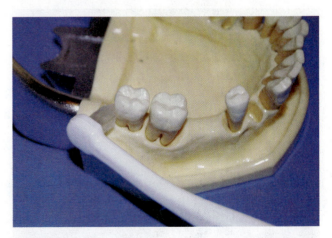

FIGURE ■ 12–25 Adaptation of a uni-tuft brush against the distal surface of the last molar.

(*Source:* Courtesy of Amy Teague.)

dental appliances, including implant abutments and prostheses, and in exposed furcations, as long as the space allows safe insertion and can be accessed by the brush.[24]

Application of the end-tuft brush starts by placing the brush into the embrasure space, furcation, or other appropriate area with gentle pressure. A combination of rotary motion and sulcular strokes with moderate pressure will result in effective cleaning.[26]

The Sulcabrush® (Figure 12–26 ■) is a specific, double-headed uni-tuft brush; the brush heads are on opposite ends of the handle and are at opposite angles. The brush heads are more finely tapered to provide better access to lingual surfaces at the gingival margin, in smaller embrasure spaces, and around crowded teeth.

Toothpick

A historical review of **toothpick** use suggests that toothpicks are one of the earliest and most persistent means of picking the teeth.[67] Use of the toothpick may date back to the days of the cave people, who probably used sticks to pick food from between the teeth. Shakespeare described its use, and writings about table manners in the 1600s include references to the use of toothpicks. Throughout history, toothpicks have been made from bronze, copper, gold, iron, silver, ivory, bone, bird claws, quills, straw, tortoise shell, whiskers, and carved wood. Today, toothpicks are made of wood and are either round or rectangular. Round toothpicks are gentler to the gingiva and more effective in removing plaque biofilm. Current recommendations to use toothpicks refer to round toothpicks.

Because improper use can result in damage to the oral tissues, proper use of the toothpick is an important aspect of oral hygiene self-care instruction. Oral injuries caused by improper use of wooden toothpicks include splintering in the gingiva, trauma to and blunting of the interdental papilla (Figure 12–27 ■), recession, and production of grooves by abrasion at the cementoenamel junction (Figure 12–28 ■).[28] Toothpick injuries in the United States have been documented by the Centers for Disease Control and Prevention and the Consumer Products Safety Commission. Injuries that have caused serious medical conditions and even death include abdominal abscess resulting

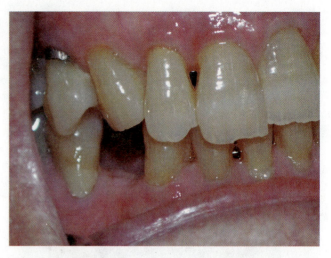

FIGURE ■ 12–27 Blunting of the interdental papilla caused by improper use of a toothpick.
(*Source:* Courtesy of Amy Teague.)

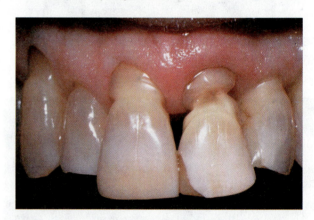

FIGURE ■ 12–28 Abrasion at the cementoenamel junction of proximal surfaces caused by improper use of a toothpick on central incissors.
(*Source:* Courtesy of Amy Teague.)

from swallowing a toothpick, poking it into the eyeball and inner ear, and lodging it in the esophagus, posterior nares, and gastrointestinal tract.[67] Patients who use wooden toothpicks should be made aware of the need for precaution to prevent serious injuries to themselves and others.

Consistent use of the toothpick can result in firm, resilient tissue. Effectiveness of toothpicks to remove plaque biofilm depends on the ability to make contact of the toothpick surface with the tooth surface. Therefore, it is more effective in smaller surface areas and from the buccal aspect compared to the lingual.[44] Today pick products that are a supple plastic material with flexible tiny bristles on the working end are available (Figure 12–29 ■).[68] Toothpicks are generally considered easier to manipulate than floss and compliance with toothpick use is greater.[54] As with all other interdental aids, motivation is a primary factor in the success of using the toothpick. The proper technique for toothpick use[44] is described in Table 12–4 ■.

Toothpick Holder

Although a toothpick may be manipulated by hand, its effectiveness, especially from the lingual aspect, is improved by

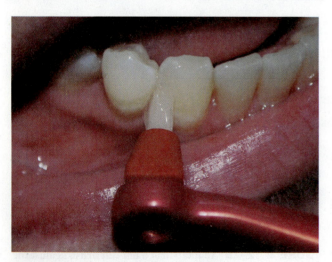

FIGURE ■ 12–26 Application of the Sulcabrush® interproximally into a small embrasure space.
(*Source:* Courtesy of Amy Teague.)

inserting it into a **toothpick holder**.[44] This handle holds a wooden toothpick securely at the proper angle in order to increase access and enhance proper adaptation of the tooth-pick in hard-to-reach areas, including subgingivally and in type II embrasures. However, the toothpick will not success-fully clean root concavities.[28] There are specific circumstances that indicate use of a toothpick holder (Box 12–5 ■). Use of the toothpick in the toothpick holder can reduce gingival bleed-ing in patients with gingivitis and slight chronic periodontitis. Nevertheless, it is important to remember that the toothpick has an increased potential to cause gingival recession, papil-lary blunting, and abrasion of the tooth surface, even when it is mounted in a toothpick holder.

Oral health professionals have recommended the Marquis Perio-Aid® toothpick holder (Figure 12–30 ■) for many years. The wooden toothpick is inserted into an adjustable plastic contra-angled handle, and the projecting end of the toothpick is broken off by snapping it in a downward direction. The broken end leaves a stem to prevent the tip from disengaging from the holder during use. The toothpick can be positioned at an acute angle (angle less than 90 degrees) on one end to access lingual surfaces and at an obtuse angle (angle greater than 90 degrees but less than 180 degrees) on the other end to adapt to buccal surfaces (Figures 12–31 ■ and 12–32 ■).

BOX 12–5	Indications for the Use of the Toothpick Holder

- Removing biofilm along the gingival margin and within the gingival sulci or periodontal pockets (Figure 12–32)
- Cleaning small concave proximal surfaces
- Cleaning exposed furcation areas that are still in contact with underlying bone
- Cleaning around orthodontic appliances and fixed prostheses
- Applying chemotherapeutic agents, such as burnishing fluoride into the tooth surface to treat hypersensitivity or delivering chlorhexidine into the gingival sulcus

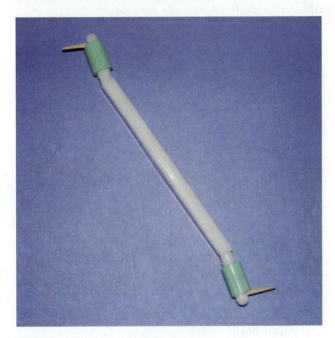

FIGURE ■ 12–30 A Perio-Aid® toothpick holder with a toothpick inserted into each end.

(*Source:* Courtesy of Amy Teague.)

Wooden or Plastic Triangular Stick

A modern adaptation of the toothpick is the **triangular wooden stick**; more recently, this device has been manufactured in a firm plastic as well (Figure 12–29 ■). Interproximal cleaning can be aided with these triangular sticks, especially in open embrasures.[28] Wooden sticks are made of balsa or birch wood; their lower surface hardness and high strength compared to

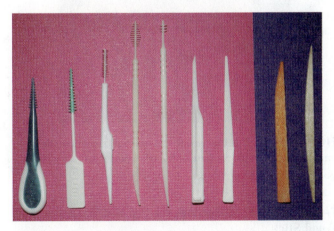

FIGURE ■ 12–29 A variety of wooden and plastic triangular sticks. The seven to the left are plastic, and the two to the right are wooden (balsa wood composition on the left and birch wood on the right). The two plastic sticks on the far left have soft, pliable plastic "bristles."

(*Source:* Courtesy of Amy Teague.)

TABLE ■ 12–4 Technique for Proper Use of a Wooden Toothpick

- Premoisten the toothpick with saliva to soften the wood.
- Place the blunt tip of the toothpick at a right angle to the buccal and lingual surfaces.
- Place it at less than a 45-degree angle to extend just below the gingival margin.
- Pull or push it across the buccal or lingual surfaces from one interproximal space to the next.
- As the tip becomes frayed from use, use it as a small cleaning "brush" to rub the tooth surfaces.
- Interproximally, angle the toothpick horizontally, and use the sides of the toothpick to clean the approximal surfaces on either side of the interdental papilla.
- Use care with subgingival insertion, and refrain from vigorous interproximal use to avoid damage to the soft and hard oral tissues.

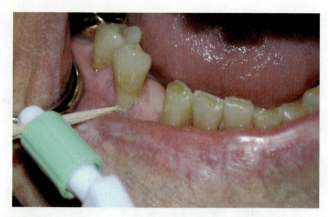

FIGURE ■ 12–31 Adaptation of a toothpick to the facial surface at the gingival margin of a premolar.

(*Source:* Courtesy of Amy Teague.)

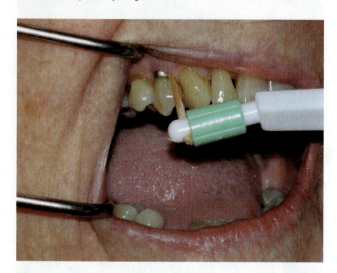

FIGURE ■ 12–32 Adaptation of a toothpick into the gingival sulcus or periodontal pocket.

(*Source:* Courtesy of Amy Teague.)

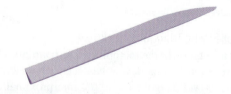

FIGURE ■ 12–33 Drawing of a triangular wood stick with the triangular cross-section showing at the bottom left of the drawing.

the round toothpick results in increased efficacy with less potential for trauma. These sticks are triangular in cross section (Figures 12–33 ■ and 12–34 ■) to slide easily between the teeth, to conform to the shape of the embrasure space, to provide gingival massage, and to reduce potential tissue trauma. Compared to the plastic triangular stick, the softer, more pliable wooden stick can be adapted more easily to the proximal surface for more effective cleaning and has less potential for gingival damage during use as well as over time.

Triangular wood and plastic sticks should be used for only type II or III embrasures where the papilla does not completely

fill the embrasure space.[28] The patient should be instructed in the correct use of these triangular sticks to prevent gingival damage caused by inappropriate use.[28] Instructions for use of the triangular wood stick are described in Table 12–5 ■ and illustrated in Figure 12–34 ■.

DID YOU KNOW ?

Triangular wooden sticks that are made of soft wood are more effective and less damaging than toothpicks.

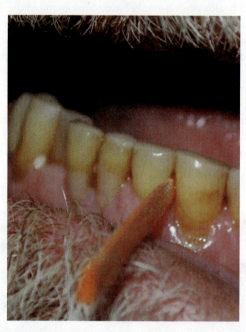

FIGURE ■ 12–34 Placement of a wooden triangular stick interproximally with the base of the triangle against the gingiva.

(*Source:* Courtesy of Amy Teague.)

TABLE ■ 12–5 Directions for Use of a Triangular Wood Stick

- Moisten the end of the triangular wood stick to soften it.
- Insert the triangular wood stick interproximally from the buccal aspect.
- Place the flat surface, or base of the triangle, on the interdental papilla.
- Use a finger rest to help prevent applying too much pressure of the tip of the stick against the gingiva.
- Press against the interdental papilla to flatten it slightly.
- Angle the tip of the stick slightly coronally or incisally.
- Move the triangular wood stick in a buccolingual direction.
- Apply approximately four burnishing strokes with moderate pressure on each side of the embrasure.
- Discard the stick when the wood becomes splayed to prevent splinters from being forced into the gingiva. Splaying will likely occur after use in one quadrant or arch.
- Plastic sticks can be thoroughly washed and reused.

Using triangular wood or plastic sticks to reduce biofilm accumulations has demonstrated a reduction in plaque biofilm, inflammation, and bleeding.[44] They reduce inflammation more in the coronal regions of interproximal pockets than in the apical regions, and more from the buccal aspect than the lingual. They also have the potential to remove biofilm 2 to 3 mm subgingivally by depressing the papilla in the presence of inflammation. Triangular wood picks are not as effective as dental floss for biofilm removal from the lingual interproximal areas but are more effective and less damaging to the tissues than round toothpicks.[44] Because wooden picks are more pliable than plastic, they can cause less gingival damage over time.

Delivery of Medicaments with Toothpicks

Traditional toothpicks, plastic picks with a tiny brush on the working end, and triangular wooden sticks have been used to deliver antimicrobials and fluoride to the interproximal areas.[68] To enhance caries control, studies have demonstrated an increase in approximal fluoride concentration after use of toothpicks impregnated with fluoride.[64] Other studies have found reductions in plaque biofilm and gingivitis with the use of toothpicks that are either impregnated with chlorhexidine or used to apply chlorhexidine gel.[69]

Rubber Tip Stimulator

Rubber tip stimulators, also referred to as rubber tips, consist of a conical, flexible rubber tip attached to a handle (Figure 12–35 ■). Rubber tips are used primarily for gingival massage and recontouring of gingival papilla after periodontal therapy. Although a possible role for the rubber tip stimulator to increase gingival circulation, keratinization, and epithelial thickening has been proposed, it has been suggested that the overall improvement

in gingival health resulting from its use is more likely due to effective removal of plaque biofilm.[28] However, the efficacy of the rubber tip stimulator in removing plaque biofilm and improving overall gingival health has been questioned because of conflicting information and lack of evidence.

Rubber tips can be used in exposed furcation areas, type II and III embrasure spaces, and along the gingival margin.[44] The rubber tip is not recommended for type I embrasures and healthy gingival contour. The tip is inserted interproximally into an open embrasure space at a 90-degree angle. The side of the rubber tip should rest on the gingiva and against the exposed proximal tooth surfaces (Figure 12–36 ■). A small circular or rolling motion against the proximal surfaces is applied from both the lingual and labial aspects. The tip can also be used on the buccal and lingual surfaces by placing it on the tooth surface, slightly beneath the gingival margin, and tracing it along the contour of the gingival margin.[28]

Aggressive application of the stimulator with heavy pressure can traumatize and destroy the soft tissues.[28] Even when used gently, these rubber tips can damage the gingiva with prolonged use because they are rigid. The use of the rubber tip should be limited and closely monitored.

DID YOU KNOW ?

When patients do not have access to expensive oral health self-care products, some nontraditional products found in the home can be adapted to clean the teeth.

Nontraditional Adjuncts

When the aforementioned products are not available, some nontraditional adjunctive aids can be applied. This may be helpful when working with certain populations that do not have access to manufactured products or cannot afford to purchase special products. The following aids can be useful when variable diameter floss is not available.

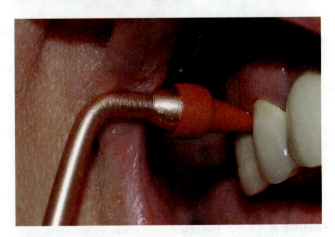

FIGURE ■ 12–36 Placement of the rubber tip stimulator interproximally in an open embrasure space at a 90-degree angle to the long axis of the tooth. It is traced along the gingival margin or moved in a buccolingual direction within the interproximal space.

(*Source:* Courtesy of Amy Teague.)

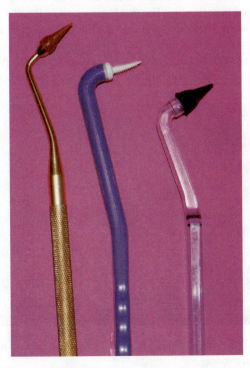

FIGURE ■ 12–35 A variety of rubber tip stimulators.

(*Source:* Courtesy of Amy Teague.)

White Knitting Yarn

An unusual application of a product found at home is the use of knitting yarn around the abutment of a fixed appliance and under pontics when the space is large enough.[70] It is also helpful in open interproximal spaces, on the distal surface of the most posterior teeth, in exposed furcations, and around malpositioned teeth or separated teeth. The increased width of the yarn provides more surface coverage and access to a shallow root concavity. When access is limited, a floss threader may be used to insert the yarn into the embrasure (Figure 12–37 ■). Once the yarn has been drawn through, the technique is the same as for dental floss with care taken not to traumatize the tissue. Because of its diameter, knitting yarn will not fit into the submarginal space. Only white knitting yarn, with no dyes, should be used. Synthetic knitting yarn is recommended because wool yarn leaves microfibers that could irritate soft tissues.

Pipe Cleaner

Another novel product for oral self-care is a pipe cleaner, which has been suggested for use in class III embrasures and class IV furcations.[29] The metal core of the pipe cleaner makes insertion

easier in open spaces, but pipe cleaners should be employed with caution to prevent damaging hard and soft tissues with this metal core. Also, because of the metal core, pipe cleaners should never be used with implants to prevent scratching of the titanium.[60]

A pipe cleaner is cut into 3-inch lengths, and a section is inserted into the embrasure space or furcation area. The pipe cleaner is wrapped around the proximal or inner root surfaces, and moved back and forth or buccolingually in a "shoeshine" motion[29] (Figure 12–38 ■). Similar to knitting yarn because of their diameter, pipe cleaners cannot be inserted into the sulcus.

Gauze Strip

One more application of an untraditional product is the use of a gauze strip to clean the proximal surfaces of teeth adjacent to edentulous areas, teeth that are widely spaced, or dental implant abutments. Gauze strips have also been recommended to clean the distal surface of the most posterior teeth in the mouth.[26]

A 1-inch-wide gauze bandage is cut into lengths of 6 to 8 inches and folded in half or in thirds. The lengthwise edge of the gauze is positioned with the fold toward the gingiva, and the edges folded inward to avoid gingival irritation. The gauze is adapted by wrapping it around the exposed proximal surface to the facial and lingual line angles of the tooth in a C-shape similar to dental floss (Figure 12–39 ■). A buccolingual shoeshine stroke is used to loosen and remove plaque biofilm and debris. The gauze strip has particular application when a significant portion of the root surface is exposed as is pictured in Figure 12–39 ■.

RINSING AND IRRIGATION

Rinsing

Vigorous rinsing of the mouth can aid in the removal of food debris and materia alba. The technique involves forcefully pushing the water back and forth through the interproximal areas of clenched teeth, using the muscles of the tongue, lips, and cheeks to force the water, and using as much pressure as possible. Although some practitioners continue to recommend mouthrinsing with

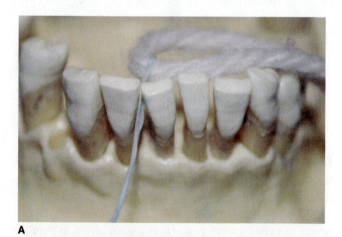

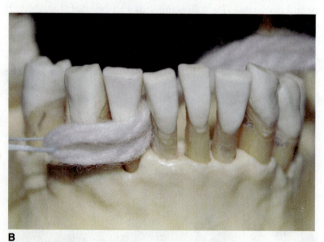

A

B

FIGURE ■ 12–37 Use of knitting yarn in a wide, open embrasure space. A. Yarn is looped through dental floss and inserted through the contact point. B. Yarn is drawn through the embrasure space.

(*Source:* Courtesy of Amy Teague.)

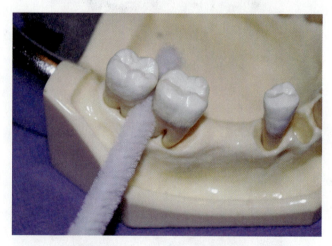

FIGURE ■ 12–38 Application of a pipe cleaner in an open embrasure space.

(*Source:* Courtesy of Amy Teague.)

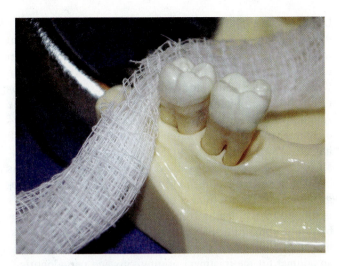

FIGURE ■ 12–39 Adaptation of a 6-inch length of 1-inch gauze bandage folded in half with the folded edge adjacent to the gingival margin.

(*Source:* Courtesy of Amy Teague.)

water after consumption of fermentable carbohydrates, national guidelines and recommendations for dental caries prevention do not include water mouthrinsing as a strategy because it does not neutralize the pH caused by the acid production.[71–74] (See Chapter 5.) On the other hand, Caries Management by Risk Assessment (CAMBRA) guidelines include rinsing with bicarbonate of soda to neutralize the oral pH.[75] In addition, while water rinsing was once recommended for patients with bulimia, the American Dental Hygienists' Association now recommends rinsing with 0.05% sodium fluoride, slightly alkaline mineral water, sodium bicarbonate, or magnesium hydroxide solution to neutralize the gastric acids following each vomiting episode.[76] The effectiveness of water rinsing to control dental caries and erosion is not supported by research results.

DID YOU KNOW ?

Water rinsing after eating fermentable carbohydrates is not an evidence-based approach to preventing dental caries.

Research has also demonstrated no effect of water rinsing on the number of bacteria present in plaque biofilm. On the other hand, various studies have shown long-lasting effects from supervised and unsupervised rinsing with chemotherapeutic agents versus water as an adjunct to oral hygiene. Effects of rinsing with antimicrobials include reduced supragingival plaque biofilm, lower bacterial counts throughout the mouth, less papillary bleeding, and fewer bacteria on the dorsum of the tongue.[77–81] The American Academy of Periodontology (AAP) recommends the use of antimicrobial agents to help reduce bacterial plaque biofilm for the prevention and treatment of gingivitis in selected patients.[3] The use of antimicrobial rinsing is included as an adjunct to oral hygiene measures in the AAP

parameters for the treatment of plaque-induced gingivitis, slight-to-moderate chronic periodontitis, refractory periodontitis, and necrotizing diseases and in periodontal maintenance when oral hygiene is only partially effective.[82] It is recommended as part of daily oral hygiene by the Academy of General Dentistry.[83] Intermittent twice daily rinsing with chlorhexidine is recommended during orthodontic treatment.[84] In addition, antimicrobial rinsing has been used as part of a full-mouth disinfection approach to improve periodontal tissue health.[85] Rinsing with 18 to 20 mg of chlorhexidine gluconate for 60 seconds twice a day is the recommended protocol to control gingivitis.[86] To avoid a strong medicinal aftertaste, the patient should not rinse with water immediately after rinsing with the CHG. In addition, the patient should wait at least 30 minutes to brush to avoid interaction of the CHG with the sodium lauryl sulfate, the detergent in toothpaste, which results in deactivation of the CHG.

Antimicrobial effects include control of bacteria associated with dental caries as well.[25] CAMBRA guidelines include rinsing and other uses of antimicrobials to control dental caries.[75] Rinsing with chlorhexidine twice daily for 1 week every 3 months has been suggested for oral disinfection to control dental caries in high-risk patients with the idea of killing bacteria in waves.[87] The reason for the quarterly repetition is that, although this procedure significantly reduces *Streptococcus mutans,* reappearance occurs, and repeated treatment is needed. A combined rinsing with chlorhexidine and fluoride has been shown to be more effective than rinsing with either compound by itself because the effect is synergistic.

Although rinsing with antimicrobials is recommended as part of a daily oral hygiene regimen, it is not recommended to take the place of oral hygiene measures to control either dental caries or periodontal diseases. It is important to stress to patients that rinsing with antimicrobials is an adjunct to toothbrushing and interdental cleaning, not a substitute. In addition, the oral health care provider should educate patients about the active ingredients and products that have been approved for rinsing and the inactive ingredients, such as alcohol, that may be contraindicated for certain individuals. See Chapter 11 for a comprehensive discussion of mouthrinses and their active and inactive ingredients.

Water rinsing is recommended for special circumstances. To neutralize the mouth acids in radiation therapy patients, the recommendation is to rinse throughout the day with saline and baking soda or with plain water and baking soda followed by plain water.[88] Water rinsing has been shown to effectively prevent the occurrence or decrease the severity of chemotherapy-induced oral mucositis in some studies. Mucositis was reduced significantly by rinsing every 10 minutes with ice cold water during and up to an hour after infusion with a chemotherapeutic drug that is excreted into the saliva.[89] Other studies have demonstrated superior results in controlling mucositis with antimicrobial rinses such as iodine and commonly used mouthwashes.[90]

Irrigation

Irrigation devices, also called *dental water jets,* are a means of irrigating specific areas of the mouth whereas rinsing is a means of flushing the entire mouth. The advantage of irrigation over rinsing is that periodontal lesions are most common interdentally; rinsing does not reach these areas of limited access, whereas irrigation does.[1] Irrigation with an antimicrobial agent has consistently achieved better results than rinsing with an antimicrobial agent.[46] Water irrigation has been recommended as an adjunct to daily oral hygiene, including toothbrushing, dental floss, and other aids as needed.[91] Because of its superior outcomes interproximally, the newest irrigation device today is promoted as a water flosser by Water Pik®.[92]

Water irrigation is not the best method to disrupt or remove plaque biofilm, is not effective without toothbrushing, and should not be used as a substitute for mechanical plaque biofilm removal.[93] However, studies have demonstrated that the regular practice of water irrigation significantly removes plaque biofilm and reduces bleeding, visual signs of gingival inflammation, and probing depth.[46,93–97] Clinicians and patients should be aware that these positive effects have been demonstrated in recent studies conducted with units that have more advanced technology; results might not generalize to older units that patients have in their possession. Dental water jets are affordable, effective with simple tap water, easy to use, can be recommended to most individuals 10 years of age and older,[58] and should be used as an alternative to flossing for individuals who will not or cannot floss effectively.[42]

? DID YOU KNOW

Oral irrigation is superior to rinsing for the delivery of antimicrobials.

According to the AAP, home irrigation is not indicated as an adjunct for those who have effective oral hygiene and have no gingival inflammation.[98] However, individuals with inconsistent or ineffective interproximal cleaning, fixed orthodontic appliances, crowns, fixed bridges, implants, and malodor may benefit from a home irrigation self-care regimen.[94,95,98] Oral irrigation may also be helpful for individuals who have their jaws temporarily wired together for stabilization after surgery or have head and neck trauma. As with other self-care measures, the benefits are derived only if self-care is practiced routinely.

The action of irrigation is the disruption of loosely attached or unattached supragingival and subgingival plaque biofilm and the removal of food debris. The action is twofold. Loosely attached microflora is disrupted when the pulsating fluid makes initial contact. There is a secondary flushing action as the irrigant is deflected from the tooth surface. The microflora is disrupted both qualitatively and quantitatively. Gingivitis reduction is a result of the alteration of subgingival microflora[99] as well as a reduction in the amount of plaque biofilm.[96]

A home-irrigation device that provides a pulsating stream of fluid versus a continuous stream is three times more effective.[58] With a pulsating stream, compression and interpulse decompression occur, allowing contaminants to escape and avoiding injury to soft tissues.[98] With a continuous flow, there is constant tissue compression, which hinders the escape of contaminants.

Use of Antimicrobials

Although supragingival irrigation with water in addition to toothbrushing contributes to the removal of plaque biofilm and reduces bleeding and gingival inflammation, irrigation with an antimicrobial instead of water increases the effectiveness of home-irrigating devices by significantly reducing the subgingival periodontopathic microflora.[91,98] On the basis of a comprehensive systematic review of the literature, the AAP has confirmed that supragingival irrigation with antimicrobials is superior to water irrigation in the treatment of gingivitis because water irrigation showed limited reduction of pathogen counts.[98] The usefulness of irrigation with antimicrobials is limited by the depth of the pocket because the antimicrobial must come in contact with the pathogens. Nevertheless, irrigation with antimicrobials is recommended by the AAP as an adjunct for the treatment of gingivitis and periodontitis.[82] Oral irrigation has been shown to be superior to rinsing for the delivery of antimicrobials to control subgingival flora.[1,46]

Chlorhexidine is the most researched antimicrobial used for irrigation.[99] Dilution of chlorhexidine to concentrations of 0.02%, 0.04%, 0.06%, and 0.1% has decreased plaque biofilm and gingival inflammation while controlling the staining that occurs with the use of chlorhexidine. Even with these lower concentrations, higher volumes of medicaments were delivered with jet irrigation than with rinsing at the normal 0.12% concentration. Other irrigants that have been tested include stannous fluoride, Listerine® antiseptic, povidone-iodine, acetylsalicylic acid (aspirin), hydrogen peroxide, sodium hypochlorite (household bleach), and herbal-based mouthrinses. Povidone-iodine is suggested by the AAP as a professional treatment for pocket disinfection and control of necrotizing ulcerative periodontitis.[3] In some cases, to reduce the risk of bacterial resistance that may occur with local antibiotic therapy, irrigation with antimicrobials has been suggested as an alternative to local delivery of antibiotics.[99]

? DID YOU KNOW

A moderate power setting is recommended for supragingival irrigation, and a lower power setting is suggested for subgingival irrigation.

Outcomes of Irrigation

Supragingival irrigation improves and prevents gingivitis but has no significant effect on periodontitis[98] although it decreases the subgingival periodontal pathogens and reduces bleeding,[46,93] inflammation and inflammatory mediators.[24] Irrigation also reduces plaque biofilm and calculus formation.[24] The fluid penetrates subgingivally 3 mm, or half the probing depth,[98] which explains why irrigation reduces gingivitis even though plaque biofilm is not eliminated. Any reduction of pocket depth that may result from irrigation is related to a reduction in inflammation and subsequent gingival shrinkage. Irrigation does not improve attachment levels of the junctional epithelium. Because supragingival irrigation also penetrates subgingivally, in a mouth without periodontal pockets, it may be as effective as subgingival irrigation to prevent the recolonization of a subgingival microflora after thorough professional debridement.

Supragingival irrigation does not project into deep pockets and has limited effect on the subgingival microflora in deep pockets. This failure to reach the base of the pocket may explain why supragingival irrigation is more effective against gingivitis than periodontitis. Irrigation has been shown to reduce proinflammatory cytokines (interleukin 1-β and prostaglandin E_2) in the gingival crevice. These cytokines lead to bone resorption when periodontal diseases are present.[100]

Home subgingival irrigation has been used to deliver medicaments further into the gingival sulcus or pockets.[98] Several studies demonstrated additional reductions in gingivitis and bleeding when an antimicrobial agent is used subgingivally. A soft latex-free rubber tip (Pik Pocket™ by Waterpik®) was tested for subgingival irrigation to deliver the antimicrobial into the pocket.[91] When the tip was placed 1 mm subgingivally, the mean pocket penetration was 90% for 4-mm to 6-mm pockets and 64% for pockets of 7 mm or deeper compared to 21% pocket penetration with rinsing.[46] Subgingival irrigation with this tip was reported to be comfortable to the patients.

The AAP recommends calculus removal along with home subgingival irrigation to further reduce bleeding and pocket depths and to allow thorough irrigation of the pockets.[98] In addition, the AAP recommends use of low irrigation forces and circumferential irrigation around teeth to ensure the delivery of the medicament throughout the periodontal pockets. Subgingival irrigation requires a good deal of dexterity combined with compliance for successful results. However, marginal irrigation results in significant subgingival penetration, has been successfully used by periodontal maintenance patients, and is an easy-to-master technique.[98]

Irrigation Tips and Units

Various irrigation tips are pictured in Figure 12–40 ■ and their identification and uses are described in Box 12–6 ■. The standard tip (B in Figure 12–40 ■) is designed for supragingival use. As was described in the previous section, supragingival irrigation also provides limited subgingival penetration. The tip is directed at the tooth at a 90-degree angle, just coronal to the gingival margin. The gingival margin is followed, stopping at each interproximal area for 5 to 6 seconds. This process is done from both the buccal and lingual aspects. For supragingival irrigation, a force of 80 to 90 pounds per square inch (psi) can be tolerated without damage to the tissues, but a psi of 60 is recommended.[98] Most units have power settings from 10 to 90, so the moderate power level should be recommended for supragingival irrigation. Supragingival irrigation has been used successfully in periodontal maintenance patients and is easier to master than subgingival irrigation.[98]

For subgingival irrigation, a rubber-tipped **cannula** (E in Figure 12–40 ■) is angled into the gingival sulcus about 2 mm, allowing a focused lavage that adds to the depth of penetration into the pockets as described in the previous section. A cannula-type tip yields results equivalent to those of a syringe.[98] A latex-free tip should be recommended. Either a side or end port cannula can be employed; each requires high dexterity and should be limited to individuals with adequate skill.[98] A low

power setting is recommended for subgingival irrigation.[98] Use of subgingival irrigation tips is recommended in deep pockets and furcation areas and around dental implants; they are also useful for areas that are difficult to access with a standard tip.[29] The routine use of home irrigation following periodontal therapy has been shown to improve outcomes of therapy.[24] Use of the cannula-type tip requires commitment on the part of the patient, and compliance may be an issue. Patient motivation is required to increase compliance with the addition of irrigation to other daily oral hygiene measures.

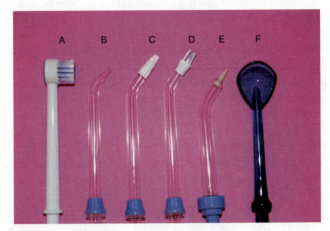

FIGURE ■ **12–40** A variety of oral irrigator tips.

(*Source:* Courtesy of Amy Teague.)

BOX 12–6   Uses of Various Irrigation Tips

TIP		USE
A.	Toothbrush tip	To brush and irrigate at the same time
B.	Classic Jet tip	To clean deep interproximally and supragingivally, also reaching slightly subgingivally
C.	Orthodontic tip	To clean around orthodontic brackets and wires
D.	Plaque Seeker™ tip	To clean around implants, crowns, bridges and other restorations
E.	Pik Pocket™ tip	To clean and deliver chemotherapeutic rinses in periodontal pockets and furcations with low pressure
F.	Tongue cleaner	To clean and irrigate the tongue

Orthodontic tips (D in Figure 12–40 ■) include a soft tapered brush end that enhances plaque biofilm removal around orthodontic appliances that are difficult to clean with a toothbrush. These tips are used in a manner similar to a standard tip by placing the tip at a 90-degree angle to the tooth surface at the neck of the tooth and following the gingival margin to trace around the teeth. Use of an orthodontic tip combined with toothbrushing has been shown to be significantly more effective at removing plaque biofilm in comparison to both toothbrushing alone and toothbrushing in combination with flossing.[29]

Various irrigation unit designs are available (Figure 12–41 ■). Although there is not much difference among the brands, results with one brand do not necessarily translate to effectiveness with another brand.[20] Evidence-based practice demands review of clinical evidence for a particular brand before recommending it. The first Waterpik® unit was patented in 1967, has been tested in more than 50 research studies, and is the number one recommended dental water jet oral irrigator.[101] The newest model is marketed as a Water Flosser.[101]

Novel irrigation unit designs have been developed, but limited research has been conducted on these units. The OxyCare® and HydroFloss® units have a magnetic device that delivers magnetized water. A research study indicated that irrigation with magnetized water more effectively reduced calculus formation by inhibiting adherence of bacteria to the tooth surface although it did not significantly reduce plaque biofilm and gingivitis.[102] Testing of a high-pressure water irrigator showed the removal of established plaque biofilm.[103] Although irrigation with the high-pressure water resulted in less gingival abrasions than the comparison electric toothbrush, care should be taken not to use too much water pressure when practicing subgingival irrigation. Another novel oral irrigator (OxyJet® by Oral B®) incorporated 5% air into the water stream, then pressurized it to form millions of long-lasting microbubbles designed to attack plaque biofilm bacteria. Its

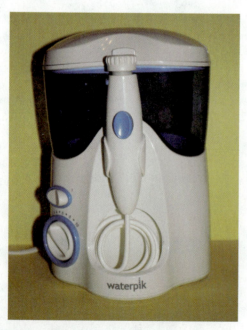

FIGURE ■ 12–41 An oral irrigator for home use.
(*Source:* Courtesy of Amy Teague.)

use reduced gingivitis, bleeding, and plaque biofilm compared to manual brushing, but the difference was not statistically significant.[104] This unit is not currently available on the market, but the technology may possibly be applied to another unit in the future.

Irrigation-Induced Bacteremias

The potential for irrigation to induce bacteremias has been studied, but it does not appear to be hazardous to healthy patients.[46] The frequency and intensity of bacteremias are believed to be related to the nature and magnitude of the tissue trauma, the density of the microbial flora, and the degree of inflammation or infection at the site of trauma.[105] Routine oral hygiene has been shown to create transient bacteremias that are dealt with swiftly by the body defenses.[39] Oral irrigators used inappropriately by individuals with poor oral hygiene have induced bacteremias, but the relationship to bacterial endocarditis is unclear.[98] The AAP suggests that supragingival and subgingival irrigation should be recommended with caution to patients who require premedication before periodontal therapy because there is no specific information on the degree of risk for bacteremia from irrigation in this population.[98]

CHEWING GUM

One of the protective factors in the prevention of dental caries is salivary flow.[106] Increasing salivary flow may be accomplished by increasing fluid intake. In addition, chewing increases salivary flow,[107] and chewing sugar-free gum after eating has especially been shown to stimulate salivary flow, which can decrease oral bacteria and reduce dental caries.[108,109] The addition of xylitol to the gum has an additional antimicrobial effect and reduces plaque pH to enhance its role in the prevention of dental caries.[110,111] Chewing gum has also been suggested as a vehicle for agents such as fluoride, chlorhexidine, and calcium phosphate to prevent caries. Patients should be counseled to chew only sugar-free gum as a means of stimulating salivary flow to prevent dental caries.

ORAL MALODOR AND THE TONGUE

Oral malodor, also referred to as bad breath and **halitosis**, is defined as an unpleasant breath emanating from the oral cavity regardless of its origin.[112] Oral malodor has been a common problem among different human populations since ancient times; Hippocrates prescribed an antidote for malodor in 400 B.C.[113] Although the true prevalence of halitosis is unknown, available evidence suggests that it is still very common today and affects people of all ages, but there is indication that it is less common in children.[114] Various studies report that 30% to more than 50% of the population have halitosis, both in the United States and globally,[115–118] and that 25% of the population experience halitosis that is severe and persistent.[119] According to the ADA, bad breath is a common chief complaint of patients in the United States.[120]

Bad breath can cause psychological distress, social handicapping, and avoidance of social situations.[121] Self-appraisal of halitosis, especially by patients who have slight or moderate oral malodor, and professional evaluation of halitosis by organoleptic (involving a sensory organ) examination are highly correlated. In a recent study, 93.9% of individuals who self-assessed that they had bad breath actually had the condition.[122]

> **DID YOU KNOW?**
>
> Tongue coating harbors bacteria that are associated with periodontal disease, dental caries, and even systemic conditions such as pneumonia.

Causes of Oral Malodor

In approximately 80–90% of cases, halitosis is caused by oral conditions.[119,123] These include tongue coating, periodontal disease, peri-implant disease, deep carious lesions, exposed necrotic tooth pulps, pericoronitis, mucosal ulcerations, healing mucosal wounds, impacted food or debris, imperfect dental restorations, unclean dentures, and factors causing decreased salivary flow rate.[123] Oral malodor has been attributed to tongue coating in 43% of cases.[124] In a study of individuals who wore dentures, the accumulation of bacterial plaque on the tongue, oral dryness, burning mouth, overnight denture wear, and lower educational levels were significantly related to oral malodor.[125]

Although it occurs in the oral cavity, the originating source of malodor can be disturbances of the upper and lower respiratory tract, disorders of the gastrointestinal tract, some systemic diseases, metabolic disorders, and carcinomas.[123] Chronically infected tonsils may be the cause if the crypts contain malodorous substrates.[112] Medications and odorous foods can also produce oral malodor, and stress is a predisposing factor.[123] A multidisciplinary approach is required by referral for a thorough physical examination to rule out a systemic disorder.[124] In a study of halitosis in healthy children, the researchers concluded that the condition does not correlate well with common oral parameters, suggesting factors other than volatile sulfur compounds (VSCs) may be associated with halitosis in children.[114]

> **DID YOU KNOW?**
>
> Periodontitis and gingivitis are associated with malodor.

The basic process of oral malodor is microbial degradation of organic substrates.[123] Sulfur-containing proteins and peptides are hydrolyzed by gram-negative bacteria in an alkaline environment resulting in putrefaction.[112] *Putrefaction* refers to a combination of protein hydrolysis by the bacteria and catabolism of the basic amino acids. The end result of putrefaction is malodor-producing VSCs. Exhaled air contains these odorous, sulfur-containing end products, including hydrogen sulfide, methyl mercaptans, and dimethyl sulfide.

The putrefaction process and its concomitant odor occur more rapidly when bacterial accumulations are high[116]; therefore, VSCs are higher in patients with periodontal disease.[126] These VSCs have been associated with the progression of periodontal disease by increasing the permeability of the mucosal membrane, which allows for invasion of bacteria into the tissue.[127] The wound-healing process can be delayed or disturbed by these compounds because they interfere with the synthesis of DNA and protein. A shift from a predominantly gram-positive to a gram-negative and anaerobic bacterial population is associated with the production of VSCs and odor production. The tongue surface provides a niche for periodontal pathogens.[116] In addition, inconsistent or ineffective interproximal plaque biofilm removal can provide a recess for gram-negative bacteria to degrade sulfur-containing amino acids, resulting in malodor. Because periodontitis and gingivitis are associated with malodor, management of periodontal disease is an important aspect in the control of malodor for some people. Treatment with nonsurgical periodontal therapy and improved oral hygiene significantly reduce VSCs.[126]

Local factors such as a rise in oral pH and reduced salivary flow accelerate this shift. Research studies have demonstrated that neutral or alkaline oral pH favors the generation of VSCs whereas an acidic oral pH inhibits their production.[128] Because the pH of plaque biofilm is at its highest in the morning, the alkalinity of the oral cavity leads to the production of unpleasant morning breath.[129] Decreased salivary flow results in reduced oral clearance, increased plaque biofilm, and higher bacterial load, amplifying the production of VSCs.[108]

People with good oral health and adequate oral hygiene can be affected by halitosis. The dorso-posterior region of the tongue is the major site for development of oral malodor in healthy individuals. This area does not benefit from the natural washing effects of the oral cavity, thus harboring bacteria that produce VSCs.[116] Therefore, regular mechanical cleaning of the tongue is important to control malodor and maintain oral health even in healthy patients.[117]

Treatment of Oral Malodor

Because of the potential overall and oral health implications of oral malodor, it is important to have a frank discussion with a patient who has the condition. Research studies support the oral health professional's approach of gently bringing the condition to the patient's attention, providing education about the causes of the condition, making appropriate referrals, and recommending treatment for and control of oral malodor based on assessment data.[119] Furthermore, patients appreciate learning about the causes and control of oral malodor.[119]

Treatment considerations can include providing professional periodontal debridement,[127] improving oral hygiene to reduce the bacterial load,[112] increasing salivary flow,[123] improving tongue hygiene,[130] and using chemotherapeutic agents to reduce gram-negative microflora and neutralize VSCs for short-term control of malodor.[117,121] Interestingly, periodontopathic bacteria were found more frequently in tongue coating samples from dentate than edentulous elderly individuals,[130] suggesting the need for a twofold approach to treatment that includes periodontal therapy and promotion of oral malodor control methods.[117] In addition, malodor in denture patients can be decreased with proper denture care and overnight removal of dentures.[125] (See Chapter 13.)

Masking products such as mouthrinses, mints, gum, sprays, and others are not effective in the management of oral malodor.[112] However, the addition of assorted chemotherapeutic agents to these products has been recommended for treatment of oral malodor with varying degrees of success. These include botanical extracts and herbal formulations; cetylpyridinium chloride contained in mouthrinses, mouth sprays, and dentifrices; 0.12% chlorhexidine mouthrinses; chlorine dioxide used in mouthwashes, dentifrices, and mouth sprays; essential oils included in mouthwashes, toothpastes, and mouth sprays; hydrogen peroxide; sodium bicarbonate; zinc salts in mouthrinses, dentifrices, and chewing gum; activated carbon in several preparations; enzymes contained in dentifrices and other products; and flavoring agents of dentifrices.[118,131,132] Chlorhexidine mouthrinses, essential oils, chlorine dioxide, and sodium carbonate in combination with either peroxide or triclosan have been shown to be the most successful in research studies.[122]

Triclosan has been shown to be effective in controlling oral mouth odor;[121] however, several recent animal studies have questioned its safety.[133] The U. S. Food and Drug Administration (FDA) has expressed "valid concerns" about possible health effects of triclosan.[134] In addition, the FDA has issued a statement that it is conducting an ongoing scientific and regulatory review of triclosan and partnering with other federal agencies to conduct research on its health effects.[133] Several oral health products that contained triclosan have been discontinued by the manufacturers.

A Cochrane review concluded that mouthrinses containing chlorhexidine and cetylpyridinium chloride may play an important role in reducing levels of halitosis-producing bacteria on the tongue, and chlorine dioxide and zinc containing mouthrinses can be effective in neutralizing malodorous VCSs.[118] Another systematic review reported that essential oils and cetylpyridinium chloride are effective only up to 2 to 3 hours; metal ions and oxidizing agents, such as hydrogen peroxide, chlorine dioxide, and iminium have a role in neutralizing VCSs and zinc is safe and effective at concentrations of at least 1%.[112] Recent studies have tested the effectiveness of a new chlorhexidine-free mouthrinse containing amine fluoride/stannous fluoride to control oral malodor. Results demonstrated that the new mouthrinse was as effective as a benchmark chlorhexidine mouthrinse.[135]

Researchers have reported that although regular use of mouthrinses may control oral malodor, single use may have only a short-term benefit.[112,117] In addition, the effectiveness of active ingredients in oral healthcare products depends on their concentration, and above a certain concentration, the ingredients can have unpleasant side effects.[112] A study of foods that are claimed to reduce halitosis demonstrated that green tea had significant temporary effectiveness, attributed to its disinfectant and deodorant properties, but other foods were not effective.[128]

Tongue Cleaning

The normal anatomical structure of the tongue contributes to the need for the regular practice of tongue cleaning. The large papillary surface area of the tongue dorsum favors the accumulation of oral microorganisms and oral debris. Anatomically, the varying heights and formations of the papillae on the tongue create elevations and depressions that can entrap debris and harbor microorganisms, making the tongue an ideal location for bacterial growth.

The tongue coating contains nutrients, desquamated epithelial cells, blood cells, and bacteria. One study reported that the bacterial load is about 25 times higher in individuals who have a coated tongue compared to those who do not.[129] Bacteria contained in the tongue coating are associated with dental caries,[4] periodontal diseases,[116] and systemic conditions such as pneumonia, especially in older adult individuals.[136] Tongue coating is associated with oral malodor in 43% of cases.[124]

Thus, reduction of the tongue coating by mechanical tongue debridement can contribute to the reduction and control of plaque biofilm accumulation, control of oral malodor, prevention and control of dental caries and periodontal diseases, and even prevention of aspiration pneumonia by reducing the oral bacterial load.[112] A systematic review concluded that tongue cleaning has the potential to successfully reduce tongue coating and breath odor associated with it.[137] However, data are insufficient to determine its effect on chronic oral malodor, which can be related to causes other than tongue coating. Another study concluded that tongue cleaning appears to be the most important hygiene procedure to reduce morning bad breath in periodontally healthy individuals.[129]

It has been suggested that although tongue cleaning reduces bacterial load on the tongue, this effect is transient, and daily tongue cleaning is required to reduce bacterial numbers long term.[138,139] The bacterial population returns within a day or less.[119] The practice of tongue cleaning is especially recommended for smokers[140] and individuals who have hairy tongue.[141]

Few patients practice tongue cleaning as an oral hygiene procedure. It has been suggested that this is due to discomfort or lack of awareness of its importance on the part of the public and the profession or both.[139] Cleaning the tongue is recommended by oral health care professional organizations as a part of daily oral hygiene practices.[138,142,143] Tongue-cleaning tools have been promoted as straightforward to use, easy to transport, inexpensively priced, and comfortable to use when used correctly. Cleaning the tongue has been endorsed as easily and quickly accomplished by individuals of all ages. Oral health care professionals should become aware of tongue-cleaning products and methods to be able to recommend the most appropriate one for the individual patient. Patients should be educated about appropriate methods of tongue cleaning to avoid gagging and prevent trauma or injury to the tongue or other oropharyngeal tissues.

When cleaning the tongue, it is important to begin at the terminal sulcus to remove the coating and bacteria from the posterior portion of the dorsal surface where they are predominant. The terminal sulcus is the V-shaped line located just posterior to the circumvallate papillae and that separates the anterior (oral or horizontal) and posterior (pharyngeal or vertical) parts of the tongue. (Figures 12–42 ■, 12–43 ■, and 12–44 ■). As with

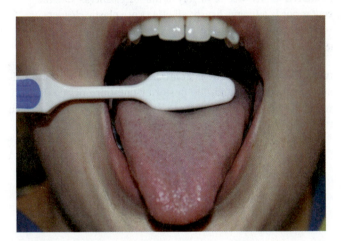

FIGURE ■ 12–42 Toothbrush placed across the tongue on the dorsal surface as far back as possible and anterior to the circumvallate papillae prior to rolling it forward to clean the dorsal surface.

(*Source:* Courtesy of Amy Teague.)

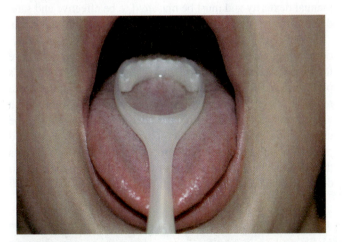

FIGURE ■ 12–43 Tongue cleaner placed on the dorsum of the tongue as far back as possible and anterior to the circumvallate papillae prior to gently pulling it forward with a sweeping motion. Serations on the rounded portion clean the surface as it is pulled forward.

(*Source:* Courtesy of Amy Teague.)

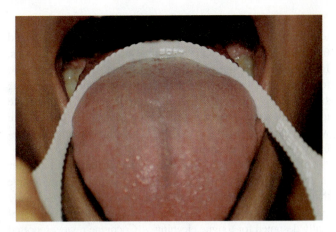

FIGURE ■ 12–44 Plastic tongue scraper used by pressing it against the dorsum of the tongue in an arc. Serrations on the tongue scraper clean the dorsal surface as it is skimmed forward on the tongue.

(*Source:* Courtesy of Amy Teague.)

toothbrushing and flossing, several strokes are required to thoroughly clean the tongue surface. Some researchers recommend repeating the tongue cleaning stroke one or two times;[144] others suggest repeating it three to four times.[145] The procedure used to clean the tongue is described in Box 12–7 ■ and illustrated in Figures 12–42 ■, 12–43 ■, and 12–44 ■.

BOX 12–7 **Procedure for Cleaning the Tongue**

With a toothbrush

1. Protrude the tongue as far as possible.
2. Hold the handle of the toothbrush at a right angle to the midline of the tongue.
3. Place the toothbrush on the terminal sulcus with the bristles directed toward the throat. (Figure 12–42 ■)
4. Roll the toothbrush forward, gently and with light pressure.
5. Repeat the procedure.
6. Take care not to scrub the tongue.
7. Avoid trauma by using gentle, forward rolling strokes, and a soft, end-rounded toothbrush.

With a tongue cleaner or tongue scraper

1. Protrude the tongue as far as possible.
2. If using a tongue cleaner, hold the handle parallel to the midline of the tongue. (Figure 12–43 ■)
3. If using a tongue scraper, hold it across the tongue. (Figure 12–44 ■)
4. Place the tongue cleaner/scraper on the dorsal surface of the tongue. (Figures 12–43 ■, 12–44 ■)
5. Pull the tongue cleaner/scraper forward with a sweeping motion to skim across the tongue surface.
6. Repeat the procedure.
7. Apply gentle pressure with each stroke.
8. Take care not to scrape the tongue with too much pressure.
9. Prevent trauma by using gentle, sweeping forward strokes and avoiding sharp metal tongue scrapers.

Some sources recommend an end-rounded soft-bristled toothbrush to clean the tongue.[142,144] It has been suggested that a tongue scraper can cause damage to the sensitive tissues. If a toothbrush is used for tongue cleaning, medium and hard toothbrushes should be avoided to prevent trauma to the tongue surface. Gagging can easily occur when trying to place the toothbrush at the posterior of the tongue, especially in people who have a propensity for gagging. These individuals may prefer using a tongue cleaner.[146]

Other sources recommend the use of a special **tongue cleaner** or **tongue scraper**,[138,143] claiming that they are more effective than the soft toothbrush for this purpose because they provide even pressure throughout the cleaning stroke. Both tools are specially designed for tongue cleaning. A Cochrane review reported that weak but unreliable evidence supports the efficacy of a tongue cleaner or tongue scraper over a soft toothbrush for tongue cleaning.[146] However, clinically, the difference is irrelevant because the reduction of VSCs is temporary for both cleaning methods. This review also reported gagging in 60% and trauma to the tongue in 10% of individuals who used the toothbrush in one study.

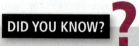

DID YOU KNOW?

If gagging occurs during tongue cleaning, use of a flat tongue cleaner will usually prevent gagging.

Various designs of tongue cleaners, scrapers, and brushes are available (Figure 12–45 ■) and are made of different materials such as plastics or stainless steel. Patients should be instructed on selection of a tongue cleaner. Plastic scrapers are gentler to the soft tissues than metal. Designs that are a combination of brush and plastic scraper may also produce more trauma in the same way a toothbrush does.[146] Gagging during tongue cleaning can be diminished by use of a flat tongue cleaner.

Still other sources indicate that tongue cleaning can be accomplished with a soft toothbrush, tongue cleaner, or tongue scraper.[147] Studies have demonstrated reduction in oral malodor and tongue coating regardless of the tool.[137] It has also been recommended that the tongue can be cleaned with a folded square of gauze.[144] Considering the disagreement among professional organizations and researchers, it seems that as long as one of the recommended tools is used, the choice of which one could be individually based on personal preferences.

Regardless of the means used to practice tongue cleaning, it is important that the concentration of cleaning be on the posterior portion of the dorsal surface of the tongue; this area has the greatest prevalence of tongue coating.[136] The anterior

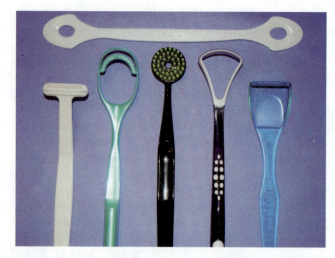

FIGURE ■ 12–45 A variety of tongue cleaners. Note the center one is a tongue brush; all others are plastic cleaners or scrapers with serrations.

(*Source:* Courtesy of Amy Teague.)

two-thirds of the tongue is continually rubbed by the hard palate. On the other hand, the posterior one-third of the dorsum, which is in contact with the soft palate that has no surface roughness, does not benefit from natural cleaning.

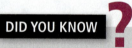

DID YOU KNOW

Malodor and tongue cleaning should be included in oral self-care instructions.

Oral health education related to tongue cleaning should include information about the ill effects of the tongue coating, safe and effective ways to clean the tongue, and guidance in selecting a toothbrush, tongue cleaner, or tongue scraper for that purpose.[144] In addition, because it is a skill that requires some manual dexterity and must be mastered to be effective and safe, demonstration and guided practice should accompany education.

It is clear that tongue cleaning helps to control oral malodor, although there is disagreement about the most effective tool to use. According to evidence-based practice, the patient's preferences should be considered as recommendations are made.[14] Especially in the absence of strong evidence that a tongue cleaner is more effective than a soft toothbrush, the choice should be based on the patient's individual needs and preferences. Additionally, the process of care model indicates the need to evaluate the patient's practice of tongue cleaning to determine that it is being accomplished effectively and safely.[11]

SUMMARY

This chapter has reviewed information about the use of dental floss, tongue cleaning, and self-care aducts for the practitioner's consideration in the development of an oral health self-care plan for the patient. In addition to oral conditions, several

factors affect the appropriate selection and use of supplemental oral hygiene devices and techniques for the oral health self care plan. The dexterity, ability and motivation for performing oral hygiene procedure and the personal preferences for specific devices should be assessed when supplemental oral hygiene aids are recommended.

When a device is introduced, it is essential that the proper application in all areas of the mouth be demonstrated, and that the potential damage with improper use is understood. To enhance compliance and skill development, dental providers should limit the number of recommended oral health devices. Personal preferences fo particular oarl hygiene aids should also be considerd. If an individual has shown a preference for a specific device, its effective use should be encouraged. It is imperative that the dental provider stay informed of the research describing all devices, as they becomes available.

PRACTICAL CONSIDERATIONS

As with all other oral health practices and recommendations, decisions about the use of oral hygiene devices and procedures must be based on principles of evidence-based practice. This requires a thorough assessment of a patient's history, oral health status, and current needs to incorporate clinical needs and preferences into the evidence-based formula.

The oral health care provider has the professional responsibility to assist patients in making decisions about oral hygiene practices and devices. The evidence of their usefulness, effectiveness, and safety is also important to ensure valid and practical recommendations.

SELF-STUDY QUESTIONS

Use the following scenario for questions 1 through 3:

A female patient presents in your office with generalized moderate clinical attachment loss, type II embrasures, and generalized bleeding points interproximally. The buccal and lingual gingiva is tight with good color and texture, and you measure a low Plaque Index score on the buccal and lingual surfaces. The patient is very motivated to practice self-care to protect the longevity of her teeth.

1. Which of the following self-care procedures should be recommended first?

   a. Daily rinse with chlorhexidine for 2 months

   b. Use of a tongue cleaner

   c. Use of unwaxed floss

   d. Use of variable-thickness (tufted) dental floss

   e. Use of triangular wood sticks

   Rationale: This patient's high level of motivation warrants trying to introduce dental floss even though the rate of compliance in the population is low. If she is unable to floss, other interproximal aids can be tried later. Because of her generalized type II embrasures, regular floss is not indicated; variable-thickness floss is better for open embrasures. Chlorhexidine rinse is not indicated because the patient does not exhibit generalized inflammation. Although a tongue cleaner is a good recommendation, the interproximal bleeding should be addressed first.

2. You find that the patient's arthritis makes flossing very difficult. What would be the best tool to recommend first?

   a. Floss holder

   b. Floss picks

   c. Interproximal brush

   d. Triangular wood sticks

   Rationale: The use of dental floss is more effective than alternative aids. Because she is highly motivated, it is best to exhaust all possibilities of her ability to floss before moving on to an alternative. Her arthritis would make floss picks as difficult to manipulate as floss. Use of a floss holder is recommended for patients who have trouble flossing as a result of arthritis.

3. The patient is noncompliant with flossing because her arthritis and other issues make it too difficult. What is the best tool to recommend as an alternative?

   a. Interproximal brush

   b. Rubber tip stimulator

   c. End-tuft brush

   d. Triangular wood sticks

   e. Toothpicks

   Rationale: The interproximal (interdental) brush is the most effective of the interproximal cleaning devices. An end-tuft brush is used interproximally only in a type III embrasure. Triangular wood sticks are not as effective as interproximal brushes but are a good alternative if a patient is an avid toothpick user and is willing to change to a safer alternative. Toothpicks are less effective and can cause trauma over time. The efficacy of the rubber tip stimulator is questionable.

4. Tongue cleaning is recommended to reduce tongue coating and the bacterial load of the mouth. The evidence shows that a tongue cleaner or tongue scraper is clearly more effective than a soft toothbrush for tongue cleaning.

   a. Both statements are true.

   b. Both statements are false.

   c. The first statement is true; the second statement is false.

   d. The first statement is false; the second statement is true.

   Rationale: The dorsum of the tongue does not benefit from self-cleansing, resulting in a coating and an accumulation of bacteria associated with oral and systemic diseases. Tongue cleaning will remove this coating and the bacteria, resulting in lower bacterial count in the mouth. There is only slight evidence that a tongue cleaner or tongue scraper is more effective than a soft toothbrush. Therefore, the recommendation can be based on the patient's needs and preference.

5. All of the following *except* one should be considered when making recommendations for self-care procedures and aids to supplement toothbrushing. Which one is the *exception*?

   a. Patient preferences

   b. Evidence of effectiveness from research studies

   c. Patient's physical condition

   d. Cost of devices that are recommended

   e. All should be considered

Rationale: Patient preferences and evidence are components of evidence-based practice which is the foundation of making sound recommendations. Cost is a factor that must be considered in all recommendations to ensure compliance. Also, cost is a component of patient preferences. Patient's physical condition, such as energy level to perform complicated oral hygiene procedures, must be considered.

REFERENCES

1. Armitage, G. C., & Robertson, P. B. (2009). The biology, prevention, diagnosis and treatment of periodontal diseases: Scientific advances in the United States. *J Am Dent Assoc,* 140:36S–43S.

2. Thomas, J. G., & Nakaishi, L. A. (2006). Managing the complexity of a dynamic biofilm. *J Am Dent Assoc,* 137 (Suppl):10S–15S.

3. American Academy of Periodontology. (2001). (Academy Report/Position Paper). Treatment of plaque-induced gingivitis, chronic periodontitis, and other clinical conditions. *J Periodontol,* 72:1790–1800.

4. Fejerskov, O., & Kidd, E. (2008). *Dental caries: The disease and its clinical management* (2nd ed.). Frederiksberg C, Denmark: Blackwell Munksgaard, XX. (Also caries bacteria on surface of tongue)

5. Tulchinsky, T. H., & Varavikova, E. (2009). *The new pubic health.* Burlington, MA: Elsevier Academic Press.

6. U. S. Department of Health and Human Services. (2000). *Oral Health in America: A Report of the Surgeon General.* Rockville, MD: USDHHS, National Institute of Dental and Craniofacial Research, National Institutes of Health.

7. Van Dyke, T. E., & Kornman, K. S. (2008). Inflammation and factors that may regulate inflammatory response. *J Periodontol,* 79:1503–7.

8. Jardim, J. J., Alves, L. S., & Maltz, M. (2009). The history and global market of oral home-care products. *Braz Oral Res,* 23(Suppl 1):e. Retrieved April 24, 2011, from SciELO at http://www.scielo.br/scielo.php?script=sci_arttext&pid=S1806-83242009000500004.

9. Reddy, S. (2008). *Essentials of clinical periodontology and periodontics* (2nd ed.). New Delhi, India: Jaypee Brothers. Retrieved February 3, 2011, from www.jaypeeonline.in.

10. Newman, M. G., Takei, H., Klokkevold, P. R., & Carranza, F. A. (2011). *Carranzas's clinical periodontology* (11th ed.). St. Louis, MO: Elsevier.

11. Mueller-Joseph, L., Homenko, D. F., Wilkins, E. M., & Wyche, C. J. (2010). The professional dental hygienist. In Wilkins, E. M., Ed. *Clinical practice of the dental hygienist* (9th ed.) Philadelphia, PA: Lippincott Williams & Wilkins, 3–17.

12. Tuthill, J. (2011). A new generation of risk assessment. *Dimen Dent Hygiene,* 9:50, 52–53.

13. Walsh, M. M., & Darby, M. L. (2010). Human needs theory and dental hygiene care. In Darby, M. L., & Walsh, M. M., Eds. *Dental hygiene theory & practice* (3rd ed.). St. Louis, MO: Elsevier, 13–23.

14. Darby, M. L., & Walsh, M. M. (2010). The dental hygiene profession. In Darby, M. L., & Walsh, M. M., Eds. *Dental hygiene theory & practice* (3rd ed.). St. Louis, MO: Elsevier, 1–12.

15. Harfst, S. A., & Vick, V. C. (2008). Individualizing preventive and therapeutic strategies. In Daniel, S. J., Harfst, S. A., & Wilder, R. S., Eds. *Mosby's dental hygiene concepts, cases, and competencies* (2nd ed.). St. Louis, MO: Mosby Elsevier, 405–16.

16. Wilkins, E. M. (2010). Health promotion and disease prevention. *Clinical practice of the dental hygienist* (10th ed.). Philadelphia, PA: Lippincott Williams & Wilkins, 381–405.

17. Harfst, S. A., & Vick, V. C. (2008). Oral risk assessment and intervention planning. In Daniel, S. J., Harfst, S. A., & Wilder, R. S., Eds. *Mosby's dental hygiene concepts, cases, and competencies* (2nd ed.). St. Louis, MO: Mosby Elsevier, 387–404.

18. Levin, R. P. (2008, October 1). Five ways to increase hygiene production. Retrieved February 4, 2011, from *Dentistry IQ* at http://www.dentistryiq.com.

19. Forrest, J. J., & Miller, S. A. (2008). Evidence-based decision making. In Daniel, S. J., Harfst, S. A., & Wilder, R. S., Eds. *Mosby's dental hygiene concepts, cases, and competencies* (2nd ed.). St. Louis, MO: Mosby Elsevier, 52–61.

20. Jahn, C. (2011). Best practices for periodontal care. In Nield-Gehrig, J. S., & Willmann, D. E., Eds. *Foundations of periodontics for the dental hygienist* (3rd ed.). Philadelphia, PA: Lippincott Williams & Wilkins, 365–80.

21. American Dental Association. (2011). *ADA Seal of Acceptance Program.* Retrieved February 4, 2011 from http://www.ada.org.

22. Gurenlian, J. A. R. (2007). The role of dental plaque biofilm in oral health. *J Dent Hygiene,* Suppl:4–12. Retrieved April 21, 2011, from http://adha.org/downloads/Antimicrobial_JDH_Supplement.pdf.

23. Bray, K. S., & Gluch, J. I. (2008). Health promotion: A basis of practice. In Daniel, S. J., Harfst, S. A., & Wilder, R. S., Eds. *Mosby's dental hygiene concepts, cases, and competencies* (2nd ed.). St. Louis, MO: Mosby Elsevier, 14–34.

24. Barnes, C. M., Gluch, J. I., Lyle, D. M., & Jahn, C. A. (2008). Devices for oral self-care. In Daniel, S. J., Harfst, S. A., & Wilder, R. S., Eds. *Mosby's dental hygiene concepts, cases, and competencies* (2nd ed.). St. Louis, MO: Mosby Elsevier, 440–70.

25. Young, D. A., Featherstone, J. D. B., & Budenz, A. W. (2008). Dental caries and caries management. In Daniel, S. J., Harfst, S. A., & Wilder, R. S., Eds. *Mosby's dental hygiene concepts, cases, and competencies* (2nd ed.). St. Louis, MO: Mosby Elsevier, 471–91.

26. Wilkins, E. M. (2010). Interdental care. *Clinical practice of the dental hygienist* (10th ed.). Philadelphia, PA: Lippincott Williams & Wilkins, 429–42.

27. Cappelli, D. P., & Mobley, C. C. (2008). *Prevention in clinical oral health care*. St. Louis, MO: Mosby Elsevier.
28. Lyle, D. M. (2010). Mechanical oral biofilm control: Interdental and supplemental self-care devices. In Darby, M. L., & Walsh, M. M., Eds. *Dental hygiene theory & practice* (3rd ed.). St. Louis, MO: Elsevier, 401–4.
29. Jahn, C., & Nield-Gehrig, J. (2011). Patient's role in nonsurgical periodontal therapy. In Nield-Gehrig, J. S., & Willmann, D. E., Eds. *Foundations of periodontics for the dental hygienist* (3rd ed.). Philadelphia, PA: Lippincott Williams & Wilkins, 433–48.
30. Hujoel, P. P., Cunha-Cruz, J., Banting, D. W., & Loesche, W. J. (2006). Dental flossing and interproximal caries: A systematic review. *J Dent Res, 85*:298–305.
31. Biesbrock, A., Corby, P. M. A., Bartizek, R., Corby, A. L., Coelho, M., Costa, S., Bretz, W. A. G., & Bretz, W. A. (2006). Assessment of treatment responses to dental flossing in twins. *J Periodontol Online, 77*:1386–91.
32. Hogan, L M. E., Daly, C. G., & Curtis, B. H. (2007). Comparison of new and 3-month old brush heads in the removal of plaque using a powered toothbrush. *J Clin Periodontol, 34*:130–36.
33. Jackson, M. A., Kellett, M., Worthington, H. V., & Clerehugh, V. (2006). Comparison of interdental cleaning methods: A randomized controlled trial. *J Periodontol, 77*:1421–29.
34. Vahabi, S., & Nazemi, B. (2008). A comparison of chlorhexidine impregnated floss vs. conventional dental floss on gingivitis. *J Dent School, Shahid Beheshti Univ Med Sci, 25*:8. Retrieved February 4, 2011, from http://journals.sbmu.ac.ir/dj/article/view/307.
35. Flatt, C. C., Warren-Morris, D., Turner, S. D., & Chan, J. T. (2008). Effects of a stannous fluoride-impregnated dental floss on in vivo salivary fluoride levels. *J Dent Hygiene, 82*:8. Retrieved February 4, 2011, from BNET Health Publications at http://findarticles.com.
36. Terezhalmy, G. T., Bartizek, R. D., & Biesbrock, A. R. (2008). Plaque-removal efficacy of four types of dental floss. *J Periodontol Online, 79*:245–51.
37. Perry, D. A., & Pattison, G. (1986). An investigation of wax residue on tooth surfaces after the use of waxed dental floss. *Dent Hygiene, 60*:16–19.
38. Dorfer, C. E., Wundrich, D., Staehle, H. J., & Pioch, T. (2001). Gliding capacity of different dental flosses. *J Periodontol, 72*:672–78.
39. Parahitiyawa, N. B., Jin, L. J., Leung, W. K., Yam, W. C., & Samaranayake, L. P. (2009). Microbiology of odontogenic bacteremia: Beyond endocarditis. *Clin Microbiol Rev, 22*:46–64.
40. Brooks, N. (2009). Prophylactic antibiotic treatment to prevent infective endocarditis: New guidance from the National Institute for Health and Clinical Excellence. *Heart Educ Heart, 95*:774–80.
41. Baby Center, LLC. (2010). *How to Brush and Floss Your Preschooler's Teeth*. Video retrieved April 28, 2011, from American Academy of Pediatric Dentistry at www.aapd.org.
42. Tilliss, T. S. I. (2009). Time for change: Oral health self-care practices based on evidence and behavior patterns. *Special Issues + Whitepapers, 30*, Aegis Communications. Retrieved April 22, 2011, from http://www.dentalaegis.com.
43. Segelnick, S. L. (2004, May/June). A survey of floss frequency, habit, and technique in a hospital dental clinic and private periodontal practice. *NY State Dent J*, 28–33. Retrieved February 4, 2011, from http://www.eperiodr.com/SegelnickFtr.pdf.
44. Melrose, D. (2005, October). Floss alternatives. *Dimen Dent Hygiene, 10*:22–26.
45. Berchier, C. E., Slot, D. E., Haps, S., & Van der Weijden, G. A. (2008). The efficacy of dental floss in addition to a toothbrush on plaque and parameters of gingival inflammation: A systematic review. *Int J Dent Hyg, 6*:265–79.
46. Van Der Weijden, F., & Slot, D. E. (2011). Oral hygiene in the prevention of periodontal diseases: The evidence, *Periodontology 2000, 55*:104–123.
47. Oliver, H. E. (2010). Communication and behavioral change theories. In Darby, M. L., & Walsh, M. M., Eds. *Dental Hygiene Theory & Practice* (3rd ed.). St. Louis, MO: Elsevier, 24–36.
48. Schuz, B., Sniehotta, F. F., Wiedemann, A., & Seeman, R. (2006). Adherence to a daily flossing regimen in university students: Effects of planning when, where, how and what to do in the face of barriers. *J Clin Periodontol, 33*:612–19.
49. American Dental Hygienists' Association. (2010). *Proper flossing*. Chicago: Author. Retrieved February 4, 2011, from www.adha.org.
50. Laing, E., Ashley, P., Gill, D., & Naini, F. (2008). An update on oral hygiene products and techniques. *Dent Update, 35*:270–79.
51. National Institute of Dental and Craniofacial Research (NIDCR). (n.d.). *Dental care every cay: A caregiver's guide*. Retrieved April 24, 2011, from NIDCR at http://www.nidcr.nih.gov/OralHealth/Topics/DevelopmentalDisabilities.
52. Carter-Hanson, C., Gadbury-Amyot, C., & Killoy, W. (1996). Comparison of the plaque removal efficacy of a new flossing aid (Quik Floss®) to finger flossing. *J Clin Periodontol, 23*:873–78.
53. Perry, D. A., & Beemsterboer, P. L. (2007). Plaque and disease control for the periodontal patient. In Perry, D. A., & Beemsterboer, P. L., Eds. *Periodontology for the dental hygienist* (3rd ed.). St. Louis, MO: Saunders Elsevier, 235–58.
54. Slim, L. H. (2007). Periodontal nitwits and flossing. *RDH, 27*. Retrieved April 19, 2011, from Dentistry IQ at http://www.rdhmag.com.
55. Collins, F. (2008). *Factoring patient compliance into oral care*. CE course from Academy of Dental Therapeutics and Stomatology, PennWell. Retrieved February 4, 2011, from http://www.ineedce.com/courses.
56. Jahn, C. (2010, August 23). Coaching: Phase II of the new revolution in patient motivation. Retrieved February 4, 2011, from *Dentistry IQ* at http://www.dentistryiq.com.
57. Jahn, C. (2011, January 1). Healthy, bright smiles during ortho. *RDH, 31*. Retrieved February 4, 2011, from http://www.rdhmag.com.
58. Lyle, D. M., & Jahn, C. A. (2011). *Prevention: The key to successful dentistry and optimal oral health*. Retrieved April 18, 2011, from Dentalaegis Continuing Education at http://cde.dentalaegis.com.
59. *The science behind Sonicare AirFloss*. Retrieved November 21, 2011, from http://www.usa.philips.com.
60. Kreismann, J., & Almas, K. (2010). Oral hygiene for the periodontal patient: Beyond the basics. In Weinberg, M. A., Westphal, C., Froum, S. J., Palat, M., & Schoor, R. S., Eds. *Comprehensive periodontics for the dental hygienist* (3rd ed.). Upper Saddle River, NJ: Prentice Hall, 285–319.
61. Slot, D. E., Dörfer, C. E., & Van der Weijden, G. A. (2008). The efficacy of interdental brushes on plaque and parameters of periodontal inflammation: A systematic review. *Int J Dent Hyg, 6*:253–64.
62. Bock, N. C., von Bremen, J., Draft, M., & Ruf, S. (2009, December 3). Plaque control effectiveness and handling of interdental brushes during multibracket treatment—A randomized clinical trial. *Eur J Orthod Advance Access*, 6p. Retrieved February 3, 2011, from http://ejo.oxfordjournals.org.
63. Imai, P. H., & Hatzimanolakis, P. C. (2010, March 1). Encouraging client compliance for interdental care with the interdental brush: The client's perspective. Retrieved February 4, 2011, from *Internet FAQ Archives Online Education* at http://www.faqs.org/periodicals.
64. Sarner, B., Birkhed, D., & Lingstrom, P. (2008). Approximal fluoride concentration using different fluoridated products alone or in combination. *Caries Res, 42*:73–78.

65. Jared, H., Zhong, Y., Rowe, M., Ebisutani, K., Tanaka, T., & Takase, N. (2005). Clinical trial of a novel interdental brush cleaning system. *J Clin Dent,* 16:47–52.

66. Hague, A. L., & Carr, M. P. (2007). Efficacy of an automated flossing device in different regions of the mouth. *J Periodontol,* 78:1529–37.

67. Petroski, H. (2007). *The toothpick: Technology and culture.* New York, NY: Random House, Vintage Books. Google eBook retrieved April 23, 2011, from http://books.google.com/books.

68. Kaiser, K. (2009). Going soft. *RDH,* 29. Retrieved April 19, 2011, from Dentistry IQ at http://www.rdhmag.com.

69. Imai, P. (2006, March 1). A review of the different methods of applying chlorhexidine in the oral cavity. *Canad J Dent Hyg,* 40. Retrieved February 4, 2011, from http://www.thefreelibrary.com.

70. Melrose, D. (2006) Improving your patient's interdental cleaning regimen. *Dimen Dent Hygiene,* 4:20,22–23.

71. Reggiardo, P. A., Feigal, R. J., Casamassimo, P. S., Chan, S. D., Ng, M. W., & Ignelzi, M. A. (2006). Clinical, research, and policy implications of the symposium on the prevention of oral diseases in children and adolescents. *Ped Dent,* 28:192–98.

72. Centers for Disease Control and Prevention, Chronic Disease Prevention and Health Promotion. (2010). *Preventing cavities, gum disease, tooth loss, and oral cancers: At A glance 2010.* Retrieved February 4, 2010, from CDC at http://www.cdc.gov/chronicdisease/resources/publications/AAG/doh.htm.

73. Kagihara, L. E., Niederhauser, V. P., & Stark, M. (2009). Assessment, management, and prevention of early childhood. *J Am Acad Nurse Prac* 21:1–10.

74. American Dental Association. (2007). For the dental patient: Braces: Straighter teeth can improve oral health. *J Am Dent Assoc,* 138:556. Retrieved April 12, 2011, from http://www.ada.org.

75. Jenson L., Budenz A. W., Featherstone, J. D., Ramos-Gomez, F. J., Spolsky, V. W., & Young, D. A. (2007). Clinical protocols for caries management by risk assessment, *Calif Dent Assoc J,* 35–7714–723. Retrieved September 24, 2010, from http://www.cda.org/library/cda.

76. American Dental Hygienists' Association. (2010). *Eating disorders.* Continuing education course #8. Retrieved April 12, 2011, from http://www.adha.org/CE_courses/index.html.

77. Addy, M., Moran, J., & Newcombe, R. G. (2007). Meta-analyses of studies of 0.2% delmopinol mouth rinse as an adjunct to gingival health and plaque control measures. *J Clin Periodontol,* 34:58–65.

78. Al-Bayaty, F. H., Al-Koubaisi, A. H., Ali, N. A. W., & Abdulla, M.A. (2010). Effect of mouth wash extracted from *Salvadora persica* (Miswak) on dental plaque formation: A clinical trial. *J Medic Plants Res,* 4:1446–54. Retrieved April 24, 2011, from http://www.academicjournals.org/JMPR. ISSN 1996-0875.

79. Albertsson, K. W., Persson, A., Lingström, P., & van Dijken, J. W. V. (2009). Effects of mouthrinses containing essential oils and alcohol-free chlorhexidine on human plaque acidogenicity. *Clin Oral Investigat,* 14:107–12.

80. Tenenbaum, H., Luc, J., Schaaf, J.-F., Federlin-Ducani, M., Cotton, C., Elkaim, R., Cuisinier, F. J. G., & Roques, C. (2011). An 8-week, randomized, controlled, clinical study of the use of a 0.1% chlorhexidine mouthwash by chronic periodontitis patients. *J Investigat Clin Dent,* 2:29–37.

81. Stoeken, J. E., Paraskevas, S., & van der Weijden, G. A. (2007). The long-term effect of a mouthrinse containing essential oils on dental plaque and gingivitis: A systematic review. *J Periodontol,* 78:1218–28.

82. American Academy of Periodontology. (2000). Parameters of care. *J Periodontol,* 71(Suppl 5):847–83.

83. Academy of General Dentistry. (n.d.) *Daily tips for good oral hygiene.* Retrieved April 13, 2011, from http://www.knowyourteeth.com.

84. Simmons, L. A. B. (2010). Persons with orthodontic appliances. In Darby, M. L., & Walsh, M. M., Eds. *Dental hygiene theory and practice* (3rd ed.). St. Louis, MO: Saunders Elsevier, 1111–36.

85. Eberhard, J., Jepsen, S., Jervøe-Storm, P-M., Needleman, I., & Worthington, H. V. (2008). Full-mouth disinfection for the treatment of adult chronic periodontitis. *Cochrane Database of Syst Rev,* 2008, (Iss. 1, Art. No. CD004622).

86. Asadoorian, J. (2010). Chemotherapy for the control of periodontal diseases. In Darby, M. L., & Walsh, M. M., Eds. *Dental hygiene theory and practice* (3rd ed.). St. Louis, MO: Saunders Elsevier, 548–60.

87. Gutkowski, S., Gerber, D., Creasey, J., Nelson, A., & Young, D. A. (2007). The role of dental hygienists, assistants, and office staff in CAMBRA. *J Calif Dent Assoc,* 35:786–93. Retrieved February 4, 2011, from California Dental Association at http://www.cda.org/library/cda.

88. Manne, D. S. (2010). The patient with cancer. In Wilkins, E. M., Ed. *Clinical practice of the dental hygienis* (10th ed.). Philadelphia, PA: Lippincott Williams & Wilkins, 858–69.

89. Takehiko, M., Hasegawa, K., Okabe, A. Tsujimura, N., Kawata, Y., et. al. (2008). Efficacy of mouth rinse in preventing oral mucositis in patients receiving high-dose cytarabine for allogeneic hematopoietic stem cell transplantion. *Int J Hematol,* 88:583–587.

90. Potting, C. M. J., Uitterhoeve, R., Scholte Op Reimer, W., & Van Achterberg, T. (2006). The effectiveness of commonly used mouthwashes for the prevention of chemotherapy-induced oral mucositis: A systematic review. *Eur J Cancer Care,*15:431–39.

91. Jahn, C. (2010). The dental water jet: A historical review of the literature. *J Dent Hygiene,* 84:114–20.

92. Jahn, C. (2010). It's a flosser with water. *RDH,* 30. Retrieved April 19, 2011, from Dentistry IQ at http://www.rdhmag.com.

93. Husseini, A., Slot, D. E., & Van der Weijden, G. A. (2008). The efficacy of oral irrigation in addition to a toothbrush on plaque and the clinical parameters of periodontal inflammation: A systematic review. *Int J Dent Hygiene,* 6:304–14.

94. Barnes, C. M., Reinhardt, R. A., Payne, J. B., & Lyle, D. M. (2005). Comparison of irrigation to floss as an adjunct to tooth brushing: Effect on bleeding, gingivitis and supragingival plaque. *J Clin Dent,* 16:71–77. Retrieved April 24, 2011, from http://www.dewittetandenwinkel.nl/docs/research/jocd/jocd_wp.pdf.

95. Sharma, N. C., Lyle, D. M., Qaquish, J. G., Galustians, J., & Schuller, R. (2008). The effect of a dental water jet with orthodontic tip on plaque and bleeding in adolescent patients with fixed orthodontic appliances. *Am J Orthod Dentofacial Orthop,* 133:565–71.

96. Gorur, A., Lyle, D. M., Schaudinn, C., & Costerton, J. W. (2009). Biofilm removal with a dental water jet. *Compend Contin Educ Dent,* 30 (Spec No 1):1–6.

97. Rosema, N. A., Hennequin-Hoenderdos, N. L., Berchier, C. E., Slot, D. E., Lyle, D. M., & van der Weijden, G. A. (2011). The effect of different interdental cleaning devices on gingival bleeding. *J Int Acad Periodontol,* 13:2–10.

98. American Academy of Periodontology. (2005). (Position Paper). The role of supra- and subgingival irrigation in the treatment of periodontal diseases. *J Periodontol,* 76:2015–27.

99. Mombelli, A., Cionca, N., & Almaghlouth, A. (2011). Does adjunctive antimicrobial therapy reduce the perceived need for periodontal surgery? *Periodontol 2000,* 55:205–16. Retrieved April 24, 2011, from http://onlinelibrary.wiley.com.

100. Deo, V., & Bhongade, M. L. (2010). Pathogenesis of periodontitis: Role of cytokines in host response. *Dent Today,* 29:60–62.

101. *About Water Pik*. Retrieved April 17, 2011, from http://www.waterpik.com.

102. Johnson, K. E., Sanders, J. J., Gellin, R. G., & Palesch, Y. Y. (1998). The effectiveness of a magnetized water oral irrigator (Hydro Floss®) on plaque, calculus and gingival health. *J Clin Periodontol,* 25:316–21.

103. Eberhard, J., Damm, S., Freitag, S., Albers, H. K., & Jepsen, S. (2004). Plaque removing capacity of a novel high pressure water irrigator. *Am J Dent,* 17:199–202.

104. Frascella, J. A., Fernandez, P., Gilbert, R. D., & Cugini, M. (2000). A randomized, clinical evaluation of the safety and efficacy of a novel oral irrigator. *Am J Dent,* 13:55–58.

105. American Heart Association. (2007). AHA guideline: Prevention of infective endocarditis. *Circulation,* 116:1736–54.

106. Modeer, T., Blomberg, C. C., Wondimu, B., Julihn, A., & Marcus, C. (2010). Association between obesity, flow rate of whole saliva, and dental caries in adolescents. *Obesity,* 18, 2367–73.

107. American Dental Association. (n.d). *Oral health topics: Saliva.* Retrieved April 13, 2011, from http://www.ada.org.

108. Dawes, C. (2008). Salivary flow patterns and the health of hard and soft oral tissues. *J Am Dent Assoc,* 139(Suppl 2):18S–24S. Retrieved February 5, 2011, from http://www.adajournal.com.

109. Stookey, G. K. (2008). The effect of saliva on dental caries. *J Am Dent Assoc,* 139(Suppl 5):11S–17S. Retrieved April 12, 2011, from http://www.adha.org/downloads/Saliva_CE.pdf.

110. Deshpande, A., & Jadad, A. R. (2008). The impact of polyol-containing chewing gums on dental caries: A systematic review of original randomized controlled trials and observational studies. *J Am Dent Assoc,* 139:1602–14.

111. Ribelles, L. M., Guinot, J. F., Mayné, A. R., & Bellet, D. L. J. (2010). Effects of xylitol chewing gum on salivary flow rate, pH, buffering capacity and presence of Streptococcus mutans in saliva. *Eur J Paediatr Dent,* 11:9–14.

112. Van Den Broek, A. M., Feenstra, L., & De Baat, C. (2008). A review of the current literature on management of halitosis. *Oral Dis,* 14:30–39.

113. Bosy, A. (2006). Managing oral malodor. *J Prac Hyg,* 15:20–21.

114. I-Hsuan Lin, M., Flaitz, C. M., Moretti, A. J., Seybold, S. V., & Chen, J.-W. (2003). Evaluation of halitosis in children and mothers. *Pediatr Dent,* 25:553–58.

115. Scully, C., & Greenman, J. (2008). Halitosis (breath odor). *Periodontology 2000,* 48: 66–75.

116. Cortelli, J. R., Barbosa, M. D., & Westphal, M. A. (2008, August). Halitosis: A review of associated factors and therapeutic approach. *Braz Oral Res,* 22(Suppl 1):44–54.

117. Hughes, F. J., & McNab, R. (2008). Oral malodour—A review. *Arch Oral Biol,* 53(Suppl 1):S1–S7.

118. Fedorowicz, Z., Aljufairi, H., Nasser, M., Outhouse, T. L., & Pedrazzi, V. (2008). Mouthrinses for the treatment of halitosis. *Cochrane Database of Syst Rev,* 2008 (Iss 4, Art. No. CD006701).

119. Lee, S. S. (2009). *Breath: Causes, diagnosis, and treatment of oral malodor* (2nd ed.). San Bernardino, CA: Culminare, Inc.

120. American Dental Association, Council on Scientific Affairs. (2003). Oral malodor. *J Am Dent Assoc,* 134:209–14.

121. Lourith, N., & Kanlayavattanakul, M. (2010). Review article: Oral malodour and active ingredients for treatment. *Int J Cosmetic Sci,* 32:321–29.

122. Romano, F., Pigella, E., Guzzi, N., & Aimetti, M. (2010). Patients' self-assessment of oral malodour and its relationship with organoleptic scores and oral conditions. *Int J Dent Hyg,* 8:41–46.

123. van den Broek, A. M. W. T., Feenstra, L., & de Baat, C. (2007). A review of the current literature on aetiology and measurement methods of halitosis. *J Dent,* 35:627–35.

124. Quirynen, M., Dadamio, J., Van den Velde, S., De Smit, M., Dekeyser, C., Van Tornout, M., & Vandekerckhove, B. (2009). Characteristics of 2000 patients who visited a halitosis clinic. *J Clin Periodontol,* 36:970–75.

125. Nalcaci, R., & Baran, I. (2008). Oral malodor and removable complete dentures in the elderly. *Oral Surg, Oral Med, Oral Pathol, Oral Radiol , Endodontol,* 105:e5–e9. Retrieved February 5, 2010, from http://www.ooooe.net.

126. Tsai, C.-C., Chou, H.-H., Wu, T.-L., Yang, Y.-H., Ho, K.-Y., Wu, Y.-M., & Ho, Y.-P. (2008). The levels of volatile sulfur compounds in mouth air from patients with chronic periodontitis. *J Periodont Res,* 43:186–93.

127. Tanabe, S.-I., Bodet, C., & Grenier, D. (2007). Treponema denticola Lippoligosaccharide activates gingival fibroblasts and upregulates inflammatory mediator production. *J Cell Physiol,* 216:727–31.

128. Lodhia, P., Yaegaki, K., Khakbaznejad, A., Imai, T., Sato, T., Tanaka, T., Murata, T., & Kamoda, T. (2008). Effect of green tea on volatile sulfur compounds in mouth air. *J Nutr Sci Vitaminol,* 54:89–94.

129. Faveri, M., Hayasibara, M. F., Pupio, G. C., Cury, J. A., Tsuzuki, C. O., & Hayacibara, R. M. (2006). A cross-over study on the effect of various therapeutic approaches to morning breath odour. *J Clin Periodontol,* 33:555–60.

130. Kishi, M., Ohara-Nemoto, Y., Takahashi, M., Kishi, K., Kimura, S., & Yonemitsu, M. (2010). Relationship between oral status and prevalence of periodontopathic bacteria on the tongues of elderly individuals. *J Med Microbiol* 59:1354–59.

131. Peruzzo, D. C., Salvador, S. L., Sallum, A. W., & da Rocha Nogueira-Filho, G. (2008). Flavoring agents present in a dentifrice can modify volatile sulphur compounds (VSCs) formation in morning bad breath. *Braz Oral Res,* 22:252–57.

132. Shinada, K., Ueno, M., Konishi, C., Takehara, S., Yokoyama, S., & Kawaguchi, Y. (2008, December 9). A randomized double blind cross-over placebo-controlled clinical trial to assess the effects of a mouthwash containing chlorine dioxide on oral malodor. *Trials,* 9:8p.

133. U. S. Food and Drug Administration. (2010, April 8). Triclosan: What consumers should know. Retrieved April 26, 2011, from http://www.fda.gov.

134. Layton, L. (2010, April 8). FDA says studies on triclosan, used in sanitizers and soaps, raise concerns. Retrieved April 25, 2011, from http://www.washingtonpost.com/wp-dyn/content/article/2010/04/07/AR2010040704621.html.

135. Wilhelm, D., Gysen, K., Himmelmann, A., Krause, C., & Wilhelm, K. P. (2010). Short-term effect of a new mouthrinse formulation on oral malodour after single use *in vivo*: A comparative, randomized, single-blind, parallel-group clinical study. *J Breath Res,* 4:7p.

136. Conti, S., Ferreira dos Santos, S. S., Koga-Ito, C. Y., & Jorge, A. O. (2009). Enterobacteriaceae and pseudomonadaceae on the dorsum of the human tongue. *J Appl Oral Sci,* 17:375–80. Retrieved February 7, 2011, from http://www.scielo.br.

137. Van der Sleen, M. I., Slot, D. E., Van Trijffel, E., Winkel, E. G., & Van der Weijden, G. A. (2010). Effectiveness of mechanical tongue cleaning on breath odour and tongue coating: A systematic review. *Int J Dent Hyg,* 8:258–68.

138. Academy of General Dentistry. (2006). *Tongue scrapers only slightly reduce bad breath.* Chicago, IL: AGD. Retrieved February 6, 2011, from http://www.agd.org.

139. Bordas, A., McNab, R., Staples, A. M., Bowman, J., Kanapka, J., & Bosma, M. P. (2008). Impact of different tongue cleaning methods on the bacterial load of the tongue dorsum. *Arch Oral Biol,* 53(Suppl 1):S13–S18. Retrieved February 6, 2011, from http://www.aobjournal.com.

140. U. K. National Health Service. (n.d.) Bad breath (halitosis). (Clinical Knowledge Summaries). London: Author. Retrieved February 5, 2011, from http://www.cks.nhs.uk.

141. Hoffman, M. (2008, July 21). *Black hairy tongue.* Retrieved February 5, 2011, from http://www.webmd.com.

142. American Dental Association. (2005). *Smile smarts! An oral health curriculum for preschool–grade 8.* Retrieved March 15, 2011, from http://www.ada.org.

143. American Dental Hygienists' Association. (2010, July 16). *Want some life saving advice? Ask your dental hygienist about understanding and eliminating bad breath.* Retrieved February 6, 2011, from http://www.adha.org (Oral Health Information).

144. Lee, S. S., Zhang, W., & Li, Y. (2007). Halitosis update: A review of causes, diagnoses, and treatments. *J Calif Dent Assoc,* 35:259–68. Retrieved February 6, 2011, from http://www.cda.org.

145. Raposa, K. A., & Ray, T. S. (2010). Oral infection control: Toothbrushes and tooth brushing. In Wilkins, E. M., Ed. *Clinical practice of the dental hygienist* (10th ed.). St. Louis, MO: Lippincott Williams & Wilkins, 406–29.

146. Outhouse, T. L., Al-Alawi, R., Fedorowicz, Z., & Keenan, J. V. (2006). Tongue scraping for treating halitosis. (Review). *Cochrane Database Syst Rev,* (Issue 2, Art. No. CD005519).

147. U. K. National Health Service. (2010). *Get rid of bad breath.* Retrieved February 6, 2010, from http://www.nhs.uk.

Implant and Denture Self-Care

Christine French Beatty
Amy Teague

OBJECTIVES

After studying this chapter, the student should be able to:

1. Identify risks for peri-implantitis and peri-implant mucositis.

2. Identify critical factors that result in implant failure.

3. Describe proper oral self-care for dental implants.

4. Describe the proper oral self-care for removable partial dentures, full dentures, and overdentures.

5. Describe the risk of *Candida* infections for denture wearers.

6. Explain the various procedures and cleansers used to prevent and control oral *Candida* infections.

KEY TERMS

INTRODUCTION

The aging trend of the U.S. population has continued with 12.3% of the population age 65 and older in 2008[1] and an expectation of a 30% increase in the number of seniors by 2050.[2] The number of dental visits among this age group is increasing,[3] and the incidence of tooth loss is decreasing in all ages.[4] Even so, 26% of seniors age 65 to 74 are completely edentulous,[5] and approximately 40% have experienced either complete or partial tooth loss[6] with a mean of 18.9 teeth present in this age group.[7] As a result of these factors in addition to the fact that tooth loss increases with age,[7] it is anticipated that edentulism rates will remain constant or increase over the next few decades, and a sizable minority of the population will need an increasing number of implants, partial dentures, and complete dentures to replace missing teeth.[8] Therefore, oral health professionals will be called upon more and more to assist patients and clients with the self-care of implants and removable prostheses. (See Chapter 12 for a discussion of the concept of self-care.)

Application of the process of care model,[9] risk assessment,[10] human needs model,[11] personalization of recommendations,[12] and principles of evidence-based practice[13] are important to be able to help patients identify appropriate products and practices for oral self-care of implants and dentures. (See Chapter 3 for discussion of these concepts.) It is important not only to teach the self-care techniques but also to communicate the reasons for recommended self-care methods and implements. Involvement of the individual in these decisions will help to ensure long-term commitment to the oral self-care plan.[12]

Valid models of communication, behavioral change, health education, and health promotion should be applied to the education of oral self-care practices.[14] Oral self-care requires a great deal of commitment on the part of the individual. Patients' compliance with recommendations will depend on their ability to master the techniques, lifestyle issues that affect time availability for a complex self-care regimen and perception of the value of performing the recommended procedures.[15] When several devices are introduced for oral self-care, patients could become overwhelmed and thus experience a reduction in motivation and compliance.[16] Repeated instructions and continual reinforcement from the oral health professional will enhance compliance.[15] Knowledge acquisition and attitude changes must occur to obtain motivation that enables the client to change behavior. Positive reinforcement can assist in motivating these behavior changes. (See Chapter 19, Health Education and Promotion Theories, for further discussion of these concepts.)

Other chapters have discussed the use of toothbrushes, dental floss, and self-care adjuncts to clean natural and restored teeth in the oral self-care plan. This chapter discusses self-care procedures and products for peri-implant cleaning and denture self-care. Some individuals require assistance with self-care because of various limitations caused by mental, physical, or medical disabilities.[17] This chapter will focus on the use of the necessary practices and aids; other chapters discuss accommodations and adaptations for individuals with special needs (see Chapters 26, 27, and 28).

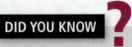

DID YOU KNOW

Routinely probing an implant during the maintenance phase is controversial unless there are visual signs of inflammation in the peri-implant tissues or the radiographs indicate bone loss around the implant.

SELF-CARE OF IMPLANTS

Overview of Implants

The use of dental implants has increased extensively in the past decade. Implants were once considered experimental.[18] However, now they are considered standard of care for single or multiple tooth replacement cases because they allow the restoration of missing teeth to optimum function and appearance without invading or damaging other teeth or tissues.[19] About 5 million people had implants placed in 2005 with an estimated increase in the market of 20% per year.[6]

With the rise in implant cases, the dental hygienist should be able to identify the parts of the dental implant to assist in patient education.[18] The **endosseous dental implant** has three components: the implant body, the implant abutment, and the prosthesis or superstructure. The **implant body** is the titanium device that is placed directly into the bone and is not visible in the oral cavity unless bone loss has occurred. The **implant abutment** is the titanium post that is attached to the implant body and is visible in the oral cavity. The **superstructure**, also referred to as the **implant prosthesis,** is the crown or denture that connects to the implant abutment (Figures 13–1 ■ and 13–2 ■).[20] The implant abutment and the implant prosthesis are exposed in the oral cavity; therefore, meticulous oral hygiene is imperative. Self-care of the implant abutment requires the use of special techniques and products that will be discussed in this chapter.

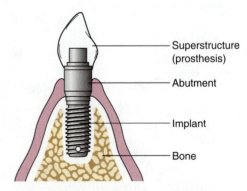

FIGURE ■ 13–1 Parts of the dental implant.

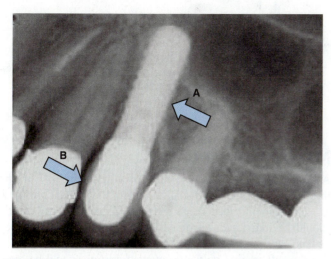

FIGURE ■ 13–2 Radiograph of fully restored implant in the premolar area. Arrow A points to the implant body, and arrow B indicates the superstructure of the implant.

(*Source:* Courtesy of Christine Beatty and Amy Teague.)

<table>
<tr><td>BOX 13–1</td><td>Factors That May Contraindicate Implant Case Selection</td></tr>
</table>

- Systemic conditions that cause immunosuppresion such as diabetes and HIV/AIDS
- Use of bisphosphonates
- Osteoporosis
- Multiple myeloma
- Social factors such as smoking, excessive alcohol use, drug abuse and stress
- Compromised blood coagulation
- Long-term use of steroids
- Cancer requiring chemotherapy

(*Source:* Based on Farrar, S. K., St. Germain, J., & Yukna, R. A. (2010). Implantology. in Weinberg, M. A., Westphal, C., Froum, S. J., Palat, M., & Schoor, R. S., Eds. *Comprehensive periodontics for the dental hygienist* (3rd ed.). Boston: Pearson Education, 413–37.)

Implant case selection is determined based on multiple factors that are associated with failure of the implant, thereby contraindicating this treatment option or requiring medical consultation prior to implant surgery (Box 13–1 ■).[20] Implant patients need to be educated on the importance of maintenance visits and about the fact that compliance with good personal self-care is a critical factor in the success of implants.[15] These specific self-care recommendations should be based on assessment of the patient's oral health status, ability, motivation, manual dexterity, and mental capacity. Accessibility and ease of cleaning are also affected by the position of the abutment, surrounding anatomy, and design of the final restoration, for example, the length of the abutment, presence of a connecting bar, and amount of space under the prosthesis.[18]

Success or failure of an implant depends on many factors, including daily self-care[21] (Table 13–1 ■). Implant failure is the result of **peri-implantitis**, which is irreversible alveolar bone loss around an osseointegrated dental implant caused by inflammation[20] and progresses more quickly than periodontitis around natural teeth.[22] A precursor to peri-implantitis is **peri-implant mucositis**, also called *peri-implant gingivitis,* which is plaque-induced reversible inflammation of the surrounding soft tissue.[22] Because microorganisms from surrounding tissues can be transmitted to the peri-implant area, meticulous daily oral hygiene must be maintained throughout the oral cavity.[18] Especially in patients who are partially edentulous, there is a potential for cross-contamination from teeth to implants.[21] Accumulation of soft and hard deposits on the abutment, connecting bar, and attached prosthesis can lead to peri-implant mucositis and peri-implantitis. The prevalence of peri-implant inflammatory problems is increasing because of the increasing number of dental implants and the aging of existing ones. Thus, it is important to learn how to assist patients in preventing and controlling these conditions to prolong the life of their dental implants.[23]

Research indicates that supragingival calculus is more prevalent on implants than subgingival deposits and that the calculus deposits on titanium implants are less tenacious than on natural teeth.[18] Calculus accumulation has contributed to the development of more severe inflammation around implants.[21] Thus, periodontal debridement is recommended as part of routine maintenance visits.[23]

TABLE ■ 13–1   Risk Factors for Peri-implantitis

History of periodontitis	Individuals who have had periodontitis are at a higher risk for developing peri-implantitis than those who have never had periodontitis.
Diabetes	Uncontrolled diabetics are at higher risk for peri-implantitis than controlled diabetics.
Genetics	Cytokine gene polymorphisms can affect the host response to peri-implantitis.
Smoking	Bone loss around implants is more likely in smokers than nonsmokers.
Oral hygiene	Poor oral hygiene increases risk for peri-implantitis.
Absence of keratinized tissue	Implants could have higher success rates in the presence of keratinized tissue; however, with optimal oral self-care, absence of keratinized tissue could be less risky.
Implant surface	Irregularities in the titanium cause the implant surface to retain plaque biofilm, which could lead to increased incidence of peri-implantitis.

(*Source:* Greenstein, G., Cavallaro, J., & Tarnow, D. (2010). Dental implants in the periodontal patient. *Dent Clin North Am,* 54:113–28.)

Adequate self-care also has a role in preventing corrosion of the titanium from which implants are manufactured. One of the potential causes of corrosion is microbial.[24] Corrosion can severely limit the fatigue life and ultimate strength of the titanium, which contributes to the implant's mechanical failure. Hence, it is important that patients practice effective oral hygiene to protect the titanium surface from corrosion.

Self-care of implants requires a variety of oral hygiene techniques and tools. Indications and contraindications for these are presented in Table 13–2 ■ and discussed in the next sections. The objectives of daily oral hygiene around implants are to minimize the supragingival and subgingival microbial accumulation and alter the pathogenesis of existing biofilm.[18] The ultimate goal is to prevent peri-implantitis that can result in the implant's failure. Although the use of multiple products could be ideal for daily self-care, the number of aids recommended should be limited because compliance decreases when too many oral self-care devices are recommended.[18]

With all oral hygiene aids, it is important to caution patients not to clean too aggressively to prevent damage to the peri-implant tissues. The mucopolysacharide bond of the implant surface to the surrounding tissues, referred to as the peri-implant seal, serves a function similar to the periodontal ligament of a natural tooth. This bond is highly vulnerable and can be severed.[25]

In the process of daily oral hygiene, protecting the surface of the implant abutment is critical to minimize surface alterations.[15] Titanium scratches easily, and a scratched surface will trap and hold biofilm that will contribute to peri-implantitis and eventual implant failure.[16] Therefore, implements and products that will maintain the smooth surface of the titanium should be selected. A soft toothbrush, an end-tuft brush, special interproximal brushes, gauze, and floss are especially recommended for mechanical debridement of implants.[26]

Manual Toothbrushing

A soft or ultrasoft toothbrush can be used effectively to brush the occlusal, lingual, and facial surfaces of the implant prosthesis. The recommended shape and size of the toothbrush head should be individualized based on the implant type and the patient's abilities.[27] To prevent scratching the titanium and protect the soft tissues, only end-rounded bristles should be recommended for use on implants (Figure 13–3 ■). The modified Bass technique of brushing is indicated for implant care.[16,28] TePe® has developed extremely soft toothbrushes, Special Care™ and Gentle Care™, that are used for the post surgery healing period.[29]

Supplementation of the toothbrush with an end-tuft brush is recommended to accomplish sulcular brushing of the peri-implant area of the abutment.[27] A flat end-tuft brush with an angled handle has been recommended to more effectively reach the facial and lingual surfaces of the abutment (Figure 13–4 ■). The angulation of the implant superstructure as it approaches the implant abutment creates a situation in which it is more difficult to access and clean the gingival margin and submarginal areas than in the case of a natural tooth (Figure 13–1 ■ and Figure 13–5A ■). TePe® has designed an implant brush that is extra narrow with only two rows of bristles to assist the patient in accessing these difficult-to-reach areas of restored implants (Figure 13–5B ■).

TABLE ■ 13–2   Home Care Indications/Contraindications for the Implant Patient

Indicated	*Contraindicated*
Twice daily cleaning of the implant	Use of abrasive toothpastes such as sodium bicarbonate and salt can scratch the titanium surface.
Use of a proxabrush with coated metal or plastic core; variable thickness floss used in a criss-cross, shoe shine manner; soft nylon multitufted toothbrush; powered multitufted toothbrush; disclosing tablets; low-abrasive toothpaste; toothpick with handle	Use of flat-ended bristles instead of round-ended bristles could cause scratching of the titanium.
	Flossing aggressively can traumatize the peri-implant tissue.
Application of chlorhexidine gluconate 0.12% (brush or variable thickness floss dipped in solution and applied to the peri-implant tissue)	Use of an uncoated metal on the implant surface can scratch the titanium surface.
Oral irrigation with chlorhexidine gluconate 0.12% on lowest setting and directed perpendicular to the implant surface	Directing the stream toward the peri-implant tissue and using a setting above "low" can traumatize the peri-implant tissue.
Written list of instructions on proper implant care provided to the patient	Use of a medium or hard-bristled toothbrush or interdental brush on the implant surface can scratch the titanium.

(*Sources:* Data from Alberto, P. L. (2007). Dental implant maintenance: The key to success. *Access,* 21:47–49; Moore, L., Cryan, L., & Starr, G. (2006). Controversy or conundrum . . . implant maintenance for the dental hygienist. *Cal Dent Hygien Assoc J,* 21(3):20–7.

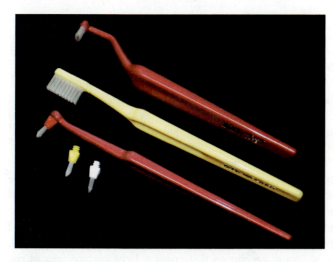

FIGURE ■ 13–3 Variety of brushes designed for implant self-care.

(*Source:* Courtesy of Christine Beatty and Amy Teague.)

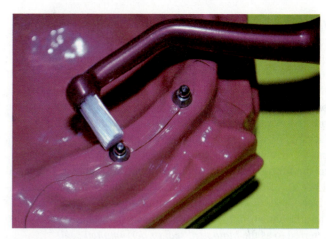

FIGURE ■ 13–4 TePe Implant Care™ end-tuft brush adapted to the lingual surface of an implant.

(*Source:* Courtesy of Christine Beatty and Amy Teague.)v

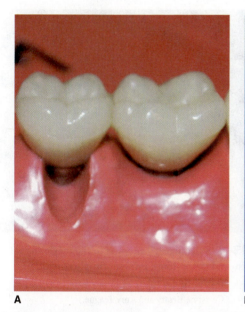

A

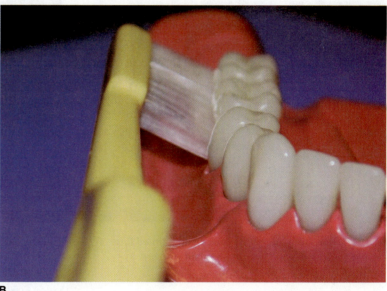

B

FIGURE ■ 13–5 A. Buccal view of a single-restored implant. Tissue removed on the model to show implant placement into the bony ridge. B. 45° angle adaptation of the TePe® implant brush.

(*Source:* Courtesy of Christine Beatty and Amy Teague.)

Powered Toothbrushes

Proper education must accompany the use of powered toothbrushes to provide maximum effectiveness.[28] A review of sonic and ultrasonic powered toothbrush studies indicated that their use by implant patients was safe, produced satisfactory results, was preferred by some patients, and resulted in more reduction of plaque biofilm and gingivitis than the use of manual toothbrushes.[30] On the other hand, a recent Cochrane review reported that there was no statistically significant evidence that sonic or powered toothbrushes were more effective than manual toothbrushes in maintaining or recovering soft tissue health around implants although sonic toothbrushes were preferred.[31] Further research is indicated in this area. In the meantime, the effectiveness of toothbrushing with either a manual or powered toothbrush should be monitored in relation to assessment of peri-implant tissues.[32] In addition, recommendations should be made and adjusted according to the patient's individual needs and successful application of the oral hygiene aids and methods employed.

Dentifrices

There is no indication that a certain dentifrice paste or gel is more effective than another to clean implants with toothbrushing.[31] However, brushing with an anticalculus dentifrice is recommended, and the use of a low-abrasive dentifrice is important to prevent scratching the titanium.[26]

Floss

Narrow dental floss is recommended for single tooth implants that have a short abutment. Tufted floss is recommended for the underside of a prosthesis that is in close proximity to the soft tissue. With a higher abutment and adequate space under the prosthesis, the abutment circumference and the underside of the prostheses can be cleaned with flossing cords, ribbon floss, dental tape, or variable thickness floss. The various types of floss can be crisscrossed on the abutment and pulled in a shoeshine method for more effective plaque removal (Figures 13–6 ■ and 13–7 ■). The patient must be instructed not to floss aggressively in an up-and-down motion in order to reduce trauma to the attachment (implant-to-tissue mucopolysacharide bond, also referred to as the *biological seal or peri-implant seal*).[25]

Interdental Aids

Daily cleaning of the collar of the abutment(s) and undersurface of the implant prosthesis is critical to prevent peri-implant disease and requires the use of supplemental interdental aids in addition to dental floss.[33] Interdental aids should be selected according to the features of the implant[27]; for example, the height of the abutment affects the best choice.

Effective interdental self-care for dental implant maintenance can include a variety of devices to supplement brushing and flossing. These include interdental brushes,[18] rubber-tip stimulators,[18] tapered rotary brushes,[18] sulcular brushes (Figure 13–8 ■),[34] toothpick with holder,[35] wooden cleaners,[27] and plastic picks.[27] An interproximal brush can be used not only to remove plaque biofilm but also to massage the mucosal tissues surrounding the implant, thus increasing blood flow.[16] Only a soft, nylon-coated interproximal brush should be used (Figure 13–9 ■). Metal-core interproximal brushes and pipe cleaners are contraindicated because of the potential to scratch the titanium.[16] In general, aids should be chosen that cover a large surface area of the abutment and are kinder to the peri-implant area, for example selection of an interproximal brush versus a wooden or plastic pick. Appropriate use of these interdental aids is described in

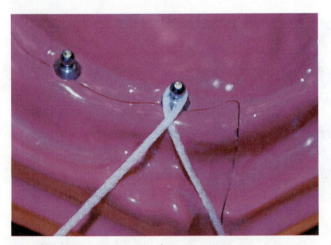

FIGURE ■ 13–6 Circumferential placement of tufted floss criss-crossed to clean denture retained implant surfaces.

(*Source:* Courtesy of Christine Beatty and Amy Teague.)

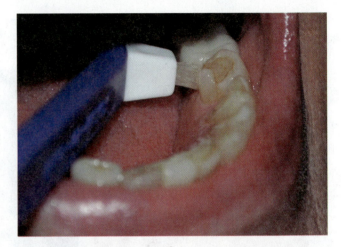

FIGURE ■ 13–8 Sulcabrush® adapted to the mesiolingual surface of a restored single-tooth implant (implant with a cemented crown on first molar).

(*Source:* Courtesy of Christine Beatty and Amy Teague.)

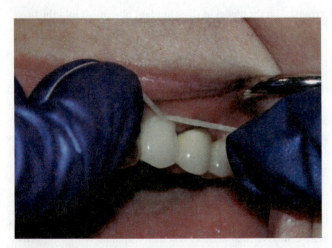

FIGURE ■ 13–7 Circumferential placement of dental floss criss-crossed to clean a single tooth implant restoration (implant with a cemented crown on the canine).

(*Source:* Courtesy of Christine Beatty and Amy Teague.)

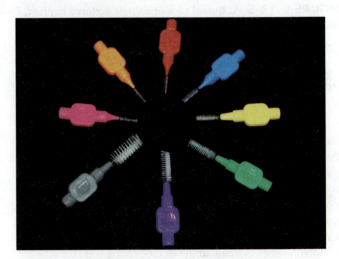

FIGURE ■ 13–9 A variety of nylon-coated interdental brushes safe for implant use.

(*Source:* Courtesy of Christine Beatty and Amy Teague.)

Chapter 12. Interdental aids should be used carefully around implants to protect the vulnerable peri-implant tissues and mucopolysacharide bond of the implant surface to the surrounding tissues.

Antimicrobials

The benefits of antimicrobial use have been discussed in Chapter 11. In addition, the benefits of rinsing and irrigating with antimicrobials were discussed in Chapter 12. The American Academy of Periodontology (AAP) suggests the use of topical antimicrobial agents with implant patients.[36] Daily rinsing with an antimicrobial mouthwash has been recommended.[22] A Cochrane review concluded that rinsing with either Listerine® or a chlorhexidine mouthwash lowered plaque biofilm and bleeding scores around implants, although the effect on maintenance and recovery of peri-implant tissue health was unclear.[31] In addition, there were no statistically significant differences in the effectiveness of different types of antimicrobials to maintain or restore soft tissue health around implants. Only nonacidic and nonfluoride agents should be used for rinsing, irrigation, peri-implant anti-infective treatment, and other reasons to prevent corrosion and etching of the implant surface.[24] Both an acidic environment and fluoride can break down the stable oxide layer that protects the titanium from corrosion. This can occur from the fluoride contained in commercial mouthwashes, toothpaste, and prophylactic gels used to prevent dental caries, kill periodontic pathogens, relieve sensitivity of retained teeth, or control malodor.

Application with an Oral Hygiene Aid

In lieu of rinsing, an antimicrobial can be applied to specific sites with an oral hygiene device. The toothbrush or interproximal brush can be dipped into 0.12% chlorhexidine gluconate as a means of applying the solution to the peri-implant area. This practice has been shown to reduce bacteria around an implant by 54% to 97% over six months of use.[16,18] Chlorhexidine can be applied to specific sites with an oral hygiene aid, cotton tip applicator, gauze, or irrigation device as a means to prevent staining that normally accompanies general chlorhexidine use.[16,22]

Irrigation

Generalized adjunctive supragingival and subgingival irrigation with antimicrobial agents can be used effectively for self-care of the dental implant[18,31] and is suggested by the AAP[36] and many authors.[13] When irrigating around a dental implant, the flow rate of an electrical irrigator should be set on the lowest setting, and the stream should not be directed subgingivally to prevent any soft tissue detachment.[16] A Cochrane review concluded that irrigation more effectively reduces the amount and pathogenesis of plaque biofilm and marginal bleeding than rinsing.[31] Compared to rinsing with chlorhexidine, irrigation with chlorhexidine

resulted in 20% more reduction of bacterial biofilm formation and 35% less peri-implant bleeding. However, evidence of superior effects on tissue health was weak. The report concluded that further research is needed and that studies should track parameters over several years to evaluate overall health of peri-implant soft tissues and bone as well as implant failure.

Other Treatment Considerations

Xerostomia must be managed carefully for an implant patient to enhance implant success. Patients with xerostomia should be monitored with a shorter maintenance interval because of their increased plaque biofilm formation. Salivary flow can be stimulated either physiologically or pharmacologically.[37]

In the event that peri-implantitis occurs, it is treated and controlled in the same manner as periodontitis because the same bacteria in plaque biofilm induce peri-implantitis.[28] Subgingival irrigation around the abutment with 0.12% chlorhexidine gluconate is recommended to reduce bacterial load for the reduction of peri-implant mucositis.[31]

Recommendations for implant self-care must begin with a thorough assessment of the implant patient's needs. Selection of a limited number of aids designed to meet those specific needs, careful instruction, and continual monitoring and reinforcement will contribute to the success of an implant.

SELF-CARE OF DENTURES

Although there are numerous innovations that are making it possible to maintain the dentition longer in this age of preventive dentistry, the need for complete dentures is likely to continue.[38] Because of the expected increase in the elderly population, the number of complete dentures in the United States is anticipated to increase from an estimated 56.5 million in 2000 to more than 61 million in 2020.[39] Oral health professionals must be familiar with the science of dentures and materials used to fabricate them in order to be able to advise and educate patients on the best methods and products to use in their daily care.

Types of Removable Prostheses

There are two types of full dentures. First is the **overdenture**, which is supported by implants or modifications to the crowns of natural teeth. The second is the **conventional denture**, which is supported by the bony ridge. It has been suggested that when possible, the two-implant overdenture should replace the conventional denture as the standard of treatment for the mandibular arch because of problems with denture fit and retention as well as patient adjustment and compliance.[38] Individuals wearing implant-assisted overdentures typically report improved oral comfort and function when compared to conventional prostheses.[39]

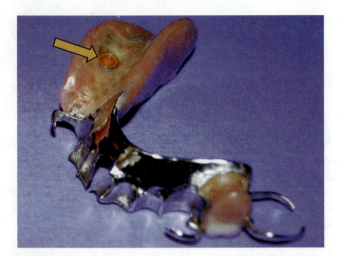

FIGURE ■ 13–10 Metal clasps present on either side of the prosthetic tooth retain this partial denture on one side of the mandibular arch. The arrow points to the locator attachment that retains this partial denture with an implant on the other side of the arch.

(*Source:* Courtesy of Christine Beatty and Amy Teague.)

There are various types of removable partial dentures.[40] Frequently referred to as *partials,* removable **partial dentures** are used if the patient still exhibits natural teeth adjacent to missing ones. These prostheses attach to the natural teeth with either clasps or precision attachments. Clasps are fabricated from metal alloy (Figure 13–10 ■) or, in the case of anterior teeth, from plastic or plasticlike materials and rest on and around remaining natural teeth. Precision attachments consist of mechanically interlocking components and are manufactured from resilient metal or nylon materials. Implants can also be used to assist in stabilizing the partial denture.

There is a variety of modes of attachment for dentures.[34,41] Overdentures can be supported by implants via locators that are placed on the implants (Figure 13–11A ■), locator attachments that are housed in the removable appliance (Figure 13–11B ■), magnets, ball attachments (Figure 13–12 ■), or clips (Figure 13–13 ■). The locator attachments must be replaced periodically when the denture becomes loosely attached to the implant. Ball attachments are not only used with implants but also attached to the crowns of existing teeth that support an overdenture, usually canines; the ball snaps into the socket, which is located on the underside of the denture. On the other hand, conventional dentures have no support other than the bony ridge of the maxilla and mandible (Figure 13–14 ■).

DID YOU KNOW

The first dentures used in Europe date back to the 1400s. They were sometimes made from teeth that had been sold by individuals who had extracted their own teeth and teeth that had been retrieved from the deceased by grave robbers.

Oral and Systemic Health of Denture Wearers

The majority of denture wearers in the United States are older than 65 years.[42] This population is at higher risk for impairment of salivary flow,[43] which contributes to the formation of plaque biofilm and calculus on prosthetic appliances.[44] The materials from which full and partial dentures are constructed, especially methacrylate, provide an irregular surface topography that enhances the attachment of these deposits. In addition, the intaglio (tissue side) surface is never polished, leaving a rougher surface to which deposits can adhere.

Deposits that form on dentures are similar to those that form on natural teeth, including pellicle, biofilm, calculus, oral debris (e.g., desquamated epithelial cells), stain, and food

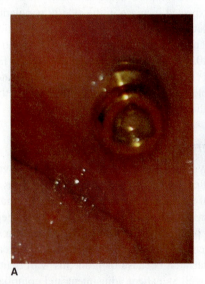

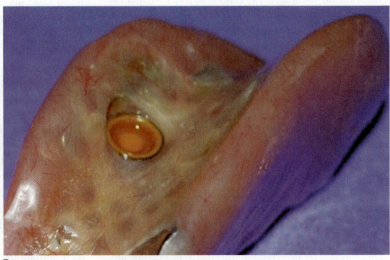

A   B

FIGURE ■ 13–11 A. Locator attached to the implant. B. Locator attachment housed in the removable appliance.

(*Source:* Courtesy of Christine Beatty and Amy Teague.)

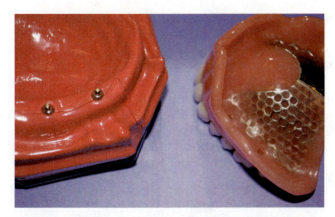

FIGURE ■ 13–12 Ball attachments placed on implant to be housed in the inner surface of the denture.

(*Source:* Courtesy of Christine Beatty and Amy Teague.)

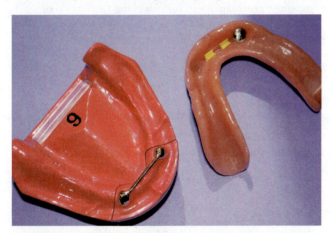

FIGURE ■ 13–13 Clips such as the one seen here aid in stabilizing the bar, which is supported with two implants on either end of the bar.

(*Source:* Courtesy of Christine Beatty and Amy Teague.)

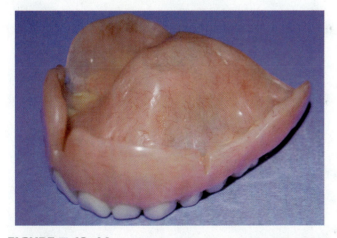

FIGURE ■ 13–14 Conventional denture that is stabilized in the oral cavity by the bony ridge.

(*Source:* Courtesy of Christine Beatty and Amy Teague.)

debris.[45] These deposits have the potential to produce tissue irritation, infection, and malodor.[46,47] The composition of denture plaque biofilm is similar to that of plaque biofilm on natural teeth. The type of bacteria can vary among individuals, among

sites in the oral cavity of the same individual, and among sites on the dentures of the same individual.[46] All of these factors contribute to the need for meticulous oral and denture hygiene for all denture wearers.

DID YOU KNOW ?

Candida species are able to adhere to the methacrylate denture surface as well as to the mucosal surfaces.

Candida organisms have a normal oral presence in healthy individuals[48] and are more prevalent in denture wearers.[49] In fact, a study of factors associated with a *Candida*-carrier state revealed that although gender, age over 60 years, low education, and xerostomia were directly and significantly associated with the intraoral presence of *Candida* yeasts ($p<.05$), denture wearing was more highly associated ($p<0.001$).[44]

Failure to adequately clean dentures can result in denture stomatitis and candidiasis, common oral conditions found in denture wearers. **Stomatitis** appears as patches of erythema (red inflamed areas) on the oral mucosa and can be caused by poor hygiene, trauma, physical irritation, irritants, allergies, infections, and systemic disorders.[46] However, the presence of *Candida* has been detected in more than 90% of denture wearers with symptoms of stomatitis.[49] Denture stomatitis is a chronic condition that tends to compromise the individual's quality of life.[46] **Candidiasis** is a *Candida*-induced stomatitis and appears as raised, white patches on the mucosa and tongue that can be painful. The patches can be easily scraped off to reveal an underlying raw, red, irritated surface that can bleed. Denture wearers are predisposed to the intraoral presence of *Candida* species and candidiasis.[44] It is estimated that up to 67% of denture wearers have *Candida*-associated stomatitis.[46]

It is well accepted that oral health is associated with overall health. Additionally, in denture wearers, oral health can significantly impact the individual's quality of life, nutrition, and social interactions.[46] Mucosal irritation can impair eating, which can have a negative nutritional impact on the individual.[50] Oral and denture plaque biofilm is not only associated with oral conditions but also can have other serious systemic consequences, especially for dependent elderly individuals.[51] Oral bacteria have been implicated in a number of serious systemic conditions, including bacterial endocarditis, aspiration pneumonia, chronic obstructive pulmonary disease, and generalized infections of the respiratory tract.[46]

Thorough weekly professional cleaning and disinfection of the oral tissues and dentures have been tested as a strategy to control aspiration pneumonia in the dependent elderly.[52] This consisted of brushing any natural teeth, ultrasonically cleaning the denture in an immersion cleanser, brushing the denture with a denture brush, and swabbing the tongue and oral mucosa with a sponge brush weekly for 5 months. The results included reduction of total oropharyngeal bacteria, staphylococci, and *Candida* species; fewer febrile days; and control of aspiration pneumonia in a nursing home population. This study demonstrated the value of good oral and denture hygiene to control medical as well as oral conditions.

Patient Education

It is the responsibility of oral health professionals to provide instructions in the proper care and cleaning of both the dentures and the underlying tissues (Box 13–2 ▪) to improve the successful maintenance of dentures and protect the oral health of denture wearers.[53] Research has shown that oral health instruction of denture patients was successful in reducing plaque biofilm on the denture and oral tissues.[54] Denture wearers need to understand the methods, products, and rationale of denture and oral care. As with other oral hygiene instructions, explanation, demonstration, and a return demonstration in which the patient performs the technique just observed will result in improved understanding and compliance.[55] Instruction should be provided verbally and supplemented with written materials for easy reference at a later time.

The denture delivery appointment is an excellent time to provide oral self-care and prosthesis-care instructions.[56] The patient's level of manual dexterity should be assessed at the time of denture delivery to provide modifications of cleaning tools and procedures if necessary. (Modifications are explained later in this chapter.) If the denture is supported by implants or retained natural teeth, the patient should be instructed to clean the implants or teeth as described in the previous section of this chapter (implants) or previous chapters (natural teeth).

The American College of Prosthodontists have developed and published evidence-based guidelines for the care and maintenance of complete dentures.[46] These guidelines are presented in Box 13–3 ▪. The rest of this chapter expands on and provides rationale for these guidelines. Additional recommended oral self-care procedures are detailed and explained in this section as well.

DID YOU KNOW ?

In England in 1791, Nicholas Dubois de Chemant patented porcelain teeth for use in the fabrication of dentures. Within 30 years, these porcelain teeth were of high quality, were natural looking, and were set into gold dentures.

Dentures and Oral Hygiene

Research has shown that a large percentage of dentures worn by the elderly are not adequately cleaned, and denture wearers are unaware of the inadequacy of their denture hygiene.[54]

BOX 13–2   Summary of Self-Care Instructions for Denture Wearers

- Remove dentures after every meal and rinse the denture and the mouth.
- Grasp denture firmly but gently and hold the denture over a towel, rubber mat, or a sink filled with several inches of water for protection while brushing or rinsing the denture.
- Soak dentures daily in an antimicrobial chemical immersion cleaning solution according to the manufacturer's directions.
- Rinse denture to remove saliva and debris before immersing in cleanser.
- Mix fresh cleanser each time you soak; do not reuse cleanser.
- Thoroughly clean container used to soak and store dentures daily.
- Rinse and brush denture carefully with a denture brush after soaking.
- If a toothbrush is used on dentures, use a soft brush that is different from the one used in the mouth.
- Moisten the brush and apply denture paste or mild hand soap; use denture paste rather than toothpaste, and avoid any other abrasives.
- Brush every surface, scrubbing gently to avoid damage, paying close attention to deep inner surfaces of the denture.
- Add the use of a clasp brush on partial dentures.
- Rinse the denture thoroughly, and use a brush to remove denture paste that could cling to the irregular denture surface.
- Check a denture for cleanliness by inspecting it visually and running a finger over it to detect slippery plaque biofilm.
- If eyeglasses are worn for close work and reading, wear them while cleaning the denture.
- Store dentures in water while they are out of the mouth.
- Use lukewarm water for rinsing and soaking a denture; never use hot water.
- Remove dentures daily for at least 6 hours or overnight.
- Observe and report irritation or other changes in oral tissues.
- Clean the soft tissues of the mouth before replacing the denture.
- Massage oral tissues daily with a soft toothbrush or the fingers.
- Keep denture in same safe, handy place to reduce likelihood of misplacement.
- If a denture adhesive is used, clean it out thoroughly before adding new adhesive.
- Make adjustments in diet, eating, speaking, and sneezing to accommodate wearing dentures.
- Return to the dentist at remmended intervals for examination of dentures and oral tissues.
- Do not attempt to self-repair a denture or use an at-home reline kit.

BOX 13–3   Guidelines for the Care and Maintenance of Dentures

1. Careful daily removal of the bacterial biofilm present in the oral cavity and on complete dentures is of paramount importance to minimize denture stomatitis and to help contribute to good oral and general health.
2. To reduce levels of biofilm and potentially harmful bacteria and fungi, patients who wear dentures should do the following:
   a. Clean dentures daily by soaking and brushing with an effective, nonabrasive denture cleanser.
   b. Use denture cleansers *only* to clean dentures outside the mouth.
   c. Always thoroughly rinse dentures after soaking and brushing with denture-cleansing solutions prior to reinsertion into the oral cavity. Always follow the product usage instructions.
3. Although the evidence regarding this is weak, have dentures cleaned annually by a dentist or dental professional by using ultrasonic cleansers to minimize biofilm accumulation over time.
4. Dentures should never be placed in boiling water.
5. Dentures should not be soaked in sodium hypochlorite bleach or in products containing sodium hypochlorite for periods that exceed 10 minutes. Doing so can damage dentures.
6. Dentures should be stored immersed in water after cleaning when not replaced in the oral cavity to avoid warping.
7. Denture adhesives, when properly used, can improve the retention and stability of dentures and help seal out the accumulation of food particles beneath the dentures, even well-fitting dentures.
8. In a quality-of-life study, patient ratings showed that denture adhesives could improve the denture wearer's perceptions of retention, stability, and quality of life; however, there is insufficient evidence that adhesives improve masticatory function.
9. Evidence regarding the effects of denture adhesives on the oral tissues when used for periods longer that 6 months is lacking. Thus, extended use of denture adhesives should not be considered without periodic assessment of denture quality and health of the supporting tissues by a dentist, prosthodontist, or dental professional.
10. Improper use of zinc-containing denture adhesives could have adverse systemic effects. Therefore, as a precautionary measure, zinc-containing denture adhesives should be avoided.
11. Denture adhesive should be used only in sufficient quantities (three or four pea-sized dollops) on each denture to provide sufficient added retention and stability to the prosthesis.
12. Denture adhesives should be compeltely removed from the prosthesis and the oral cavity on a daily basis.
13. If increasing amounts of adhesives are required to achieve the same level of denture retention, the patient should see a dentist or dental professional to evaluate the fit and stability of the dentures.
14. Although existing studies provide conflicting results, it is not recommended that dentures be worn continuously (24 hours per day) in an effort to reduce or minimize denture stomatitis.
15. Patients who have dentures should be checked annually by the dentist, prosthodontist, or dental professional for maintenance of optimum denture fit and function, for evaluation of oral lesions and bone loss, and for assessment of oral health status.

(*Source:* Felton, D., Cooper, L., Duqum, I., Minsley, G., Guckes, A., Haug, S., Meredith, P., Solie, C., Avery, D., & Chandler, N. D. (2011). Evidence-based guidelines for the care and maintenance of complete dentures. A publication of the American College of Prosthodontists. *J Am Dent Assoc,* 142(Suppl): 1S–20S. Retrieved May 25, 2011, from http://jada.ada.org/content/142/suppl_1/1S.full.pdf+html.)

Many do not use proper methods and products to clean their dentures, possibly because they have not been instructed in denture care[57] or do not follow the advice. Frequently, denture wearers are aware of only the aesthetic benefits of maintaining cleanliness. Cleaning the tissue-bearing side of the denture, which is critical to control candidiasis, is often overlooked.[58] Oral health professionals need to stress the numerous benefits of consistent, effective denture cleaning. These include enhancing a sense of oral cleanliness; preserving the aesthetic appearance of the denture[56]; preventing oral malodor,[45] denture stomatitis, and other tissue irritations and infections[46]; and contributing to overall oral health.[46]

Self-Care of Oral Soft Tissues

Daily oral hygiene should also include immaculate cleaning of the intraoral soft tissues to help prevent denture stomatitis and control candidiasis. Lack of mucosal care has been associated with higher rates of opportunistic infections with *Candida* species.[44] At least once a day, a face cloth, gauze squares, or a soft toothbrush should be used to clean the intraoral tissues.[59,60] In addition, after eating, the dentures and mouth should be rinsed thoroughly to remove food particles that can cause irritation and malodor.[60]

Massaging the oral mucosa under a denture will stimulate circulation and increase resistance to trauma.[60] These tissues can be cleaned and massaged simultaneously by brushing with a soft end-rounded toothbrush or a powered brush twice a day. Massage of the mucosa can also be accomplished by placing the thumb and index finger over the ridge to apply a press-and-release stroke and by rubbing the palate with the ball of the thumb.

Regular oral self-examinations should be performed to observe and report any irritation or chronic changes in appearance of the tissues.[56] Because denture wearers are primarily in the age group that is at higher risk for oral cancer than other age groups, they should be taught and encouraged to perform routine self-examination for oral cancer.

Daily Removal of Dentures

Dentures should be removed daily for at least 6 hours during the day or overnight to allow the bearing tissues to rest[56] as well as to allow the tongue and saliva to stimulate and cleanse the tissue.[61] Failure to remove the denture daily can result in oral malodor, excessive alveolar ridge resorption, denture stomatitis, candidiasis, epulis fissuratum, and other oral pathology, lesions, and infections.[46,56,62] Research has shown that continuously wearing dentures is associated with patients' developing denture stomatitis and increased growth of *Candida* species intraorally.[46] A denture should be stored out of the reach of children and pets to keep it safe while it is out of the mouth.[63] It is commonly recommended that dentures be stored in solution while out of the mouth to prevent warping[56] and stored in the same place to prevent loss.[61] The solution should be changed daily and the container washed thoroughly to enhance denture cleanliness.[63] While the dentures are out of the mouth, other important self-care procedures can be performed, such as the recommended daily cleaning and massaging of the tissues under the denture. Also, denture wearers should be taught to perform oral cancer self-examination during this time.

Diet and Eating

Denture wearers need assistance with food selections that are nutritionally sound because they accommodate the limitations that result from their dentures. Practice and patience are important during the adjustment to eating with new dentures.[63] Especially new denture wearers can have problems with foods that require incising, raw vegetables, fibrous meats, and sticky foods. Food should be cut into small pieces, and small portions should be chewed slowly. If possible, distributing food on both sides of the mouth during chewing to stabilize the denture will help. When biting food, the canine and premolar areas should be used, and food should be inserted at the angle of the mouth. In addition, the food should be pushed back as it is incised rather than pulling or tearing the food in a forward direction as is normally done.

Speaking and Making Other Accommodations Related to Denture Wearing

Practice is required to learn to speak with a new denture.[63] The patient should be advised to practice in front of a mirror, repeat and practice words that are the most difficult to say, and speak slowly and quietly. Patients should also be advised to cover the mouth when sneezing because doing so can cause loss of retention.

DID YOU KNOW ?

Denture wearers are at a higher risk for undetected oral cancer because of poor compliance with routine dental visits.

Regular Examinations

It is also important that denture patients understand the need to return for regular oral examinations based on their individual needs.[56] No studies have evaluated appropriate continuing care intervals for denture wearers,[46] although 6 months has been suggested.[60] Denture wearers must be informed of the importance of this health-protective practice. The Centers for Disease Control and Prevention reported in 2009 that although 69% to 73% of dentate adults age 65 and over had visited the dentist within the previous year, only 17% to 21% of edentate older persons had a dental visit in the past year.[5]

DID YOU KNOW ?

Caregivers of institutionalized and homebound elderly individuals need to be instructed in the importance and skills of denture care.

At these regular follow-up appointments, the dental professional can check residual ridge resorption; denture fit and retention vertical dimension; integrity of denture bases, prosthetic tooth wear, and phonetics; and can make adjustments or follow-up recommendations as needed. In addition, the oral health professional can monitor the effectiveness of daily denture and oral care, reinforce instructions, and clean dentures as well as natural teeth or implants professionally if necessary.[60] Also, biologic health parameters can be monitored, such as general systemic health and condition of oral soft tissues, and oral cancer and blood pressure screening can be performed.[46] The majority of denture wearers are over age 65, so performing oral cancer examinations for this population is critical to increase oral cancer survival rates[64] because 95% of oral cancers occur over age 40, and age 60 is the average age at diagnosis.[65]

Assistance with Self-Care

Dependent elderly usually require assistance with their denture and oral self-care.[66] This becomes a significant problem for elderly persons who are homebound or in long-term care settings. Because these individuals are medically compromised, their oral and denture hygiene is even more important.[51] Caregivers need to be trained in oral and denture hygiene for denture wearers as well as infection control during these procedures to prevent cross contamination in nursing homes and other institutionalized settings.[67] In addition, cognitively impaired patients should not have access to dentures that are soaking in a chemical denture cleansing solution. This is to prevent their inadvertently reinserting the denture without rinsing it properly.[68]

Another problem in long-term care and residence facilities is loss and mix-up of dentures.[63] To prevent this, dentures should be marked with the resident's name or some other identification. This is required at the time of denture fabrication in some countries and states in the United States. Various methods have been described to mark existing dentures that were not marked during fabrication.[63] Marking dentures can also be helpful to identify individuals who are unconscious or suffering from amnesia.

Self-Repair of Dentures

Patients should be advised never to use "do-it-yourself" repair kits and over-the-counter glues to repair, adjust, or reline a denture.[60] They can do permanent damage to a denture, making professional repair more expensive or replacement necessary. These do-it-yourself products also sometimes contain chemicals that may be harmful to oral tissues.

Denture Cleaning

All types of dentures, including partials, should be removed from the mouth for thorough cleaning at least once a day.[56,60] Commonly practiced cleaning methods include immersion, brushing, or a combination of both. The majority of denture wearers use either brushing or immersion in a cleanser. There is no evidence that any denture-cleaning method is superior for the health of the denture-bearing tissues or patient satisfaction.[46] However, studies have demonstrated that different biofilms respond differently to various cleaning methods.[69] Therefore, a combination of methods is recommended to attack the various biofilms that can be present.[70]

Whichever method is used to clean the denture, it should be thoroughly rinsed under running, tepid water according to the manufacturer's instructions before reinsertion into the mouth.[71] This step will remove any cleaning substances to avoid damage to the denture acrylic and prevent tissue irritation, inflammation, allergic reactions, or swallowing traces of caustic agents.[56] Both the ADA and Academy of General Dentistry recommend that only tepid water be used because hot water will warp the acrylic denture material.[61,71]

Many chemical immersion cleansers leave an unpleasant taste.[72] Soaking overnight in water or briefly in a mouthwash can be recommended to improve the taste of the denture before reinsertion. Overnight soaking in mouthwash is not recommended because prolonged contact with alcohol, essential oils, or other chemicals found in commercial mouthrinses can dry, bleach, or stain the denture acrylic.[73] In addition, soaking overdenture locator attachments in Cool Mint Listerine according to manufacturer's instructions resulted in their discoloration in one study.[74]

Denture cleansers are creams, pastes, gels, and solutions. See Box 13–4 ■ for characteristics of the ideal denture cleanser. Denture cleansers contain chemicals that can be harmful to the soft tissues. Therefore, they should never be applied while the denture is still in the mouth.[71]

DID YOU KNOW ?

Using toothpaste rather than denture paste to clean a denture will scratch the surface of the synthetic denture materials and is not recommended.

Brushing Dentures

Brushing the denture more effectively removes plaque biofilm from the surface than immersion in a chemical solution.[72] All surfaces of the denture should be brushed. Special care should

BOX 13–4 | **Characteristics of an Ideal Denture Cleanser**

- Antibiofilm activity to remove biofilm and stains
- Antibacterial and antifungal
- Nontoxic
- Compatible with denture materials; should not roughen, degrade, or discolor the acrylic resin, denture base, or prosthetic teeth
- Short acting ($\leq$8 hours)
- Easy to use by the patient and caregiver
- Acceptable or no taste
- Cost effective

(*Source:* Based on Felton, D., Cooper, L., Duqum, I., Minsley, G., Guckes, A., Haug, S., Meredith, P., Solie, C., Avery, D., & Chandler, N. D. (2011). Evidence-based guidelines for the care and maintenance of complete dentures. A publication of the American College of Prosthodontists. *J Am Dent Assoc*, 142(2 Suppl):1S–20S. Retrieved May 25, 2011, from http://jada.ada.org/content/142/suppl_1/1S.full.pdf+html.)

be taken to brush the intaglio surface and thoroughly rinse the denture after brushing. During brushing, the wet denture is slippery and can be dropped and broken easily.[75] A denture can break if it is dropped even a few inches. To avoid this, it should be held over a sink filled with water, a rubber mat, or a folded towel to cushion the fall.

Creams, pastes, and gels Denture materials are easily scratched with abrasive compounds. This will dull the surface and remove anatomic and aesthetic details from it, creating a rougher surface that will more easily trap plaque biofilm and other deposits.[56] Therefore, only products designed for use on dentures should be used when brushing them. A **denture paste** is recommended rather than toothpaste to protect the acrylic surface from scratching; denture paste is harmless to the denture when used properly.[56]

Brushes Most researchers recommend a specially designed **denture brush** rather than a toothbrush to access all surfaces of a denture[60] (Figure 13–15 ■). Denture brushes feature stiff bristles. The bristles are all one length on one side in order to brush the flat parts of the denture such as the facial, lingual, and palatal surfaces. On the other side, the bristles are set in a pyramid shape in order to brush the recessed intaglio surface of the denture (Figure 13–16 ■). These special brushes have a wide handle for easy gripping. A clasp brush (Figure 13–15 ■) is recommended to reach the inner surfaces of partial dentures clasps (Figure 13–17 ■).[76] Because the locator attachment of an overdenture is recessed, a sulcular or other small brush can be used to clean it more easily.

A hand or nail brush is adequate to clean a denture. A soft toothbrush is also recommended to clean dentures.[59] If a toothbrush is used, it should not be the same one used to brush any natural teeth still present in the mouth. This precaution is to maintain the condition of the toothbrush for adequate oral hygiene of the natural teeth. When brushes other than denture brushes are used, sometimes bristles cannot reach into the depressions of

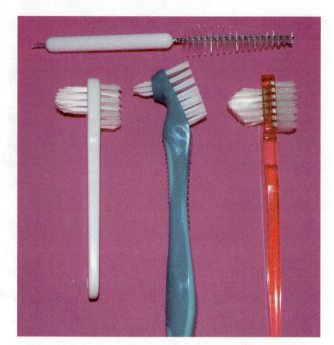

FIGURE ■ 13–15 Sample denture brushes. The brush positioned horizontally is a clasp brush. The vertically positioned brushes are denture brushes with even-cut bristles on one side and tapered-cut bristles on the other side.

(*Source:* Courtesy of Christine Beatty and Amy Teague.)

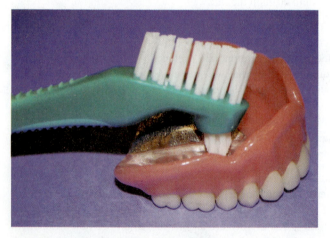

FIGURE ■ 13–16 Pyramid-shaped bristles of a denture brush applied to the inner surface of a denture.

(*Source:* Courtesy of Christine Beatty and Amy Teague.)

the intaglio surface. Application of undue pressure by the brush handle to some areas of the denture surface to allow the bristles to reach other areas can damage the denture over time. In this case, a denture brush should be used to avoid the damage. Hard-bristled brushes should not be used on dentures because they will damage the acrylic surface.[60]

Brush modifications   Although denture brushes are designed with large handles for easy grip, some older denture wearers could require further modifications to their brushes to accommodate arthritis and other disabilities.[77] For patients who are limited in the use of one hand or one arm, a hand or nail brush

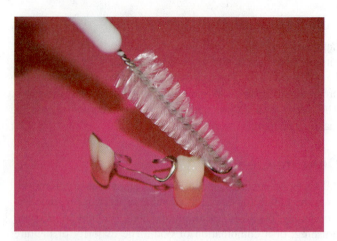

FIGURE ■ 13–17 Clasp brush applied to the inner surface of a partial denture clasp.

(*Source:* Courtesy of Christine Beatty and Amy Teague.)

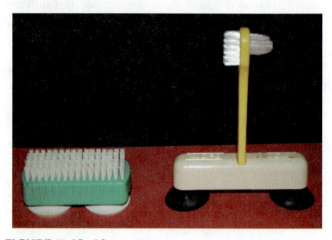

FIGURE ■ 13–18 A nail brush and a denture brush stabilized to the countertop with suction cups for use by a patient who has the use of only one arm or hand.

(*Source:* Courtesy of Christine Beatty and Amy Teague.)

can be modified (Figure 13–18 ■) so that it can be attached to the countertop or side of the sink with suction cups. A denture brush, clasp brush, or any self-care aid with a handle can be inserted into a ball, bicycle grip or other holder to accommodate a patient with limited grasp caused by arthritis or other reasons. (Figure 13–19 ■). These and other modified aids are available from suppliers of rehabilitation services. They can also be created in the dental office or at home.

Denture Cleaning Products

Immersion of the denture in a **commercial chemical cleanser solution** is recommended daily to supplement brushing as long as manufacturers' instructions are followed (Box 13–5 ■).[71] Some microbial species are resistant to mechanical cleaning.[46] Therefore, using a combination of brushing and immersion is more effective than brushing alone to remove plaque biofilm, debris, and stain. Brushing should follow immersion to brush away deposits that are loosened by the chemical cleanser.

Compared to brushing, the use of these commercial immersion chemical solutions has the additional benefits of providing

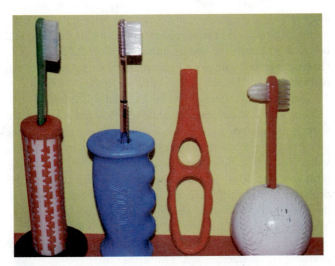

FIGURE ■ 13–19 A self-care aid can be modified for use by a patient with limited grasp by inserting the handle of the aid into a variety of handles.

(*Source:* Courtesy of Christine Beatty and Amy Teague.)

antimicrobial effects on the denture surface[72] and controlling malodor more effectively.[56] It is important to remember, however, that although these cleansers can reduce the biomass on the denture, they are not bactericidal.[46] Other advantages of immersion cleaning are that it reaches all areas of the denture, it is easier for denture wearers who have difficulty handling a brush, it offers safe storage, it requires minimum handling of the denture, it reduces the risk of dropping the denture during cleaning, and it is significantly less abrasive than denture paste. A Cochrane review revealed that only limited research has been conducted on adverse effects of these commercial chemical immersion products on acrylic denture material.[72] Although one study found adverse effects,[78] other studies revealed no such results,[79,80,81] and the American

Academy of General Dentistry, the American Dental Association, and professionals recommend the products.[46,56,58,60,61,71,82] Continual studies are needed to ensure their safety.[72]

Several chemicals are used to compound immersion cleanser solutions. To guide their patients' selection, oral health professionals need to be familiar with these cleaning products and stay up-to-date with continual research conducted to test the effectiveness and safety of existing and new products. No one product is best in all situations. The advantages and disadvantages must be weighed in relation to an individual patient's needs. Selecting an immersion cleanser requires consideration of the type of denture material and the desired outcome. For example, when killing microorganisms such as *Staphylococcus* and *Candida* species is the goal, it is necessary to use a special chemical that is not normally utilized daily. Also, the use of some chemical solutions can tarnish metal commonly used to fabricate partials.[58]

Alkaline peroxide Industry estimates are that 80% of denture wearers use effervescent commercial alkaline peroxide denture-cleaning products, which form bubbles when dissolved in water as a result of the release of a gas. These products include compounds for oxidizing (usually an alkaline perborate), effervescing (perborate and/or carbonate), and chelating (ethylenediaminetetraacetic acid [EDTA]). When dissolved in water, the compounds decompose and release oxygen bubbles, which mechanically loosen plaque and debris on the denture surface. The alkaline substances and detergent enhance the mechanical effect of the bubbles. However, because cleaning with these solutions is superficial, mechanical cleaning with a denture brush and paste or an ultrasonic is also required.[58] These effervescent alkaline peroxide solutions also have an antibacterial effect, but they are not bactericidal, do not affect *Candida* species, and are ineffective in removing calculus.[59]

BOX 13–5   Instructions for Use of a Chemical Immersion Cleanser

- Use a plastic container with a fitted cover that is not used for any other purpose.
- Use warm (not hot) water to promote the action of the cleanser.
- Fill the container with enough warm (not hot) water to submerge the denture.
- Mix the cleansing solution; follow the manufacturer's instructions for correct dilution of cleanser.
- Place the denture in the solution; confirm that the solution covers the denture.
- Soak the denture for the time recommended by the manufacturer.
- To remove loosened deposits, brush the denture with a denture brush after it has soaked the recommended time, brush all surfaces including the inner surface.
- Rinse the denture thoroughly under lukewarm running water.
- Empty and wash the container after each use; dispose of the cleansing solution and use new solution each time the denture is cleaned.
- Fill the container with lukewarm water for storage of the denture if it will not be re-inserted into the mouth right away.

(*Sources:* Academy of General Dentistry. (2008). *What is a denture?* Chicago, IL: Author. Retrieved February 6, 2011, from For the Public, http://www.agd.org; American Dental Association. (n.d.) *Denture cleansers.* Chicago, IL: Author. Retrieved February 6, 2011, from Oral Health Topics, http://www.ada.org; Felton, D., Cooper, L., Duqum, I., Minsley, G., Guckes, A., Haug, S., Meredith, P., Solie, C., Avery, D., & Chandler, N. D. (2011). Evidence-based guidelines for the care and maintenance of complete dentures. A publication of the American College of Prosthodontists. *J Am Dent Assoc,* 142(2 Suppl):1S–20S. Retrieved May 25, 2011, from http://jada.ada.org/content/142/suppl_1/1S.full.pdf+html; Rhan, A. O., Ivanhoe, J. R., & Plummer, K. D. (2009). *Textbook of complete dentures* (6th ed.). Shelton, CT: People's Medical Publishing House. Retrieved February 6, 2010, from http://books.google.com; Tonn, E. M. (2009, February 8). *Caring for your dentures.* Retrieved February 6, 2010, from http://www.webmd.com.)

They have been shown to effectively achieve a 99% kill rate of most organisms in the recommended 10- to 20-minute soaking time, and their effects are enhanced by using water at 50°C (122°F).[82] Alkaline peroxide solutions should not be used with soft denture liners because they will cause the denture liner to harden.[58]

DID YOU KNOW ?

If used too often, commercial acid cleansers that are used to professionally clean dentures in the dental office can corrode and weaken any metal parts of a complete or partial denture.

Alkaline hypochlorite Alkaline hypochlorite is recommended for 20 minutes of soaking daily followed immediately by rinsing and soaking the denture in water.[83] This agent has superior action in cleaning dentures, dissolving mucin and plaque biofilm matrix, inhibiting calculus formation, and bleaching stains. In addition, alkaline hypochlorite has more bactericidal and fungicidal effects than alkaline peroxide,[58] although it still does not eradicate *Candida* species.[84] Because the active ingredient is dilute sodium hypochlorite, which is the chemical used in household bleach, it has a tendency to corrode metal-based dentures and fades the color of the pink denture acrylic.[58] It has been suggested that this can be controlled by not using the product daily[58] and by soaking for periods not to exceed 10 minutes, immediately followed by thorough rinsing and soaking in water.[83] Corrosion can occur not only to exposed metal but also to the metal pins that retain the porcelain denture teeth. Research has been done to reduce the corrosive quality of sodium hypochlorite products by the addition of additives.[85] An alkaline hypochlorite solution is safe to use with denture liners provided the denture is not soaked longer than the recommended time.[86]

Acids Commercial acid cleansers are 3% to 5% solutions of hydrochloric acid alone or in combination with phosphoric acid.[58] They are effective in removing resistant stains and calculus.[58] Because these compounds must be handled with extreme care, they are primarily recommended for use by dental office personnel and should not be used routinely to clean metal prostheses because of their corrosive nature.[58]

Other chemicals Proteolytic enzymes have been added to various commercial immersion cleansers to break down mucin deposits on dentures, thus breaking up the plaque biofilm and allowing it be flushed away more easily.[82] However, these enzymes are inferior to alkaline peroxide compounds against *Candida* species.[82] A new silicone polymer cleanser has been tested with promising results to prevent readherence of bacteria to the denture surface.[82]

Ultrasonic cleaners The use of a tabletop ultrasonic cleaner is less common but highly effective in cleaning and disinfecting a denture.[58] These small units for individual use at home employ a cleaning solution in conjunction with agitation. Only a cleaning solution that is recommended for dentures should be used. Although the use of ultrasonic cleaning has demonstrated remarkably improved bacterial kill rates, its use is still not bactericidal.[46]

An ultrasonic cleaner can be especially helpful for individuals with limited dexterity although they are not designed to replace daily brushing of the denture.[59] Use of an ultrasonic cleaner can be impractical and expensive for use by some individual patients at home but can be especially useful in long-term care facilities.[70] It is important that facility personnel protect owner identification and control cross contamination of dentures during ultrasonic cleaning. This can be accomplished by placing the denture into the cleaning solution in a sealed plastic bag or secure cup before agitation.[87] Various units are available on the Internet at an affordable cost.

Although the evidence is limited, the successful use of ozone for disinfection of acrylic resin dentures has been reported in a systematic review of ozone use in dentistry.[88] Application of ozone to the cleaning solution used for ultrasonication has improved the bactericidal effects of this treatment. In addition, use of ozonated water combined with ultrasonication has been found to be more effective than either treatment alone although the use of ozone as an immersion solution without ultrasonication has been shown to effectively kill *Candida* species and other microbes. Ozone gas has also been suggested as a bactericidal treatment for acrylic dentures. Further research on ozone use to disinfect dentures was suggested by this systematic review.

Household products Many denture wearers clean their dentures with a household product not specifically designed for that purpose. Patients need guidance in how to use these products effectively and safely. Nonabrasive agents such as hand soap and mild dishwashing liquid are safe to use for cleaning but have no antimicrobial effect.[75] Toxic and abrasive cleansing agents such as scouring powders will scratch or otherwise damage the synthetic denture surfaces and should never be used.[71] Both salt and bicarbonate of soda are mildly abrasive.[75]

Vinegar is acetic acid and can dissolve and soften calculus deposits although not as effectively as commercial acid cleansers.[75] It also has disinfectant properties.[89] As an acid, it is corrosive to metal parts of a denture,[75] has an aftertaste, and can be irritating to the soft tissues if not thoroughly rinsed.[72]

Some denture wearers soak their dentures in an antimicrobial mouthrinse. Studies have shown disinfectant properties of these products,[90] but they do not act as cleansers that loosen deposits.

DID YOU KNOW ?

Dentures today are fabricated from synthetics such as acrylic and other plastics that will lose their natural pink color when cleaned with household bleach.

Sodium hypochlorite   The most common household product used to clean dentures is household bleach (sodium hypochlorite) diluted 1:10 in tap water. Research has shown that it is the most effective disinfecting chemical solution, but it is only safe when used properly.[46] It is recommended for only 10 minutes of soaking daily followed by thorough rinsing to avoid tissue reaction when the denture is reinserted into the mouth.[72] It is more effective than commercial cleansers against *Candida* species. It is also capable of killing *Staphylococcus aureus* (MRSA), which has become a major issue in hospitalized patients and increases mortality rates significantly, but it is not effective against other opportunistic or pathogenic microorganisms.[46] On the other hand, sodium hypochlorite has several disadvantages, negative effects, and safety issues (Box 13–6 ■).[46,58,59,72] Although overnight soaking of nonmetal prostheses sodium hypochlorite has been recommended in textbooks, evidence suggest that it should not be practiced routinely.[46,59,72]

It has been suggested that adding Calgon® to the bleach enhances its ability to penetrate the denture surface and detach the deposits.[75] The recommended formula for the solution is 15 ml (1 T) bleach, 8 ml (2 T) Calgon, and 114 ml (4 ounces) water. This immersion solution can be especially effective to kill *Candida* species but must be used with great care because of the harmful effects of the bleach.

BOX 13–6   Disadvantages of Sodium Hypochlorite Denture Cleanser

- It corrodes, pits, and reduces the reflectance of the metal of partial dentures.
- Prolonged use or soaking for longer than the recommend 10 minutes will degrade the acrylic resin components, which causes fading of the pink acrylic.
- Discoloration, softening, and reduced retentive values of locator attachments (employed for retention of overdentures) can result.
- The evident aftertaste could influence its acceptability and thus reduce its effectiveness in daily use.
- Severe tissue reaction can occur when the denture is reinserted into the mouth if the bleach has not been completely removed with thorough rinsing.

(*Sources:* de Souza, R. F., de Freitas Oliveiras Paranhos, H., Lovato da Silva, C. H., Abu-Naba'a, L., Fedorowicz, Z., & Gurgan, C. A. (2009). Interventions for cleaning dentures in adults (Review). *Cochrane Datab Syst Re* (Iss. 4, No. CD007395). Retrieved February 5, 2011, from http://www.cfah.org/hbns/archives/viewSupportDoc.cfm?supportingDocID=839; Felton, D., Cooper, L., Duqum, I., Minsley, G., Guckes, A., Haug, S., Meredith, P., Solie, C., Avery, D., & Chandler, N. D. (2011). Evidence-based guidelines for the care and maintenance of complete dentures. A publication of the American College of Prosthodontists. *J Am Dent Assoc,* 142(Suppl 2):1S–20S. Retrieved May 25, 2011, from http://jada.ada.org/content/142/suppl_1/1S.full.pdf+html; Rhan, A. O., Ivanhoe, J. R., & Plummer, K. D. (2009). *Textbook of complete dentures.* (6th ed.). Shelton, CT: People's Medical Publishing House. Retrieved February 6, 2010, from http://books.google.com; Nguyen, C. T., Masri, R., Driscoll, C. F., & Romberg, E. (2010). The effect of denture cleansing solutions on the retention of pink locator attachments: An in vitro study. *J Prosthodont,* 19:226–30.)

Precautions with Denture Cleansers

The misuse of denture-cleansing products can cause adverse reactions, including damage to the esophagus, abdominal pain, burns, breathing problems, hypotension, seizures, bleaching of tissues, internal bleeding, and vomiting.[46] In 2008, the U.S. Food and Drug Administration (FDA) issued a requirement for manufacturers of denture cleansers to revise their labeling to include product ingredients and instructions for the product's proper use.[91] This action was precipitated by adverse effects of **persulfates**, an ingredient in some effervescent alkaline peroxide cleansers and a known allergen. At least 73 injuries and 1 death were linked to the use of denture cleansers containing persulfates. These adverse events occurred both when the product had been used properly as well as when improperly used. At the same time, the agency recommended that manufacturers consider alternatives to the use of persulfates. The FDA also recommended that oral health professionals take the initiative to instruct patients never to ingest or use immersion denture cleansers intraorally, to recognize allergic reactions, and to review labeling information and follow manufacturers' instructions when using these products. This professional responsibility should be taken seriously to avoid allergic reactions and adverse effects caused by improper use. Symptoms of an allergic reaction to persulfates include irritation of the tissues, tissue damage, gingival tenderness, rash, hives, breathing problems, and hypotension.[46]

DID YOU KNOW ?

Treatment of candidiasis is challenging because it involves disinfection of the denture as well as removal of the *Candida* yeasts from the mucosal tissue; sometimes the only solution is to reline or replace an infected denture.

Treatment of Candidiasis

When a patient's denture becomes contaminated with *Candida* yeasts, the surface is not only contaminated but also the depths of the porosity within the denture material become contaminated.[46] The same types of microorganisms found within the oral mucosa of patients with candidiasis are also impregnated in the denture.[48] Management of this condition requires disinfection of the denture at the same time as treatment of the mucosa.[46] Treatment is extremely challenging because of the potential for reinfection by the denture. Elimination of *Candida* species from a denture is difficult. Sometimes, the only solution is to reline or replace the denture to prevent re-contamination of the mucosal tissues.

Although commercial immersion-type denture cleansers disinfect dentures when they are used on a daily basis, they are not effective in killing *Candida* yeasts or *Staphylococcus* when the mucosa and denture are infected.[46] Therefore, in addition to immaculate denture hygiene, various other therapeutic strategies have been recommended to eliminate *Candida* species from the denture, although there is not a standard of treatment. Soaking the denture for 5 minutes daily in full-strength household bleach has been suggested for disinfection of a *Candida*-infected denture. The soak must be carefully timed because of the problem of bleaching the pink acrylic and must be followed by thorough rinsing to avoid tissue reaction upon reinsertion.[72] The new guidelines for care and management of complete dentures do not address the treatment of candidiasis but do suggest that sodium hypochlorite can be used to disinfect a denture as long as the time is kept to 10 minutes or less.[46] However, although soaking in sodium hypochlorite provides a stronger bacterial kill, it still does not achieve sterilization: *Candida* species are not completely eliminated.[46] Other denture disinfectant treatments that have been used are soaking dentures in antifungal suspensions or chlorhexidine.[92]

The only apparently safe treatment to sterilize a denture is microwave irradiation of the denture immersed in sterile water at 650 watts for 3 minutes.[46] This treatment does not seem to adversely affect the denture material.[79] The long-term effects of microwave irradiation of denture materials have not been studied; this question is suggested for future research.[46]

Elimination of *Candida* yeasts from the mucosal tissues is accomplished with topical and/or systemic antifungal agents in combination with meticulous oral and denture hygiene.[48] Topical antifungal agents come in a variety of delivery forms (liquids, pastiles, and troches) designed to maintain the medication in contact with the infected tissues.[93] Nystatin and clotrimazole are common topical antifungal drugs used to treat oral candidiasis.[93] When a severe infection is not responding to topical treatment, systemic antifungal agents can be used. These drugs should be employed cautiously because of their interactions with commonly prescribed medications and the emergence of resistant fungal organisms after their repeated use.[93] Commonly used systemic antifungal drugs used to inhibit oral *Candida* species are ketoconazole, fluconazole, and itraconazole.[44,93]

Various antiseptics are also used to kill oral *Candida* species, and it appears that antiseptics that contain chlorine are more effective.[94] Angular cheilitis, possibly caused by loss of vertical dimension of the denture, can be present in the denture wearer. This condition can be complicated with *Candida* infection.[63] A combination of antifungals and steroids can be used to treat the fungal infection and the inflammation associated with the angular cheilitis.[93]

In addition, proper oral hygiene is fundamental in treating candidiasis to prevent reinfection. Because denture wearers are predisposed to *Candida* species intraorally, meticulous daily self-care cleaning of the denture and oral tissues is required to control candidiasi.

DID YOU KNOW?

Additives to denture products can cause allergic reactions or other ill effects; the FDA has recommended that manufacturers label denture products and that oral health professionals instruct patients to read labels and exercise caution when using these products.

Denture Liners

Constant, ongoing changes in hard and soft tissues over time are normal and expected, resulting in compromised denture fit.[95] Denture relining and rebasing are solutions used when hard- and soft-tissue changes reduce denture retention and stability.[46] The life span of complete dentures is 5 to 7 years of continuous use,[59] after which relining or remaking the denture is necessary due to these tissue changes or wearing of denture materials.[39] When hard-tissue changes are significant, the denture must be remade rather than relined.[95] Patients should be advised never to use home relining products,[56] which are not suitable for improvement of denture fit because of inferior physical properties[96] and can exert adverse pressures that are capable of damaging hard and soft tissues.[56]

Denture liners that are used to permanently fix the problem of denture fit and stability are hard liners and can be cleaned in the same manner the original dentures were cleaned. Sometimes a soft temporary liner is placed to address soft tissue problems. Soft reliners can be damaged by commercial cleansers and brushing.[97] These reliners should be rinsed thoroughly with water after eating and soaked daily in alkaline hypochlorite solution but not in an effervescent product or in household bleach. A soft cloth or cotton can be used to gently wipe the surface as well. Other commercial cleansers will damage a soft liner and should be avoided.[83]

Denture Adhesives

Denture adhesives are recommended for denture wearers.[39] Denture adhesive is a nontoxic, water-soluble material that is placed on the inner surface of the denture and is in contact with the soft tissues when the denture is in place. A denture adhesive enhances the normal physiological forces that hold dentures in place. Dentures adhere to the soft tissue because saliva adheres to both the denture and the tissue. Denture adhesives improve retention because they adhere better to both the denture surface and the soft tissue.[56]

Only soluble denture adhesives should be used.[56] Soluble creams and powders, once wet, flow under pressure to evenly spread over the inner denture surface, providing even distribution of occlusal forces on tissue-bearing surfaces. Insoluble denture adhesives such as denture liners, pads, and wafers should be avoided.[56] These products are unable or limited in their ability to flow under pressure. As a result, they add thickness of the unyielding material, contribute to uneven load on tissue-bearing surfaces, and exert adverse tissue pressures, thus producing trauma to the tissues.[56] Insoluble adhesives are usually next to the soluble adhesives on the shelf at the store, so patients need to be advised to read labels carefully when selecting an adhesive.[56]

Compared with older products, adhesives today are safer and improved, providing a stronger, longer hold. Advantages of the use of denture adhesives include increased sense of security and confidence; enhanced psychological well-being; improved comfort, bite force, chewing rates, retention, and stability of the dentures; reduction of tissue irritation under the denture; and less food-particle collection under the dentures.[39,46,56] Many of these advantages are true even for denture wearers who have good-quality denture support tissues.[46] Improved retention and stability have been demonstrated with the use of denture adhesives for both ill-fitting and well-fitting dentures.[95]

Few negative effects have been attributed to the use of denture adhesives although no longitudinal studies have been conducted to test the effects of long-term use.[46] It is a fallacy that the correct use of denture adhesives causes tissue irritation, mucosal infection, and bone resorption.[56] Their use can safely enhance denture performance, but they should not be used to compensate for denture deficiencies.[39] It is especially important to stress the need for regular annual examinations to patients who use denture adhesives because adhesives can obscure the usual signs of looser denture fit that trigger a visit to the dental office.[56]

DID YOU KNOW ?

Denture adhesives should be used with all conventional dentures (those that are not overdentures) to improve retention and stability and are not a solution for ill-fitting dentures.

A potential problem with denture adhesives is that they leach out sodium, which can cause a problem for patients on a sodium-free diet. Because powder-based adhesives leach out more sodium than paste-form adhesives, the paste form should be recommended to these patients.[58] The most serious consequence of chronic and excessive use of denture adhesives is potential neurotoxicity caused by **zinc** as an adhesive component,[98] which has resulted in lawsuits filed by individuals who claim injury.[99] The FDA issued a recommendation to label adhesive product ingredients and replace zinc with a safer ingredient.[100] At least one manufacturer has discontinued the manufacture of zinc-containing products and has plans to reformulate the products without zinc.[101]

Adhesives are especially beneficial to musicians, public speakers, and those who feel the need for the additional sense of security.[46] They are also helpful to those who have very little alveolar ridge, suffer from xerostomia, have undergone maxillofacial jaw resection, and are neurologically compromised because of stroke, multiple sclerosis, or closed-head injury.[56] Contraindications for the use of denture adhesives include open sores or cuts in the mouth, ill-fitting dentures, dentures that have not been evaluated recently, poor oral and denture hygiene, and allergic reactions to adhesive product ingredients.[56]

Patients should be instructed in the appropriate use of denture adhesive (Box 13–7 ■) to prevent the patient acquiring incomplete or inaccurate information from other, less reliable sources.[56] There are recommended rules and procedures for the application of the denture adhesive to the dentures (Box 13–8 ■). It is essential that patients understand how much adhesive to use, and that the concept of "more is better" does not hold true.[39] Use of excessive amounts of adhesive is never indicated. Additionally, patients should be informed that the necessity of using higher amounts of adhesive over

BOX 13–7   Patient Education Topics Needed Relative to Denture Adhesives

- What denture adhesive is and its role in satisfactory denture wearing
- What products are acceptable to use (soluble adhesives such as powders and creams)
- What products should be avoided (insoluble wafers and pads)
- How to apply soluble denture adhesives
- How to remove dentures that contain adhesive
- Denture hygiene when adhesive is being used
- Importance of regular continuing care

(*Source:* Shay, K., Grasso, J. E., & Barrack, K. S. (2010). The complete denture prosthesis: Clinical and laboratory applications—insertion, patient adaptation, and post-insertion care. Two-hour CE course retrieved February 6, 2011, from http://www.dentalcare.com.)

time could indicate an inadequate fit and the need for a reline or remake of the denture.[39] Although it is important to provide guidelines for patients, each person will need to experiment to determine the right amount of adhesive needed to meet individual needs.[56] Patients should be given a sample of adhesive and told where they can purchase it locally to encourage its use.[39]

A denture adhesive should be completely cleaned out of the denture daily and prior to supplementation with more adhesive during the day.[58] This can be accomplished by brushing the adhesive off the denture surface under running warm water. Use of a power toothbrush while the denture is submerged in water has also been suggested.[39] An alternative is to soak the denture overnight in water to loosen the adhesive, allowing it to be more easily brushed and rinsed off.[56] The adhesive must also be removed from the oral tissues, which can be accomplished with a power or manual soft toothbrush with frequent rinsing of warm water.[39] This will clean and massage the oral tissues at the same time. Studies have shown that patients perceive that adhesive is difficult to remove from the denture,[46] possibly indicating their lack of knowledge in its proper removal.

A denture adhesive can make it difficult to remove the denture from the mouth. Denture adhesives are intended to provide all-day hold.[56] An adhesive used for short time periods can make denture removal even more difficult. In this event, the patient should swish vigorously with warm water for a minute or more. Another technique is to alternately puff the cheeks and firmly pull downward with the fingers on the most distofacial flange.[56]

DID YOU KNOW ?

Xerostomia will reduce the retention, stability and comfort of a denture.

BOX 13–8   How to Apply the Denture Adhesive

Four rules of application

1. Less is better: Use the minimum amount necessary to provide the maximum benefit. The denture should not be filled. If excessive denture cream oozes out from under denture after biting on it, too much was used.
2. Spread the wealth: Distribute the adhesive evenly on the tissue-bearing surface of the denture.
3. Clean it up: Always apply the denture adhesive to a thoroughly clean denture.
4. Keep it up: Apply or reapply when necessary to provide the desired effect.

Cream adhesive application

1. Clean and dry the intaglio surface of the denture.
2. On maxillary denture, apply a series of three or four very small (size of a pea or a pencil eraser) dots of adhesive evenly spaced on the anterior ridge, midline of the palate, and posterior border; adhesive should be placed no closer than 5 mm to a denture border.
3. On mandibular denture, apply a series of three or four small dots (size of a pea or a pencil eraser) evenly around the entire ridge area.
4. Evenly disperse the adhesive with a clean dry finger to produce a thin, even layer of adhesive.
5. Submerge the denture in cool water for 20 to 30 seconds to hydrate the adhesive.
6. Insert the denture, press it firmly in place, and hold it in place for approximately 10 seconds, causing the adhesive to flow throughout the interfacial space between the denture base and the denture bearing soft tissues.
7. Wait briefly (10–20 minutes) before drinking hot liquids or chewing to allow the adhesive to attain its full strength.

Powder adhesive application

1. Clean the intaglio surface of the denture.
2. Wet the base of the intaglio surface of the denture.
3. Sprinkle a thin uniform layer of powder to the entire tissue-bearing surface of the clean denture.
4. Shake off any excess powder.
5. Follow the steps for cream adhesive to insert the denture.

(*Sources:* American College of Prosthodontists. (2010). *Dentures: How to properly apply denture adhesive.* Chicago, IL: Author. Retrieved February 6, 2011, from Public & Patients, http://www.prosthodontics.org; Cagna, D. R., & Massad, J. J. (2010). Prosthesis retention and effective use of denture adhesive in complete denture therapy. Two-hour CE course retrieved May 13, 2011, from http://www.dentalcare.com; Shay, K., Grasso, J. E., & Barrack, K. S. (2010). The complete denture prosthesis: Clinical and laboratory applications—Insertion, patient adaptation, and post-insertion care. Two-hour CE course retrieved February 6, 2011, from http://www.dentalcare.com; Shay, K. (2008). Care of appliances and dental prostheses. In Daniel, S. J., Harfst, S. A., & Wilder, R. S., Eds. *Mosby's dental hygiene concepts, cases, and competencies* (2nd ed.). St. Louis, MO: Mosby Elsevier, 558–69.)

Xerostomia and the Denture Patient

Saliva is critical for retention of and comfort in wearing removable prostheses.[102] Most denture wearers are in the age group with higher prevalence of **xerostomia** (dry mouth) caused by local factors, systemic diseases, head and neck irradiation and/or multiple medications.[43] The prevalence of xerostomia is associated with age, female status, and smoking.[103] It is the most commonly occurring drug-related adverse oral event.[93] Xerostomia and salivary hypofunction can have a devastating effect for the denture-wearing edentulous patient because of numerous compounding factors that affect chewing, swallowing, tasting and speaking.[102] Results of inadequate saliva in denture wearers include poor retention, denture sores and traumatic ulcerations, which can lead to epulis fissuratum if left unchecked.[63] Also, individuals who suffer from hyposalivation will experience more and more rapid plaque biofilm accumulation on the denture as well as an increase in *Candida* presence in the mouth.[44] Use of saliva substitutes, artificial saliva and saliva stimulants, along with practicing immaculate denture hygiene self-care more frequently, will help to compensate for the effects of inadequate saliva. In addition, only alcohol-free antimicrobials should be used to prevent further drying.

It is important to keep the denture moist to improve retention and prevent mucosal irritation and ulcerations caused by the denture.[102] Lack of saliva in the denture-mucosa interface can produce denture sores as the denture rubs against the mucosal tissues. The denture should be wet prior to insertion and again before eating. An alcohol-free rinse containing aloe or lanolin or water-soluble lubricating jelly can help patients who suffer with dry mouth. The lubricating jelly can be placed in the base of the denture and will release over time. Increasing water intake, especially with meals, will improve chewing and swallowing. Saliva substitutes can only improve patient comfort without a significant effect on retention,[104] in which case denture adhesives are recommended to improve retention.[46] Use of a denture adhesive by the patient with hyposalivation also reduces frictional tissue irritation and prevents further tissue dehydration.[39] Wetting the denture prior to placement of the denture adhesive is recommended, and combining saliva substitutes with a denture adhesive will be beneficial.[102]

Patients with severe xerostomia caused by a systemic condition or multiple medications can benefit from salivary stimulation by pharmacologic intervention if they can tolerate the side effects.[93] Use of pilocarpine (5 mg three times per day) has been suggested for denture wearers with dry mouth.[41]

SUMMARY

This chapter discusses self-care procedures and products for peri-implant cleaning and denture self-care. It should be noted that some individuals require assistance with self-care because of various limitations. When appropriate, accommodations and adaptations for individuals with special needs can be applied. Dental providers and oral health educators should keep abreast of the research on these devices and products, so patients and the public will receive evidence-based information.

PRACTICAL CONSIDERATIONS

Teaching proper self-care of dental implants and full and partial dentures is necessary in the planning and delivery of the dental and dental hygiene care plan. Long-term maintenance is imperative to achieve longevity of the restorations and prostheses and to maintain the health of the patient. Motivating patients for behavior change proves to be one of the major challenges for the oral health practitioner. Limiting the oral hygiene aids to the fewest number necessary to achieve optimum results will provide the best compliance among patients. In addition, it is important to remember that all patients are different, and oral hygiene instruction cannot be a "one size fits all" approach. The oral hygiene instructions planned and given to the patient must fit the individual's abilities, needs and limitations in order to maintain health and achieve success. Products and procedures should be recommended based on current evidence and the professional expertise of the professional. Additionally, patients should be educated about the advantages and ill effects of various denture products.

SELF-STUDY QUESTIONS

1. Which of the following is contraindicated for self-care of an implant?

   a. Brushing with a power toothbrush

   b. Daily rinsing with an antimicrobial

   c. Self-application of fluoride

   d. Use of floss and other interdental aids

   Rationale: Both acidic products and fluorides are contraindicated because they can break down the stable oxide layer that protects the titanium from corrosion. All other answers are recommended to clean and reduce bacterial attack of implants.

2. Use of metal on an implant, for example, a metal-core interproximal brush, is contraindicated because a scratched titanium surface traps plaque biofilm that can contribute to peri-implantitis and implant failure.

   a. Both statements are true and related.

   b. Both statements are true but unrelated.

   c. The first statement is true, and the second is false.

   d. The first statement is false, and the second is true.

   e. Both statements are false.

Rationale: The use of metal on an implant is contraindicated because it can scratch the implant surface. A scratched implant provides a rough surface that can trap plaque biofilm. A primary risk factor for peri-implantitis and implant failure is bacteria in the plaque biofilm. Therefore, it is critical that the implant surface be maintained as smooth and is easily cleaned. Also, bacteria can cause corrosion of the titanium surface, which can cause fatigue and weakening of the titanium, contributing to the implant's mechanical failure.

3. Which of the following is the most likely result of practicing oral hygiene of an implant too aggressively?

   a. Corrosion of the titanium surface of the implant abutment that can eventually lead to implant failure

   b. Missing plaque biofilm on the gingival area of the abutment that is angled and difficult to reach

   c. Severing the mucopolysacharide bond of the implant surface to the surrounding tissues

   d. Tenderness of the peri-implant tissues, which will contribute to reduced compliance of self-care

Rationale: This mucopolysacharide bond of the implant surface to the surrounding tissues is more vulnerable to damage from aggressive oral hygiene than the periodontal ligament of a natural tooth. The bond is easily severed by mechanical trauma.

4. Patients with dentures are at a higher risk for candidiasis than nondenture-wearers. Treatment of candidiasis requires treating the denture as well as the mouth.

   a. Both statements are true.

   b. Both statements are false.

   c. The first statement is true, and the second is false.

   d. The first statement is false, and the second is true.

   Rationale: Denture wearers are predisposed to the intra-oral presence of *Candida* species and candidiasis with an estimated 67% having *Candida*-associated stomatitis. The *Candida* species impregnate the oral soft tissues as well as the surface of the denture. Therefore, treatment of candidiasis requires addressing both to kill the *Candida* yeasts.

5. Toothpaste is contraindicated to clean a complete denture because the acrylic denture material scratches more easily than enamel.

   a. Both statements are true and related.

   b. Both statements are true but unrelated.

   c. The first statement is true, and the second is false.

   d. The first statement is false, and the second is true.

   e. Both statements are false.

   Rationale: Toothpaste is more abrasive than denture paste and can scratch the denture surface. The surface of synthetic denture materials is more easily scratched than enamel.

Therefore, toothpaste is contraindicated to clean synthetic denture materials. Special denture creams, pastes, and gels are manufactured for this purpose.

6. All of the following *except one* is an advantage of using immersion cleansers to clean a denture. Which one is the exception?

   a. The solution reaches all areas of the denture.

   b. Immersion agents are more abrasive than denture paste.

   c. It is easier for denture wearers who have difficulty handling a brush.

   d. It offers safe storage.

   Rationale: Chemical immersion cleansing agents are not abrasive although some have other potential ill effects on the denture surface. All other answers are advantages of immersion cleansers.

7. Which of the following chemical cleansers has the potential to whiten an acrylic denture?

   a. Alkaline hypochlorite

   b. Alkaline peroxide

   c. Commercial acid solutions

   d. Denture paste

   Rationale: The active ingredient of alkaline hypochlorite is dilute sodium hypochlorite (bleach), which can fade the pink color of acrylic denture material. The products in the other answers do not bleach acrylic. Denture paste has no ill effects, but the other products can cause a potential allergic reaction to perborates in some alkaline peroxide products and corrosion of metal resulting from commercial acid solutions.

REFERENCES

1. U.S. Census Bureau. (2007, March 26). *Age and sex in the United States: 2008*. Washington, DC: Author. Retrieved May 3, 2011, from http://www.census.gov.

2. Centers for Disease Control and Prevention. (2006, December). *Oral health for older Americans*. Atlanta: Author. Retrieved May 10, 2011, from http://www.cdc.gov/OralHealth/publications/factsheets/adult_older.htm.

3. Centers for Disease Control and Prevention, National Center for Health Statistics. *FastStats:Oral and dental health*. Atlanta: Author. Retrieved May 3, 2011, from http://www.cdc.gov/nchs/fastats/dental.htm.

4. Centers for Disease Control and Prevention. (2007, August 17). QuickStats: Prevalence of complete tooth loss among older adults. *Morbid Mortal Week Rep,* 56:823. Retrieved May 3, 2011, from http://www.cdc.gov/mmwr,

5. Centers for Disease Control and Prevention. (2011). *Oral health: Preventing cavities, gum disease, tooth loss, and oral cancers: At a glance 2010*. Atlanta: Author. Retrieved May 8, 2011, from http://www.cdc.gov/chronicdisease/resources/publications/AAG/doh.htm.

6. Astra Tech Dental. (2005, April 12). (Press Release). *Background information: Astra Tech and dental implantation*. Waltham, MA: Author. Retrieved May 8, 2011, from http://www.astratechdental.com/Library/396636.pdf.

7. National Institute of Dental and Craniofacial Research. (2011). *Tooth loss in seniors (age 65 and over)*. Bethesda, MD: Author. Retrieved May 8, 2011, from http://www.nidcr.nih.gov/DataStatistics/FindDataByTopic/ToothLoss/ToothLossSeniors65andOlder.

8. American College of Prosthodontists. (2006, June). *Reframing the future of prosthodontics. Mega issue*. Chicago, IL: Author. Retrieved May 3, 2011, from http://www.prosthodontics.org/pdf/summit-report.pdf.

9. Mueller-Joseph, L., Homenko, D. F., Wilkins, E. M., & Wyche, C. J. (2010). The professional dental hygienist. In Wilkins, E. M., Ed. *Clinical practice of the dental hygienist* (9th ed.). Philadelphia, PA: Lippincott Williams & Wilkins, 3–17.

10. Harfst, S. A., & Vick, V. C. (2008). Oral risk assessment and intervention planning. In Daniel, S. J., Harfst, S. A., & Wilder, R. S., Eds. *Mosby's dental hygiene concepts, cases, and competencies* (2nd ed.). St. Louis, MO: Mosby Elsevier, 387–404.

11. Walsh, M. M., & Darby, M. L. (2010). Human needs theory and dental hygiene care. In Darby, M. L., & Walsh, M. M., Eds. *Dental hygiene theory & practice* (3rd ed.). St. Louis, MO: Elsevier, 13–23.

12. Harfst, S. A., & Vick, V. C. (2008). Individualizing preventive and therapeutic strategies. In Daniel, S. J., Harfst, S. A., & Wilder, R. S., Eds. *Mosby's dental hygiene concepts, cases, and competencies* (2nd ed.). St. Louis, MO: Mosby Elsevier, 405–16.

13. Jahn, C. (2011). Best practices for periodontal care. In Nield-Gehrig, J. S., & Willmann, D. E., Eds. *Foundations of periodontics for the dental hygienist* (3rd ed.). Philadelphia, PA: Lippincott Williams & Wilkins, 365–80.

14. Oliver, H. E. (2010). Communication and behavioral change theories. In Darby, M. L., & Walsh, M. M., Eds. *Dental hygiene theory & practice*. St. Louis, MO: Elsevier, 24–36.

15. Allen, E., Ziada, H., Irwin, C., Mullally, B., & Byrne, P. J. (2008). Periodontics: 10. Maintenance in periodontal therapy. *Dent Update,* 35:150–56.

16. Kracher, C. M., & Smith, W. S. (2010). Oral health maintenance of dental implants. *Dent Assist,* 79:27–35.

17. Oczakir, C., Balmer, S., & Mericske-Stern, R. (2005). Implant-prosthodontic treatment for special care patients: A case series study. *Int J Prosthodont,* 18:383–89.

18. Draper, C. (2007). The dental hygienist's role in implant therapy: From treatment to maintenance. *Contemp Oral Hygiene,* 7(5):14–24.

19. American College of Prosthodontists. (2011) *Dental implants and dental implant surgery*. Chicago, IL: Author. Retrieved May 10, 2011, from http://www.prosthodontics.org/patients/implants.asp.

20. Farrar, S. K., St. Germain, J., & Yukna, R. A. (2010). Implantology. In Weinberg, M. A., Westphal, C., Froum, S. J., Palat, M., & Schoor, R. S., Eds. *Comprehensive periodontics for the dental hygienist* (3rd ed.). Boston: Pearson Education, 413–37.

21. Greenstein, G., Cavallaro, J., & Tarnow, D. (2010). Dental implants in the periodontal patient. *Dent Clin North Am,* 54:113–28.

22. Jones, A. (2011). Maintenance for the dental implant patient. In Nield-Gehrig, J. S., & Willmann, D. E., Eds. *Foundations of periodontics for the dental hygienist* (3rd ed.). Philadelphia, PA: Wolters Kluwer Health/Lippincott Williams & Wilkins, 579–96.

23. Shumaker, N. D., Metcalf, B. T., Toscano, N. T., & Holtzclaw, D. J. (2009). Periodontal and periimplant maintenance: A critical factor in long-term treatment success. *Compend Cont Educ Dent,* 30:388–390,392. Retrieved April 17, 2011, from http://cde.dentalaegis.com

24. Chaturvedi, T. P. (2009). An overview of the corrosion aspect of dental implants (titanium and its alloys). *Indian J Dent Res,* 20:-91–08. Retrieved May 27, 2011, from http://www.ifdr.in/article.asp?issn=0970-9290;year=2009;volume=20;issue=1;spage=91;epage=98;aulast=Chaturvedi.

25. Moore, L., Cryan, L., & Starr, G. (2006). Controversy or conundrum . . . implant maintenance for the dental hygienist. *Cal Dent Hygien Assoc J,* 21(3):20-7.

26. Alberto, P. L. (2007). Dental implant maintenance: The key to success. *Access,* 21:47–49.

27. Kreismann, J., & Almas, K. (2010). Oral hygiene for the periodontal patient: Beyond the basics. In Weinberg, M. A., Westphal, C., Froum, S. J., Palat, M., & Schoor, R. S., Eds. *Comprehensive periodontics for the dental hygienist* (3rd ed.). Boston: Pearson Education, 285–319.

28. Silverstein, L. H., & Kurtzman, G. M. (2006). Oral hygiene and maintenance of dental implants. *Dent Today,* 25(3):70–75.

29. Caring for implants and peri-implantitis. (2009, March/April). A*uxillary,* 26. Retrieved May 3, 2011, from EBSCO HOST.

30. Costa, M. R., Marcantonio, R. A. C., & Cirelli, J. A. (2007). Comparison of manual versus sonic and ultrasonic toothbrushes: A review. *Int J Dent Hygiene,* 5:75–81.

31. Grusovin, M. G., Coulthard, P., Worthington, H. V., George, P., & Esposito, M. (2010). Interventions for replacing missing teeth: Maintaining and recovering soft tissue health around dental implants. *Cochrane Datab Syst Rev.* 2010. (Iss. 8, Art. No. CD003069).

32. Serio, F. G. (2008). Periodontal examination. In Daniel, S. J., Harfst, S. A., & Wilder, R. S. Eds. *Mosby's dental hygiene concepts, cases, and competencies* (2nd ed.). St. Louis, MO: Mosby Elsevier, 307–334.

33. Mercer, L. T. (2008). Implications for the dental hygienist when dealing with dental implants. *J Prac Hygiene,* 17(2):14–16.

34. Young-McDonald, V. L. (2010). Dental implant maintenance. In Darby, M. L., & Walsh, M. M., Eds. *Dental hygiene theory & practice* (3rd ed.). St. Louis, MO: Elsevier, 1076–1110.

35. Matsuda, S. A. (2009). The patient with dental implants. In Wilkins, E. M., Ed. *Clinical practice of the dental hygienist* (9th ed.). Philadelphia, PA: Lippincott Williams & Wilkins, 489–500.

36. American Academy of Periodontology. (2003). (Position Paper). Periodontal maintenance. *J Periodontol,* 74:1395–1401.

37. Spolarich, A. E. (2010). Pharmacologic history. In Darby, M. L., & Walsh, M. M., Eds. *Dental hygiene theory and practice*. St. Louis, MO: Saunders Elsevier, 195–204.

38. Carlsson, G. E., & Omar, R. (2009). The future of complete dentures in oral rehabilitation. A critical review. *J Oral Rehab,* 37:143–56.

39. Cagna, D. R., & Massad, J. J. (2010). Prosthesis retention and effective use of denture adhesive in complete denture therapy. Two-hour CE course retrieved May 13, 2011, from http://www.dentalcare.com.

40. Shay, K. (2008). Care of appliances and dental prostheses. In Daniel, S. J., Harfst, S. A., & Wilder, R. S. *Mosby's dental hygiene concepts, cases, and competencies* (2nd ed.). St. Louis, MO: Mosby Elsevier, 558–69.

41. Craig, B. (2010). Persons with fixed and removable dentures. In Darby, M. L., & Walsh, M. M., Eds. *Dental hygiene theory and practice*. St. Louis, MO: Saunders Elsevier, 1044–60.

42. Skarnulis, L. (2007, January 27). *7 Health challenges of aging*. Retrieved February 28, 2007, from http://theheadliners.wordpress.com.

43. Towle, J. H. (2009). The elderly patient. In Wilkins, E. M., Ed. (2010). *Clinical practice of the dental hygienist* (10th ed.). Philadelphia, PA: Lippincott Williams & Wilkins, 818–31.

44. Lyon, J. P., Costa, S. C., Totti, V. M. G., Munhoz, M. F. V., & Resende, M. A. (2006). Predisposing conditions for *Candida* spp. carriage in the oral cavity of denture wearers and individuals with natural teeth. *Canad J Microbiol,* 52:462–67.

45. Lee, S. S. (2009). *Breath: Causes, diagnosis, and treatment of oral malodor* (2nd ed.). San Bernardino, CA: Culminare, Inc.

46. Felton, D., Cooper, L., Duqum, I., Minsley, G., Guckes, A., Haug, S., Meredith, P., Solie, C., Avery, D., & Chandler, N. D. (2011). Evidence-based guidelines for the care and maintenance of complete dentures. A publication of the American College of Prosthodontists. *J Am Dent Assoc,* 142(2 Suppl):1S–20S. Retrieved May 25, 2011, from http://jada.ada.org/content/142/suppl_1/1S.full.pdf+html.

47. Nalcaci, R., & Baran, I. (2008). Oral malodor and removable complete dentures in the elderly. *Oral Surg, Oral Med, Oral Pathol, Oral Radiol, Endod,* 105:e5–9. Retrieved February 5, 2010, from http://www.ooooe.net.

48. Salerno, C., Pascale, M., Contaldo, M., Esposito, V., Busciolano, M., Milillo, L., Guida, A. Petruzzi, M., & Serpico, R. (2011). *Candida-associated denture stomatitis. Med Oral Patol Oral Cir Bucal,* 16:-e139–43. Retrieved May 2, 2011, from http://www.medicinaoral.com/pubmed/medoralv16_i2_p139.pdf.

49. Anaissie, E. J., McGinnis, M. R., & Pfaller, M. A. (2009). *Clin mycol* (2nd ed.). St. Louis, MO: Elsevier.

50. Gonsalves, W. C., Chi, A. C., & Neville, B. W. (2007, February 15). Common oral lesions: Part I. Superficial mucosal lesions. *Am Fam Physic,* 75:501–7.

51. Coulthwaite, L., & Verran, J. (2007). Potential pathogenic aspects of denture plaque. *Brit J Biomed Sci,* 64:180–89.

52. Ishikawa, A., Yoneyama, T., Hirota, K., Miyake, Y., & Miyake, K. (2008). Professional oral care reduces the number of oropharyngeal bacteria. *J Dent Res,* 87:594–98.

53. Sadig, W. (2010). The denture hygiene, denture stomatitis and role of dental hygienist. *Int J Dent Hygiene* 8:227–31.

54. Paranhos, H. F. O., da Silva, C. H. L., Venezian, G. C., Macedo, L. D., & de Souza, R. F. (2007). Distribution of biofilm on internal and external surfaces of upper complete dentures: The effect of hygiene instruction. *Gerodontol,* 24:162–68.

55. Kimbrough, V. J., & Henderson, K. (2006). *Oral health eduction.* Upper Saddle River, NJ: Pearson Prentice Hall.

56. Shay, K., Grasso, J. E., & Barrack, K. S. (2010). The complete denture prosthesis: Clinical and laboratory applications—insertion, patient adaptation, and post-insertion care. Two-hour CE course retrieved February 6, 2011, from http://www.dentalcare.com.

57. Peracini, A., Andrade, I. M., Paranhos, H. F., da Silva, C. H. L., & de Souza, R. F. (2010). Behaviors and hygiene habits of complete denture wearers. *Braz Dent J,* 21:247–52.

58. Rhan, A. O., Ivanhoe, J. R., & Plummer, K. D. (2009). *Textbook of complete dentures* (6th ed.). (e book). Shelton, CT: People's Medical Publishing House. Retrieved February 6, 2010, from http://books.google.com.

59. American Dental Association. (n.d.) *Oral longevity outline for consumer presentation.* Chicago, IL: Author. Retrieved February 6, 2011, from Oral Health Topics, http://www.ada.org.

60. Tonn, E. M. (2009, February 8). Caring for your dentures. Retrieved February 6, 2010, from http://www.webmd.com.

61. Academy of General Dentistry. (2008). *What is a denture?* Chicago, IL: Author. Retrieved February 6, 2011, from For the Public, http://www.agd.org.

62. Garrett, N. R. (2010). Poor oral hygiene, wearing dentures at night, perceptions of mouth dryness and burning, and lower educational level may be related to oral malodor in denture wearers. *J Evid Based Dent Prac,* 10:67–69.

63. Ragalis, K. (2009). The edentulous patient. In Wilkins, E. M., Ed. *Clinical practice of the dental hygienist* (10th ed.). Philadelphia, PA: Lippincott Williams & Wilkins, 832–44.

64. Centers for Disease Control and Prevention, Division of Oral Health. (2009, March 30). *Oral cancer.* Retrieved May 9, 2011, from http://www.cdc.gov/OralHealth/topics/cancer.htm.

65. Centers for Disease Control and Prevention, Division of Oral Health. (2009, March 23). *Oral cancer: Deadly to ignore.* Retrieved May 9, 2011, from http://www.cdc.gov/OralHealth/publications/factsheets/oc_facts.htm.

66. Wyche, C. J., & Wilkins, E. M. (2009). The patient who is homebound. In Wilkins, E. M., Ed. *Clinical practice of the dental hygienist* (10th ed.). Philadelphia, PA: Lippincott Williams & Wilkins, 899–910.

67. Fuzy, J., & Leahy, W. (2006). *The home health aide handbook* (2nd ed.). (e book). Albuquerque: Hartman. Retrieved February 6, 2011, from http://books.google.com.

68. Frazer, C., Frazer, R. Q., & Raymond, J. (2009). Prevent infections with good denture care. *Nurs,* 39(8):50–53.

69. Paranhos, H. F. O., da Silva-Lovato, C. H., de Souza, R. F., Cruz, P. C., Freitas-Pontes, K. M., & Watanabe, E. (2009). Effect of three methods for cleaning dentures on biofilms formed in vitro on acrylic resin. *J Prosthodont,* 18:427–31.

70. Paranhos, H. F. O., da Silva-Lovato. C. H., de Souza, R. F., Cruz, P. C., Freitas, K. M., & Peracini, A. (2007). Effects of mechanical and chemical methods on denture biofilm accumulation. *J Oral Rehab,* 34:606–12.

71. American Dental Association. (n.d.) *Denture cleansers.* Chicago, IL: Author. Retrieved February 6, 2011, from Oral Health Topics), http://www.ada.org.

72. de Souza, R. F., de Freitas Oliveiras Paranhos, H., Lovato da Silva, C. H., Abu-Naba'a, L., Fedorowicz, Z., & Gurgan, C. A. (2009). Interventions for cleaning dentures in adults (Review). *Cochrane Datab Syst Rev* (Iss 4.). Retrieved February 5, 2011, from http://www.cfah.org/hbns/archives/viewSupportDoc.cfm?supportingDocID=839.

73. Cal, E., Guneri, P., & Kose, T. (2007). Digital analysis of mouthrinses' staining characteristics on provisional acrylic resins. *J Oral Rehab,* 34:297–303.

74. Nguyen, C. T., Masri, R., Driscoll, C. F., & Romberg, E. (2010). The effect of denture cleansing solutions on the retention of pink locator attachments: An in vitro study. *J Prosthodont,* 19:226–30.

75. Ragalis, K. (2009). Care of dental prostheses. In Wilkins, E. M., Ed. *Clinical practice of the dental hygienist* (10th ed.). Philadelphia, PA: Lippincott Williams & Wilkins, 472–88.

76. Lyle, D. M. (2010). Mechanical oral biofilm control: Interdental and supplemental self-care devices. In Darby, M. L., & Walsh, M. M., Eds. *Dental hygiene theory and practice.* St. Louis, MO: Saunders Elsevier, 401–16.

77. Ragalis, K. (2009). Care of patients with disabilities. In Wilkins, E. M., Ed. *Clinical practice of the dental hygienist* (10th ed.). Philadelphia, PA: Lippincott Williams & Wilkins, 870–98.

78. Peracini, A., Davi, L. R., Ribeiro, N. Q., de Souza, R. F., da Silva, C. H. L., & Paranhos, H. F. O. (2010). Effect of denture cleansers on physical properties of heat-polymerized acrylic resin. *J Prosthodont Res,* 54:78–82. Retrieved May 2, 2011, from http://www.sciencedirect.com/science/article/pii/S188319580900139X.

79. Machado, A. L., Breeding, L. C., Vergani, C. E., & Perez, L. E. C. (2009). Hardness and surface roughness of reline and denture base acrylic resins after repeated disinfection procedures. *J Prosthet Dent,* 102:115–22. Retrieved May 24, 2011, from http://www.ncbi.nlm.nih.gov/pubmed/19643225.

80. Paranhos, H. F. O., Resende, L., Peracini, A., Soares, R. B., Lovato, C. H. S., & de Souza, R. F. (2009). Comparison of physical and mechanical properties of microwave-polymerized acrylic resin after disinfection in sodium hypochlorite solutions. *Braz Dent J,* 20:331–35.

81. Paranhos, H. F. O., Orsi, I. A., Zaniquelli, O., Zuccolotto, M. C. C., & Magalhães, F. (2008). Effect of chemical denture cleansers on flexural resistance and color changes of microwave-polymerized acrylic resins. *Braz J Oral Sci,* 7(26):1580–84.

82. Garg, R. (2010). Denture hygiene, different strategies. *WebmedCentral Dent,* 1:WMC00932. Retrieved May 23, 2011, from http://www.webmedcentral.com/article_view/932.

83. Cosme, D. C., Baldisserotto, S. M., Fernandes, E. D. L., Rivaldo, E. G., Rosing, C. K., & Shinkai, R. S. A. (2006). Functional evaluation of oral rehabilitation with removable partial dentures after five years. *J Appl Oral Sci,* 14:1–12. Retrieved February 28, 2007, from http://www.scielo.br/scielo.php.

84. Vieira, A. P. C., Senna, P. M., da Silva, W. J., & Del Bel Cury, A. A. (2010). Long-term efficacy of denture cleansers in preventing *Candida* spp. biofilm recolonization on liner surface. *Braz Oral Res,* 24(3):e.

85. McIsaac, J. H. (2006). Decontamination and personal protection. In McIsaac, J. H. *Hospital preparation for bioterror: A medical and biomedical systems approach.* London: Elsevier Academic Press, 89–118.

86. Pavan, S., Filho, J. N. A., Dos Santos, P H., Nogueira, S. S., & Batista, A. U. D. (2007). Effect of disinfection treatments on the hardness of soft denture liner materials. *J Prosthodont,* 16:101–6.

87. Bhat, V. S., Shetty, M. S., & Shenoy K. K. (2007). Infection control in the prosthodontic laboratory. *J Indian Prosthodont Soc,* 7:62–65. Retrieved May 23, 2011, from http://www.adldental.com/resources/Infection%20Control.pdf?phpMyAdmin=qk%2Cl9c-CLBG-A3l-ODiEAfRI2I1.

88. Azarpazhooh, A., & Limeback, H. (2008). The application of ozone in dentistry: A systematic review of literature. *J Dent,* 36:104–16. Retrieved May 24, 2011, from http://www.sciencedirect.com.

89. Johnston, C. S., & Gaas, C. A. (2006, May 30). Vinegar: Medicinal uses and antiglycemic effect. *MedGenMed,* 8(2):e. Retrieved May 24, 2011, from http://www.ncbi.nlm.nih.gov/pmc/articles/PMC1785201/.

90. Uludamar, A., Ozkan, Y. K., Kadir, T., & Ceyhan, I. (2010). *In vivo* efficacy of alkaline peroxide tablets and mouthwashes on *Candida albicans* in patients with denture stomatitis. *J Appl Oral Sci,* 18(3)e.

91. U.S. Food and Drug Administration. (2008, February 14). *FDA public health notification: Denture cleanser allergic reactions and misuse.* Retrieved May 23, 2010, from http://www.fda.gov/MedicalDevices/Safety/AlertsandNotices/PublicHealthNotifications/ucm062012.htm.

92. Pusateri, C. R., Monaco, E. A., & Edgerton, M. (2009). Sensitivity of *Candida albicans* biofilm cells grown on denture acrylic to antifungal proteins and chlorhexidine. *Archiv Oral Biol,* 54:588–94. Retrieved May 24, 2011, from http://www.aobjournal.com/article/S0003-9969%2809%2900035-1/.

93. Spolarich, A. E., & Gurenlian, J. A. (2008). Drug-induced adverse oral events. In Daniel, S. J., Harfst, S. A., & Wilder, R. S., Eds. *Mosby's dental hygiene concepts, cases, and competencies.* St. Louis, MO: Mosby Elsevier, 259–76.

94. Atayese, A. O., Effedua, H. I., Oritogun, K. S., Kareem, K. T., & Ogunledun, A. (2010). Comparative study of the antimicrobial activity of chlorinated and non-chlorinated antiseptics against *C. albicans. Acad Arena,* 2:35–40. Retrieved May 24, 2011, from http://sciencepub.net/academia/aa0209/07_2699aa0209_35_40.pdf.

95. American College of Prosthodontists. (2010). *Dentures: How to properly apply denture adhesive.* Chicago, IL: Author. Retrieved February 6, 2011, from Public & Patients, http://www.prosthodontics.org.

96. Murata, H., Hong, G., Yamakado, C., Kurogi, T., Kano, H., & Hamada, T. (2010). Dynamic viscoelastic properties, water absorption, and solubility of home reliners. *Dent Mater J,* 29:554–61. Retrieved May 21, 2011, from http://www.jstage.jst.go.jp/article/dmj/29/5/554/_pdf.

97. Pisani, M. X., da Silva, C. H. L., Paranhos, H. F. O., de Souza, R. F., & Macedo, A. P. (2010). The effect of experimental denture cleanser solution *ricinus communis* on acrylic resin properties. *Mater Res,* 13:e.

98. Nations, S. P., Boyer, P. J., Love, L. A., Burritt, M. F., Burz, J. A., Wolfe, G. I., Hynan, L. S., Reisch, J., & Trivedi, J. R. (2008). Denture cream: An unusual source of excess zinc, leading to hypocupremia and neurologic disease. *Neurol,* 71:639–43.

99. Hope, J. (2010, February 19). Drug firm removes zinc from denture glue over health fears. *MailOnline.* London: Associated Newspapers, Ltd. Retrieved May 24, 2011, from http://www.dailymail.co.uk/health/article-1252051/Poligrip-remove-zinc-denture-adhesive-concerns-triggers-health-problems.html#ixzz1NQCRnuXs.

100. U.S. Food and Drug Administration. (2011, February 23). *Letter sent to denture adhesive manufacturers.* Washington DC: Author. Retrieved May 24, 2011, from http://www.fda.gov/downloads/MedicalDevices/ResourcesforYou/Industry/UCM244652.pdf.

101. Wilson, D. (2010, February 18). Glaxo plans to remove zinc from Poligrip denture adhesive. *NY Times.* (Online). Retrieved May 24, 2011, from http://www.nytimes.com/2010/02/19/business/19grip.html.

102. Turner, M., Jahangiri, L., & Ship, J. A. (2008). Hyposalivation, xerostomia and the complete denture: A systematic review. *J Am Dent Assoc,* 139:146–50.

103. So, J. S., Chung, S. C., Kho, H. S., Kim, Y. K., & Chung, J.W. (2010). Dry mouth among the elderly in Korea: A survey of prevalence, severity, and associated factors. *Oral Surg Oral Med Oral Pathol Oral Radiol Endod,* 110:475–83.

104. Sipahi, C., Beyzadeoglu, M., Demirtas, S., & Ozen, J. (2007). Effect of different mucosal and acrylic resin surface treatments in a denture retention model for patients with radiotherapy-induced xerostomia. *Int J Prosthodont,* 20:405–8.

PEARSON **myhealthprofessionskit™**

Visit www.myhealthprofessionskit.com to access the interactive Companion Website for this textbook. Simply select "Dental Hygiene" from the choice of disciplines. Find this book and log in by using your user name and password to access additional learning tools.

The authors extend their gratitude to Elaine R. Schilling, D.D.S., M.S. in Prosthodontics, North Texas Dental Specialists PC, Sherman, Texas, for her consultation and assistance with patient photographs during the preparation of this chapter.

Community Water Fluoridation

Howard F. Pollick

OBJECTIVES

After studying this chapter, the student should be able to:

1. Define *community water fluoridation*.

2. Describe the four historical periods in the evolution and development of community water fluoridation.

3. Explain the role of community water fluoridation and the impact of multiple sources of fluoride on the decline of dental caries.

4. Describe the effect of the discontinuation of water fluoridation in a community on caries prevalence.

5. Describe fluorosis classifications and characteristics by severity and the need to monitor exposure to fluoride.

6. Describe the economic aspects of water fluoridation.

7. State the optimal fluoride concentration for drinking water in the United States, in parts per million (ppm F), for maximum caries protection with minimal risk of fluorosis.

8. List the additives used for water fluoridation and briefly describe the technical aspects of fluoridation, including monitoring and surveillance of water fluoridation in the United States.

9. Describe the regulatory standards and policies for naturally occurring fluoride in drinking water.

10. State the daily Adequate Intake and Tolerable Upper Limit of fluoride for different age groups.

11. Summarize the current status of fluoridation in other countries and describe alternatives to water fluoridation.

INTRODUCTION

Community water fluoridation, also referred to as **fluoridation**, is defined as the upward adjustment of the natural fluoride level in a community's water supply to a level optimal for dental health. It is a population-based method of primary prevention that uses piped water systems to deliver a low concentration of fluoride over frequent intervals during the day. By consuming the water directly or indirectly through incorporation in foods and beverages, consumers accrue preventive benefits regardless of age or socioeconomic status. Fluoridation has been cited by the Centers for Disease Control and Prevention (CDC) as one of the 10 great public health achievements of the 20th century. Extensive research spanning more than 65 years has consistently supported the effectiveness, safety, and cost-effectiveness of fluoridation. Fluoridation contributed to a dramatic decline in dental caries from the 1950s to the 1980s and continues to effectively reduce and prevent tooth decay today when multiple sources of fluoride, such as fluoride toothpaste, are readily available. Continued monitoring of fluoride exposure from all sources, especially from discretionary sources such as fluoride-containing toothpaste, is important to achieve the appropriate balance between maximum caries-preventive benefit and minimal risk of enamel fluorosis. Fluoridation has been shown to be an effective intervention and sound public policy; however, vocal opponents have challenged the practice of fluoridating community water supplies (CWS) since its inception.

Fluoridation can be enacted at the state level by legislative action but more commonly is implemented at the local level through administrative action or a vote of the electorate. Communities often become embroiled in hard-fought, emotional fluoridation referenda that attract significant media attention. Initiation of a fluoridation campaign requires careful planning and coordination, which includes conducting an assessment to determine a community's readiness. Support for fluoridation can be influenced by public opinion; the political climate; the media; voter turnout; knowledge, skills, and political savvy of the campaign committee; external forces; key community leaders; and other factors. Oral health professionals need to remain well informed about issues and events affecting fluoridation by keeping abreast of the scientific literature as well as relevant state and community policy decisions. Dentists and dental hygienists should be able to provide accurate information to their patients and address questions about fluoridation benefits or risks. This duty requires not only a grasp of the science but also an understanding of the forces that affect public attitudes, the policy process, and the strategies employed by the opposition. This chapter defines community water fluoridation, reviews its history, and provides information about effectiveness, cariostatic mechanisms of action, safety, cost-effectiveness, engineering aspects, and strategies used by proponents and opponents of fluoridation. The principles of risk communication are important to educational and promotional efforts for fluoridation.

DEFINITION AND BACKGROUND

The American Dental Association (ADA) officially defines **community water fluoridation** as the adjustment of the natural fluoride concentration in water up to the level recommended for optimal dental health.[1] In 2011, the U.S. Department of Health and Human Services (HHS) proposed "new guidance to update and replace the 1962 U.S. Public Health Service Drinking Water Standards related to recommendations for fluoride concentrations in drinking water. The U.S. Public Health Service recommendations for optimal fluoride concentrations were based on ambient air temperature of geographic areas and ranged from 0.7–1.2 mg/L. HHS proposed that community water systems adjust the amount of fluoride to 0.7 mg/L to achieve an optimal fluoride level. For the purpose of this guidance, the optimal concentration of fluoride in drinking water is that concentration that provides the best balance of protection from dental caries while limiting the risk of dental fluorosis. Community water fluoridation is the adjusting and monitoring of fluoride in drinking water to reach the optimal concentration."[2] Parts per million (ppm) and milligrams/liter (mg/l) are essentially equivalent, and the terms are used interchangeably. One part per million is the same concentration as 1 mg/l. Some documents refer to concentrations used in water fluoridation as parts per million; others use milligrams per liter. In this chapter, parts per million will be used.

Fluoride is the reduced or ionic form of fluorine, the 13th most abundant element on earth. This naturally occurring substance is found in water, soil, plants, and even in air. Certain foods, such as tea and fish, contain significant amounts of fluoride.[3] Oceans of the world contain fluoride at concentrations equal to or above levels used for community water fluoridation.[4] Virtually all water sources contain some naturally occurring fluoride; surface water such as rivers, lakes, and reservoirs normally contain lower amounts of fluoride than ground water, which is obtained from wells that draw water from beneath the earth's surface. Because most freshwater sources contain natural levels of fluoride at concentrations below those recommended for optimal dental health, the amount of fluoride is adjusted upward to the optimal level (Figure 14–1 ■).

The Institute of Medicine and the World Health Organization (WHO) identify fluoride as a nutrient important for health.[5,6] Fluoridation can be thought of as a form of nutritional supplementation in which fluoride is added to the drinking water. Nutritional supplementation frequently is used to prevent diseases; examples include the addition of vitamin C to fruit juices to prevent scurvy; vitamin D to milk and breads to prevent rickets; iodine to table salt to prevent goiter; folic acid to

Naturally occurring F in water + Added F = 0.7 ppm F ↑ Optimal Level

FIGURE ■ 14–1 Adjustment of fluoride concentration in water.

grains, cereals, and pastas to prevent birth defects, including spina bifida; and other vitamins and minerals to breakfast cereals to promote normal growth and development. The treatment of water for public consumption is a primary public health activity that has been used by public health agencies to prevent diseases since the 1840s. Water treatment prevents diseases such as amoebic dysentery, cholera, enteropathogenic diarrhea (*Escherichia coli*), giardiasis, hepatitis A, leptospirosis, paratyphoid fever, schistosomiasis, typhoid fever, and many other diseases including dental caries.[7,8]

Fluoridation is an example of an ideal public health intervention in that it (1) benefits people of all ages, (2) is socially equitable and does not exclude any group, (3) imparts continuous protection with no compliance or conscious effort required by consumers other than drinking optimally fluoridated water, (4) works without requiring individuals to access care or gather in a prescribed location as with other disease-prevention strategies or programs such as immunizations, (5) does not require the costly services of health professionals, (6) requires no daily-dosage schedules, (7) does not involve taking painful inoculations or oral medicines, and (8) is remarkably cost effective.

Every U.S. Surgeon General since 1950 has advocated the adoption of water fluoridation by communities. Dr. Luther Terry, U.S. Surgeon General, 1961 to 1965, described water fluoridation as one of the four great advances in public health, calling it one of the "four horsemen of public health," along with chlorination, pasteurization, and immunization. Dr. C. Everett Koop, U.S. Surgeon General, 1981 to 1989, stated, "Fluoridation is the single most important commitment that a community can make to the oral health of its children and to future generations."[9] In 1992, U.S. Surgeon General Antonia Novello stated, "the optimum standard for the success of any prevention strategy should be measured by its ability to prevent or minimize disease, ease of implementation, high benefit-to-cost ratio, and safety. Community water fluoridation to prevent tooth decay clearly meets this standard."[10] U.S. Surgeon General David Satcher stated, "Community water fluoridation remains one of the great achievements of public health in the twentieth century" and "an inexpensive means of improving oral health that benefits all residents of a community, young and old, rich and poor alike."[11] In the first-ever report on oral health in the United States, released in May 2000, *Oral Health in America: A Report of the Surgeon General,* Dr. Satcher noted that "one of my highest priorities as Surgeon General is reducing the disparities in health that persist among our various populations. Fluoridation holds great potential to contribute toward elimination of these disparities."[12] U.S. Surgeon General Richard Carmona issued a strong endorsement stating, "Policymakers, community leaders, private industry, health professionals, the media, and the public should affirm that oral health is essential to general health and well being and take action to make ourselves, our families, and our communities healthier. I join previous Surgeons General in acknowledging the continuing public health role for community water fluoridation in enhancing the oral health of all Americans."[13]

Fluoridation is a population-based method of primary prevention designed to serve as the cornerstone for the prevention of dental caries, one of the most prevalent childhood diseases. In 2010, 18,427 community water systems serving U.S. communities had fluoridated water, and 73.9% of the U.S. population using public water systems, or a total of 204,283,554 people, had access to fluoridated water.[14]

HISTORY OF COMMUNITY WATER FLUORIDATION

The history of community water fluoridation in the United States can be traced back to the first decade of the 20th century and may be categorized into four separate periods or phases: (1) clinical discovery phase, (2) epidemiologic phase, (3) demonstration phase, and (4) technology transfer phase.[15–18]

The first period, the **clinical discovery phase**, 1901 to 1933, was characterized by the pursuit of knowledge to determine the cause of developmental enamel defects present in people exposed to naturally occurring high levels of fluoride in drinking water in certain western areas of the United States. In 1901, Dr. Frederick McKay, a recent dental school graduate, moved west and set up a dental practice in Colorado Springs, Colorado. He noticed that some of his patients presented with discolored enamel that sometimes exhibited surfaces that were rough, uneven, or even pitted. Local residents called this condition "Colorado Brown Stain." McKay made two important observations about this enamel defect: (1) The stains could not be polished away, meaning that they were intrinsic, or incorporated into the enamel structure, and (2) not everyone's enamel had these characteristics; only a small portion of patients had it, and they were limited to a subgroup of patients who had either been born in Colorado Springs or moved there at a very young age. The fact that this uncharacteristic enamel condition was not present among individuals who had not lived in the vicinity as young children led McKay to believe that the etiologic or causal agent was environmental in nature and was incorporated into the enamel structure at the time of tooth formation.

McKay named this condition "mottled enamel" and noted that it appeared to be under-mineralized, or hypomineralized, enamel.[19] McKay sought the consultation of Dr. G. V. Black, one of the most well-known and respected researchers, and together they notified the dental profession about this condition by publishing their observations in *Dental Cosmos,* the premier national dental journal of the time[20] (Figure 14–2 ■). Over several decades, McKay examined children in various nearby communities and other states to determine the extent of the condition in the population. He was able to demonstrate that mottled enamel was confined to specific geographic areas, and he hypothesized and demonstrated that this condition was directly related to something in the drinking water in these areas.[18,21] In 1927, McKay published an important corollary finding: People who had enamel fluorosis also experienced less dental decay.[22]

Around the same time period, in the early 1930s, H. V. Churchill, a chemist with the Aluminum Company of America, used a new method of spectrographic analysis to examine the water in the town of Bauxite, Arkansas, known to have residents with high levels of mottled enamel. He identified high levels of

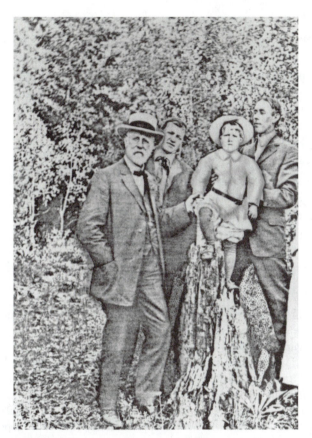

FIGURE ■ 14–2 In 1909, Dr. G. V. Black (left) visited Dr. F. McKay (right) in Colorado Springs to investigate the Colorado brown stain phenomenon.

(*Source:* Courtesy of the Centers for Disease Control and Prevention (CDC).)

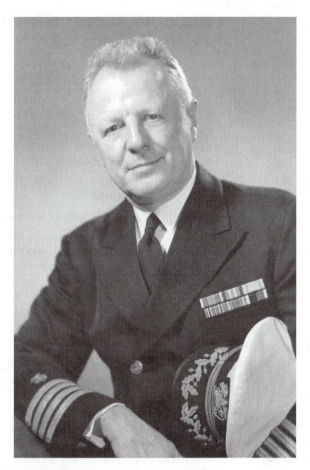

FIGURE ■ 14–3 Dr. H. Trendley Dean.

(*Source:* Courtesy of the Centers for Disease Control and Prevention (CDC).)

naturally occurring fluoride in the drinking water supply.[19,23] McKay contacted Churchill and sent him samples of water from Colorado Springs and other areas he had observed to have a high prevalence of mottled enamel. The results showed fluoride concentrations ranging from 2 ppm F to 12 ppm F.[24] McKay had identified his etiologic agent. The high level of fluoride in the water was associated with mottled enamel.

The search for additional information about the role of fluoride in the cause of enamel fluorosis and the prevention of dental caries led to the second period, known as the **epidemiologic phase**, which lasted from 1933 to 1945. Concern about the discovery of fluoride in the water led to the appointment of Dr. H. Trendley Dean, a commissioned officer in the U.S. Public Health Service. Dean was the sole person in what was called the Dental Hygiene Unit, part of the newly established National Institutes of Health (Figure 14–3 ■).

Dean's job was to map out the prevalence of mottled enamel across the country and to look for a way to reduce or eliminate it. He wrote to dental societies across the country asking for their input regarding fluorosis in their locale; in 1933, he published his first map showing the prevalence of mottled enamel in the United States.[25] Although this era predated databases or computers, Dean showed remarkable organizational and epidemiologic prowess in collecting, sorting, and mapping data. By the mid-1930s, he began using the term *fluorosis* to replace *mottled enamel*. In 1934, Dean developed the Community Fluorosis Index that allowed collection and mapping of severity data in addition to prevalence data.[26] This index assessed not only the location of the condition but also its severity. Dean later modified the index to classify the full range of enamel conditions from fine, lacy markings to stained, pitted, damaged enamel (Table 14–1 ■).

DID YOU KNOW

The Dental Hygiene Unit evolved over time into the National Institute of Dental Research, which later became the National Institute of Dental and Craniofacial Research.

DID YOU KNOW ?

Dean's Fluorosis Index has been the most widely used fluorosis index in the world and is still used today, especially for surveillance and research activities.

TABLE ■ 14–1   Dean's Fluorosis Index

Diagnosis	Criteria
Normal	Usual translucent semivitriform type of structure; smooth, glossy, usually a pale creamy-white color
Questionable	Slight deviation from normal translucency ranging from a few white "flecks" to occasional white spots
Very mild	Less than 25% of tooth's surface affected; small, opaque, paper-white areas scattered irregularly over the tooth; tips of cusps often show "snow capping"
Mild	More than 25% but less than 50% of tooth's surface affected; more extensive, opaque, paper-white areas
Moderate	All enamel surfaces affected, frequently with brown staining
Severe	All enamel surfaces affected with widespread brown staining and discreet or confluent pitting; teeth can exhibit a "corroded" appearance

In addition to studying fluorosis during the epidemiologic phase, researchers began looking at the relationship of fluoride in the water and tooth decay. With assistance from colleagues at the U.S. Public Health Service's National Institutes of Health, Dean conducted some impressive epidemiologic studies, including the "4 city study" and "Dean's 21-Cities Study." The 4 city study highlighted the difference in dental health and fluorosis among four Illinois cities with differing concentrations of fluoride in the water supply[27] (Table 14–2 ■).

In the 21-city study, Dean examined the data collected by teams of researchers who had examined the teeth of children residing in 21 different communities that had varying levels of naturally occurring fluoride in the drinking water.[28,29] Dean and his team documented the number of carious lesions and fluorosed teeth observed in each of the 21 communities and compared the findings with the fluoride concentration in the respective water supplies. The findings from Dean's 21-City Study showed that (1) higher concentrations of fluoride in the water correlated with fewer teeth affected by dental caries in children, constituting an inverse relationship between the level of natural fluoride in the water and the prevalence of dental caries and (2) higher levels of fluoride were associated with more children with fluorosis of the teeth, meaning that

a direct relationship existed between the level of natural fluoride in the water and the prevalence of enamel fluorosis (Figure 14–4 ■).

Dean's results showed that both a reduction of dental caries and an acceptable level of enamel fluorosis could be attained with water containing fluoride levels at approximately 1 ppm of fluoride. At this level, substantial reductions in dental caries of up to 60% were observed with approximately 10% of the population exhibiting very mild enamel fluorosis. The unattractive form of fluorosis, often called *mottling,* that was associated with higher levels of fluoride was not observed to occur at the level of 1 ppm F. Consequently, 1 ppm F became the benchmark level, and was used by the U.S. Public Health Service in 1962 in establishing the optimal range: 0.7 ppm F to 1.2 ppm F. The optimal fluoride level seeks to maximize the benefits of dental caries reduction and minimize the probability of enamel fluorosis (Figure 14–5 ■).

The third period, known as the **demonstration phase,** began in January 1945 and was characterized by a series of community trials in which fluoride levels were adjusted in the public drinking water supply. On January 25, 1945, Grand Rapids, Michigan, became the first city in the world to fluoridate its drinking water as a measure to promote dental health and

TABLE ■ 14–2   Dean's "4 City" Study

City	Fluoride (ppm) in Water	Number of Children[a]	Caries Free (%)	Mean DMFT	Prevalence of Mottled Enamel
Quincy	0.2	291	4.1	6.28	0.0
Macomb	0.2	63	14.3	3.68	1.6
Monmouth	1.7	99	36.4	2.08	67.7
Galesburg	1.8	243	36.2	1.94	46.9

DMFT: decayed, missing, filled teeth.

[a]Children ages 12–14 years with a history of continuous use of the public water supply.

(*Source:* Dean, H. T., Jay P., Arnold, Jr., F. A., McClure, F. J., & Elvove, E. (1939). Domestic water and dental caries, including certain epidemiological aspects of oral *L. Acidophilus. Public Health Rep,* 54:862–88.)

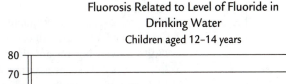

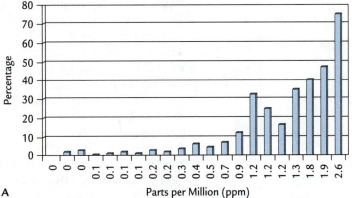

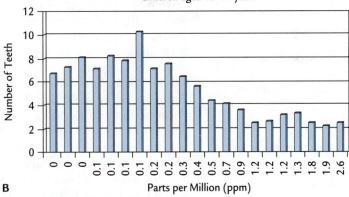

FIGURE ■ 14–4 Findings from 21 cities studied by Dean and colleagues in the 1930s showing the prevalence of dental caries and enamel fluorosis.

(*Source:* Data from Dean, H. T., Jay P., Arnold, Jr., F. A., McClure, F. J., & Elvove, E. (1939). Domestic water and dental caries, including certain epidemiological aspects of oral L. Acidophilus. *Public Health Rep*, 54:862–88.)

prevent disease. Grand Rapids was the test, or intervention, city; Muskegon, Michigan, whose water was not fluoridated, was the control city. These cities were the first of four pairs of demonstration cities; the others were (listed by intervention and control) Newburgh and Kingston, New York; Evanston and Oak Park, Illinois; and Brantford and Sarnia, Ontario, Canada. The demonstration cities allowed a comparison of dental and medical observations collected over time from children living in communities with community water fluoridation and those in communities with negligible levels of naturally occurring fluoride. The results were impressive. Sequential cross-sectional surveys conducted in these communities over 13 to 15 years showed reductions in dental caries of 50% to 70% among children in the communities with fluoridated water[30] (Table 14–3 ■).

The demonstration phase lasted until about 1954; at that time, the benefits of the optimal adjustment of fluoride levels in drinking water became so apparent that many U.S. cities began fluoridation programs for their citizens. Thus, the

demonstration phase overlapped slightly with the fourth period in the history of community water fluoridation, known as the *technology transfer phase.*

The **technology transfer phase** began about 1950 when planning began in earnest for the implementation of fluoridation in many large U.S. cities. Continuing to this day, the technology transfer phase is characterized by the establishment of a set of national health goals, which include fluoridation. The year 2020 health objectives for the nation call for increasing the proportion of the U.S. population served by community water systems with optimally fluoridated water. The Healthy People 2020 target goal for fluoridation is that 79.6% of the U.S. population on community water systems should be served with fluoridated water, which represents a 10% increase over the 2008 statistic.[31]

In 2010, 73.9% of the U.S. population on community water systems received fluoridated water (more than 204 million people).[14] This percentage has increased every year since 1945 when fluoridation began in Grand Rapids, Michigan. See

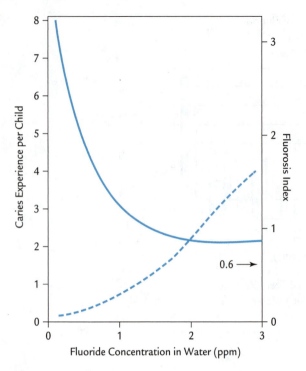

FIGURE ■ 14–5 Dean's Fluorosis Index/caries/fluorosis curve.

Dean considered a Community Fluorosis Index above 0.6 to be of public health significance

(*Source:* Data from Dean, H. T., Jay P., Arnold, Jr., F. A., McClure, F. J., & Elvove, E. (1939). Domestic water and dental caries, including certain epidemiological aspects of oral L. Acidophilus. *Public Health Rep*, 54:862–88.)

Figure 14–6 ■ for trends in total U.S. population growth, people on public water systems, and people who have optimally fluoridated water.[32] Interestingly, the number of people drinking *naturally* fluoridated water has not increased as explained by the fact that most *naturally* fluoridated waters are groundwater systems serving small populations. About 10 million people in the United States are served by drinking water with optimal levels of *naturally* occurring fluoride.

In total, in 2010, 66.2% of the entire U.S. population and 73.9% of the population served by centralized piped-water systems received drinking water with optimal fluoride concentrations.[14] State rankings show wide variations in the percentage of the population receiving fluoridation (Table 14–4 ■). Between 2000 and 2010, the U.S. population on community water systems served by water fluoridation increased from 65.8% to 73.9%, advancing toward the Healthy People 2010 target of 75%. Twenty-six states have met or exceeded the Healthy People 2010 goal of 75% of the population being served by community water fluoridation. Of the nation's largest cities, 45 of 50 have adopted fluoridation. Of the five largest U.S. cities that are not fluoridated—Fresno, Portland, San Jose, Tucson, and Wichita—Fresno and Tucson have partially fluoridated water; Portland and San Jose made decisions to fluoridate in 2012. The most recent and largest U.S. city to fluoridate is San Diego, which began fluoridation in 2011. In 2010, the United States had more than 18,427 public water systems with optimal levels of fluoride. Of these water systems, 6,042 have fluoride levels adjusted to optimal levels, more than 5,590 water systems have natural fluoride levels at or above optimal levels, and approximately 6,795 water systems are consecutive with optimal systems.[14]

The technology transfer phase has extended fluoridation worldwide with Singapore implementing fluoridation in 1958, serving 100% of the population.[19] The Republic of Ireland became the first country to actually legislate mandatory nationwide fluoridation in 1960. Israel initiated its mandatory universal fluoridation program in 1981. Countries offering water fluoridation include the United Kingdom, Chile, South Korea, Singapore, Spain, Ireland, Israel, the United States, Canada, Brazil, Malaysia, Vietnam, Australia, and New Zealand.[13] The WHO issued the following statement in 2005: "Fluoridation of water supplies, where possible, is the most effective public health measure for the prevention of dental decay."[32] Advocated by the WHO, fluoridation benefits over 405 million people in 60 countries worldwide.[13]

Because of its history of effectiveness in reducing the prevalence of dental caries in the United States, the U.S. CDC has cited water fluoridation as one of the 10 great public health achievements of the 20th century.

MECHANISMS OF ACTION OF FLUORIDE

Fluoride works in three ways to reduce and prevent tooth decay: (1) systemically by being ingested and incorporated into the enamel structure during tooth development,[33] (2) topically by

TABLE ■ 14–3   Classic Fluoridation Studies of Paired Cities

Fluoridated Cities	Demonstration Phase	
	Year of Study[a]	Decrease in DMFT of Children Ages 12–14 Years
Grand Rapids, MI	1959	55.5%
Newburgh, NY	1960	70.1%
Evanston, IL	1959	48.4%
Brantford, ON	1959	56.7%

DMFT: Decayed, Missing (extracted due to caries), and Filled permanent teeth.
[a]All four communities began fluoridating in 1945–1946.
(*Source:* Based on Burt, B. A., & Eklund, S. A. (2005). *Dentistry, dental practice, and the community* (6th Ed.). St. Louis, Mo: Elsevier Saunders.)

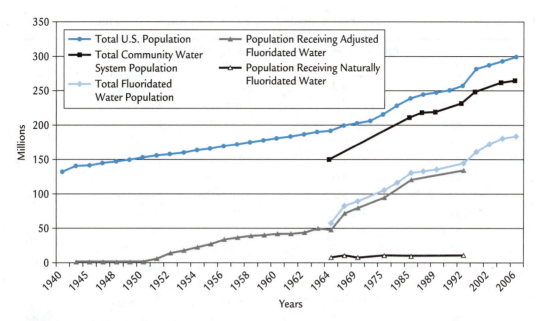

FIGURE ■ 14–6 **Fluoridation chart.**

(*Source:* National Center for Chronic Disease Prevention and Health Promotion. National Oral Health Surveillance System. Fluoridation Growth by Population, United States 1940–2006. Accessed at http://www.cdc.gov/nohss/FSGrowth.htm on 9/23/2013.)

promoting remineralization and inhibiting demineralization of tooth surfaces after eruption,[34,35] and (3) topically by inhibiting glycolysis in microorganisms, thereby hindering the ability of bacteria to metabolize carbohydrates and produce acid.[36] The greatest effect on reducing and preventing decay is topical[34]; however, both systemic and topical mechanisms are important.

Systemic fluoride is ingested, or taken into the body, during consumption of foods or beverages. Systemic fluoride can be incorporated directly into the hydroxyapatite crystalline structure of the developing tooth with the smaller fluoride ions replacing hydroxyl ions in the crystalline structure of the tooth and producing a less-soluble apatite crystal.[37,38] In the years before water fluoridation was initiated and for several decades afterwards the caries-preventive properties of fluoride were attributed almost exclusively to the systemic, or pre-eruptive, effects on the developing teeth. Because it was known that enamel fluorosis could occur only by incorporating fluoride into the structure of developing teeth, this assumption was reasonable. Today it is accepted that the systemic effect on caries prevention is the lesser effect compared to the topical effect[34]; however, there is current evidence that systemic exposure to fluoride during tooth formation reduces tooth decay.[39,40]

Topical fluoride concentrates in the plaque and saliva,[34,41] thereby enabling it to come into frequent contact with the surfaces of the teeth. These posteruptive effects can benefit people of nearly all ages by reducing decay on both the coronal and root surfaces.[42,43] The decay process is a continuum that involves both demineralization and remineralization and can move in either direction. Just as tooth structure can be lost through demineralization, the enamel can reform through remineralization. Cycles of demineralization and remineralization continue throughout the lifetime of the tooth (Figure 14–7 ■). Fluoride, especially that held in plaque, is an essential nutrient in the remineralization of teeth.[34]

Cariogenic bacteria residing in dental plaque metabolize sugars and other carbohydrates, producing acid that begins to dissolve, or demineralize, the tooth's enamel crystal surface. Calcium, phosphate, and carbonate are lost from the enamel and can be captured in the adjacent plaque. The lowered pH caused by the acid also releases fluoride contained in the plaque. Then the fluoride from the plaque and available saliva is taken up by the demineralized enamel along with calcium and phosphate; this results in remineralization as the ions reform into an improved enamel crystal structure that contains more fluoride and less carbonate and is more resistant to acid.[37,38] Fluoride also inhibits the process that bacteria use to metabolize carbohydrates, thus reducing bacterial acid production and reducing dissolution of tooth enamel.[24,44–49]

One reason that water fluoridation is the most effective method of fluoride delivery is that populations consume small quantities of water, directly or indirectly, throughout the day, not just a couple of times when they brush their teeth or eat. Fluoride from the water is also incorporated into manufactured beverages; absorbed into foods, such as vegetables while growing; and through cooking, such as soups, and foods that swell with water, such as rice and pasta. Therefore, on a regular basis, water fluoridation replenishes small quantities of fluoride to the plaque and saliva, which contributes to reduced tooth decay and good oral health.

Systemic fluorides also provide a topical effect because saliva contains some fluoride from ingestion, is continually available at the tooth surface, and becomes concentrated in dental plaque where it inhibits acid-producing cariogenic bacteria from demineralizing tooth enamel.[1,44] Fluoride concentration in the plaque is 50 to 100 times higher than in the whole saliva.[19,50]

TABLE ■ 14–4 State Fluoridation Percentage Calculations and States Ranked by Fluoridation Percentage, 2010

State	%	Persons Receiving Fluoridated Water	Persons Served by CWS	State	Rank
United States	73.9	204,283,554	276,607,387	Kentucky	1
Alabama	80.0	3,821,766	4,779,736	Maryland	2
Alaska	62.8	404,039	643,373	Illinois	3
Arizona	56.7	3,114,799	5,493,584	Minnesota	4
Arkansas	64.7	1,724,131	2,666,306	North Dakota	5
California	62.1	22,812,721	36,756,666	Virginia	6
Colorado	70.1	3,523,554	5,029,196	South Dakota	7
Connecticut	91.0	2,370,423	2,604,427	Indiana	8
Delaware	86.2	705,344	818,110	West Virginia	9
District of Columbia	100	595,000	595,000	Iowa	10
Florida	78.0	13,377,651	17,156,553	Georgia	11
Georgia	92.1	8,924,598	9,687,653	Michigan	Tied for 12
Hawaii	10.8	139,598	1,290,549	Tennessee	Tied for 12
Idaho	30.5	335,127	1,099,561	Connecticut	14
Illinois	99.3	11,325,132	11,403,176	Wisconsin	15
Indiana	94.4	4,326,732	4,582,296	Ohio	16
Iowa	92.3	2,344,818	2,541,455	North Carolina	17
Kansas	65.1	1,155,071	1,775,588	South Carolina	18
Kentucky	99.9	4,334,223	4,339,367	Delaware	19
Louisiana	40.7	1,846,149	4,533,372	Rhode Island	20
Maine	79.0	521,414	660,367	Texas	21
Maryland	99.8	5,140,618	5,151,947	Alabama	22
Massachusetts	70.7	4,626,859	6,547,629	Missouri	23
Michigan	91.6	7,322,410	7,996,744	Maine	24
Minnesota	98.8	4,117,266	4,166,424	Florida	25
Mississippi	55.2	1,639,348	2,967,297	New Mexico	26
Missouri	79.8	3,966,102	4,966,951	New York	27
Montana	29.6	233,221	788,705	Nevada	28
Nebraska	70.2	1,001,665	1,425,929	Massachusetts	29
Nevada	72.9	1,855,460	2,544,079	Nebraska	30
New Hampshire	42.9	357,262	832,631	Colorado	31
New Jersey	13.5	1,111,624	8,221,293	Kansas	32
New Mexico	77.0	1,210,777	1,571,600	Arkansas	Tied for 33
New York	74.7	14,468,141	19,378,102	Oklahoma	Tied for 33
North Carolina	87.3	6,174,598	7,072,012	Washington	35
North Dakota	96.9	559,246	577,325	Alaska	36
Ohio	87.7	8,772,683	10,005,412	California	37
Oklahoma	64.7	2,296,459	3,547,668	Arizona	38
Oregon	22.6	833,227	3,688,540	Vermont	39
Pennsylvania	54.6	5,802,260	10,636,421	Mississippi	40
Rhode Island	85.3	853,580	1,000,413	Pennsylvania	41
South Carolina	87.1	3,434,565	3,944,594	New Hampshire	42
South Dakota	94.8	642,942	678,028	Louisiana	43
Tennessee	91.6	5,336,600	5,827,549	Wyoming	44
Texas	80.4	19,362,219	24,080,084	Utah	45
Utah	33.2	918,473	2,763,885	Idaho	46
Vermont	56.6	256,006	452,116	Montana	47

TABLE ■ 14–4 (Continued)

State	%	Persons Receiving Fluoridated Water	Persons Served by CWS	State	Rank
Virginia	95.6	6,124,274	6,403,141	Oregon	48
Washington	64.6	3,490,031	5,402,328	New Jersey	49
West Virginia	92.4	1,208,015	1,307,369	Hawaii	50
Wisconsin	87.9	3,300,037	3,755,613		
Wyoming	36.8	165,296	449,223		

(*Source:* Centers for Disease Control and Prevention. 2010 Water Fluoridation Statistics. Retrieved September 23, 2012 from http://www.cdc.gov/fluoridation/statistics/2010stats.htm.)

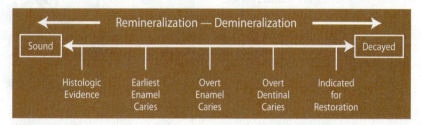

FIGURE ■ 14–7 Remineralization and demineralization of teeth.

In summary, fluoridation has been found to reduce dental decay by three mechanisms: (1) systemic ingestion of fluoride, which is incorporated into the developing tooth structure and converts hydroxyapatite into fluorapatite, thus reducing the solubility of tooth enamel in acid and making it more resistant to decay, (2) topical action of fluoride in the plaque and saliva, which enhances remineralization of tooth enamel that has been demineralized by acids produced by decay-causing bacteria, and (3) topical interaction with bacteria in the plaque, which reduces the acid production by dental-plaque organisms.

BENEFITS AND EFFECTIVENESS OF FLUORIDATION

Determination of the benefits and effectiveness of community water fluoridation should consider the state of the population's oral health before fluoridation. It may be difficult to imagine that, during the 1940s in the United States, extractions of first molars in young children were routine; complete dentures were the norm for older adults; 10% of recruits into World War II were rejected because of poor oral health, which meant those recruits did not have six opposing teeth; 40% needed immediate treatment for relief of pain; and dowries of new brides sometimes included dentures.

Over the past 65+ years, numerous studies have been conducted on the effectiveness of fluoridation and fluorides in preventing dental caries and decreasing caries rates. When Grand Rapids, Michigan, decided to fluoridate its water supply in 1945, a long-term study of schoolchildren was initiated to determine the effectiveness of fluoridation in decreasing dental caries rates; the study found that, after 11 years of fluoridation, dental caries rates had declined by 50% to 63%.[51,52]

Corroborative studies in the same era conducted in New York (Newburgh, Kingston) and Illinois (Evanston, Oak Park) reported reductions in caries rates from 57% to 70%.[53,54] Of 73 studies published between 1956 and 1979, the most frequently reported rate of caries reduction was 50% to 60%; it was generally acknowledged that fluoridating a community's water supply would reduce dental decay by half.[19]

Community water fluoridation has continued to play a dominant role in the decline in caries, even though the absolute differences in caries prevalence that once were observed between fluoridated and nonfluoridated communities appear to be diminishing.[27] During the early years of fluoridation, its primary source was the drinking water because there were no other discretionary sources of fluoride available, such as fluoride toothpaste. Consequently, the reductions in dental caries rates attributed to water fluoridation were easily measurable and significant. By 1980, 98% of the available toothpastes contained fluoride.[13,36] As more professional and consumer products containing fluoride came on the market, it was increasingly difficult to measure what portion of the caries reduction was attributable solely to water fluoridation. However, the impact of fluoridation remains evident.

The reduction in the absolute measurable benefits of water fluoridation has been attributed to the dilution and diffusion effects.[19] **Dilution** results from the increased availability of fluoride from multiple sources, diluting the impact of any one source of fluoride, including water.[55–57] Dilution is the apparent reduction in the measurable water fluoridation benefits resulting from the ubiquitous availability of fluoride from other sources in both the fluoridated and the fluoride-deficient comparison community.[15] Today the most universally available source of fluoride in the United States is a fluoride-containing toothpaste.[17,57] All fluoride-containing toothpastes have very high concentrations of fluoride, from 1,100 ppm F to 1,500 ppm F, and are a significant potential source of fluoride overexposure and fluorosis in young children. Moreover, toothpastes are not meant to be swallowed, especially during the years when the crowns of teeth are forming.[58] The other major modifying factor regarding the effectiveness of fluoridation is the diffusion effect. **Diffusion** is described as the extension of benefits of community water fluoridation to residents of fluoride-deficient communities.[19] Diffusion results from the consumption of commercial foods and beverages that were processed in a fluoridated community and transported to fluoride-deficient communities, making fluoride available to consumers in the fluoride-deficient community.[59] Just as ripples in a lake affect water many feet away from the center, foods and beverages produced in fluoridated cities can reach nonfluoridated cities that are hundreds or thousands of miles distant.

Diffusion has also been called the "halo effect." The differences in caries-prevalence rates between fluoridated and nonfluoridated communities are diminishing.[6] According to Ripa, the weaker association reported by contemporary studies between exposure to fluoridated drinking water and caries experience, therefore, is not due to a lessening of the effects of waterborne fluoride but is actually caused by the extension of those effects through a process of diffusion of fluoride into fluoride-deficient areas[19] (Figure 14–8 ■). Increased mobility of the population with travel to fluoridated communities impacts the effect of diffusion as well. Also, residents who live in a fluoride-deficient community and work on a military base in the same community may be exposed to fluoridated water because most military bases have it.

In 1986–1987, decades after the initiation of community water fluoridation, the National Institute of Dental Research (NIDR) conducted an epidemiologic study of more than 39,000 children ages 5–17 years.[55,60] This study determined that younger children who had lived all their lives in optimally fluoridated communities experienced fewer carious lesions and fillings compared with children who had lived in nonfluoridated communities. The impact of water fluoridation and other sources of fluoride on dental caries is apparent from examination of the

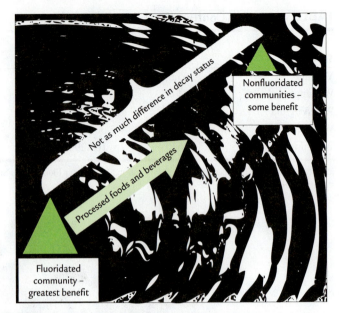

FIGURE ■ 14–8 Diffusion of fluoridation benefits.

(*Source:* National Survey Findings.)

findings of national surveys assessing the oral health status of school-age children in the United States, which show a steady decline in rates of caries prevalence and increasing percentages of children who are caries free (Figure 14–9 ■). With this decline is the recognition that socioeconomic status has a profound influence on caries severity. In U.S. surveys from 1988 to 1994 and 1999 to 2004, the number of filled tooth surfaces in young children (Figure 14-10■) has also increased. Although this has been described as an increase in caries severity, it is noted that the mean number of untreated carious surfaces for these children has not increased, so it could instead represent an increase in access to care and dental treatment.[61]

In separate studies, Brunelle and Carlos (1990) and Murray and colleagues (1991) found higher percentages of caries-free children and lower caries-prevalence rates in fluoridated

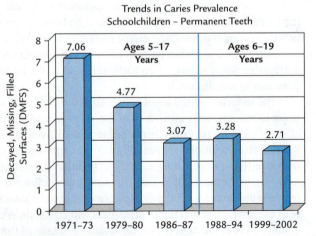

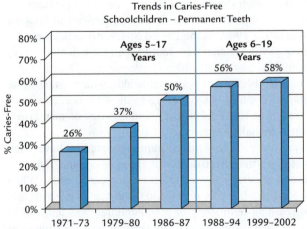

FIGURE ■ 14–9 Decline in prevalence rates of caries in U.S. schoolchildren.

(*Source:* National Survey Findings.)

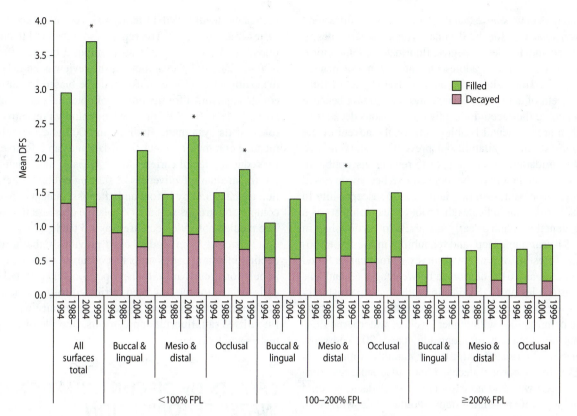

FIGURE ■ 14–10 **The relationship between poverty and pediatric dental decay.**

Difference in mean Decayed, Missing due to caries and Filled Permanent Tooth Surfaces (DMFS) between children with continuous exposure to water fluoridation and those with no such exposure.

(*Source:* Data from Table 6 of Brunelle, J. A., & Carlos, J. P. (1990).)

communities where other sources of fluoride were also available.[55,62] The findings of these two studies emphasize that water fluoridation remains an important contributor to caries prevention.[17,55] Analyzing the 1986–1987 NIDR data, Brunelle and Carlos found that when excluding children with a reported history of exposure to supplemental or topical fluorides, there was a 25% lower mean number of Decayed, Missing due to caries and Filled Permanent Tooth Surfaces (DMFS) among a sample of 3574 children ages 5–17 who were continuously exposed to water fluoridation compared to 2380 children with no fluoridation exposure.

In the 1986–1987 NIDR study, for all children ages 5–17 years, there was a lower mean difference of 0.6 DMFS for those in fluoridated area with an increasing benefit for the older children. Because the permanent teeth do not erupt into the mouth until 5–6 years of age, there are fewer teeth and tooth surfaces available to become decayed. By age 17, there was a mean 1.5 surface benefit.

Newbrun reported that surveys conducted in the 1980s reported less tooth decay in communities that were fluoridated; fluoridation was credited for preventing 30% to 60% of dental caries in the primary dentition, 20% to 40% in the mixed dentition, and 15% to 35% in the permanent dentition.[63] The decline in percentages of caries reduction has been found in both fluoridated and nonfluoridated communities with children who had always been exposed to community water fluoridation

demonstrating mean scores for decayed, missing, and filled tooth surfaces that ranged from 18% to 40% lower than those who had never lived in fluoridated communities.[63–65] Griffin estimated that fluoridation was responsible for a 27% reduction in tooth decay for adults.[66]

As described, the decline in dental caries rates was highest, up to 65% to 70%, in the earlier years (1940s–1960s) of fluoridation when water was the primary source of fluoride and the availability of other sources was limited. The caries-inhibition effectiveness of fluoride in water resulted in a parallel rush to develop other sources of fluorides, resulting in (1) licensed health professionals dispensing to the public adjunctive systemic fluorides, such as tablets, drops, lozenges, and vitamins with fluoride meant to be swallowed and (2) topical fluorides, which were intended for only topical application.[67] Dental providers use some topical fluorides in the office whereas others are used in public health programs and schools. In addition, consumers use over-the-counter fluoride products. As more cities adopted fluoridation and as the ingestion of dietary fluoride supplements increased in fluoride-deficient communities, consumer use of fluoride-containing products such as toothpastes, mouthrinses, and gels also increased. As a result, exposure to fluoride from numerous sources has become more widespread with benefits accruing at varying levels. At the same time, it is becoming more difficult to accurately determine the level of reduction in caries rates attributed to fluoridated water alone versus other sources.

Most researchers now believe that the "dilution" and "diffusion" effects are responsible for the decline in dental caries rates in nonfluoridated and, to a lesser degree, fluoridated communities.

Although children and adolescents are the major beneficiaries of fluoridation, adults also benefit. The impact of fluoride on the teeth of adults has become more important because they are retaining their teeth longer than in previous decades as a result of improved dental health practices, the advent of the dental hygienist, and availability of preventive interventions, especially fluoridation. With aging, teeth remain susceptible to coronal caries,[68] and more of the root surfaces become exposed to the oral environment, resulting in increased susceptibility to root caries.[69] Research indicates that root caries manifests as a significant dental problem as early as ages 35 to 44, doubling in the 45- to 54-year age group, and redoubling in the 55- to 66-year group.[70] Results of a national survey of root caries found that 67% of men and 61% of women between ages 65 and 84+ had root-surface lesions.[71] Studies in adults have consistently reported fewer coronal and root caries in the teeth of adults residing in communities with higher levels of waterborne fluoride.[8] Results of one study of young adults ages 20 to 34 years who resided in fluoridated (adjusted or natural) communities showed 25% fewer coronal decayed and filled surfaces compared with those who had no exposure to fluoridated water.[72] Similar findings were noted in a study of older adults with mean ages of 40 and 43 years; residents of communities with 1.6 ppm fluoride in the water had 28% less coronal caries and 17% less root caries than residents of communities with 0.2 ppm fluoride. Newbrun has estimated that the reduction in caries attributable to water fluoridation for adults ages 20 to 44 years is between 20% and 30% for coronal caries and 20% to 40% for root caries.[63] A recent examination of studies published during or after 1980 found that any fluoride (self-applied and professionally applied or from fluoridated water) annually averted 0.29 carious coronal surfaces and 0.22 carious root surfaces in adults.[43] The same study found that the prevention attributable to water fluoridation was 27%.[43]

Historically, assessments of effectiveness depended on interpretation of individual studies. In recent years, however, the scientific and health communities have conducted systematic reviews, summarizing the available evidence on a given topic. Systematic reviews use a rule-based process to summarize existing knowledge about the effectiveness of an intervention—in this case, fluoridation. The review process is established before the review begins. This rule-based process increases the likelihood that the review captures available knowledge and objectively summarizes methods and results. This objective process seeks to diminish the likelihood of bias that can be introduced by investigators. As such, the systematic review provides the strongest evidence of effectiveness of an intervention.

Several systematic reviews have been conducted on both the safety and effectiveness of fluoridation. The University of York review on fluoridation effectiveness published in 2000 found that fluoridation of drinking water supplies reduced caries prevalence in variable ranges with a median of 14.6% reduction in rates as measured by the change in the decay, extracted, filled primary teeth (deft)/decayed, missing, and filled permanent teeth (DMFT) indices scores and the proportion of caries-free children.[73] The report also attempted to address the impact of fluoride-containing toothpaste on the effectiveness of fluoridation.[74] The authors of the review acknowledged that the estimates of effectiveness could be biased because of inadequate adjustment for the impact of potential confounding variables.[73] The U.S. Task Force on Community Preventive Services released its systematic findings in 2002 and strongly recommended community water fluoridation as an effective measure for reducing dental caries. On the basis of their included studies, the median effectiveness of starting or continuing fluoridation as measured by before and after assessments of concurrent comparison groups was a 29% relative decrease in tooth decay. The median absolute decrease was 1.3 teeth.[75,76]

It is clear from studies cited previously that a worldwide decline in dental caries rates has occurred even though certain population groups are still disproportionately affected by dental caries. This decline has been attributed to the widespread use of fluorides from various sources: community water supplies, fluoridated salt, fluoride supplements, fluoride rinses, gels, varnishes and toothpastes.

EFFECTS OF DISCONTINUATION OF WATER FLUORIDATION

During the early years of fluoridation when fluoride in the water supply was the primary source of fluoride, studies showed that dental caries rates increased dramatically when fluoridation was discontinued. In 1960, the city of Antigo, Wisconsin, discontinued community fluoridated water after having had it for 11 years. Six years later, when Antigo elementary school children were found to have substantial increases in caries rates, ranging from 70% to 200%, fluoridation was reinstated.[77] Similar findings occurred in Scotland upon cessation of fluoridation: In the town of Wick, caries rates increased by 40% in primary teeth and by 27% in permanent teeth. This dramatic increase in dental caries rates occurred despite ready availability of fluoride toothpaste and a continuing decline in national caries rates in Scotland.[78] Moreover, 5 years after fluoridation was discontinued in the town of Stranraer, caries rates increased to levels approaching those found in the nonfluoridated town of Annan. In Stranraer, restorative dental treatment costs for decay alone rose by 115%.[79]

Similar results can occur if a city changes its water source from one that is optimally fluoridated to one that is fluoride deficient. The impact would be equivalent to discontinuation of fluoridation, as in the case in Galesburg, Illinois, which in 1959 switched from a water source that was naturally fluoridated to a nonfluoridated source. In 2 years, the caries-prevalence rate increased by 38%.[80] A U.S. Public Health Service Report on risks and benefits of fluoride stated that "one way to demonstrate the effectiveness of a therapeutic agent, such as fluoride, is to observe if the benefits are lost when the agent is removed."[81] One of the more notable systematic reviews in recent years was completed in 2002 by the U.S. Task Force on Community Preventive Services, made up of a non federal group of health experts. The task force found that communities that stopped community water fluoridation, on average, experienced an 18% increase in dental caries after discontinuation.[76]

Although these studies serve to demonstrate that the discontinuation of community water fluoridation has resulted in the significant loss of the benefits of dental caries prevention, some more recent studies cannot replicate these results,[82,83] most probably because of the dilution and diffusion effects that introduce fluoride to citizens living in nonfluoridated cities. Still, water fluoridation remains the most efficient way for a community to provide fluoride to its citizens.

Individuals using bottled water as their primary drinking source could lessen the benefits imparted by fluoridation. Although the fluoride concentrations in bottled water can vary considerably,[84,85] most bottled water contains low fluoride concentrations,[86] which are shown on labels only if fluoride is added during the bottling process.[87] The CDC recommended in 2001 that manufacturers include fluoride concentrations on labels.[88] Because fluoridation works by replenishing fluoride concentrations in the plaque and saliva on a frequent basis, substituting optimally fluoridated drinking water with low-fluoride bottled water reduces the overall preventive effect.

ENAMEL FLUOROSIS

Fluoridation has risks as well as benefits. As mentioned earlier in the historical background section, fluoride in water can cause a dental condition known as *enamel fluorosis,* also referred to as *dental fluorosis* or *fluorosis.* Although the mild and very mild forms of fluorosis can be so minimally apparent that individuals might not even realize their teeth are affected,[89] moderate and severe forms of fluorosis result in stained and pitted teeth that are cosmetically objectionable.[90] Regulations, guidelines, and expert panels make this distinction and normally develop and promote recommendations that protect individuals against the development of moderate and severe but not lower fluorosis types. Although the goal should be to eliminate all moderate and severe fluorosis, it is improbable to expect elimination of the less objectionable forms of very mild and mild fluorosis. Decades before community water fluoridation began, investigators such as McKay and Dean found that fluorosis was prevalent in many communities across the country from natural sources of fluoride.[21,25,26] It should also be noted that, when adjusted fluoridation was initiated in 1945, it was accepted that a portion of the population would develop very mild fluorosis, which was considered an acceptable trade-off for the increased caries protection and improved dental health. Fluoridation involves finding the appropriate balance between the benefits of caries prevention and improved oral health and the potential for cosmetic conditions associated with very mild and mild fluorosis.

Enamel fluorosis results from hypomineralization in enamel surfaces of teeth that have been exposed to fluoride ingested during enamel formation. Enamel fluorosis can present in a number of ways from barely discernible, white, lacy lines to the most severe form that could be classified as a developmental defect of the enamel.[19,89] The degree of fluorosis depends on the total dose of fluoride from all sources as well as on the timing and duration of fluoride exposure. Enamel fluorosis occurs in children who consume fluoride when their teeth are developing; it cannot occur once enamel formation is complete and the teeth have erupted regardless of intake; therefore, older children and adults are not at risk for enamel fluorosis.[1,91,92] Children ages 8 years or younger are at risk for developing fluorosis, but children ages 6 years and older are considered safe from developing objectionable fluorosis that will show when they speak or smile because the anterior permanent teeth have formed.[88]

Excessive levels of exposure, those that exceed levels set to protect against moderate and severe fluorosis, can occur in various ways, such as consuming drinking water that contains higher-than-optimal fluoride levels as can happen with private wells or community water systems with high levels of naturally occurring fluoride. In 1986, the U.S. Environmental Protection Agency (EPA) considered the fluoride content of drinking water that was higher than 2 ppm F a cosmetic influence and required public water systems reaching or exceeding this level to issue a public notification. In 2011, the EPA announced a change to the Maximum Contaminant Level (MCL) of naturally occurring fluoride in drinking water following an extensive review by a committee of the National Academy of Sciences.[93] The findings of the 2006 National Research Council (NRC) panel diverged from those of the 1993 panel in categorizing severe dental fluorosis resulting in pitting of the tooth enamel as the health endpoint that should be evaluated. The 2006 panel also concluded that the present MCL of 4 mg/L was not protective for severe dental fluorosis and might not be protective for the skeletal fracture endpoint. The NRC report does not question the beneficial effects for fluoride at levels practiced for fluoridation programs.[93,94]

The Institute of Medicine (IOM) established a **Tolerable Upper Intake** Level (UL) for fluoride in different age, life stage, and/or gender groupings.[5] A UL is defined as the maximum level of a total chronic daily intake of a nutrient that is unlikely to pose risks of adverse health effects for almost all individuals in the general population. In the case of fluoride, the UL for infants and children up to age 9 was selected based on prevention of moderate dental fluorosis; for all other age groups, the UL was selected based on the prevention of skeletal fluorosis. In the derivation of the UL for children, IOM[5] used the Dean[29] data and considered that there was a less than a 5% prevalence of moderate dental fluorosis at a 2 mg/L drinking water concentration. At this concentration, IOM estimated that fluoride intakes would range from 0.08 to 0.12 mg/kg/day but did not provide the body weight and water intakes used for this estimate. The middle of the range (0.1 mg/kg/day) was identified as a lowest-observed-adverse-effect level (LOAEL) for moderate dental fluorosis "the threshold beyond which moderate enamel fluorosis appears in some children"[5] The LOAEL was divided by an uncertainty factor of 1 to establish a dose of 0.1 mg/kg as the UL for infants and children through 8 years of age. Based on reference weights of 7 kg and 9 kg, respectively, the UL for infants in the first 6 months of life is 0.7 mg/day and that for the second 6 months is 0.9 mg/day. Children were divided into two age groups, 1 to 3 years old (body weight[bw] = 13 kg) and those 4 through 8 years old (bw = 22 kg). The UL for the first group of children is 1.3 mg/day and that for the second group is 2.2 mg/day. The UL for all other age groups is 10 mg/day and was based on a no-observed-adverse-effect level (NOAEL) of 10 mg/day for the development of skeletal fluorosis.[95]

After evaluation of the available literature, U.S. EPA identified a study conducted by Dean[29] using data from 1930 to early 1940 as that providing the most useful information on the association of fluoride intake from drinking water and the development of dental fluorosis in children. Although Dean's study has some limitations, its value lies in the fact that it is relatively free of confounding factors associated with the widespread use of fluoride-containing consumer products introduced after that time. Dean's study documented the prevalence and severity of dental fluorosis in 5,824 children in 22 U.S. communities in 10 states where fluoride levels in drinking water ranged from 0.0 to 14.1 mg/L. The Dean study provides baseline data from which a statistically sound estimate of the threshold for severe dental fluorosis was derived.

NRC (2006) identified severe dental fluorosis, a condition defined by Dean as pitting of the enamel of the teeth, as a condition that could lead to an increased risk for dental caries by diminishing the protective function of the enamel. The threshold for severe dental fluorosis in the children studied by Dean was derived statistically as the concentration in drinking water associated with the lower bound confidence limit for a prevalence rate of 0.5% (i.e., the concentration at which no more than 0.5% of exposed children in the susceptible age groups would develop any signs of severe dental fluorosis—pitting of one or more teeth). This threshold fluoride concentration (for Dean's study populations) is 1.87 mg/L.[96]

In 2006, the American Dental Association issued an interim guidance advising, "If liquid concentrate or powdered infant formula is the primary source of nutrition, it can be mixed with water that is fluoride free or contains low levels of fluoride to reduce the risk of fluorosis."[97] The greatest likelihood of exposure to excess fluoride in children results from (1) inadvertent ingestion of toothpaste containing very high concentrations of fluoride and (2) ingestion of inappropriately prescribed dietary fluoride supplements.[1,98]

As a follow-up in 2011, the ADA convened an expert panel to review the literature on the subject. The panel suggested that when dentists advise parents and caregivers of infants who consume powdered or liquid concentrate infant formula as the main source of nutrition, they can suggest the continued use of powdered or liquid concentrate infant formulas reconstituted with optimally fluoridated drinking water while being cognizant of the potential risks of enamel fluorosis development.[99]

Data from the National Health and Nutrition Examination Survey (NHANES) 1999–2002 indicated that approximately 23% of persons ages 6 to 39 years in the United States exhibited fluorosis.[100] This represents an increase of 9 percentage points in fluorosis prevalence in the United States since the previous national survey.[100] Both national surveys classified the majority of identified fluorosis cases as being very mild or mild. The minor forms of fluorosis (questionable, very mild, or mild) are

not considered to be abnormal, nor are they considered to constitute an adverse health effect. However, both researchers and practitioners should continue to monitor and assess the risk of enamel fluorosis to ensure that the more severe forms of fluorosis do not occur. Although the authors of the NHANES 1999–2002 survey report could not specifically identify the factors responsible for the rise in fluorosis prevalence, they noted, "a potentially important source is toothpaste." In 1936, Dean estimated that approximately 10% of children who drank optimally fluoridated water would develop very mild enamel fluorosis.[101] More recent studies have shown that enamel fluorosis attributed to fluoridation is around 13%.[102] It is probable that about 10% of children will develop a mild form of fluorosis if exposed only to optimally fluoridated drinking water and no other sources of fluoride.[1]

University of Iowa researchers who have followed a cohort of children from birth through adolescence and documented fluoride intake as reported by parents on questionnaires have determined that the first 3 years of life are critical to the development of fluorosis.[103] They also found much variation with regard to intake and individual response.[104,105] Even though fluorosis is determined by fluoride exposure and is related to dose and duration, some children will develop fluorosis and some will not even when they are exposed to the same level of fluoride. The Iowa researchers have also noted a positive association between fluorosis in the primary and secondary dentition even when they adjust for fluoride exposure.

The Safe Drinking Water Act enacted by Congress in 1986 established primary and secondary standards for natural fluoride levels in public drinking water in the United States. The legislation set the **primary standard** (the maximum concentration of fluoride allowed in public drinking water systems) at 4.0 ppm F to protect the public against unwanted health effects such as skeletal fluorosis. A **secondary standard** of 2.0 ppm F was set to protect children from moderate/severe enamel fluorosis. The report *Fluoride in Drinking Water: A Scientific Review of EPA's Standards,*[105] issued by the NRC in 2006, examined the current EPA water standards. For the first time, the NRC separated severe and moderate enamel fluorosis and considered each separately. In doing so, the committee determined that the current maximum contaminant level goal of 4 ppm F in drinking water was not protective against severe enamel fluorosis. The NRC stated that communities with fluoride concentrations in the public water supply at or near 4 ppm F can expect a 10% frequency of severe enamel fluorosis. For the first time, this expert panel considered severe enamel fluorosis an adverse health effect instead of a cosmetic effect.[65,79,106] Of note, this effect applies to severe enamel fluorosis only, not the other forms of fluorosis. Previous assessments considered all forms of enamel fluorosis to be esthetically displeasing but not adverse to health because of the lack of direct evidence that severe enamel fluorosis results in tooth loss, loss of tooth function, or psychologic, behavioral, or social problems. However, in this report, the NRC committee noted suggestive but inconclusive evidence that severe enamel fluorosis increased the risk of developing caries.[104] Severe enamel fluorosis results in discrete and confluent pitting and structural damage to the tooth's enamel surface.

The committee determined that this damage compromises the function of the tooth surface to protect the dentin and pulp from decay and infection. The report states that the hypothesis of a causal link between severe enamel fluorosis and increased caries risk is plausible and that the evidence for this link is mixed but supportive. In addition, the report acknowledged that restorative dental treatment is often considered for children with the enamel pitting that characterizes this condition.

The NRC report also noted strong evidence of a true population threshold for severe fluorosis at 2 ppm F in the water supply.[105] In other words, severe enamel fluorosis essentially is absent when the water supply contains less than 2 ppm F. Strong evidence exists that lowering the maximum contaminant level goal for fluoride to a level below 2 ppm F will effectively eliminate severe enamel fluorosis. This observation is supported by an intervention study conducted by Horowitz and others in North Dakota where partial defluoridation of drinking water from 6 ppm F to slightly below 2 ppm F prevented severe fluorosis.[107]

The differential diagnosis of dental fluorosis can be difficult.[108] Not all enamel opacities or irregularities are caused by fluorosis. The commonly accepted diagnostic criteria for fluorosis discriminate between nondiscrete symmetrical and asymmetrical distributions of opacities of dental enamel. These criteria appear to identify most cases of dental fluorosis. However, it is not yet confirmed that the pattern and distribution of dental fluorosis are unique phenomena. Metabolic, physiological, other trace elements, and malnutrition have been reported to induce bilateral symmetrical developmental enamel opacities. Misdiagnosis of nonfluoride-induced opacities remains a possibility. Reports of unexpectedly high population prevalence and individual cases of fluorosis where such diagnoses are incompatible with the known fluoride history indicate the need for a positive identification of the levels of fluoride available to communities and individuals before a diagnosis of fluorosis is confirmed. Diseases and conditions, such as celiac disease, can result in enamel hypoplasia, which may be mistaken for fluorosis.[109] Idiopathic opacities for which the cause is currently unknown also exist.

As previously mentioned, questionable, very mild, and mild stages of fluorosis often result from very young children swallowing too much fluoride-containing toothpaste or from inappropriate supplementation with prescription fluoride

products such as physicians or dentists independently prescribing (1) fluoride supplements or (2) fluoride supplements without checking the fluoride content of the child's water supply. In either case, a child gets a "double" dose of fluoride on a daily basis. Monitoring total fluoride intake is complicated, considering the availability of multiple sources of fluoride. Also, fluoride from tablets/drops is ingested and absorbed at one time of day as opposed to fluoride in water in which the ingestion and absorption of low-dose fluoride is distributed throughout the day. These factors have been considered in the establishment of fluoride dosage schedules, which were adjusted downward in the 1990s, particularly for children in the first 6 months of life. The dietary fluoride supplement schedule approved by the American Dental Association,[110] the American Academy of Pediatrics,[111] and the American Academy of Pediatric Dentistry[112] should be followed when fluoride supplements are prescribed (Table 14–5 ■). In 2010, an expert panel convened by the American Dental Association recommended that dietary fluoride supplements should be prescribed only for children who are at high risk of developing caries.[113]

Fluoride ingestion should be reduced during the ages of tooth development, particularly under the age of 2 years. Parents need to assist in attaining this goal by supervising young children during toothbrushing to ensure that they use only a small amount of toothpaste (smear or pea-sized) and do not swallow it.[88]

REDUCTION OF THE RISK FOR ENAMEL FLUOROSIS

In 2011, U. S. Department of Health and Human Services (HHS) proposed its recommendation to standardize the fluoride concentration for fluoridated water for the entire United States at the level of 0.7 mg/L. Prior to that, the CDC had in 2001 developed recommendations to reduce the risk for enamel fluorosis. The CDC report *Recommendations for Using Fluoride to Prevent and Control Dental Caries in the United States* contains the following as well as other recommendations:[88]

- All persons should know whether the fluoride concentration in their primary source of drinking water is below optimal (less than 0.7 ppm F), optimal (0.7–1.2 ppm F),

TABLE ■ 14–5   **Dietary Fluoride Supplement Schedule, 1994**

Age	Fluoride Ion Level in Drinking Water (ppm)[a]		
	< 0.3 ppm F	*0.3–0.6 ppm F*	*> 0.6 ppm F*
Birth–6 months	None	None	None
6 months–3 years	0.25 mg/day[b]	None	None
3–6 years	0.50 mg/day	0.25 mg/day	None
6–16 years	1.0 mg/day	0.50 mg/day	None

[a]1.0 part per million (ppm) = 1 milligram/liter (mg/l).
[b]2.2 mg sodium fluoride contains 1 mg fluoride ion.
(*Source:* Meskin, 1995[105]; American Academy of Pediatrics Committee on Nutrition, 1995[106]; and American Academy of Pediatric Dentistry, 1995[107].)

or above optimal (higher than 1.2 ppm F). This knowledge is the basis for all individual and professional decisions regarding use of other fluoride modalities (e.g., fluoride toothpaste for children under 2 years of age, mouthrinses, or supplements).

• Parents of children younger than 6 years should brush the child's teeth (recommended particularly for preschool children) or supervise the toothbrushing. Parents should encourage the child to spit excess toothpaste into the sink to minimize the amount swallowed.

• Parents and caregivers should consult a dentist or other health care provider before introducing a child younger than 2 years to fluoride toothpaste.

• For children younger than 6 years who use fluoride toothpaste, parents and caregivers should follow the directions on the label and place no more than a pea-sized amount (0.25 grams) of toothpaste on the toothbrush.

• Where community water supply systems and home wells contain a natural fluoride concentration of more than 2 ppm F, children younger than 9 years should have an alternative source of drinking water that preferably contains fluoride at the recommended optimal level.

• Use of other discretionary forms of fluoride, including fluoride mouthrinses and dietary fluoride supplements, should be limited to children who are at a high risk for developing tooth decay. Supplements should be used for only high-risk children living in areas where the drinking water has a low concentration of fluoride. Supplements should be prescribed judiciously and in accordance with the dietary fluoride supplement schedule (Table 14–5).

• Parents of formula-fed infants should weigh the balance between a child's risk for very mild or mild enamel fluorosis and the benefit of fluoride for preventing tooth decay and the need for dental fillings.

Groups opposing fluoridation initiatives frequently exhibit photographs of children and/or adults with severe fluorosis in which pitting or mottling of the enamel and brown stains are evident. Attributing these manifestations directly to water fluoridation is misleading. Fluoridation opponents may also describe enamel fluorosis as a major risk factor for people of all ages, which is not accurate. Severe fluorosis does not occur from fluoridated water alone but most frequently occurs when too much naturally occurring fluoride is in water. In making dental health decisions, patients depend on the dental professional team to assist them in evaluating the risks versus the benefits of a given procedure or public health measure. To do this, dentists and dental hygienists need to stay current with scientific literature and to use this knowledge as a basis for educating themselves and their patients. The risk of developing very mild fluorosis versus the benefit of decreased dental caries and attendant treatment costs should be communicated to patients who express concern.

OPTIMAL FLUORIDE LEVELS

Prior to 2011, the U.S. Public Health Service had established nonregulatory standards for optimal concentrations of fluoride in the drinking water in the United States in 1962. Those standards were derived from the annual average of maximum daily air temperatures based on the work of Dean, Galagan, and others and was founded on the principle that water consumption is higher in hotter climates and less in colder climates (see Figure 14–11 ■).[25,27,28,113–117] Consequently, the higher the average temperature in a community, the lower the recommended water fluoride level.[118]

Much has changed in the United States since the recommendations for optimal fluoride levels were issued in 1962.

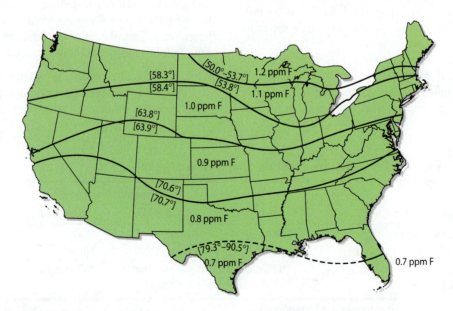

FIGURE ■ **14–11** Optimal fluoride concentrations in the United States.

(*Source:* Centers for Disease Control. (1991). *Dental disease prevention activity, 1991.* Atlanta, GA: Centers for Disease Control, National Center for Prevention Services.)

Some studies have examined fluid intake and questioned whether temperature influences the amount people drink as it once did because of the widespread use of air conditioning in homes, automobiles, and workplaces.[119,120] Modern consumption patterns of bottled water and other beverages, such as soft drinks and fruit juices, also complicate the matter because fluoride levels in them vary greatly.[6,121] In addition, optimal fluoride concentrations were recommended at a time before there were other regular sources of fluoride exposure, such as discretionary fluoride toothpaste, mouthrinses, and dietary supplements. Other factors such as consumer use of home distillation and reverse-osmosis water treatment systems, which can remove significant amounts of fluoride from the water supply, influence the determination of daily fluoride intake. In 2001, the CDC recommended review of the methodology used to determine optimal levels to determine whether it was still relevant.[88] Ten years later, the CDC and the U.S. HHS have proposed a uniform optimal fluoride concentration of 0.7 ppm for all community water supplies, a change from the range of 0.7 to 1.2 ppm.

Optimal fluoride concentrations in other countries are not identical to those in the United States; however, most values were originally based on the U.S. methodology. Some countries (Hong Kong, Singapore) have optimal levels as low as 0.5 ppm F. A 1994 WHO report recommended that some regions, especially tropical and subtropical areas, revise the optimal range to establish appropriate higher and lower limits.

ENGINEERING ASPECTS: CHEMICALS AND TECHNICAL SYSTEMS

Three additives are used for water fluoridation in the United States, sodium fluoride (NaF), sodium fluorosilicate (Na_2SiF_6), and hydrofluosilicic acid (H_2SiF_6), also known as *fluorosilicic acid*. States require these additives to meet the standards, testing, and certifications set by the American Water Works Association (AWWA) and the National Sanitation Foundation (NSF) International.[122] The AWWA sets minimum requirements for a product's design, installation, performance, and manufacturing. NSF International sets criteria on the purity of drinking water additives or products and for protection of the integrity of additives during transport. Fluoridation additives represent just one kind of chemical used in the water supply. Water treatment chemicals are used for a number of reasons including disinfection, absorption, algae control, decolonization, oxidation, metal coagulation, water softening, filtration, pH control, iron control, coagulation, corrosion control, chlorination, and fluoridation.[123,124,]

Sodium fluoride (granular or powder) and sodium fluorosilicate (granular) are used in distribution systems that use "dry" compounds, whereas fluorosilicic acid, a liquid, is used in solution or "wet" systems.[125] Sodium fluoride was the first compound used in controlled water fluoridation programs and is still used in many water systems in smaller communities, usually those serving fewer than 5,000 people.[123] Sodium fluorosilicate is substantially less expensive than sodium

fluoride and tends to be used in community water systems serving between 5,000 and 50,000 people. Today, the most frequently used compound for water fluoridation in the United States is fluorosilicic acid because of its low cost and ease of handling; it is used primarily in larger communities with water distribution systems serving 50,000 or more people; this represents approximately 57% of all fluoridation systems in the United States.[126]

Opponents of fluoridation often attempt to distinguish between sodium fluoride and the hexafluorosilicates, sodium fluorosilicate and fluorosilicic acid, in terms of availability of the fluoride ion. Those groups opposing fluoridation suggest that hexafluorosilicates are industrial waste dumped into the drinking water and that they contaminate the water with a harmful residue. However, according to EPA scientists, no hexafluorosilicate remains in drinking water at equilibrium, which is readily achieved.[127] This statement has been verified by other research,[128] which implies that there is no difference in the source of fluoride ions from the three chemicals used in fluoridation as the detractors would have one believe.

The CDC Engineering and Administrative Recommendations for Water Fluoridation and the AWWA Water Fluoridation Principles and Practices are two credible sources for guidelines related to the engineering aspects of water fluoridation, including administration, monitoring, and surveillance; technical requirements; and safety procedures.[129]

Determination of the appropriate compound to use in fluoridation depends largely on the type of distribution system used by the individual water plant. The most common methods by which fluoride is added to water supplies in the United States are (1) the volumetric dry-feeder system, which delivers a predetermined quantity of dry fluoride chemical, (2) the acid-feed system, in which a small metering pump is used to add fluorosilicic acid to the water supply system, and (3) the saturator-feed system, a system unique to water fluoridation that uses an up-flow saturator to provide saturated solutions of sodium fluoride in constant strengths of 4%, which are pumped into the water system via a small metering pump.[123,124]

THE MONITORING AND SURVEILLANCE OF FLUORIDATION

The process of adding fluoride to drinking water supplies to the level recommended to achieve the maximum dental therapeutic benefits is technically simple, uncomplicated, and similar to the processes used when dealing with chlorine and other water treatment chemicals.[123,124] All three types of fluoride additives used in the water fluoridation process are certified as to their purity and safety when used appropriately; fluoride is just one of nearly 50 additional substances approved by the EPA and is certified as safe for addition to drinking water by the AWWA and NSF International. Contrary to popular perception, fluoride does not affect the taste, odor, color, or turbidity of the water at the levels used for water fluoridation.[123,124]

For fluoridation to be properly implemented, a number of factors should be considered. Of prime importance is the compatibility of the fluoride additive to be used with the existing water treatment and distribution system. Other factors that influence the technical engineering aspects of fluoridation include (1) source of water—underground or surface, (2) size of the water plant, (3) number and types of point sources of water—one or many treatment plants with water coming from wells, reservoirs, rivers, aqueducts, or desalination plants, (4) number of injection points at which fluoride is introduced into the water, (5) fluoride additive costs, including transportation, (6) modification of existing plant versus construction of a new plant, (7) need to train water plant operators, and (8) type of monitoring and surveillance system to be used.

Modern water plant design includes engineering controls that ensure the prevention of excessive amounts of fluoride entering the water supply. Properly designed fluoridation systems prevent the addition of excess fluoride to the water system in several ways: (1) Maintaining only a limited amount of fluoride in the day tanks (or hoppers), effectively limiting the bulk amount that could be put into the water system even in the event of a system failure, (2) installing positive controls for feeding fluoride from the hoppers into the dissolving tanks, and (3) electrically connecting metering pumps to the water pump in a manner ensuring that failure of one pump stops operation of all pumps—and stops addition of fluoride to the system.[124] Many water plants today use in-line fluoride monitors that give continuous readings of the fluoride concentration in the water supply, providing the ability to assess the fluoride level at any time, not just when the water is tested. In addition to regular testing and documenting fluoride levels in the water, utilities should have a quality assurance program in place that includes monthly split sampling.[125] This procedure involves taking two samples of water: One is tested at the water plant by normal testing procedures (e.g., ion meter, colorimeter), and the other is sent to a reference laboratory, often at the state department of health. The reference laboratory tests the water and compares its results with those from the water plant; if there is a discrepancy, the water plant reviews and adjusts its testing procedures until the results are in agreement. To be certain the results of the reference laboratories are accurate, CDC maintains a national program for proficiency testing, which compares water plants' results to reference standards with known fluoride concentrations.[130]

Maintaining a constant level of fluoride in the water supply is the responsibility of the water plant operators. Variation in the adjusted water fluoride levels has occurred in water plants where the operators were not properly trained and/or operator turnover was high.[131] Variability in water fluoride concentration could also occur if a water plant fails to provide adequate and appropriate storage facilities, if the feed equipment malfunctions, or if proper water analysis equipment is lacking, all of which are readily avoidable with proper planning and implementation. Most of the variances in fluoride concentrations that have occurred were due to poor monitoring at water treatment facilities, resulting in fluoride levels below the recommended level (hypofluoridation). For this reason, communities that have implemented fluoridation must continue to monitor the

fluoride levels to ensure that the full benefits of fluoridation will accrue in a community. Hyperfluoridation occurs when an excess amount of fluoride is added to the drinking water over several days, usually secondary to an overfeed from malfunctioning equipment and/or maintenance errors.[132,133] Between 1977 and 2002, nine instances of hyperfluoridation that resulted in outbreaks of acute fluoride poisoning occurred in the United States, all of which could have easily been prevented.[134] When a community decides to fluoridate its public water supplies, it also must assume the responsibility for monitoring the equipment, training the water plant operators, and implementing performance reviews to ensure that a process is in place to protect the public from an overfeed. The CDC offers national fluoridation training for state fluoridation program managers and has developed a 6-hour training module designed to assist plant operators in sustaining and monitoring their fluoridation systems.[135]

COST OF COMMUNITY WATER FLUORIDATION

The cost of water fluoridation should be put into perspective with overall cost of water treatment. According to the EPA,

it costs less for our drinking water than it does for most other goods and services, such as cable television, telephone service, and electricity. On average, tap water costs are slightly more than $2 per 1,000 gallons, although the costs tend to be lower for large water systems, and higher for small systems. Treatment accounts for about 15 percent of that cost. Other costs are for equipment (such as the treatment plants and distribution systems), and labor for operation and maintenance of the system. Yet think about how important water is to our daily lives. The average person uses over 100 gallons of water per day for everything from drinking and bathing to watering gardens. This equates to an average annual water bill of about $300 per household, though costs vary considerably across the country.[136]

Community water fluoridation provides significant cost savings for a community and has been described as "the most cost-effective, practical and safe means for reducing and controlling the occurrence of tooth decay in a community."[137] Estimates of the cost of water fluoridation vary depending on the factors included in the calculations. The size and complexity of the water system, including the number of systems, the number of wells, the use of a dry feeder versus a solution (wet) feeder system, purchase of equipment and installation, purchase of fluoride, labor, and maintenance, as well as the number of service connections and size of the population all factor into the cost of fluoridation.[138-140]

The cost of water fluoridation is usually expressed as the annual cost per person of the population being served.[19] An inverse relationship exists between the cost per person and the size of the population of a community. Consequently, the cost per person is lower in larger communities and higher in smaller communities where the actual cost of fluoridation may approach that of other methods of caries prevention.[139] Fluoridation also eliminates or diminishes additional costs incurred through other forms of fluoride administration, such as costs incurred when accessing professionals to obtain provider-prescribed fluoride products and the lower effectiveness of other forms of fluoride distribution. Fluoridation is the most cost-efficient and cost-effective method of prevention of dental caries for almost all communities.[12]

Another way to look at cost-saving benefits is to determine the dental treatment cost savings of beneficiaries. Employers who pay prepaid dental care fringe benefits for their employees save on costs. Hidden production or service costs caused by dental-related missed workdays by employees are also minimized through fluoridation. Taxpayers who support public programs also benefit from dental treatment cost savings. In fact, skyrocketing dental Medicaid expenditures in California (a state with a low percentage of the population having access to fluoridation) provided the impetus for enactment of a state-wide mandatory fluoridation bill in 1995.[141,142] Sudies comparing dental Medicaid expenditures in Louisiana and Texas also demonstrated that treatment costs were significantly higher in nonfluoridated communities than in fluoridated communities.[143,144] Patients can also be expected to benefit from lower health care bills, lower dental care costs, and lower insurance premiums because of lower costs incurred by providers for uncompensated care.

With the availability of baseline levels of dental caries rates and treatment costs, two different types of analyses can be done to determine (1) the effectiveness of fluoridation as a measure to prevent dental caries (a cost-effectiveness analysis), and (2) associated cost savings (a cost-benefit analysis). It has been postulated that the higher the initial caries prevalence and treatment costs, the higher will be the potential benefits realized by the introduction of fluoridation.[19] Using Florida data from 1988, the cost of water fluoridation was converted to 1995 dollars and calculated by size of community.[139] The annual costs per person varied from about $3.17 for communities with less than 5,000 people, to about $0.50 for communities with more than 20,000. An average fee of $72 (in 1995 dollars) for an amalgam restoration for a single tooth surface was used and various factors were considered when estimating the cost savings from water fluoridation alone. The authors concluded that the annual per person cost savings resulting from fluoridation ranged from $15.95 for very small communities to $18.62 in large communities. These cost savings could well have increased because the treatment for dental caries can vary from a single surface restoration to a multiple surface filling, to a crown and root canal treatment, or extraction and replacement by a bridge or implant. For every carious lesion initially prevented, the need for repeated restorations and treatment of recurrent carious lesions is reduced over a lifetime.[145] Different studies have shown that the replacement rates for amalgam restorations caused by recurrent decay vary between 38% and 50%; the savings to be realized from prevention are substantial. In New Zealand, cost savings were in part based on replacement of amalgam restorations every 8 years.[143,146]

Two published studies on the economics of fluoridation conducted by CDC found that for large communities of more than 20,000 people fluoridating the water costs about 50 cents per person, every $1 invested in this preventive measure yields approximately $38 savings in dental treatment costs.[147] Other studies also demonstrate the substantial cost benefits generated through community water fluoridation. In a comprehensive study for the Texas Department of Health, Brown and colleagues demonstrated cost savings for the publicly funded Texas Health Steps Program when they compared program costs for clients from fluoridated communities with those from nonfluoridated communities.[148] Similarly, Barsley and colleagues demonstrated that the costs for hospital-based treatment of acute dental conditions to Louisiana's publicly funded Medicaid program were much less for residents of fluoridated communities than for residents of nonfluoridated communities.[149] In Colorado, costs and savings associated with community water fluoridation programs (CWFPs) were calculated.[150] The authors estimated that Colorado CWFPs were associated with annual savings of $148.9 million (credible range, $115.1 million to $187.2 million) in 2003, or an average of $60.78 per person (credible range, $46.97 to $76.41). Using 2006 Medicaid claims data in New York state, Kumar et al. found that compared with the predominantly fluoridated counties, the mean number of restorative, endodontic, and extraction procedures per recipient was 33.4% higher in less fluoridated counties. The mean number of claims per child for caries-related services was inversely correlated with the extent of fluoridation in a county but claims for noncaries related services were not.[151] Finally, Wright and colleagues established conclusively that fluoridation remains an extremely cost-effective public health program in New Zealand in their comprehensive 1999 report for the New Zealand Ministry of Health.[146]

OTHER FLUORIDE VEHICLES

Many countries without centralized water distribution systems have chosen to add fluoride to table salt, a process known as **salt fluoridation**, to provide primary benefits of dental caries prevention to their populations. Although it is difficult to obtain a verifiable accounting of usage, estimates say as many as 300 million people in the world use fluoridated salt.[152,153]

Using salt as a vehicle of fluoride supplementation is similar to the concept of iodine supplementation and is a relatively inexpensive method of fluoride delivery. Similar to water fluoridation, salt fluoridation results in small amounts of fluoride being released from plasma throughout the day.[154] To achieve dental caries reductions at levels comparable to water fluoridation, the level of fluoride supplementation of refined salt should be at least 200 mg F/kg as sodium fluoride or potassium fluoride.[155,156] Salt fluoridation requires centralized salt production as well as monitoring.[157] Because the consumption of high quantities of sodium is a risk factor for hypertension, the use of fluoridated salt is not recommended for those at risk.[157,158] Countries using salt fluoridation include Switzerland, France, Costa Rica, Jamaica, Germany, Mexico, Colombia, Ecuador, Venezuela, and Uruguay. It has also been introduced in a number of other countries.[23] Salt fluoridation is not appropriate for countries where water fluoridation is widely used because the additional source of fluoride would make management of intake levels difficult.

Milk fluoridation, the addition of 5 mg of fluoride to 1 liter of milk, has been introduced as a vehicle of school-based fluoride delivery in some countries (Bulgaria, Chile, China, Russia, and the United Kingdom).[5] According to the WHO report, "The distribution of fluoridated milk can be more complicated than that of fluoride supplements (tablets or drops)."[5] The existence of an established distribution system that includes provisions for pasteurization and refrigeration is a limiting factor in milk-fluoridation programs. A Cochrane review in 2005 found that there is insufficient evidence to show the effectiveness of fluoridated milk in preventing tooth decay. The authors concluded there were insufficient studies with good quality evidence examining the effects of fluoridated milk in preventing dental caries. However, the included studies suggested that fluoridated milk was beneficial to schoolchildren, especially their permanent dentition. The data need to be supplemented by further RCTs to provide the highest level of evidence for practice.[159]

SUMMARY

Community water fluoridation is the prime example of community-based prevention in which the benefits accrue to all individuals consuming drinking water that is optimally fluoridated without regard to socioeconomic status. Fluoridation remains a safe, effective health measure to prevent dental caries and makes an excellent public policy.

PRACTICAL CONSIDERATIONS

A historical understanding of the scientific evidence on benefits, safety, and cost-effectiveness as well as knowledge of ethical considerations, legal rulings, and social implications are important in advocating for community water fluoridation. Maintaining up-to-date information on fluoridation and fluoride from authoritative and reliable sources, such as the CDC and ADA, is vital in communicating to professional and community groups and leaders to maintain and expand fluoridation. Furthermore, experience in community organization and building community support for fluoridation can be acquired along with expertise in risk communication. Although general principles apply to every community, remember that all politics is local when pursuing the maintenance or initiation of community water fluoridation.

SELF-STUDY QUESTIONS

1. What is the sequence of the four phases of the development and implementation of community water fluoridation?

   a. Clinical discovery phase, epidemiologic phase, demonstration phase, and technology transfer phase

   b. Epidemiologic phase, clinical discovery phase, technology transfer phase, and demonstration phase

   c. Epidemiologic phase, demonstration phase, technology transfer phase, and clinical discovery phase

   d. Clinical discovery phase, demonstration phase, epidemiologic phase, and technology transfer phase

   Rationale: Individual dentists, notably Dr. McKay in Colorado, discovered and described their clinical findings of caries and mottled enamel (the *clinical discovery phase* prior to the 1930s), which led to the suggestion of an optimal fluoride concentration of 1 ppm to minimize dental caries and dental fluorosis. The investigation of caries and fluorosis prevalence and severity in multiple communities with varying fluoride concentration of the water supplies occurred in the *epidemiologic phase* of the 1930s. The *demonstration phase* that began in 1945–1946 to adjust the fluoride concentration of water supplies in Grand Rapids, Michigan; Newburgh, New York; Evanston, Illinois; and Brantford, Ontario, Canada. The results of these community trials produced clear evidence of the benefit of that optimal fluoride concentration as well as the safety and lack of negative health effects in the 1950s, resulting in many communities deciding to fluoridate their water supplies thereafter (the *technology transfer phase*).

2. Evidence provided even further confirmation that water fluoridation is responsible for the reduction of the prevalence and severity of dental caries?

   a. Increases in the prevalence and severity of enamel fluorosis in the NHANES

   b. Cross-sectional studies of caries prevalence and severity

   c. Increases in prevalence and severity of dental caries where fluoridation was discontinued.

   d. Reductions in caries prevalence and severity in nonfluoridated communities

Rationale: An increase in the severity and prevalence of dental caries following reduction in the fluoride concentration of community water supplies provides additional robust evidence of the cause-and-effect relationship between fluoride in water and dental caries. This was demonstrated in the 1960s in Antigo, Wisconsin, where fluoridation was discontinued after having it for 11 years. Six years later, when Antigo elementary schoolchildren were found to have substantial increases in caries rates, ranging from 70% to 200%, fluoridation was reinstated. Other similar studies have generally supported these findings.

Cross-sectional studies of caries prevalence and severity since the demonstration phase of fluoridation have supported the fluoride–caries hypothesis but cannot claim to prove cause and effect.

Reductions in caries prevalence and severity in nonfluoridated communities are considered to be due to the use of fluoride toothpaste and other dental sources of fluoride in addition to the diffusion effect of water fluoridation.

3. Why is the difference found in caries prevalence and severity between fluoridated and nonfluoridated communities much reduced since the demonstration phase of fluoridation?
   a. Diffusion effect of fluoridated and nonfluoridated processed foods and beverages transported from one to the other
   b. Measurement of difference in children who could have very few permanent teeth at risk for tooth decay because they have not yet erupted in the mouth
   c. Provision of the nearly ubiquitous use of fluoride toothpaste giving additional source of fluoride that did not exist in the 1940s and early 1950s.
   d. All the above.

Rationale: The analysis of the 1986–1987 survey of schoolchildren where a region had about 75% fluoridation showed no detectable difference in dental caries severity between fluoridated and nonfluoridated areas although there was 60% less caries severity in children in fluoridated areas that had less than 20% fluoridation. This was considered to be due to the diffusion effect of fluoridated and nonfluoridated processed foods and beverages being transported from one area to the other. That same survey found a benefit of 0.6 DMFS in children aged 5–17 years from fluoridated areas across the United States. This small difference, however, increased from age 5 to age 17 years as a result of an increasing number of tooth surfaces at risk and the effect of time on the development of caries. The dilution effect of fluoridation is the increased use of fluoride toothpaste and has provided an additional source of fluoride that did not exist in the 1940s and early 1950s. This is an additional reason that the difference found in caries prevalence and severity between fluoridated and nonfluoridated communities is much reduced since the demonstration phase of fluoridation.

REFERENCES

1. American Dental Association Council on Access, Prevention and Interprofessional Relations. (2005). *Fluoridation facts 2005.* Chicago, IL: American Dental Association.
2. Federal Register/Vol. 76, No. 9/Thursday, January 13, 2011/ Notices. Page 2384
3. U.S. Department of Agriculture. (2005). *USDA national fluoride database of selected foods and beverages, Release 2.* Retrieved January 17, 2011, from http://www.ars.usda.gov/Services/docs.htm?docid=6312.
4. Whitford, G. M. (1989). The metabolism and toxicology of fluoride. *Monogr Oral Sci, 13:*1–160.
5. Institute of Medicine, Food and Nutrition Board. (1997). *Dietary reference intakes: Calcium, phosphorus, magnesium, vitamin D, and fluoride.* Washington, DC: National Academy Press, 288–313.
6. World Health Organization. (1994). *Fluorides and oral health.* (Technical Report Series 846). Geneva, Switzerland: Author.
7. Easley, M. (2000). Opposition to community water fluoridation and connections to the "alternative medicine" movement. *Sci Rev Altern Med, 5:*24–31.
8. Easley, M. W. (1995). Celebrating 50 years of fluoridation: A public health success story. *Br Dent J, 21:*72–75.
9. U.S. Department of Health and Human Services. (1983, February 8). *Surgeon General statement on community water fluoridation* (Dr. C. Everett Koop). Washington, DC: U.S. Department of Health and Human Services, Public Health Service.
10. U.S. Department of Health and Human Services. (1995, December 14). *Surgeon General statement on community water fluoridation* (Dr. Antonio Novello). Washington, DC: U.S. Department of Health and Human Services, Public Health Service.
11. U.S. Department of Health and Human Services. (2000, March 25). *First-ever Surgeon General's report on oral health finds profound disparities in nation's population.* Bethesda, MD: U.S. Department of Health and Human Services, National Institute of Dental and Craniofacial Research, National Institutes of Health.
12. U.S. Department of Health and Human Services. (2000). *Oral health in America: A report of the Surgeon General.* (NIH Publication No. 00-4713). Rockville, MD: U.S. Department of Health and Human Services, National Institute of Dental and Craniofacial Research, National Institutes of Health.
13. U.S. Department of Health and Human Services. (2004, July 28). *Surgeon General statement on community water fluoridation* (Dr. R. Carmona). Washington, DC: U.S. Department of Health and Human Services, Public Health Service.
14. Centers for Disease Control and Prevention. 2010 Water Fluoridation Statistics. Retrieved September 23, 2012, from http://www.cdc.gov/fluoridation/statistics/2010stats.htm.
15. Ripa, L. W. (1999). Water fluoridation. In Harris, N. O., & Garcia-Godoy, F., Eds. *Primary preventive dentistry* (5th ed.). Stamford, CT: Appleton and Lange, 658.
16. McClure, F. J. (1970). *Water fluoridation. The search and the victory.* Washington, DC: U.S. Government Printing Office.

17. Murray, J. J., Rugg-Gunn, A. J., & Jenkins, G. N. (1991). *Fluorides in caries prevention* (3rd ed.). Oxford, UK: Butterworth-Heinemann, Ltd.

18. Leske, G. S. (1983). Water fluoridation. In Mellberg, J. R., & Ripa, L. W., Eds. *Fluoride in preventive dentistry.* Chicago, IL: Quintessence Publishing, 290.

19. Harris, N. O., & Garcia-Godoy, F., Eds. (1999). *Primary preventive dentistry* (5th ed.). Stamford, CT: Appleton and Lange, 658.

20. Black, G. V., & McKay, F. S. (1916). Mottled teeth—An endemic developmental imperfection of the teeth heretofore unknown in the literature of dentistry. *Dent Cosmos,* 58:129–56.

21. McKay, F. S. (1933). Mottled enamel: The prevention of its further production through a change of water supply at Oakley, Idaho. *J Am Dent Assoc,* 20:1137–49.

22. McKay, F. S. (1928). The relation of mottled enamel to caries. *J Am Dent Assoc,* 15:1429–37.

23. Burt, B. A., & Eklund, S. A. (2005). *Dentistry, dental practice, and the community* (6th ed.). St. Louis, MO: Elsevier Saunders.

24. Centers for Disease Control and Prevention. (1999). Achievements in public health, 1900–1999: Fluoridation of drinking water to prevent dental caries. *MMWR Morb Mortal Wkly Rep,* 48:933–40. Retrieved from http://www.cdc.gov/mmwr/preview/mmwrhtml/mm4841a1.htm.

25. Dean, H. T. (1993). Distribution of mottled enamel in the United States. *Public Health Rep,* 48:703–34.

26. Dean, H. T., Dixon, R. M., & Cohen, C. (1935). Mottled enamel in Texas. *Public Health Rep,* 50:424–42.

27. Dean, H. T., Jay P., Arnold, F. A., Jr., McClure, F. J., & Elvove, E. (1939). Domestic water and dental caries, including certain epidemiological aspects of oral *L. acidophilus. Public Health Rep,* 54:862–88.

28. Dean, H. T., Jay, P., Arnold, F. A., Jr., & Elvove, E. (1941). Domestic water and dental caries. II. A study of 2,832 white children aged 12–14 years, of eight suburban Chicago communities, including *L. acidophilus* studies of 1,761 children. *Public Health Rep,* 56:761–92.

29. Dean, H. T., Arnold, F. A., Jr., & Elvove, E. (1942). Domestic water and dental caries. V. Additional studies of the relation of fluoride domestic waters to dental caries experience in 4,425 white children aged 12–14 years of 13 cities in 4 states. *Public Health Rep,* 157:1155–79.

30. Ast, D. B., & Fitzgerald, B. (1962). Effectiveness of water fluoridation. *J Am Dent Assoc,* 65:581–87.

31. U.S. Department of Health and Human Services. *Healthy People 2020 Topics & Objectives: Oral Health. Oral Health Interventions.* Retrieved from http://www.healthypeople.gov/2020/topicsobjectives2020/objectiveslist.aspx?topicid=32 on 1/17/11.

32.

33. Groeneveld, A., Van Eck, A. A., & Backer Dirks, O. (1990, February). Fluoride in caries prevention: Is the effect pre- or post-eruptive? *J Dent Res,* 69 (Spec No):751–55; (discussion):820–23.

34. Featherstone, J. D. (1999). Prevention and reversal of dental caries: Role of low level fluoride. *Community Dent Oral Epidemiol,* 27:31–40.

35. Rolla, G., & Edstrand, J. (1996). Fluoride in oral fluids and dental plaque. In Fejerskov, O., Ekstrand, J., & Burt, B. A., Eds. *Fluoride in dentistry* (2nd ed.). Copenhagen, Denmark: Munksgaard, 215–19.

36. Hamilton, I. R. (1990). Biochemical effects of fluoride on oral bacteria. *J Dent Res,* 69 (Spec Iss):660–67.

37. Chow, L. C. (1990). Tooth-bound fluoride and dental caries. *J Dent Res,* 69 (Spec Iss):595–600.

38. Kidd, E. A., Thylstrup, A., Fejerskov, O., & Bruun, C. (1980). Influence of fluoride in surface enamel and degree of dental fluorosis on caries development in vitro. *Caries Res,* 14:196–202.

39. Singh, K. A., Spencer, A. J., & Brennan, D. S. (2007). Effects of water fluoride exposure at crown completion and maturation on caries of permanent first molars. *Caries Res,* 41:34–42.

40. Singh, K. A., Spencer, A. J., & Armfield, B. A. (2003). Relative effects of pre- and post-eruption water fluoride on caries experience of permanent first molars. *J Public Health Dent,* 63:11–19.

41. Koulourides, T. (1990). Summary of session II: Fluoride and the caries process. *J Dent Res,* 69 (Spec Iss):558.

42. Newbrun, E. (1989). Effectiveness of water fluoridation. *J Public Health Dent,* 49 (Spec Iss):279–89.

43. Griffin, S. O., Regnier, E., Griffin, P. M., & Huntley, V. (2007). Effectiveness of fluoride in preventing decay in adults. *J Dent Res,* 86:410–15.

44. Lambrou, D., Larsen, M., Fejerskov, O., & Tachos, B. (1981). The effect of fluoride in saliva on remineralization of dental enamel in humans. *Caries Res,* 15:341–45.

45. Backer-Dirks, O., Kunzel, W., & Carlos, J. P. (1978). Caries-preventive water fluoridation. In Ericcson, Y., Ed. Progress in caries prevention. *Caries Res,* 12 (Suppl 1):7–14.

46. Silverstone, L. M. (1983, May). Remineralization and enamel caries: New concepts. *Dent Update,* 10:261–73.

47. Featherstone, J. D. (1987). The mechanism of dental decay. *Nutr Today,* 22:10–16.

48. Fejerskov, O., Thylstrup, A., & Larsen, M. J. (1981). Rational use of fluorides in caries prevention. *Acta Odontol Scan,* 39:241–49.

49. Silverstone, L. M., Wefel, J. S., Zimmerman, B. F., Clarkson, B. H., & Featherstone, M. J. (1981). Remineralization of natural and artificial lesions in human dental enamel in vitro. *Caries Res,* 15:138–57.

50. Bowen, W. H., & Geddes, D. A. M. (1990). Summary of Session III: Fluoride in saliva and dental plaque. *J Dent Res,* 69 (Spec Iss):637.

51. Arnold, F. A., Jr., Likins, R. C., Russell, A. L., & Scott, D. B. (1962). Fifteenth year of the Grand Rapids fluoridation study. *J Am Dent Assoc,* 65:780–85.

52. Arnold, F. A., Jr., Dean, H. T., & Knutson, J. W. (1953). Effect of fluoridated public water supplies on dental caries incidence. Results of the seventh year of study at Grand Rapids and Muskegon, Mich. *Public Health Rep,* 68:141–48.

53. Ast, D. B., Finn, S. B., & McCaffrey, I. (1950). The Newburgh-Kingston Caries Fluorine Study. I. Dental findings after three years of water fluoridation. *Am J Public Health,* 40:716–24.

54. Blaney, J. R., & Tucker, W. H. (1948). The Evanston dental caries study. II. Purpose and mechanism of the study. *J Dent Res,* 27:279–86.

55. Brunelle, J. A., & Carlos, J. P. (1990). Recent trends in dental caries in U.S. children and the effect of water fluoridation. *J Dent Res,* 69 (Spec Iss):723–27.

56. Rozier, R. G. (1995). The effectiveness of community water fluoridation: Beyond dummy variables for fluoride exposure. *J Public Health Dent,* 55:195.

57. Horowitz, H. S. (1996). The effectiveness of community water fluoridation in the United States. *J Public Health Dent,* 56 (5 Spec):253–58.

58. Stookey, G. K. (1994). Review of fluorosis risk of self-applied topical fluorides: Toothpastes, mouthrinses and gels. *Community Dent Oral Epidemiol,* 22:181–86.

59. Griffin, S. O., Gooch, B. E., Lockwood, S. A., & Tomar, S. L. (2001). Quantifying the diffused benefit from water fluoridation in the United States. *Community Dent Oral Epidemiol,* 29:120–29.

60. Newbrun, E. (1992). Current regulations and recommendations concerning water fluoridation, fluoride supplements, and topical fluoride agents. *J Dent Res,* 67:1255–65.

61. Shenkin, J. D. (2011, Winter) An increase in caries rate or an increase in access to care: Data show mixed results. *J Public Health Dent,* 71:1–5.

62. Murray, J. J., Breckon, J. A., Reynolds, P. J., Tabari, E. D., & Nunn, J. H. (1991). The effect of residence and social class on dental caries experience in 15–16-year-old children living in three towns (natural fluoride, adjusted fluoride and low fluoride) in the north east of England. *Br Dent J,* 10:319–22.

63. Newbrun, E. (1989). Effectiveness of water fluoridation. *J Public Health Dent,* 49 (Spec Iss):279–89.

64. Kaminsky, L. S., Mahoney, M. C., Leach, J., Melius, J., & Miller, M. J. (1990). Fluoride: Benefits and risks of exposure. *Crit Rev Oral Biol Med,* 1:261–81.

65. Barnard, P. D., & Sivaneswaran, S. (1990). Oral health of Tamworth schoolchildren 24 years after fluoridation. *J Dent Res,* 69 (Div Abstr):934.

66. Griffin, S. O., Regnier, E., Griffin, P. M., & Huntley, V. N. (2007). Effectiveness of fluoride in preventing caries in adults. *J Dent Res,* 86:410–14.

67. Burt, B. A. (1985). Fluoride: How much of a good thing? *J Public Health Dent,* 5:37–38.

68. Griffin, S. O., Griffin, P. M., Swann, J. L., & Zlobin, N. (2005). New coronal caries in older adults: Implications for prevention. *J Dent Res,* 84:715–20.

69. Griffin, S. O., Griffin, P. M., Swann, J. L., & Zlobin, N. (2004). Estimating rates of new root caries in older adults. *J Dent Res,* 83:634–38.

70. Stamm, J. W., Banting, D. W., & Imrey, P. B. (1990). Adult root caries survey of two similar communities with contrasting natural water fluoride levels. *J Am Dent Assoc,* 120:143–49.

71. U.S. Department of Health and Human Services. (1987). *Oral health of United States adults. The national survey of oral health in U.S. employed adults and seniors: 1985–1986. National findings.* (NIH Publication No. 87-2868). Bethesda, MD: U.S. Department of Health and Human Services, National Institutes of Health.

72. Grembowski, D., Fiset, L., & Spadafora, A. (1992). How fluoridation affects adult dental caries. *J Am Dent Assoc,* 123:49–54.

73. McDonagh, M., Whiting, P., Bradley, M., Cooper, J., Sutton, A., Chestnutt, I., Misso, K., Wilson, P., Treasure, E., & Kleijnen, J. (2000). *A systematic review of public water fluoridation.* York, UK: University of York, NHS Centre for Reviews and Dissemination.

74. Morris, J., & White, D. (2000, December). The York review of water fluoridation—Key points for the busy practitioner. *Dent Update,* 474–75.

75. Centers for Disease Control and Prevention. (2001). Promoting oral health: Interventions for preventing dental caries, oral and pharyngeal cancers, and sports-related craniofacial injuries: A report on the recommendations of the Task Force on Community Preventive Services. *MMWR Morb Mortal Wkly Rep,* 50(RR-14):1–42.

76. Truman, B. I., Gooch, B. F., Sulemana, I., Gift, H. C., Horowitz, A. M., Evans C. A., Jr., Griffin, S. O., & Carande-Kulis, V. G. (2002). The task force on community preventive services. Reviews of evidence on interventions to prevent dental caries, oral and pharyngeal cancers, and sports-related craniofacial injuries. *Am J Prev Med,* 23(1S):21–54.

77. Lemke, C. W., Doherty, J. M., & Arra, M. C. (1970). Controlled fluoridation: The dental effects of discontinuation in Antigo, Wisconsin. *J Am Dent Assoc,* 80:782–86.

78. Stephen, K. W., McCall, D. R., & Tullis, J. I. (1987). Caries prevalence in Northern Scotland before and 5 years after water defluoridation. *Brit Dent J,* 163:324–26.

79. Attwood, D., & Blinkhorn, A. S. (1991). Dental health in schoolchildren 5 years after water fluoridation ceased in south-west Scotland. *Int Dent J,* 41:43–48.

80. Way, R. M. (1964). The effect on dental caries of a change from a naturally fluoridated to a fluoride-free communal water. *J Dent Child,* 31:151–57.

81. U.S. Department of Health and Human Services. (1991). *Public Health Service committee to coordinate environmental health and related programs. Review of fluoride: Benefits and risk.* Washington, DC: U.S. Department of Health and Human Services, Public Health Service.

82. Maupome, G., Clark, D. C., Levy, S. M., & Berkowitz, J. (2001). Patterns of dental caries following the cessation of water fluoridation. *Community Dent Oral Epidemiol,* 29:37–47.

83. Burt, B. A., Keels, M. A., & Heller, K. E. (2000). The effects of a break in water fluoridation on the development of dental caries and fluorosis. *J Dent Res,* 79:761–69.

84. Flaitz, C. M., Hill, E. M., & Hicks, M. J. (1989). A survey of bottled water usage by pediatric dental patients: Implications for dental health. *Quintessence Int,* 20:847–52.

85. Bartels, D., Haney, K., & Khajotia, S. S. (2000, Summer). Fluoride concentrations in bottled water. *J Okla Dent Assoc,* 91:18–22.

86. Tate, W. H., & Chen, J. T. (1994). Fluoride concentrations in bottled and filtered waters. *Gen Dent,* 42:362–66.

87. Food and Drug Administration. (1995). Beverages: Bottled water; final rule. 21 CFR 103, 60, 57075–57130.

88. Centers for Disease Control and Prevention. (2001). Recommendations for using fluoride to prevent and control dental caries in the United States. *MMWR Morb Mortal Wkly Rep,* 50:1–42.

89. Dean, H. T. (1942). The investigation of physiological effects by the epidemiological method. In Mouton, F. R., Ed. *Fluorine and dental health.* Washington, DC: American Association for the Advancement of Science, 19:23–31.

90. Fejerskov, O., Manji, F., & Baelum, V. (1990). The nature and mechanisms of dental fluorosis in man. *J Dent Res,* 69 (Spec Iss):692–700.

91. Whitford, G. M. (1996). *The metabolism and toxicity of fluoride* (2nd rev. ed.). (Monographs in Oral Science). Basel, Switzerland: Karger, 16.

92. Horowitz, H. S. (1986). Indexes for measuring dental fluorosis. *J Public Health Dent,* 46:179–83.

93. National Research Council. (2006). *Fluoride in drinking water. A scientific review of EPA's standards.* Washington, DC: National Academy Press.

94. U.S. EPA, Office of Water. New fluoride risk assessment and relative source contribution documents. EPA 822-F-11-001.

95. U.S. EPA. Health and Ecological Criteria Division, Office of Water. (2010, December). Fluoride: Dose-response analysis for non-cancer effects. EPA 820-R-10-019. http://water.epa.gov/action/advisories/drinking/upload/Fluoride_dose_response.pdf).

96. U.S. EPA. Health and Ecological Criteria Division, Office of Water. (2010, December). Fluoride: Dose-response analysis for non-cancer effects. EPA 820-R-10-019. http://water.epa.gov/action/advisories/drinking/upload/Fluoride_dose_response.pdf).

97. American Dental Association. (2006, November). ADA offers interim guidance on infant formula and fluoride. Retrieved March 12, 2008, from http://www.ada.org/prof/resources/positions/statements/fluoride_infants.asp.

98. Pendrys, D. G. (2000). Risk of enamel fluorosis in nonfluoridated and optimally fluoridated populations: Considerations for the dental professional. *J Am Dent Assoc,* 131:746–55.

99. Berg, J., Gerweck, C., Hujoel, P. P., King, R., Krol, D. M., Kumar, J., Levy, S., Pollick, H., Whitford, G. M., Strock, S., Aravamudhan, K., Frantsve-Hawley, J., & Meyer, D. M. (2011, January). Evidence-based clinical recommendations regarding fluoride intake from reconstituted infant formula and enamel fluorosis: A report of the American Dental Association Council on Scientific Affairs. *J Am Dent Assoc,* 142:79-87.

100. Beltran-Aguilar, E. D., Barker, L. K., Canto, M. T., Dye, B. A., Gooch, B. F., Griffin, S. O., Hyman, J., Jaramillo, F., Kingman, A., Nowjack-Raymer, R., Selwitz, R., & Wu, T. (2005). Surveillance for dental caries, dental sealants, tooth retention, edentulism, and enamel fluorosis. *MMWR CDC Suveill Summ,* 54 :1–44.

101. Dean, H. T. (1936). Chronic endemic dental fluorosis. *J Am Med Assoc,* 107:1269–73.

102. Lewis, D. W., & Banting, D. W. (1994). Water Fluoridation: Current effectiveness and dental fluorosis. *Community Dent Oral Epidemiol,* 22:153–58.

103. Hong, L., Levy, S. M., Broffitt, B., Warren, J. J., Kanellis, M. J., Wefel, J. S., & Dawson, D. V. (2006). Timing of fluoride intake in relation to development of fluorosis on maxillary central incisors. *Community Dent Oral Epidemiol,* 34:299–305.

104. Levy, S. M., Warren, J. J., Davis, C. S., Kirchner, H. L., Kanellis, M. J., & Wefel, J. S. (2001). Patterns of fluoride intake from birth to 36 months. *J Public Health Dent,* 61:70–77.

105. National Academy of Sciences, National Research Council. (2006). Fluoride in drinking water: A scientific review of EPA's standards. Washington, DC: National Academies Press.

106. Clark, D. C., Hann, H. J., Williamson, M. F., & Berkowitz, J. (1993). Aesthetic concerns of children and parents in relation to different classifications of the Tooth Surface Index of Fluorosis. *Community Dent Oral Epidemiol,* 21:360–64.

107. Horowitz, H. S., Heifetz, S. B., & Driscoll, W. S. (1972). Partial defluoridation of a community water supply and dental fluorosis. *Health Serv Rep,* 87:451–55.

108. Cutress, T. W., & Suckling, G. W. Differential diagnosis of dental fluorosis. (1990, February) *J Dent Res,* 69 (Spec No): 714–20; (discussion): 721.

109. National Institutes of Health. Consensus Development Conference Statement, NIH Consensus Development Conference on celiac disease. (2004, June). Retrieved March 12, 2008, from.

110. Meskin, L. H., Ed. (1995). Caries diagnosis and risk assessment: A review of preventive strategies and management. *J Am Dent Assoc,* 126 (Suppl):1S–24S.

111. American Academy of Pediatrics Committee on Nutrition. (1995). Fluoride supplementation for children: Interim policy recommendations. *Pediatrics,* 95:777.

112. American Academy of Pediatric Dentistry. (1995). Reference manual 1994–95. *Pediatr Dent,* 16 (Spec Iss):1–96.

113. Rozier, R. G., Adair, S., Graham, F., Iafolla, T., Kingman, A., Kohn, W., Krol, D., Levy, S., Pollick, H., Whitford, G., Strock, S., Frantsve-Hawley, J., Aravamudhan, K., & Meyer, D. M. (2010, December). Evidence-based clinical recommendations on the prescription of dietary fluoride supplements for caries prevention: A report of the American Dental Association Council on Scientific Affairs. *J Am Dent Assoc,* 141:1480–89. Retrieved from http://jada.ada.org/cgi/reprint/141/12/1480.

114. Galagan, D. J. (1953). Climate and controlled fluoridation. *J Am Dent Assoc,* 47:159–70.

115. Galagan, D. J., & Vermillion, J. R. (1957). Determining optimum fluoride concentrations. *Public Health Rep,* 72:491–93.

116. Galagan, D. J., Vermillion, J. R., Nevitt, G. A., Stadt, Z. M., & Dart, R. E. (1957). Climate and fluid intake. *Public Health Rep,* 72:484–90.

117. U.S. Public Health Service. (1962). *Public Health Service drinking water standards 1962* (PHS Publication No. 956). Washington, DC: Government Printing Office.

118. Heller, K. E., Sohn, W., Burt, B. A., & Eklund, S. A. (1999). Water consumption in the United States in 1994–96 and implications for water fluoridation policy. *J Public Health Dent,* 59:3–11.

119. Sohn, W., Heller, K. E., & Burt, B. A. (2001). Fluid consumption related to climate among children in the United States. *J Public Health Dent,* 61:99–106.

120. Levy, S. M., Kiritsy, M. C., & Warren, J. J. (1995). Sources of fluoride intake in children. *J Public Health Dent,* 55:39–52.

121. Kiritsy, M. C., Levy, S. M., Warren, J. J., Guha-Chowhury, N., Heilman, J. R., & Marshall, T. (1996) Assessing fluoride concentrations of juices and juice-flavored drinks. *J Am Dent Assoc,*1 27:895–902.

122. Reeves, T. G. (1996). Technical aspects of water fluoridation in the United States and an overview of fluoridation engineering world-wide. *Community Dent Health,* 13 (Suppl 2):21–26.

123. U.S. Department of Health and Human Services. (1986). *Water fluoridation. A manual for engineers and technicians 1986.* Bethesda, MD: U.S. Department of Health and Human Services, U.S. Public Health Service, Centers for Disease Control.

124. Centers for Disease Control and Prevention. (1995). Engineering and administrative recommendations for water fluoridation, 1995. *MMWR Morb Mortal Wkly Rep,* 44:1–40. Retrieved March 15, 2011, from http://www.cdc.gov/mmwr/preview/mmwrhtml/00039178.htm.

125. Hinman, A. R., Sterritt, G. R., & Reeves, T. G. (1996). The U.S. experience with fluoridation. *Community Dent Health,* 13 (Suppl 2):5–9.

126. Urbansky, E. T., & Schock, M. R. (2000). Can fluoridation affect lead (II) in potable water? Hexafluorosilicate and fluoride equilibria in aqueous. *Intern J Environ Studies,* 57:597–637.

127. Finney, W. F., Wilson, E., Callendar, A., Morris, M. D., & Beck, L. W. (2006, April). Reexamination of hexafluorosilicate hydrolysis by 19F NMR and pH measurements. *Environ Sci Technol,* 40:2572–77.

128. American Water Works Association. (2004). *Water fluoridation principles and practices. Manual of Water Supply Practice–M4* (5th ed.) USA.

129. Centers for Disease Control and Prevention. (2009, August). *Water fluoride laboratory proficiency testing program.* Retrieved January 30, 2011, from http://www.cdc.gov/fluoridation/fact_sheets/engineering/pt_factsheet.htm.

130. Lalumandier, J. A., & Jones, J. L. (1999). Fluoride concentrations in drinking water. *J Am Water Works Assoc,* 91:42–51.

131. Leland, D. E., Powell, K. E., & Anderson, R. S. (1980). A fluoride overfeed incident at Harbor Springs, Michigan. *J Am Water Works Assoc,* 72:238–43.

132. Petersen, L. R., Denis, D., Brown, D., Hadler, J. L., & Helgerson, S. D. (1998). Community health effects of a municipal water supply hyperfluoridation accident. *Am J Public Health,* 78:711–13.

133. Gessner, B. D., Beller, M., Middaugh, J. P., & Whitford, G. M. (1994). Acute fluoride poisoning from a public water system. *N Engl J Med,* 330:95–99.

134. Centers for Disease Control and Prevention. (2007, September). Oral health resources: Community water fluoridation. December 11, 2007, from .

135. CDC-Sponsored Water Fluoridation Training. Available at http://www.cdc.gov/fluoridation/engineering/training.htm

136. U.S. EPA, & Ground Water & Drinking Water—Customer Service. Frequent questions. How much does it cost to treat and deliver drinking water? Retrieved March 13, 2011, from http://safewater.supportportal.com/ics/support/default.asp?deptID=23015.)

137. Surgeon General's Statement on Community Water Fluoridation (2001). Retrieved from http://www.cdc.gov/fluoridation/fact_sheets/sg01.htm.

138. Ringelberg, M. L., Allen, S. J., & Jackson Brown, L. (1992). Cost of fluoridation: 44 Florida communities. *J Public Health Dent,* 52:75–80.

139. Griffin, S. O., Jones, K., & Tomar, S. L. (2001). An economic evaluation of community water fluoridation. *J Public Health Dent,* 61:78–86.

140. Neenan, M. E. (1996). Obstacles to extending fluoridation in the United States. *Community Dent Health,* 13 (Suppl 2):10–20.

141. Speier and Brown, W., Assembly members; & Maddy, Senate member. (1995, February 22). California Legislature Assembly bill 733.

142. Brown, J. P. (2000, May) Water fluoridation costs in Texas: Texas Health Steps (EPSDT-Medicaid)

143. Centers for Disease Control and Prevention. (1999). Water fluoridation and the costs of medicaid treatment for dental decay, Louisiana, 1995–1996. *MMWR Morb Mortal Wkly Rep,* 48:753–57.

144. Mjor, I. A. (1989). Amalgam and composite resin restorations: Longevity and reasons for replacement. In Anusavice, K. J., Ed. *Quality evaluations of dental restorations.* Chicago, IL: Quintessence Publishing, 61–72.

145. Qvist, J., Qvist, V., & Mjor, I. A. (1990). Placement and longevity of amalgam restorations in Denmark. *Acta Odontol Scand,* 48(5):297–303.

146. Wright, J. C., Bates, M. N., Cutress, T., & Lee, M. (2001, April). The cost-effectiveness of fluoridating water supplies in New Zealand. *Aust N Z J Public Health,* 25:170–78.

147. Centers for Disease Control and Prevention. (). Cost Savings of Community Water Fluoridation. Retrieved March 15, 2011, from http://www.cdc.gov/fluoridation/fact_sheets/cost.htm)148

148. Texas Department of Health. (2000, May). *Water fluoridation costs in Texas: Texas health steps. (EPSDT-Medicaid).* Retrieved from http://www.tdh.state.tx.us/dental/flstudy.htm.

149. Centers for Disease Control and Prevention. (1999). Water fluoridation and the costs of medicaid treatment for dental decay, Louisiana, 1995–1996. *MMWR Morb Mortal Wkly Rep,* 48:753–57.

150. O'Connell, J. M., Brunson, D., Anselmo, T., & Sullivan, P. W. (2005, November). Costs and savings associated with community water fluoridation programs in Colorado. *Prev Chronic Dis.* Retrieved from http://www.cdc.gov/pcd/issues/2005/nov/05_0082.htm.

151. Kumar, J. V., Adekugbe, O., & Melnik, T. A. (2010) Geographic variation in medicaid claims for dental procedures in New York State: Role of fluoridation under contemporary conditions. *Public Health Rep,* 125:647–54. Erratum in: Public Health Rep. 2010 Nov-Dec;125(6):788.)

152. World Health Organization. (2003). *World oral health report 2003.* Geneva, Switzerland: Author.

153. Estupiñán-Day, S. (2005). *Promoting oral health: The use of salt fluoridation to prevent dental caries.* Pan American Health Organization.

154. Bergmann, K. E., & Bergmann, R. L. (1995). Salt fluoridation and general health. *Adv Dent Res,* 9:138–43.

155. Mejia, R., Espinal, F., Velez, H., & Aguirre, M. (1976). Estudio sobre la fluoruracion de la sal. VIII Resultados obtenidos de 1964 a 1972. *Boll of Sanit Panam,* 80:67–80.

156. Kunzel, W. (1993). Systemic use of fluoride—Other methods: Salt, sugar, milk, etc. *Caries Res,* 27 (Suppl 1):16–22.

157. Review of water fluoridation and fluoride intake from discretionary fluoride supplements. Review for the National Health and Medical Research Council by the Royal Melbourne Institute of Technology-Key Centre for Applied and Nutritional Toxicology in conjunction with the Monash University Medical School's Centre for Epidemiology and Preventive Medicine, Melbourne, Australia, 15 April 1999.

158. Intersalt Cooperative Research Group. (1988). Intersalt: An international study of electrolyte excretion and blood pressure. Results for 24 hour urinary and potassium excretion. *Br Med J,* 297:319–28.

159. Yeung, A., Hitchings, J. L., Macfarlane, T. V., Threlfall, A., Tickle, M., & Glenny, A.-M. (2005). Fluoridated milk for preventing dental caries. *Cochrane Datab Syst Rev* (Iss 3. Art. No. CD003876).

Topical Fluoride Therapy

Howard F. Pollick

OBJECTIVES

After studying this chapter, the student should be able to:

1. List the fluoride compounds used to control caries and indicate their relative effectiveness.

2. Describe how topical fluorides work to prevent caries.

3. Identify what percentages of sodium fluoride, acidulated phosphate fluoride and stannous fluoride are available for office and home use.

4. Describe how topical fluoride is applied to the teeth.

5. Describe safety considerations with topical fluoride.

6. State the expected decreases in caries formation following use of dentifrices and mouthrinses containing fluoride.

7. Describe fluoridated varnishes and fluoride-releasing dental restorative materials and the potential of these materials to inhibit demineralization and enhance remineralization.

8. Describe safety considerations with topical fluoride.

INTRODUCTION

When public water supplies are available, community water fluoridation clearly represents the most effective, efficient, and economical of all known measures for preventing dental caries, although similar results have been observed with fluoridated salt in many countries. Unfortunately, fluoridated water is available to only about two-thirds of the U.S. population. Thus, it is obvious that additional measures are needed for the dental profession to provide more protection against caries to as many segments of the population as possible.

The term **topical fluoride therapy** refers to the use of systems containing relatively high concentrations of fluoride that are applied locally, or topically, to erupted tooth surfaces to prevent the formation of carious lesions requiring surgical treatment. This term encompasses the use of fluoride rinses, dentifrices, pastes, gels, foams, and varnishes, which are applied in various ways.

This chapter will focus on professionally applied topical fluoride; another chapter addresses self-applied topical fluoride, such as toothpastes (dentifrices) and rinses.

MECHANISM OF ACTION OF TOPICAL FLUORIDE TREATMENTS

Recent reviews of the mechanism of action of fluoride for caries control reveal a complex interaction over time between the fluoride concentration, the basic chemical building blocks of tooth enamel and dentin, saliva, dental plaque, and dietary sugars.[1] Permanent enamel is an acellular tissue composed chiefly of minerals (calcium-deficient carbonated hydroxyapatite, 85% in volume—$(Ca_{10-x}Na_x(PO_4)_{6-y}(CO_3)_z(OH)_{2-u}F_u)$).[2] The scientific evidence on the structure of the apatite portion of enamel has been the subject of discovery since the 1940s.[3] Hydroxyapatite molecules are arranged in long and thin apatite crystals, which in turn are organized into the resulting enamel prisms. Despite the high mineral content, the space between the crystals is occupied by water (12% by volume) and organic material (3% by volume). It is in this space filled with the enamel fluid that the de- and remineralization reactions take place. Upon a cariogenic challenge, hydroxyapatite crystals are dissolved from the subsurface while fluorapatite crystals are deposited at the surface, thus resulting in a subsurface lesion. The dissolution process of enamel is therefore a chemical event. On the other hand, permanent dentin contains (by volume) 47% apatite, 33% organic components, and 20% water. Fluoride concentrations as small as 1 ppm present in an acid solution can reduce the solubility of carbonated hydroxyapatite to that equivalent to hydroxyapatite. Higher concentrations of fluoride in solution decrease the solubility following a logarithmic pattern. To interfere in the dynamics of dental caries formation, fluoride must be constantly present in the oral environment at low concentrations. CaF_2-like globules deposited on enamel and biofilm after application of highly concentrated fluoride products act as a pH-controlled fluoride and calcium reservoir.

CaF_2 forms when the fluoride concentrations in the solution bathing enamel are higher than 100 ppm.

After an acidic challenge that causes demineralization of tooth surfaces, salivary flow buffers the acids produced by the bacterial breakdown of dietary sugars in dental plaque. When the pH is higher than 5.5, remineralization will naturally occur because saliva is supersaturated with respect to the dental mineral. Fluoride will adsorb to the surface of the partially demineralized crystals and attract calcium ions. Because carbonate-free or low-carbonate apatite is less soluble, these phases will tend to form preferentially instead of the original mineral coating and will be less soluble due to the exclusion of carbonate and incorporation of fluoride, rendering the enamel more resistant to future acidic challenges

Clinical studies indicate that fluoride has an antimicrobial effect that depends on factors such as the fluoride concentration applied and associated antibacterial components. With regard to fluoride concentration, studies with different research protocols have shown significantly lower plaque scores in subjects using a 5,000 ppm fluoride toothpaste in comparison with formulations containing 500, 1,100, and 1,500 ppm fluoride.

If low concentrations of fluoride applied with high frequency appear to be the most desirable for caries control, why are these professionally applied high-fluoride-concentration topical agents successful?[4] The discussion surrounding the desirability of producing more tightly bound fluoride (predominantly fluorhydroxyapatite) and less tightly bound calcium fluoride reaction products has continued for decades. In the 1940s and 1950s, when these high-fluoride-concentration/low-frequency-of-application compounds were developed, fluorhydroxyapatite was thought to be the most desirable reaction product from topical agents. This was because it mimicked what was achieved when systemic fluoride either substituted for the OH ion or occupied the "ionic gaps" in the hydroxyapatite lattice, therefore apparently making the tooth less vulnerable to caries by reducing its enamel solubility. Such reasoning has been disputed, and more emphasis has been placed on the desirable properties of having fluoride in a soluble (less tightly bound) form. Certainly, calcium fluoride can be formed on the surfaces of teeth from the high fluoride concentration/low pH, and probably from high-fluoride-concentration, neutral pH, topical agents. It is less certain whether such a reaction product can result from fluoride toothpaste that contains 1000 ppm or less. The rationale for the aim to form a sparingly soluble reaction product is that, as it dissolves in saliva and/or plaque fluid, it is available to supply low concentrations of ambient fluoride that can interfere with demineralization and promote remineralization at the tooth surface during the initial caries process. Fluoride could still be detected as leaving both sound and carious enamel surfaces 2 and 3 months after a topical fluoride application. Judging from *in vitro* experiments, these low levels of fluoride should have a marked effect on the mineral kinetics during enamel dissolution. However, such fluoride concentration can also be reached during the dissolution of fluorhydroxyapatite, thus again influencing the demineralization/remineralization of enamel. Therefore, the desirability of producing soluble versus insoluble reaction products relates not only to which is the *most* desirable because both would appear to be effective anticaries reaction products but also to whether fluorhydroxyapatite can be formed in or on tooth surfaces other than through systemic fluoride administration.

Whether fluoride is optimally positioned either in or on the tooth surface, as opposed to in the plaque or plaque fluid, is debatable and could be irrelevant as long as ionic fluoride is available at the site of the developing lesion. This hypothesis is supported by a number of studies reviewed by Ripa that showed the same caries reduction after topical fluoride applications with and without the prior removal of dental plaque.[5]

Individual patients should expect to see inter- and intraoral differences in the effectiveness of fluoride. Fluoride distribution in the mouth can differ in an individual and among individuals. Fluoride from a mouthrinse can be distributed proportionally in the mouth during the rinse, but its retention will be different at different intraoral sites. The effectiveness of either a passively dissolving fluoride tablet or a fluoridated dentifrice can also differ, depending on the intraoral distribution and retention of fluoride. There is subject-to-subject variability and site-to-site variability within the same mouth.

Clarkson proposed that "fluoride *controls* the progression of caries rather than *prevents* its initiation.[6] Clarkson proposed this based on a reevaluation of the Tiel-Culemborg study (which compared the prevalence of caries in two Dutch cities, one fluoridated and one nonfluoridated) and showed that if white spots were incorporated into both sets of prevalence data, there was no difference in caries activity between the fluoridated town of Tiel and the nonfluoridated town of Culemborg. However, if the classic epidemiological diagnosis of caries was used, the fluoridated town of Tiel showed a 50% decline in caries activity compared with the nonfluoridated town of Culemborg. Thus, the re-interpretation of these data suggests that fluoride does not prevent the initiation of the disease but, in fact, controls its progression.[7]

The concept of posteruption enamel maturation was postulated in the 1960s.[8] If no visible change in the enamel on permanent smooth tooth surfaces took place within 1½ years after eruption, it was found unlikely that any visible change would occur before the age of 15. In pits and fissures, the caries process starts early, and the first visible changes are soon followed by the formation of cavities. Up to 50% of incipient caries on proximal surfaces diagnosed only on radiographs did not progress within 4 to 8 years. Throughout these early posteruptive years, called the period of posteruption **enamel maturation**, fluoride and other elements continue to accumulate in the more superficial portions of enamel. This fluoride is derived from the saliva as well as from the exposure of the teeth to fluoride-containing water, food, and dental products. Following the period of enamel maturation, relatively little additional fluoride is incorporated from such sources into the enamel surface.[9] Thus, most of the fluoride that is incorporated into the developing enamel occurs during the preeruptive period of enamel formation and the posteruptive period of enamel maturation.

Most of the initial studies concerning topical fluoride applications were conducted with **sodium fluoride (NaF)**. At that time, it was recognized that prolonged exposure of the teeth to low concentrations of fluoride in the dental office was not practical. To overcome this problem, researchers explored two approaches: increasing the fluoride concentration and decreasing the pH of the application solution. Although it was initially proposed that the effectiveness of topically applied NaF was due to the formation of a fluorhydroxyapatite, subsequent investigations indicated that the primary reaction product involved the transformation of surface hydroxyapatite to calcium fluoride.[10]

The use of acidic fluoride solutions greatly favored the formation of calcium fluoride.[11] Neutral NaF solutions with fluoride concentrations of 100 ppm or less resulted primarily in the formation of fluorapatite whereas higher fluoride concentrations resulted in the formation of calcium fluoride.[12] Because topical applications of NaF involve the use of 2.0% solutions (slightly more than 9,000 ppm), the use of these solutions essentially involves the formation of calcium fluoride.[13]

The second fluoride compound developed for topical use in the dental office during the 1950s was **stannous fluoride (SnF_2)**.[14–16] Compared with NaF, the reaction of SnF_2 with enamel is unique because both the cation (stannous) and the anion (fluoride) react chemically with enamel components. Formation of stannous fluorophosphate prevents, at least temporarily, the phosphate loss typical of NaF applications. The exact nature of the tin-containing reaction products varies depending on reaction conditions, including pH, concentration, and length of exposure (or reaction time).[17,18]

A third topical fluoride system for professional use was developed during the 1960s and is widely known as **acidulated phosphate fluoride (APF)**. This system was developed by Brudevold and co-workers in an effort to achieve higher amounts of fluorhydroxyapatite and lower amounts of calcium fluoride formation.[19,20] These investigators reviewed the various chemical reactions of fluoride with hydroxyapatite and concluded that (1) if the pH of the fluoride system was made acidic to enhance the rate of reaction of fluoride with hydroxyapatite and (2) if phosphoric acid was used as the acidulant to increase the concentration of phosphate present at the reaction site, it should be possible to obtain higher amounts of fluoride deposited in surface enamel as fluorhydroxyapatite with minimal formation of calcium fluoride and minimal loss of enamel phosphate. On the basis of this chemical reasoning, APF systems were developed and shown to be effective for caries prevention.

Subsequent independent studies of the reactions of APF with enamel indicated, however, that the original chemical objectives were only partially achieved. The major reaction product of APF with enamel is also calcium fluoride although a higher amount of fluorhydroxyapatite is formed than is with the previous topical fluoride systems.[21–23] The primary chemical reaction product with all three types of topical fluoride systems (i.e., NaF, SnF_2, and APF) is the formation of calcium fluoride on the enamel surface.

The initial deposition of calcium fluoride on the treated tooth surfaces is by no means permanent; a relatively rapid loss of fluoride occurs within the first 24 hours with some continued loss occurring during the following 15 days.[24–28] The rate of loss varies among patients and is influenced by the nature of the fluoride treatment.[29,30] Nevertheless, it is known that professionally applied fluoride treatment in each individual results in an increase in the permanently bound fluoride content of the outermost layers of the enamel with a subsequent decrease in the susceptibility of the enamel for caries initiation and progression.

DID YOU KNOW ?

Numerous investigations of professional fluoride applications have focused on the role that calcium fluoride deposits on the enamel surface play in providing the observed cariostatic benefits, that is, preventing formation of dental caries.

The most desirable form of fluoride in enamel for caries prevention is fluorhydroxyapatite, and the most efficient means of forming this reaction product occurs with prolonged exposure of the enamel to low concentrations of fluoride. Calcium fluoride can serve as a fluoride source for enamel remineralization, and calcium fluoride dissolves much more slowly in the oral environment than in an aqueous solution because of the presence of a phosphate or protein-rich coating of the globular deposits of calcium fluoride on the enamel surface.[31–34] As a result of continued research, a growing body of convincing evidence suggests that the deposits of calcium fluoride serve as an important fluoride reservoir and that these phosphate-coated globules are dissolved in the presence of plaque acids, providing an available source of both fluoride and phosphate to facilitate the remineralization of decalcified areas.[35]

Regardless of the mechanism of action of professionally applied topical fluoride treatments, the results of clinical trials clearly indicate that the benefits are related to the number of treatments. (Table 15–1 ■) summarizes a clinical study in which schoolchildren were given a dental prophylaxis and a topical application of 8% SnF_2 at 6-month intervals throughout a 3-year period.[36] Dental caries examinations were performed initially and each year thereafter. It is apparent from these data that the caries-preventive benefits increased in relation to the number of treatments. Similar observations have been noted with the other two fluoride systems used for professional applications. The original NaF topical application procedure developed by Knutson specified a series of four treatments during a 2-week period.[37] Mellberg and co-workers have also indicated the need for repeated topical applications of APF to obtain maximal benefits.[38,39,43] Thus, it is apparent that maximal patient benefits can be obtained only with repeated topical applications regardless of the nature of the fluoride system used.

It was noted earlier that the reaction of SnF_2 with enamel resulted in the formation of tin-containing compounds. Although much less is known about the precise nature and ultimate fate of these compounds, it appears that they contribute significantly to the cariostatic activity of SnF_2. The tin reaction products formed on sound enamel surfaces appear to be leached from the enamel in a manner similar to that for calcium fluoride.[40] The most accumulation of stannous complexes occurs in circumscribed areas of enamel defects; typically, such areas are hypomineralized and are frequently the result of decalcification associated with the initiation of the caries process. Extremely high concentrations of tin, about 20,000 ppm, have been reported in these locations.[41] Clinically, these areas, which have been described as *frank carious areas,* become pigmented (presumably because of the presence of the tin complexes) and appear to be more calcified following the application of SnF_2. This pigmentation has thus been suggested as indicative of the arrest of carious lesions and is typically retained for 6 to 12 months or longer, implying that these stannous reaction products are of considerably greater significance than those formed on sound enamel.

It has become increasingly apparent that application of fluoride to sound, fully matured enamel results in very little fluoride deposition that lasts more than 24 hours. This situation apparently occurs regardless of the nature of the fluoride compound, the concentration of fluoride, or the manner of application. Thus, there appears to be no preventive benefits from the application of fluoride to maturated, sound enamel. However, where the enamel is demineralized, fluoride application is of benefit.

EFFECTS OF FLUORIDE ON PLAQUE AND BACTERIAL METABOLISM

Thus far, the assumption has been that the cariostatic effects of fluoride are mediated through a chemical reaction between this ion and the outermost portion of the enamel surface. Overwhelmingly, data support this view. A growing body of

TABLE ■ 15–1   Clinical Reductions in Incremental Caries as a Function of the Number of Topical Fluoride Applications

Study Period (Years)	Total Number of Topical Applications	Caries Reduction (%)	
		DMFT	DMFS
1	2	2.8	12.6
2	4	29.2	34.1
3	6	47.4	51.5

DMFT, decayed, missing, or filled permanent teeth; DMFS, decayed, missing, or filled surfaces.
(*Source:* Data from values calculated from data presented by Beiswanger, B. B., Mercer, V. H., Billings, R. J., & Stookey, G. K. (1980).)

information suggests, however, that the caries-preventive action of fluoride can also include an inhibitory effect on the oral flora involved in the initiation of caries. The ability of fluoride to inhibit glycolysis (breaking down of glucose) by interfering with the enzyme enolase has long been known; concentrations of fluoride as low as 50 ppm have been shown to interfere with bacterial metabolism. Moreover, fluoride can accumulate in dental plaque in concentrations higher than 100 ppm. Although the fluoride normally present in plaque is largely bound and thus unavailable for antibacterial action, it dissociates to ionic fluoride when the pH of plaque decreases (i.e., when acids are formed). Thus, when the carious process starts and acids are formed, plaque fluoride in ionic form could serve to interfere with further acid production by plaque microorganisms. In addition, it could react with the underlying layer of dissolving enamel, promoting its remineralization as fluorhydroxyapatite. The end result of this process is a biochemical restoration of the initial lesion by remineralization of enamel and the formation of a more resistant enamel surface. The ability of fluoride to promote the reprecipitation of calcium phosphate solutions in apatitic forms has been repeatedly demonstrated.

In addition to these possible effects of fluoride, several investigators have reported that the presence of tin, especially as provided by stannous fluoride, SnF_2, is associated with significant antibacterial activity, which has been reported to decrease both the amount of dental plaque and gingivitis in both animals and adult humans.[42,43] Existing evidence suggests that these antibacterial effects of fluoride and tin can also contribute to the observed cariostatic activity of topically applied fluorides.

TOPICAL FLUORIDE APPLICATIONS

A recent review of professionally applied fluoride was undertaken as part of the IoM report.[44] Fluorides can be professionally applied in the form of varnish or gel. Varnishes are brushed onto clean, dry teeth. The application takes about 1 minute, and the varnish sets quickly. To keep the varnish on the teeth for a number of hours, patients are told to eat soft foods and avoid brushing and flossing for the remainder of the day. Gels are applied to the teeth using gel trays, which must stay on the patient's teeth for approximately 4 minutes Increasingly, varnishes are used instead of gels due to the ease of application and low risk of ingestion, especially for younger children Varnishes and gels are equally effective at preventing caries.[45]

Fluoride varnish has been shown to be effective in the prevention of caries in both primary and permanent teeth.[46] The interval for frequency of application of fluoride varnish varies depending on the risk of the patient—more frequently for children with higher risk.[47] Although use of fluoride varnish for caries prevention is technically considered an "off-label" use, there is a robust evidence base for the efficacy of varnish at preventing caries.[46,48,49]

Given the longer period of time that is required for such studies, the large numbers of subjects required and the need to target high caries risk patients, these are not studies easily undertaken. Future clinical trials are needed to evaluate whether the modality of fluoride administration in moderate versus high caries risk adults makes a difference in the reduction or remineralization of caries, and whether multiple modalities of fluoride versus use of a single modality are more effective for these patients.

Although the reviewed clinical trials varied greatly in design, conduct, and quality scores, all demonstrated that the use of supplemental and professionally applied fluoride in moderate and high caries risk adults is effective in preventing and/or remineralizing dental caries.

Low dose daily NaF rinses had the most generalizable results for adults at risk for caries. This was followed by evidence for 1.1 percent NaF paste/gel, although these studies are more targeted to root caries lesions. Finally, while small in numbers of participants, 5 percent NaF varnish had two studies with high quality ratings and showing moderate magnitude in controlling root caries.[50]

A pragmatic trial of fluoride varnish applied three times a year for three years with children aged 7–8 years at baseline failed to demonstrate prevention of caries (DMFT) in the first permanent molar teeth. Similar results have been reported by Tagliaferro et al., when not accompanied by the application of sealants.[51] Based on the results of the systematic review alone, school varnish programs are likely to be implemented without rigorous evaluation, but the findings of this trial suggest that programs to prevent caries in the permanent dentition are not an efficient use of resources.[46, 52]

Considering the currently available evidence and risk-benefit aspects, it seems justifiable to recommend the use of fluoridated dentifrices to individuals of all ages, and additional fluoride therapy should also be targeted toward individuals at high caries risk.[53]

The use of concentrated fluoride solutions (see Table 15–2 ■) applied topically to the dentition for the prevention of dental caries has been studied extensively during the past 60 years, although few studies have been conducted since the 1970s. This procedure results in a significant increase in the resistance of the exposed tooth surfaces to the development of dental caries and, as a result, has become a standard procedure in most dental offices.

At present, three different fluoride systems have been adequately evaluated and approved for use in this manner in the United States. These three systems are 2% sodium fluoride (NaF) containing 9000 ppm fluoride, 8% stannous fluoride (SnF_2) containing 19,400 ppm fluoride, and acidulated phosphate fluoride (APF) systems containing 1.23% fluoride or 12,300 ppm fluoride.

Available Forms

When topical fluoride applications became available to the profession, the fluoride compounds, NaF and SnF_2, were obtained in powder or crystalline form, and aqueous solutions were prepared immediately prior to use. Subsequently, it was realized that NaF solutions were stable if stored in plastic containers, and this compound became available in liquid, gel, and powder form. Several factors resulted in a trend toward the use of ready-to-use, stable, flavored preparations in gel and

TABLE ■ 15–2   **Fluoride Concentration and Total Amounts in Fluoride Products**

Agent	Fluoride Concentration	ppm F	Volume or Weight	Total F Dose	Comments	Time/ Frequency
F varnish (5% NaF)	2.2500%	22,600	0.25 ml	5.65 mg		1 min; 3/yr
F varnish (5% NaF)	2.2500%	22,600	0.4 ml	9 mg		1 min; 3/yr
8% SnF_2	1.9360%	19,360	5 ml	96.8 mg	Seated, suction, spit	4 min; 2/yr
APF office gel	1.2300%	12,300	5 ml	61.5 mg	Seated, suction, spit	4 min; 2/yr
NaF gel/foam (2%)	0.9000%	9,000	5 ml	45 mg	Seated, suction, spit	4 min; 2/yr
Toothpaste (0.22% NaF)	0.1000%	1000	1 g	1 mg		2/day
Home gel (0.4% SnF_2)	0.0970%	970	1 g	1 mg		1/day
Mouthinse (0.05% NaF)	0.0250%	225	10 ml	2.25 mg		1/day
Fluoridated water	0.0001%	1	1 liter	1 mg		Several/day

foam form: continued research of different types of agents; professional recognition of disadvantages of existing forms with regard to patient acceptance and stability; and the need to use professional time more efficiently. The "one-minute foams" are also popular, but research supports use of only the 4-minute foams.

Sodium Fluoride

This material is available as a powder, gel, foam, liquid, and varnish. The compound is recommended for use in a 2% concentration (9000 ppm fluoride), which can be prepared by dissolving 0.2 g of powder in 10 ml of distilled water. The prepared solution or gel has a basic pH and is stable if stored in plastic containers. The lack of acidity makes this product preferable when there are composite and porcelain restorations because they can be etched by acidic solutions. Ready-to-use 2% solutions and gels of NaF are commercially available. Because of the relative absence of taste considerations with this compound, these solutions generally contain little flavoring or sweetening agents.

Stannous Fluoride

This compound is available in powder form, either in bulk containers or pre-weighed capsules. The recommended and approved concentration is 8%, which is obtained by dissolving 0.8 g of the powder in 10 ml of distilled water. Stannous fluoride solutions are quite acidic with a pH of about 2.4 to 2.8. Aqueous solutions of SnF_2 are not stable because of the formation of stannous hydroxide and, subsequently, stannic oxide, which is visible as a white precipitate. As a result, solutions of this compound must be prepared immediately prior to use. As will be noted later, SnF_2 solutions have a bitter, metallic taste. A stable, flavored solution can be prepared with glycerin and sorbitol to retard hydrolysis of the agent and with any of a variety of compatible flavoring agents, thus eliminating the need to prepare this solution from the powder and improving patient acceptance.

Acidulated Phosphate Fluoride

This treatment system is available as a solution, foam, or gel; all forms are stable and ready to use.[54,55] All contain 1.23% fluoride, generally obtained by the use of 2.0% NaF and 0.34%

hydrofluoric acid. Phosphate is usually provided as orthophosphoric acid in a concentration of 0.98%. The pH of true APF systems should be about 3.5. Gel preparations feature a greater variation in composition, particularly with regard to the source and concentration of phosphate. In addition, the gel preparations generally contain thickening (binders), flavoring, and coloring agents.

Another form of APF for topical applications, namely thixotropic gels, is also available. The term **thixotropic** denotes a solution that sets in a gel-like state but is not a true gel. With application of pressure, thixotropic gels behave like solutions; it has been suggested that these preparations are more easily forced into the interproximal spaces than conventional gels. The active fluoride system in thixotropic gels is identical to conventional APF solutions. Although the initial thixotropic gels exhibited somewhat poorer biologic activity in in vitro studies, subsequent formulations were at least equivalent to conventional APF systems. Even though few clinical efficacy studies have been reported, the collective data were considered adequate evidence of activity.[56]

A foam form of APF is also available. Laboratory studies indicate that the amount of fluoride uptake in enamel after applications using the foam is comparable to that observed with conventional APF gels and solutions.[57,58] The primary advantage of foam preparations is that appreciably less material is used for a treatment; therefore, lesser amounts are likely to be inadvertently swallowed by young children during professional application.[59] Equally important, foam applications are better tolerated by patients owing to the pleasant taste imparted by the flavoring agents.

Application Procedures

In essence, three procedures are available for administering topical fluoride treatments. One procedure, in brief, involves the isolation of teeth and continuously painting the liquid solution onto the tooth surfaces. The second, and more popular, procedure involves the use of fluoride foams or gels applied with a disposable tray. Most recently, fluoride varnish has been used for young children and individuals with developmental disabilities; it is easily painted on the tooth surfaces without the need for isolation.

In the past, it was assumed that it was necessary to administer a thorough dental prophylaxis prior to the topical application of fluoride. This hypothesis was supported by the results of an early study that suggested topically applied NaF was more effective if a prophylaxis preceded the treatment.[60] The results of four clinical trials have indicated that a prophylaxis immediately prior to the topical application of fluoride is not necessary.[61–64] In these studies, the children were given topical applications of APF in the conventional manner, except that three different procedures were used to clean the teeth immediately prior to each treatment: a dental prophylaxis, toothbrushing and flossing, or no cleaning procedure. The results indicated that the cariostatic activity of the APF treatment was not influenced by the different pre-application procedures.

DID YOU KNOW

Thus, the administration of a dental prophylaxis prior to the topical application of fluoride must be considered optional; it should be performed if there is a general need for a prophylaxis, but it need not be performed as a prerequisite for topical fluoride applications.

It should be stressed that various precautions should be taken routinely to minimize the amount of fluoride that is inadvertently swallowed by the patient during the application procedure. A number of reports have shown that 10 to 30 mg of fluoride can be inadvertently swallowed during the application procedure, and it has been suggested that the ingestion of these quantities of fluoride by young children can contribute to the development of dental fluorosis in teeth that are unerupted and in the developmental stage.[65–71] Precautions that should be undertaken include (1) using only the required amount of the fluoride solution or gel to perform the treatment adequately, (2) positioning the patient in an upright position, (3) using efficient saliva aspiration, or suctioning, apparatus, and (4) requiring the patient to expectorate thoroughly on completion of the fluoride application. The use of these procedures has been shown to reduce the amount of inadvertently swallowed fluoride to less than 2 mg, which can be expected to be of little consequence.[72]

After the topical application is completed, the patient is advised not to rinse, drink, or eat for 30 minutes. This recommendation is supported by a 1986 study that measured the amount of fluoride deposition in incipient lesions (subsurface enamel demineralization) in patients who either were, or were not, permitted to rinse, eat, or drink during this 30-minute post-treatment period.[73] It was found that significantly higher fluoride deposition occurred when the patients were not permitted to rinse, eat, or drink following the fluoride treatment.

Whichever fluoride system is used for topical fluoride applications, the teeth should be exposed to the fluoride for 4 minutes for maximal cariostatic benefits.[46,74–76] This treatment time has

consistently been recommended for both NaF and APF. Some confusion has arisen, however, with regard to SnF_2 because shorter application periods of 15 to 30 seconds with SnF_2 have been reported to result in significant cariostatic benefits. Nevertheless, the collective results of these and subsequent clinical investigations indicate that maximum caries protection is achieved only with the use of the longer exposure period. Thus, although reduced exposure periods of 30 to 60 seconds are frequently advised as a fluoride maintenance or preventive measure, the use of the longer, 4-minute application should be required for patients. The 1-minute time period advertised by some companies on available fluorides is not adequate for most patients because more time is needed for the product to be maximally effective.

Application of Fluoride Gels and Foams

The commonly used and convenient technique for providing treatments with fluoride gels and foams involves the use of a soft, styrofoam tray. These trays can be bent to insert in the mouth and are soft enough to produce no discomfort when they reach the soft tissues. These trays, as well as some of the previous types of trays, allow simultaneous treatment of both arches.

As with the use of topical fluoride solutions, the treatment can be preceded by a prophylaxis if indicated by existing oral conditions. With the tray application technique, the armamentarium (equipment and pharmaceutical agents) consists simply of a suitable tray and the fluoride gel or foam.

Many different types of trays are available; selection of a tray adequate for the individual patient is an important part of the technique.[77] Most manufacturers offer sizes to fit patients of different ages. An adequate tray should cover all the patient's dentition; it should also have enough depth to reach beyond the cementoenamel junction and to contact the alveolar mucosa to prevent saliva from diluting the fluoride gel or foam.

If a prophylaxis is given, the patient is permitted to rinse, and the teeth of the arch to be treated are dried with compressed air. A ribbon of gel or foam is placed in the trough portion of the tray and the tray seated over the entire arch. The method used must ensure that the gel/foam reaches all of the teeth and flows interproximally. If, for instance, a soft pliable tray is used, the tray is pressed or molded against the tooth surfaces, and the patient can also be instructed to bite gently against the tray. Some of the early trays contained a sponge-like material that "squeezed" the gel against the teeth when the patient was asked to bite lightly or to simulate a chewing motion after the trays were inserted. It is recommended that the trays be kept in place for a 4-minute treatment period for optimal fluoride uptake, even though some systems recommend a 1-minute application time. As noted previously, the patient is advised not to eat, drink, or rinse for 30 minutes following the treatment.[73] Figure 15–1 ■ illustrates the tray technique of fluoride gel application.

Application of Fluoride Varnish

Teeth should be relatively dry before applying fluoride varnish. The paint brush that comes with the product is used to paint the varnish on all selected tooth surfaces (see Figure 15–2 ■). Patients should be instructed that some varnishes leave a temporary, yellow stain that can last for 24 hours. In addition,

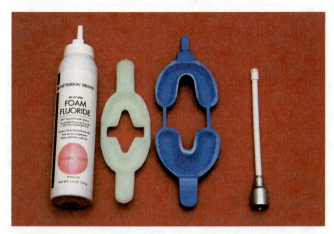

FIGURE ■ 15–1 Fluoride trays. Appropriate-size soft styrofoam trays are used to avoid pinching the soft tissues. A ribbon of gel is dispensed into the trough of the tray. Enough gel should be used to cover all tooth surfaces, but care should be used to avoid an excess that will flow into the mouth. (Experience will teach the operator how much gel to use.) A saliva ejector is also needed during fluoride application.

(*Source:* M. Sigman-Grant & J. Morita, Defining and interpreting intakes of sugars, *American Journal of Clinical Nutrition,* 2003.)

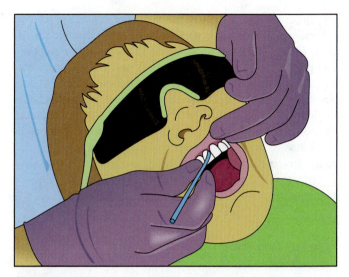

FIGURE ■ 15–2 Fluoride Varnish Application. Operator should paint on fluoride varnish to areas at high caries risk.

patients should not eat abrasive food or brush their teeth until the next morning for optimum effectiveness. Fluoride varnish has shown promising results in preventing early childhood caries in young children and in treating exposed root surfaces in adults. It has also been recommended that adults not drink alcohol for the first 4 hours following fluoride varnish application as it dissolves the varnish. Hypersensitive reactions have infrequently been reported to the wood rosin used in the varnish.

Application Frequency

As previously mentioned, although a single, topical application is accepted as not being able to impart maximal caries protection, considerable confusion has arisen regarding the preferred frequency for administering topical fluoride treatments. Much of this confusion is caused by the absence of controlled, clinical evaluations of this variable, particularly with the most commonly used agent APF.

The original Knutson technique for the topical application of NaF consisted of a series of four applications provided at approximately 1-week intervals with only the first application preceded by a prophylaxis.[37] It was further suggested that this series of applications be administered at ages 3, 7, 10, and 13 years with these ages selected, or varied, in accordance with the eruption pattern of the teeth.[78] The objective of the timing was to provide protective benefits to the permanent teeth during the period of changing dentition. Because this treatment sequence did not coincide with the common patient-recall pattern in the dental office, Galagan and Knutson explored the possible use of longer intervals of 3 or 6 months between the individual applications in each treatment series.[79] The results of their work indicated that although significant benefits were obtained with single applications provided at 3- or 6-month intervals, maximal benefits were obtained only with a series of treatments. Nevertheless, the administration of single applications of NaF at 3- to 6-month intervals became a common practice because these intervals were more convenient to the dentist's normal recall system.

When SnF_2 and APF were subsequently developed and evaluated, apparently little, if any, attempt was made to determine the optimal treatment frequency. Instead, the treatments were administered as single applications provided at 6- or 12-month intervals, which were convenient to the normal office schedules. Because these treatment intervals resulted in significant cariostatic benefits, the procedure that was ultimately approved and recommended involved this application frequency.

In view of this background, it seems that the frequency of topical applications should be dictated by the conditions and needs presented by each patient and not by the convenience of the dental office. This conclusion is supported by the data cited earlier, which reveal that a series of applications is required to impart maximal caries resistance to the tooth surface. Current studies support this recommendation.[80–82]

Thus, it is recommended that new patients, regardless of age, with active caries be given an initial series of four topical fluoride applications within a period of 2 to 4 weeks. If desired, the initial application can be preceded by a thorough prophylaxis and the remaining three applications of the initial treatment series should be preceded by toothbrushing to remove plaque and oral debris. It should be obvious that this series of treatments can be very conveniently combined with plaque control, dietary counseling, and initial restorative programs that the dental provider has devised for these patients. Following this initial series of treatments, the patient should be given single, topical applications at intervals of 3, 6, or 12 months, depending on the patient's caries status. There was insufficient evidence to recommend that adult patients with little evidence of existing or anticipated caries, at low risk for caries, should be given single applications every 12 months as a preventive measure.[76]

Special effort should be made by the dental provider to schedule topical fluoride applications so as to provide treatment to newly erupted teeth within 12 months after eruption, and preferably as close to eruption as possible. As noted earlier, an approximate 2-year enamel maturation period occurs immediately following tooth eruption. The preventive benefits of fluoride are invariably much higher on newly erupted teeth than on previously erupted teeth.[83–86] This finding is apparent regardless of the fluoride system used and is presumably due to the greater reactivity, permeability, and ease of formation of fluorhydroxyapatite in enamel still undergoing calcification (or maturation).

DID YOU KNOW?

Fluoride varnish application is more appropriate than other topical fluoride modalities for newly erupted primary teeth. Children at this young age could swallow too much of a topical fluoride gel or foam and might have pre-cooperative behavior, making it difficult to use typical topical fluoride gels or foams.

EFFICACY OF TOPICAL FLUORIDE THERAPY

Clinical studies demonstrate that topical fluoride therapy contributes significantly to the partial control of dental caries. Unfortunately, the practitioner is frequently concerned, and sometimes confused, about which procedure or agent should be used in a given situation to provide a maximal degree of dental caries protection for the patient. Such concern and confusion are understandable when it is realized that dental caries investigators themselves frequently do not agree on these matters.

The results of the numerous clinical investigations of various topical fluoride agents and treatment procedures have been the subject of several reviews.[86–100] The recommendations based on those reviews provide excellent guidance to practitioners. Adair summarized his recommendations in Table 15–3 ■.

As noted earlier, the Food and Drug Administration (FDA) has evaluated and approved three different types of fluoride systems (NaF, SnF_2, and APF) as safe and effective for topical fluoride applications.[101] To determine which of these systems could be the most effective, practitioners would have to compare the results of independent clinical studies in which all three systems have been tested when used in the recommended manner. Unfortunately, such data are not available, and alternative procedures must be sought.

Different approaches have been taken to estimate the magnitude of the cariostatic benefits that can be expected from topical applications of the different approved fluoride systems. One approach is simply to list all of the pertinent clinical trials and then determine the arithmetic mean of the reported caries reduction. This approach has been used by several investigators who observed the results for children residing in a nonfluoridated community.[102–104] Another approach is to use an empirically based procedure with existing clinical data to predict the efficacy of different systems.[105] Whatever the approach, study designs varied in a number of ways, such as the number and frequency of topical applications and the study duration. These variations serve to confound estimates of cariostatic efficacy. Over 4400 children were included in the trials comparing a fluoride gel with a placebo and over 2700 in those comparing fluoride gel with no treatment. For the great majority of children the fluoride gel they received was Acidulated Phosphate Fluoride (APF). There is clear evidence that fluoride gel has a caries-inhibiting effect. Basing the estimate on those trials with placebo rather than no-treatment controls, provides a more conservative estimate of treatment effect and suggests that use of this intervention is associated with a 21% (95% CI, 14% to 28%) reduction in decayed, missing and filled tooth surfaces. This would correspond to a number needed to treat (NNT) of 2 to avoid one D(M)FS per year in a child population with a caries increment of 2.2 D(M)FS per year (in the middle range of control group rates for included studies), or an NNT of 24 for children from a population with a caries increment of 0.2 D(M)FS/year (at the lowest end of the observed range).

Considerably less information is available to document the efficacy of topical fluoride applications in adults. A total of 14 clinical trials were conducted in adults during the period 1944–1974, but the studies used a wide variety of experimental conditions, including the type of topical fluoride system, frequency of applications, and duration of the test period.[106–118] Although most of the methods resulted in a significant cariostatic benefit, the magnitude of this effect varied considerably, as might be expected. Furthermore, none of these studies used the application frequency suggested earlier for children.

Dental scientists generally recognize that the dental caries process is fundamentally the same in both children and adults, although the rate of progression in young and middle-age adults is frequently much slower) because of a variety of factors, including more efficient oral hygiene and fewer between-meal snacks. Conversely, in older adults, the rate of progression can increase because of medications that reduce salivary flow and root exposure. A common assumption is that topical fluoride applications are effective for preventing coronal caries regardless of the age of the patient. Root caries will be discussed later. Once again, the frequency of application should be dictated by the patient's needs; in the presence of frank or incipient caries activity, an initial series of applications should be given followed by maintenance applications at 3, 6, or 12 months, depending on patient needs (i.e., evidence and extent of caries activity).

The choice of the fluoride system can be at the discretion of the dentist and be based on personal experience. All professionally applied fluoride systems have been demonstrated to be effective. Factors to consider are ease of application for the operator, including time, cost, materials, potential for swallowing, and availability of adequate suction. For the patient, the factors include comfort, taste, staining, frequency, and fee.

TABLE ■ 15–3   Fluoride Regimens in Contemporary Pediatric Dental Practice[a]

Dietary supplements (0.25, 0.5 or 1.0 mg F/day)

- Allow no dietary supplements where the drinking water for the child's residence has more than 0.6 ppm fluoride.
- Assay patient's primary source of drinking water; consider other sources of fluoride intake.
- Prescribe fluoride for children considered at high risk for caries between 6 months and 16 years of age.
- Consider delaying supplementation until after eruption of permanent first molars for all children to reduce the risk for development of dental fluorosis.
- Ensure that parents understand risks/benefits of supplementation.
- Ensure that parents and older children understand the need to adhere to a daily routine for many years.
- Instruct patient to chew/swish supplement for 1 minute prior to swallowing the supplement every evening.
- Prescribe no more than 120 mg F in the bottles of tablets/lozenges to protect against severe symptoms of acute overdose in the event that all tablets are inadvertently consumed at one time
- Administer no prenatal administration because it has no benefit.

Fluoride toothpaste/dentifrice (1000 ppm F)

- Use in children less than 2 years old should be based on caries risk assessment. For those at high risk, parents should apply a thin smear on an infant toothbrush up to age 2 years once a day.
- Have an adult brush teeth of a young child and supervise brushing by older child.
- Use pea-sized dab of dentifrice in children age 2–6 years of age (those with immature swallowing reflexes); older children can use larger amounts
- Brush with fluoride toothpaste twice daily.

Mouthrinses (225 ppm F)

- Reserve for use in children with moderate/high caries risk.
- Reserve for use in children more than 6 years of age who have mastered swallowing reflex and can spit out the rinse.
- Recommend alcohol-free preparations.

Self-applied gels/pastes (5000 ppm F)

- Reserve for patients in fluoride-deficient communities who are at increased risk for caries.
- Have adult apply for young child and supervise for older child.
- Use 4 minutes for application period.
- Allow patient to expectorate freely after application; postpone eating/drinking for 30 minutes
- Use with caution in children who have not mastered swallowing reflex.
- Monitor effectiveness; terminate regimen when feasible.

Professionally applied gel/foam (12,300 ppm F)

- Determine application frequency based on caries risk assessment.
- Follow a pumice prophylaxis with fluoride application.
- Use minimum amount of gel/foam necessary to cover teeth.
- Seat patient upright and use suction to reduce swallowing of product.
- Apply for 4 minutes.
- Allow patient to expectorate freely after application; postpone eating/drinking for 30 minutes

Fluoride varnish (22,600 ppm F)

- Use after pumice prophylaxis as noted for gel/foam application.
- Use in alternative restorative technique to arrest lesions in young, precooperative patients.
- Have patient refrain from eating/drinking for 30 minutes after application,
- Have patient postpone brushing teeth until following morning.

[a]Table assumes that the baseline recommendation for all patients is twice daily use of a fluoridated dentifrice coupled with once- or twice-yearly professional application of fluoride gel/foam/varnish. Use of all regimens except fluoride dentifrice should be based on a caries risk assessment.
(*Source:* Based on Adair, S. M. (2006). Evidence-based use of fluoride in contemporary pediatric dental practice. *Pediatr Dent*, 28:133–42.)

On occasion it has been suggested that present topical fluoride treatment systems involve the use of excessive concentrations of fluoride. For example, some have suggested that the use of 0.4% rather than 8% SnF_2 is adequate to obtain maximal benefits from topical applications of this compound. The basis for such suggestions invariably rests with the results of in vitro studies, quite commonly enamel-solubility studies, in which maximal effects are achieved with lesser concentrations of fluoride. Unfortunately, in vitro data do not necessarily predict clinical effects, and the results of a clinical investigation clearly contradict these suggestions.[119] The use of lower concentrations of SnF_2 resulted in smaller caries-preventive benefits in children. Thus, until considerably more clinical data to the contrary become available, there is no legitimate basis for using concentrations of fluoride for topical applications other than those that have been adequately evaluated clinically and approved by review groups.

The relative superiority of APF gel or solution systems has been a frequent topic for research. Five clinical trials directly investigated this question, and the results are summarized in Table 15–4 ■. Four of these studies involved single annual applications; another one involved semiannual treatments.[120–122] These data suggest that the two forms are quite comparable, particularly when applied semiannually. In practice, the gels are greatly preferred over the solutions because of their ease of application, reduced chair time when trays are used, and safety.[53]

ROOT CARIES

Due to increased retention of permanent teeth because of various caries-preventive measures and the increase in life expectancy, root caries is prevalent in adults. The 1985–1986 U.S. Public Health Service (U.S. PHS) survey of adults found about one-half of U.S. adults were afflicted with root caries by age 50 with an average prevalence of about three lesions by age 70.[123] However, more recent evidence has shown a decline in the prevalence of root caries among U.S, dentate adults more than 20 years of age, from 23.3% in the NHANES survey of 1988-1994, to 17.5% in 1999–2002.[124] There was a higher decline for those 60 years of age and older in those two time periods from 43.2% to 31.6%.

TABLE ■ 15–4   **Comparative Effectiveness of Topically Applied APF Gels and Solutions**

Clinical Trial	Reduction in Caries Incidence	
	APF Solution (%)	APF Gel (%)
Ingraham and Williams[120]	11	41
Cons et al.[121]	0	22
Horowitz and Doyle[122]	28	24
Szwejda[203]	28	4
Cobb et al.[56]	34	35

APF, acidulated phosphate fluoride

Interestingly, a study conducted at the University of Iowa has indicated that adults older than 65 can expect an incidence of about 0.9 newly decayed, missing, or filled (DMF) coronal surfaces per year as well as about 0.6 new DMF root surfaces per year.[125] A more recent study reported similar results on the incidence of coronal and root caries in elderly Iowans between 1987 and 1998.[125] Thus, this form of caries has received increased attention from dental scientists with investigations covering both its cause and measures for prevention.[127] For the nine studies from Australia, Canada, Sweden, and the United States that reported root caries incidence, the summary measure of annual root caries incidence equaled 23.7% (CI = 17.1–30.2%). For the nine studies reporting root caries increment, the summary measure was 0.47 surfaces per person per year (CI = 0.34–0.61). These authors concluded that the annual root caries increment and root + coronal increment were 0.47 and 1.31 surfaces, respectively. A review of studies conducted in the late 1970s and 1980s among children aged 5 to 15 years found that, among children living in fluoride-deficient communities, the mean annual coronal caries increment was 1.4 surfaces, and among children living in fluoridated communities, it was 0.8 surfaces.[127] Thus, older adults could experience similar or higher levels of new caries than do schoolchildren, the primary recipients of caries-prevention programs.

A systematic review of 20 studies on the effectiveness of self- and professionally applied fluoride and water fluoridation among adults was conducted. Among studies published after/during 1980, any fluoride (self- and professionally applied or water fluoridation) annually averted 0.29 (95%CI: 0.16–0.42) carious coronal and 0.22 (95%CI: 0.08–0.37) carious root surfaces. The prevented fraction for water fluoridation was 27% (95%CI: 19%–34%). These findings suggest that fluoride prevents caries among adults of all ages.[128]

Quite clearly, fluoride is very effective for the prevention of root caries as evidenced by a limited number of clinical trials and numerous in vitro as well as in situ studies. For example, the results of several epidemiologic studies and reports have demonstrated that the presence of fluoridated drinking water throughout the lifetime of an individual prevents the development of root caries.[129–133] The magnitude of this effect is consistently higher than 50%. Furthermore, it has been observed that the use of NaF dentifrice significantly results in a decrease in root caries (more than 65%).[13,29]

Much less information is available, however, to document the effect of topical fluoride applications on the prevention of root caries and particularly the relative efficacy of different fluoride systems. Nyvad and Fejerskov reported the arrest of root caries following the topical application of 2% NaF and the daily use of a fluoride dentifrice.[135] Wallace and co-workers reported a 70% reduction in the incidence of root caries following semiannual applications of an APF gel during a 4-year study period.[136] To obtain some perspective on the potential efficacy of different topical fluoride systems, an established animal root caries model was used.[13,138] The results of this investigation are summarized in (Table 15–5 ■). From these data, it is apparent that all three approved topical fluoride systems decreased

TABLE ■ 15–5 **Effect of Professional Topical Fluoride Systems on Root Caries in Hamsters**

Topical Fluoride System	Root Caries Score	Percent Reduction
Control (water)	8.2	NA
Stannous fluoride (0.4%) + acidulated phosphate fluoride (0.3%)	4.9	40.2
Acidulated phosphate fluoride (1.2%)	3.0	63.4
Sodium fluoride (2.0%)	2.3	72.0
Stannous fluoride (8.0%)	2.0	75.6

(*Source:* Data from Stookey, G. K., Rodlun, C. A., Warrick, J. M., & Miller, C. H. (1989). Professional topical fluoride systems vs root caries in hamsters. *J Dent Res,* 68:372. Abstract 1521.)

the formation of root caries by 63% to 76% in this preclinical model. In the absence of the results of similar clinical data and with the recognition that the application of 8% SnF_2 imparts a brown pigmentation to exposed dentin, it seems appropriate to recommend the topical use of 2% NaF for the prevention of root caries.

RECOMMENDATIONS: TOPICAL FLUORIDE TREATMENTS

On the basis of the foregoing discussion, it is apparent that although periodic topical applications of any of the three approved agents provide protection against dental caries, maximal patient benefits can be expected only through the use of selected procedures previously mentioned.

FLUORIDE VARNISHES

Fluoride varnish has been shown to be effective in the prevention of caries in both deciduous and permanent teeth.[46] The interval for frequency of application of fluoride varnish varies depending on the risk of the patient—more frequently for children with higher risk.[47] Although use of fluoride varnish for caries prevention is technically considered an "off-label" use, a robust evidence base supports the efficacy of varnish at preventing caries.[46,48,49] Fluoride-containing varnishes are available in the United States and are being recommended to provide topical fluoride treatments, particularly for very young children. Most varnishes contain 5.0% NaF (2.26% fluoride or 22,600 ppm); a typical application requires only 0.3 to 0.5 ml of the varnish, which contains 3 to 6 mg of fluoride. The application procedure involves cleaning the tooth surfaces by toothbrushing and painting the varnish on the teeth. The varnish is retained for 24 to 48 hours, during which time fluoride is released for reaction with the underlying enamel.[139–141] It is recommended that the applications be repeated at 3- to 6-month intervals.

The efficacy of fluoride varnishes for caries prevention has been repeatedly demonstrated in Europe, where they have been in common use for many years; the results of these studies have been summarized in recent reviews.[142,143] These studies have consistently demonstrated a significant reduction in the incidence of dental caries and have indicated that the magnitude of the benefit is related to the frequency of application, particularly in children at high risk for caries. Research specifically aimed at using fluoride varnishes as a preventive agent for children at high risk for early childhood caries has been conducted in the United States.[49]

Although there is convincing evidence of benefit and safety with the use of fluoride varnish for caries prevention, the FDA has not approved fluoride varnish for this purpose but has approved it for treating dental hypersensitivity. This issue has been addressed by several organizations. The ASTDD has stated that FDA approval is not required to use fluoride varnish off-label.[146] Many medications are currently prescribed and administered for off-label use, and many drugs used in medical practice for children have never been tested on children. The FDA regulation states,

> Good medical practice and the best interests of the patient require that physicians use legally available drugs, biologics and devices according to their best knowledge and judgment. If physicians use a product for an indication not in the approved labeling, they have the responsibility to be well informed about the product, to base its use on firm scientific rationale and on sound medical evidence, and to maintain records of the product's use and effects.[144]

The American Public Health Association has also supported the use of fluoride varnish in the prevention of dental caries.[145]

Because of the adoption of water fluoridation and widespread use of fluoride toothpaste, approximately 75% of the U.S. public is at low risk for dental caries. Therefore, the use of any professionally applied fluoride, including fluoride varnish, should be limited to those individuals and communities deemed to be at moderate to high risk for developing dental caries. A targeted approach offers additional opportunities toward improving the prevention and control of dental caries. The use of fluoride varnish to prevent and control dental caries in young children and seniors is expanding in both public and private dental practice settings and in nondental settings that incorporate health risk assessments and counseling. These settings include Head Start programs and Special Supplemental Nutrition Programs for Women, Infants, and Children; medical offices; well-child clinics and home visits conducted by public health nurses; child care programs; and other, sometimes overlapping, community programs.[146]

Fluoride varnish is generally preferred as the topical fluoride of choice by panels of experts. In 2007, the U.S. Maternal and Child Health Bureau convened a panel of experts and produced a report.[147] Recommendations were made for two groups—children under 2 years and children aged 2–6 years. The panel noted that community water fluoridation is a part of a comprehensive population-based strategy to prevent or control dental caries in communities. The panel recommended a "smear" of toothpaste for children under 2 years and a "pea-size" amount of toothpaste for children 2–6 years and suggested that photographs would be helpful in differentiating these amounts. The panel also recommended that:

- Children should spit out excess toothpaste.
- Children should not rinse after brushing.

The panel agreed that fluoride varnish should be recommended for high-risk children and on the adoption of the ADA recommendation that fluoride varnish be applied every 3–6 months. The panel also indicated that rinses, gels, or foams not be recommended for children under 6 years because the ability to control the swallowing reflex is not fully developed in preschool-aged children, increasing the likelihood that children younger than 6 years of age can inadvertently ingest excess fluoride.

The application of fluoride varnish is a prime example for the potential expanded role of nondental health care professionals. Fluoride varnish is increasingly being applied by nondental health care professionals and in community-based settings through county and city health departments, state public health dental programs also provide fluoride varnish, mouthrinse, and fluoride tablets. The Division of Oral Health of the Indian Health Service (IHS) provides oral health care and promotes oral health improvements for Native Americans and Alaska Natives (NA/AN). In early 2010, the IHS began an early childhood caries (ECC) initiative Through the initiative, the IHS is working with community partners such as Head Start; the Women, Infants, and Children Program; and nurses, doctors, and community health representatives to reduce the prevalence of ECC in AI/AN children by 25% by fiscal year (FY) 2015. Other goals of the initiative are to increase access to dental care for 0- to 5-year old AI/AN children by 10 percent in FY 2010 and 50 percent by FY 2015; to increase the number of children 0–5 years old who receive a fluoride varnish treatment by 25 percent by FY 2015.

Little information is available to compare the effectiveness of fluoride varnishes with professionally applied topical fluoride solutions or gels. The results of a clinical study conducted on children in India, comparing the efficacy of a fluoride varnish with topical applications of an APF gel, indicated that the fluoride varnish was more effective, although both treatments resulted in a significant reduction in caries.[148] Seppä and co-workers reported the results of a clinical trial comparing semiannual applications of the NaF varnish with similar applications of an APF gel in 12- and 13-year-old children with a history of caries and observed no significant differences between the two treatment regimens.[45] Fluoride varnish intervention had greatest efficacy on surfaces that were sound at baseline and among those sound surfaces, maxillary anterior facials received most caries-preventive benefit.[149]

A 2004 Cochrane review found that fluoride toothpastes in comparison to mouthrinses or gels appear to have a similar degree of effectiveness for the prevention of dental caries in children. There was no clear suggestion that fluoride varnish is more effective than mouthrinses, and the evidence for the comparative effectiveness between fluoride varnishes and gels and between mouthrinses and gels was inconclusive. No conclusions about adverse effects could be reached because no data were reported on in the trials. Acceptance is likely to be higher for fluoride toothpaste.[150] In 2006, a study of 376 caries-free children (mean age 1.8 years at baseline) from low-income Chinese or Hispanic San Francisco families was reported. All families in the study received counseling, and children were randomized to the following groups: no fluoride varnish, fluoride varnish once/year, or fluoride varnish twice/year. Analyzing the number of actual, active fluoride varnish applications received resulted in a dose-response effect, $p < 0.01$. Caries incidence was higher for "counseling only" vs. "counseling + fluoride varnish assigned once/year" (OR = 2.20, 95%CI 1.19-4.08) and "twice/year" (OR = 3.77, 95%CI 1.88-7.58). No related adverse events were reported. The authors concluded that fluoride varnish added to caregiver counseling was efficacious in reducing early childhood caries incidence.[151]

In the absence of additional clinical data, various topical fluoride procedures appear to be equivalent in efficacy.

INITIATION OF THERAPY

Practitioners frequently wonder when they should recommend and initiate a topical fluoride application program. All too frequently, they tend to defer such treatments until the child is older and a majority of the permanent dentition has already erupted.

As discussed earlier, it is well established that the enamel surface of a newly erupted tooth is not completely mineralized; therefore, the period when the tooth is most susceptible to carious attack is the first few months after eruption. Furthermore, it has been shown that topical fluoride treatments are effective for both the deciduous and permanent dentitions. Several dental organizations have promoted a recommendation that parents should take their 12-month-old infants to the pediatrician or dentist to receive guidance on the prevention of early childhood caries, including the application of fluoride varnish. Several websites provide clear instructions on how to do this.[152] Early childhood caries, ECC, is the presence of one or more decayed, missing (because of caries), or filled tooth surfaces in any primary tooth in a child age 71 months or younger.[153] Thus, it follows that topical fluoride therapy should be initiated when the child is about 12 months of age when the primary maxillary incisors should have erupted. The treatment regimen should be maintained at least on a semiannual basis throughout the period of increased caries susceptibility, which persists for about 2 years after eruption of the permanent second molars (i.e., until the child is about 15 years old).

Susceptibility of the dentition to dental caries does not end at 15 years of age. It is probable, however, that the gradual decrease in caries susceptibility with increasing age will permit a less frequent topical application program to maintain cariostasis in many patients; annual fluoride treatments might suffice. However, according to evidence-based recommendations by a scientific panel convened by the American Dental Association, no evidence supports a benefit from professionally applied topical fluoride for patients considered to be at low risk for dental caries. The ADA has developed a chairside guide for professionally applied topical fluoride that presents different strategies for low, moderate, and high caries risk as well as for different age groups: < 6 years, 6–18 years, and older than 18 years.[154]

DISADVANTAGES OF FLUORIDE TREATMENTS

Some clinical situations can alter the selection of the treatment agent. For example, the use of SnF_2 could be contraindicated for aesthetic reasons in specific instances. The reaction of tin ions with enamel, particularly carious enamel, results in the formation of tin phosphates, some of which are brown in color. Thus, the use of this agent produces a temporary brownish pigmentation of carious tooth structure. This stain could exaggerate existing aesthetic problems when the patient has carious lesions in the anterior teeth that will not be restored. Stannous fluoride, however, has not been found to discolor composite restorative materials.

Another problem frequently raised, particularly by pediatric dentists (formerly known as **pedodontists**), concerns the strong, unpleasant, metallic taste of SnF_2. Although experienced practitioners can handle this problem, children without question accept flavored APF preparations much better. Acidulated phosphate fluoride systems have the disadvantage of possibly etching ceramic or porcelain surfaces. As a result, porcelain veneer facings and similar restorations should be protected with cocoa butter or petroleum jelly or should be isolated prior to applying APF. NaF gel, foam, or varnish are preferred to APF because NaF has a neutral pH and will not etch restorations.

The tendency in many dental offices is to use a specific topical fluoride system and treatment regimen for every patient. It should be emphasized, however, that specific patient needs should be determined initially and a specific treatment program developed to fulfill those needs.[154] For example, the use of a series of four or more topical fluoride applications within a 4-week period followed by repeated single applications at 3- to 6-month intervals should be considered for a patient with a severe caries problem. A reduced topical application time of 30 seconds as opposed to 4 minutes could be adequate to maintain a patient with little or no current caries activity. In other words, the practitioner should be familiar with the indications and contraindications for using various approaches and should select the treatment system and conditions that best meet the needs of the patient as well as the need to be efficient.

FLUORIDE-CONTAINING PROPHYLACTIC PASTES

Fluoride-containing prophylactic pastes have been available and widely used in dental offices for many years to clean and polish accessible tooth surfaces and restorations. Abrasives are needed to clean and polish teeth efficiently. Because the abrasives are harder than enamel, they inevitably removed a small amount of the enamel surface by abrasion during the prophylaxis. The actual amount of enamel removed during a prophylaxis is very small and has been shown to involve the loss of surface enamel to a depth of about 0.1 to 1.0 microns during a 10-second polishing.[155,156] Because it has been noted that the highest concentrations of fluoride in enamel occur in the outermost surface layers, it follows that the loss of even a small amount of surface enamel during a prophylaxis causes the exposed enamel surface to have a lower concentration of fluoride than was present prior to polishing.[157,158]

When fluoride-containing prophylactic pastes first became available in the 1950s, the use of the preparations to perform a routine dental prophylaxis was thought to result in a significant reduction in the subsequent development of dental caries. Consequently, a number of clinical trials were conducted to determine the magnitude of this benefit. The results of these investigations, considered collectively, indicated that although the use of fluoride-containing pastes resulted in a very modest increase in the resistance of the tooth surfaces to the development of dental caries, the magnitude of the effect of using the pastes was not statistically significant. As a result, the FDA has never accepted fluoride-containing prophylactic pastes as therapeutic agents. However, the pastes are commonly recommended for use during tooth polishing to at least replace the fluoride lost from the enamel surface by abrasion during the procedure. In summary, the following recommendations are proposed:

- When a simple prophylaxis that will not be followed by a topical fluoride application is administered, fluoride-containing prophylactic pastes should be used to replenish the fluoride lost during the procedure.

- When a topical fluoride application is given to a caries-susceptible patient and a prophylaxis is deemed to be necessary, it is advisable to administer the prophylaxis with a fluoride-containing paste. Although no definitive proof of the additive benefits of both procedures exists as yet, some studies have shown an increased benefit. Even when doubt exists, it is preferable to give the patient the possible benefit of any increased protection.

MULTIPLE FLUORIDE THERAPY

From the previous discussions of various measures to apply fluoride to erupted teeth, it is apparent that no single fluoride treatment provides total protection against dental caries. Recognition of this fact led early investigators to evaluate the use of combinations of fluoride measures.

Multiple fluoride therapy describes fluoride combination programs. As originally developed, this program included the application of fluoride in the dental office in the form of both a fluoride-containing prophylactic paste and a topically applied fluoride solution, in addition to self-care using an approved fluoride dentifrice. In addition, some form of systemic fluoride, preferably community water fluoridation, was included.

The only published reports of clinical investigations that attempted to assess the total effect of this type of multiple

TABLE ■ 15–6   Results of Older Clinical Studies Using Multiple Fluoride Therapy Involving Stannous Fluoride-Containing Prophylactic Paste, Topical Fluoride, and Dentifrice

Clinical Investigation	Study Population	Fluoride in Water	Study Duration	Caries Reduction (%)
Gish and Muhler[146]	Children	Yes	3 years	55
Bixler and Muhler[147]	Children	No	3 years	58
Muhler et al.[148]	Adults	Yes	30 months	64
Scola and Ostrom[149]	Adults	No	2 years	58[a]
Scola[150]	Adults	No	2 years	56[a]
Obersztyn et al.[151]	Adults	No	1 year	60

[a]Average reduction for similar multiple groups

fluoride therapy on dental caries involved the use of SnF_2 topical systems in the 1960s.[159–164] Each of these studies administered the topical fluoride treatments semiannually; the results are summarized in Table 15–6 ■. The results of these investigations indicate that the combination of topical fluoride applications and self-care using a fluoride dentifrice resulted in approximately 59% fewer carious lesions.

The fact that the magnitude of this benefit is somewhat less than that of the sum of the components evaluated individually indicates that the caries-protective effects of the individual components (i.e., prophylactic paste, topical solution, and dentifrice) are only partially additive. Nevertheless, it is important to note that the combination of SnF_2 treatments not only reduced the incidence of caries by more than 50% in both children and young adults but also did so in both the presence and absence of community water fluoridation. Clinical investigators have explored combinations of fluoride treatments using agents other than SnF_2 with variable success. For example, Beiswanger and co-workers in 1978 reported that additive benefits were observed with topical applications of APF and self-care using an SnF_2 dentifrice.[165] However, neither Downer et al. nor Mainwaring and Naylor were able to demonstrate additive benefits from the combined use of an MFP dentifrice and topical application of APF.[166,167]

The available data relating to multiple fluoride therapy thus suggest additive benefits from the use of either SnF_2 or APF in the dental office and self-care using dentifrices containing fluoride.[168] This finding does not necessarily mean that other combinations of fluoride treatments cannot provide additive benefits but merely that they have not yet been evaluated. In the meantime, the dental practitioner is strongly advised to use combinations of fluoride treatments to provide maximal caries protection for patients.

FLUORIDE RINSES

In 1960, reports indicating that the regular use of neutral NaF solutions decreased the incidence of caries began to appear. In an attempt to identify topical fluoride measures especially appropriate for use in dental public health programs, the use of neutral NaF solutions was studied extensively during the subsequent 15 years. Although these studies used a wide variety of

experimental conditions, a number of investigations involved either the daily use of solutions containing 200 to 225 ppm or the weekly use of solutions containing about 900 ppm fluoride. The majority of these studies were conducted in schools with supervised use of the rinse throughout the school year.

The results of these investigations have been summarized on several occasions and will not be repeated here.[168–172] In general, both types of fluoride rinses resulted in significant caries reduction of about 30% to 35%. On the basis of these findings, the simplicity of administration, and the lack of need for professional dental supervision, weekly fluoride rinse programs in schools became increasingly popular. The September 1986 issue of the *Journal of the American Dental Association* included "Guide to the Use of Fluoride." See Table 15–6 for the composition of and recommended use of approved fluoride mouthrinses.

Nearly all of the investigations in the 1960s using fluoride rinses involved children residing in areas in which the drinking water was deficient in fluoride. As a result, the approvals given to fluoride rinses were related to their use in nonfluoridated communities. Reports in 1970s indicated, that significant benefits from fluoride rinses used in the presence of an optimal concentration of fluoride in the drinking water.[173,174] Results from three additional reports concerning the use of fluoride rinses in children residing in fluoridated communities indicate that cariostatic benefits provided by fluoride rinses are additive to those derived from community water fluoridation.[175–177] In view of these collective observations, there appeared to be no reason to restrict the use of fluoride rinses to nonfluoridated communities.

The FDA's approval of fluoride rinses for use in public health programs opened the door for self-care with these products as a component of multiple fluoride preventive programs. Although the approved preparations were intended to be available strictly by prescription, a 0.05% neutral NaF rinse (Fluorigard®) containing about 225 ppm fluoride was subsequently introduced for over-the-counter (OTC) sale. Ultimately, approval was given to OTC fluoride rinses for oral self-care, although some restrictions applied. These restrictions included the distribution of quantities containing no more than 300 mg fluoride in a single container and a label cautioning users to avoid swallowing the product and indicating that

TABLE ■ 15–7   **Composition and Frequency of Approved Fluoride Rinses**

Source of Fluoride	Fluoride Content		Recommended Frequency
	Percent	*Parts Per Million*	
Sodium fluoride	0.20	900	Weekly
Sodium fluoride	0.02	100	Twice daily
Sodium fluoride	0.05	225	Daily
Acidulated phosphate fluoride	0.02	200	Daily
Stannous fluoride	0.10	243	Daily

children younger than 6 years of age should not use the preparations. At present, several fluoride rinse products distributed containing about 225 ppm fluoride are intended for daily use (see Table 15–7 ■).

Answers to the question of additive effects of fluoride rinses to those obtained using other fluoride vehicles have been contradictory. Two studies conducted in the 1970s found a modest additive benefit from the supervised daily rinsing in school with an APF rinse coupled with supervised brushing in school plus normal self-care using an MFP dentifrice.[178,179]On the other hand, in the 1970s, Blinkhorn et al. failed to observe any indication of additive caries protection between the similar supervised daily use of a neutral 0.05% NaF and self-care using the same dentifrice.[180] Likewise, Ringelberg et al. failed to find an additive effect of a daily NaF rinse and self-care using an SnF_2 dentifrice.[181] Similarly, Horowitz et al. studied the supervised weekly use of an NaF rinse and a daily NaF tablet plus self-care with approved fluoride dentifrices and observed a caries reduction comparable in magnitude to that reported earlier by investigators with fluoride tablets or rinses used individually.[182]

Additive effects can also be inferred from the numerous school fluoride rinse studies in which caries reductions from 30% to 35% were observed. Because the majority of these children in both the control and experimental groups used fluoride-containing dentifrices, it follows that the benefits observed in those studies were greater than those provided by the fluoride dentifrices alone. The same conclusion can be reached from the data reported by Birkeland and co-workers in Norway, a country where more than 90% of the children use fluoride dentifrices.[169] After 10 years of a mouthrinsing program, these authors found a caries reduction of more than 50% and reduction in the need for restoration of more than 70%.

It can thus be concluded that fluoride rinses have a place as a component of a preventive program along with but not as substitutes for other modalities of fluoride use. Fluoride rinses are used mainly for patients with a high caries risk. Although existing evidence could lead some to doubt whether additional benefits for the patients accrue from the use of rinses, it is preferable in these instances to give the patients the benefit of the doubt. Fluoride rinses should be recommended, for example, for the following:

- Patients who because of medication, surgery, or radiotherapy have reduced salivation and increased caries risk.

- Patients who have orthodontic appliances or removable prostheses that act as traps for plaque accumulation.

- Patients who are unable to achieve acceptable oral hygiene.

- Patients who have extensive dental restorations and multiple restorative margins that represent sites of high caries risk.

- Patients who need fluoride in their self-care regimen but cannot tolerate a custom-fitted tray.

- Patients who have gingival recession and susceptibility to root caries.

- Patients who have evidence of active caries or rampant caries.

As a general rule, daily rinses should be recommended rather than a weekly regimen; the daily procedure appears not only to be slightly more effective, but, as a practical consideration, also is easier for patients to remember and comply with. In all these instances, it is important to remember that the rinses should not be used in place of any of the other modalities of fluoride use but as part of a comprehensive, preventive program that should also include plaque control, regular professional dental hygiene appointments, frequent fluoride topical applications, self-care use of a fluoride dentifrice, diet control, and tests to determine whether and when the oral environment is no longer conducive to caries. For children living in nonfluoridated areas, daily use of prescription fluoride supplements should also be considered.[183]

FLUORIDE GELS FOR ORAL SELF-CARE

A number of fluoride gels have become available as additional measures available to help achieve caries control. These products contain 0.4% SnF_2 (1,000 ppm fluoride) or 1.0% NaF (5,000 ppm) and are formulated in a nonaqueous gel base that does not contain an abrasive system. Their recommended method of use involves toothbrushing with a gel (similar to using a dentifrice), allowing the gel to remain in the oral cavity for 1 minute, and then expectorating thoroughly.

Even though no controlled clinical trials have been conducted on the products used in this manner, the ADA's Council on Dental Therapeutics has approved a number of them as an additional caries-preventive measure for use in patients with rampant caries. The basis for the approval of these products has been the numerous prior clinical caries studies using dentifrices that contain the same amount of SnF_2, coupled with analytic data demonstrating the stability of these preparations.

From a practical point of view, the recommended use of fluoride gels is generally similar to that cited earlier for fluoride rinses. In other words, they can be considered as an alternative to the use of fluoride rinses and an adjunct to the use of professional, topical fluoride applications, and fluoride dentifrices as a collective means of achieving caries control in patients who are especially prone to caries formation. Like fluoride rinses, the use of these gels is generally restricted to the period required to achieve caries control. Compared with fluoride rinses, however, fluoride gels appear to have an advantage in terms of patient compliance. Because only dental clinics can distribute these preparations to patients, it is commonly thought that patients are more likely to use them in compliance with the recommendations of their dentist or dental hygienist.

It should be stressed that fluoride gels should not be used in place of fluoride dentifrices. Because the gels contain no abrasive system to control the deposition of pellicle, their use in place of a dentifrice results in the accumulation of stained pellicle in the majority of patients within a few weeks. Nevertheless, the proper use of these preparations in combination with professional topical fluoride applications and self-care with fluoride dentifrices can be expected to help achieve caries control in caries-active patients.

To combine the benefits of a high fluoride gel and a dentifrice, products that contain both include PreviDent® 5000 plus™, Control Rx™, Clinpro™ 5000, and others containing 5000 ppm fluoride.

FLUORIDE-RELEASING DENTAL MATERIALS

Fluoride-releasing dental restorative materials can provide an additional benefit in preventive dentistry. Although not currently available in the United States, a fluoride-releasing amalgam has demonstrated recurrent caries inhibition at enamel and dentin restoration margins.[184] Likewise, both chemical-cured and light-cured glass ionomer cements have demonstrated caries inhibition at these restoration margins.[185–188] Fluoride-releasing resin composites and sealants have also consistently demonstrated recurrent caries inhibition at enamel margins, yet there are conflicting results concerning whether caries inhibition occurs at dentin margins.[189–191] Preliminary studies indicate that glass ionomer cement and fluoride-releasing resin composite have synergistic effects with fluoride rinses and fluoridated dentifrices in the remineralization of incipient enamel caries.[192,193] The materials could act as a fluoride delivery system. Upon exposure to additional external fluoride, the material surface undergoes an increase in fluoride. This fluoride is subsequently released and has demonstrated inhibition of demineralization and even the occurrence of remineralization at the adjacent tooth structure. Further clinical research to evaluate these fluoride-releasing restorative materials should provide more information for clinical recommendations.

TOXICOLOGY OF FLUORIDE

The FDA and occupational safety health legislation carefully regulates the handling of fluorides in industry and in the marketplace. Commercial dental fluoride products and professional practices can be toxic and even lethal when used inappropriately. The lethal dose for an adult is somewhere between 2.5 and 10 g with the average lethal dose being 4 to 5 g. The use of the term *average lethal dose* is a very imprecise designation that makes it difficult to predict the outcome of an accidental swallowing of an excess of fluoride. To correct this problem, investigators have recommended a probable toxic dose (PTD) standard based on body weight as a more practical approach to making treatment decisions. With it, the urgency for first aid and more definitive emergency treatment can be determined rapidly. The PTD approach, first reported by Bayless and Tinanoff,[194] bases the level and urgency of treatment on the number of multiples of 5 mg/kg of fluoride ingested (Table 15–8 ∎).

If the amount ingested is less than 5 mg/kg, the office use of available calcium, aluminum, or magnesium products as first aid antidotes should suffice. If the amount is more than 5 mg/kg, first aid measures should be expeditiously applied followed by hospital observation for the need for further care. Finally, if the amount of fluoride ingested approaches or exceeds 15 mg/kg, the immediate first aid treatment should be followed by a most urgent action to move the patient swiftly into a hospital emergency room where cardiac monitoring, electrolyte evaluation, and shock support are available. Ingestion of 15 mg/kg fluoride can be lethal.

Excessive exposure to fluoride results in four general reactions (1) when a concentrated fluoride salt contacts moist skin or mucous membrane, hydrofluoric acid forms, causing a chemical burn, (2) inhibition of enzyme systems, (3) binding calcium needed for nerve action, and (4) hyperkalemia (excessive amount of phosphate in the bloodstream) contributing to cardiotoxicity (damage to the heart muscle).

When dry fluoride powder contacts the mucous membrane or the moist skin, a reddened lesion occurs and later becomes swollen and pale; still later, ulceration and necrosis can occur. In past years, skin burns of this type were common for many water engineers who emptied drums of fluoride agents into the hoppers feeding water supplies. Federal and state occupational safety acts have greatly reduced this risk.

Following excessive ingestion of fluoride, nausea and vomiting can occur. The vomiting is usually caused by the formation of hydrofluoric acid in the acid environment of the stomach, causing damage to the lining cells of the stomach wall. Local or general signs of muscle tetany (intermittent, prolonged spasms) ensue from a drop in blood calcium (hypocalcemia). Abdominal pain can accompany this effect. Finally, as the hypocalcemia and hyperkalemia intensify, the severity of the condition becomes ominous with the onset of the three C's that can indicate death—coma, convulsions, and cardiac

TABLE ■ 15–8   Emergency Treatment for Fluoride Overdose

Milligrams Fluoride Ion Per Kilogram Body Weight[a]	*Treatment*
Less than 5 mg/kg	1. Give calcium (milk) orally to relieve gastrointestinal symptoms. Observe for a few hours. 2. Do not induced vomiting.
More than 5 mg/kg	1. Empty stomach by inducing vomiting with emetic. For patients with depressed gag reflex caused by age (<6 months old), Down syndrome, or severe mental retardation, induced vomiting is contraindicated and endotracheal intubation[b] should be performed before gastric lavage. 2. Give orally soluble calcium in any form (e.g., milk, 5% calcium gluconate, or calcium lactate solution). 3. Admit to hospital and observe for a few hours.
More than 15 mg/kg	1. Admit to hospital immediately. 2. Induce vomiting. 3. Begin cardiac monitoring—especially for peaking T waves and prolonged intervals—and be prepared for cardiac arrhythmias. 4. Slowly administer intravenously 10 ml of 10% calcium gluconate solution. Give additional doses if clinical signs of tetany or QT interval prolongation develops. As necessary, monitor and correct electrolytes, especially calcium and potassium. 5. Ensure that adequate urine output is maintained; use diuretics if necessary. 6. Use general supportive measures for shock.

[a] Average weight per age: 1–2 years = 10 kg; 2–4 years = 15 kg; 4–6 years = 20 kg; 6–8 years = 23 kg
[b] Insertion of an endotracheal tube through the mouth into the trachea to aspirate fluoride secretions
(*Source:* Data from Bayless, J. M., & Tinanoff, N. (1985). Diagnosis and treatment of acute fluoride toxicity. *J Am Dent Assoc,* 110:209–11.)

arrhythmias (irregular heartbeat). Generally, death from ingestion of excessive fluoride occurs within 4 hours; if the individual survives for 4 hours, the prognosis is guarded to good.

Despite all precautions, potential for signs and symptoms of acute fluoride toxicity could exist in dental office misuse of excess amounts of professionally applied topical fluoride. To be prepared for such an unlikely emergency, the professional staff should be trained to institute emergency procedures if necessary.

Emergency Treatment

Four actions are especially significant in treating fluoride poisoning: (1) immediate treatment, (2) induced vomiting, (3) protection of the stomach by binding fluoride with orally administered calcium or aluminum preparations, and (4) maintenance of blood calcium levels with intravenous calcium. Urgent and decisive treatment is mandatory once the PTD of 15 mg/kg has been approached or exceeded. The speed of initiating proper treatment can be critical to a person's chance for survival.[195] The blood level of fluoride reaches its maximum from one-half to 1 hour after the fluoride is ingested; by that time treatment could be too late.

If an excessive amount of NaF is ingested, first aid treatment can be initiated. Milk or, better yet, milk and eggs should be given, for two reasons: (1) as demulcents, they help protect the mucous membrane of the upper gastrointestinal tract from chemical burns and (2) they provide the calcium that acts as a binder for the fluoride. Lime water (calcium hydroxide) or Maalox (an aluminum preparation) can be ingested to accomplish the same purpose. Plenty of fluid, preferably milk, should be ingested to help dilute the fluoride compound in the stomach. Vomiting is beneficial and often occurs spontaneously. When vomiting does occur, the majority of the ingested fluoride is often expelled. Preferably, the patient should be taken directly to a hospital emergency room. Otherwise, the closest emergency medical service unit or physician capable of dealing with fluoride toxicity is an alternative. Once in a well-equipped medical facility, several options are possible, such as gastric lavage (use of a fluid to wash fluoride out of the stomach), blood dialysis (diffusion of blood across a semipermeable membrane to remove the fluoride), or intravenous delivery of calcium gluconate to maintain blood calcium levels. Every effort should be made to rid the body rapidly of the fluoride or to negate its toxicity before refractory (resistant to treatment) hyperkalemia and cardiac fibrillation (rapid, irregular contraction of muscle fibers in the heart) become a more serious problem than the fluoride intoxication.[196]

Chronic Excessive Fluoride Exposure

At high levels of industrial fluoride exposure as experienced by cryolite and bauxite workers prior to the era of occupational safety regulations, the combined intake of fluoride through inhalation, ingestion, and water consumption often resulted in a daily dose of more than 20 mg. This exceedingly high level of continual intake for 10 to 20 years resulted in a severe skeletal fluorosis characterized by osteosclerosis (abnormal increase in thickness and density of bone), calcification of the tendons, and the appearance of multiple exostoses (bony growths that arise from the bone's surface). This same crippling bone fluorosis can also occur in some parts of the world from long-term consumption of naturally fluoridated waters that contain 14 ppm or more of fluoride. Other factors that increase the severity of bone fluorosis are high temperatures with a concomitant increase in drinking episodes, an elevated intake of fluoride in food, nutritional diseases, and low-calcium diets. No cases of skeletal fluorosis have been reported in the United States where water-fluoridation concentrations at that time were under 3.9 ppm.[197]

Home Security of Fluoride Products

The lack of secure home storage of OTC and prescription fluoride products poses hazards to consumers. As presently packaged, the fluoride content of OTC fluoride products can exceed the PTD for children.[198] Two deaths of children, one in Austria and the other in Australia, attest to the real danger at home after swallowing fluoride tablets.[199] In one year (1986–1987), 13 cases of fluoride poisoning were reported to the North Carolina Poison Center. The poison center noted that no health care providers who contacted the center were familiar with the treatment of the gastrointestinal symptoms induced by fluoride poisoning.[200] Clearly, parents need to be educated about the hazards of fluoride-containing dental products. Dentifrices, mouthrinses, and fluoride supplements need to be securely stored when young children are in the home. Also, health professionals need to be educated about the emergency treatment protocol for excessive intake of fluoride.

In 2004, the American Association of Poison Control Centers reported the occurrence of 24,180 exposures involving toothpaste with fluoride. Of these, only 440 cases were actually treated in an emergency department.[201] Children younger than 6 years of age accounted for 21,890 of these exposures. No deaths from fluoride exposure were reported in 2004; however, one death from ingestion of fluoride toothpaste had occurred in 2002.[202]

SUMMARY

A number of different aspects of topical fluoride therapy have been reviewed in the material presented here. Without a doubt, the use of topical fluoride therapy contributes significantly to the control of dental caries; however, one cannot expect to control dental caries completely through the use of fluorides alone. Furthermore, because no single fluoride treatment procedure provides the maximal degree of caries protection possible with fluoride, multiple fluoride therapy is advocated. In particular, the dentist should identify each patient's needs and caries risk status and institute a multiple fluoride treatment program designed specifically to fulfill those needs.

PRACTICAL CONSIDERATIONS

Determination of the caries risk for each patient is required prior to application of professionally applied topical fluoride because those at low risk might not need, or benefit from, this preventive treatment. For those at higher risk for caries, the trend in professionally applied topical fluoride is to use 5% fluoride varnish in most situations for all age groups. After reviewing the available evidence, several dental and medical organizations have concluded that fluoride varnish provides the longest lasting and highest fluoride concentration that is the safest due to a low overall fluoride dose and prolonged time of ingestion.

SELF-STUDY QUESTIONS

1. What factors contribute to the decision to apply topical fluoride in a dental office?

   a. Age of the patient

   b. Number of teeth

   c. Caries risk status

   d. All the above

   Rationale: Age, number of teeth present and caries risk status are all indicators when topical fluoride should be used.

2. What additional factors contribute to the decision to apply topical fluoride in a dental office?

   a. Dental insurance coverage

   b. Patient's informed consent

   c. Recommendations and guidelines of professional organizations

   d. All the above

   Rationale: Dental insurance coverage may determine whether a patient will decide to receive a fluoride application. All patients must provide informed consent for fluoride treatment and recommendations help providers make decisions about fluoride application.

3. What factors contribute to the type of topical fluoride applied in a dental office?

   a. Evidence of efficacy

   b. Cost

   c. Ability to control swallowing

   d. All the above

   Rationale: Topical fluoride application should be determined on the basis of efficacy.

4. What additional factors contribute to the type of topical fluoride applied in a dental office?

   a. Presence of composite or porcelain restorations

   b. Time it takes to apply the topical fluoride

   c. Evidence of safety

   d. All the above

Rationale: All of the above including safety, time allowance, and restorations help determine which type of application should be used.

5. Without a doubt, the use of topical fluoride therapy contributes significantly to the control of dental caries; however, one cannot expect to control dental caries completely through the use of fluorides alone.

   a. The first statement is true, the second statement is false

   b. The first statement is false, the second statement is true

   c. Both statements are true

   d. Both statements are false

Rationale: The use of topical fluoride therapy contributes significantly to the control of dental caries; however, one cannot expect to control dental caries completely through the use of fluorides alone.

REFERENCES

1. Buzalaf, M. A., Pessan, J. P., Honório, H. M., & ten Cate, J. M. (2011). Mechanisms of action of fluoride for caries control. *Monogr Oral Sci,* 22:97–114.

2. Featherstone J. D., & Lussi, A. (2006). Understanding the chemistry of dental erosion. *Monogr Oral Sci,* 20:66–76.

3. McConnell, D. (1952). The crystal chemistry of carbonate apatites and their relationship to the composition of calcified tissues. *J Dent Res,* 31:53–63.

4. Clarkson, B. H. (1991, December). Caries prevention—fluoride. *Adv Dent Res.* 5:41–45.

5. Ripa LW. Need for prior toothcleaning when performing a professional topical fluoride application: review and recommendations for change. *J Am Dent Assoc.* 1984 Aug;109(2):281–5.

6. Clarkson, J. J., Ed. (2000). International collaborative research on fluoride. *J Dent Res* 79:893–904.

7. Groeneveld, A., Van Eck, A. A., & Backer Dirks, O. (1990, February). Fluoride in caries prevention: Is the effect pre- or posteruptive? *J Dent Res,* 69 (Spec No):751–55.

8. Backer Dirks, O. (1966). Posteruptive changes in dental enamel. *J Dent Res* 45:503-11.

9. Weatherall, J. A., Hallsworth, A. S., & Robinson, C. (1973). The effect of tooth wear on the distribution of fluoride in the enamel surface of human teeth. *Arch Oral Biol,* 18:1175–89.

10. Joost-Larsen, M., & Fejerskov, O. (1978). Structural studies on calcium fluoride formation and uptake of fluoride in surface enamel in vitro. *Scand J Dent Res,* 86:337–45.

11. Fischer, R. B., & Muhler, J. C. (1952). The effect of sodium fluoride upon the surface structure of powdered dental enamel. *J Dent Res,* 31:751–755.

12. McCann, H. G. & Bullock, F. A. (1955). Reactions of fluoride ion with powdered enamel and dentin. *J Dent Res,* 34:59–67.

13. Joost-Larsen, M., & Fejerskov, O. (1978). Structural studies on calcium fluoride formation and uptake of fluoride in surface enamel in vitro. *Scand J Dent Res,* 86:337–45.

14. Scott, D. B., Picard, R. G., &Wyckoff, W. G. (1950). Studies of the action of sodium fluoride on human enamel by electron microscopy and electron diffraction. *Public Health Rep,* 65:43–56.

15. Muhler, J. C., & Van Huysen, G. (1947). Solubility of enamel protected by sodium fluoride and other compounds. *J Dent Res,* 26:119–27.

16. Muhler, J. C., Boyd, T. M., & Van Huysen, G. (1950). Effects of fluorides and other compounds on the solubility of enamel, dentin, and tricalcium phosphate in dilute acids. *J Dent Res,* 29:182–93.

17. Jordan, T. H., Wei, S. H. Y., Bromberger, S. H., & King, J. C. (1971). $Sn_3F_3PO_4$: The products of the reaction between stannous fluoride and hydroxyapatite. *Arch Oral Biol,* 16:241–46.

18. Wei, S. H. Y., & Forbes, W. C. (1974). Electron microprobe investigations of stannous fluoride reactions with enamel surfaces. *J Dent Res,* 53:51–56.

19. Brudevold, F., Savory, A., Gardner, D. E., Spinelli, M., & Speirs, R. (1963). A study of acidulated fluoride solutions. *Arch Oral Biol,* 8:167–77.

20. Wellock, W. D., & Brudevold, F. (1963). A study of acidulated fluoride solutions. II. The caries inhibition effect of single annual topical applications of an acidic fluoride and phosphate solution, a two year experience. *Arch Oral Biol,* 8:179–82.

21. Frazier, P. D., & Engen, D. W. (1966). X-ray diffraction study of the reaction of acidulated fluoride with powdered enamel. *J Dent Res,* 45:1144–1148.

22. DeShazer, D. O., & Swartz, C. J. (1967). The formation of calcium fluoride on the surface of fluorhydroxyapatite after treatment with acidic fluoride-phosphate solution. *Arch Oral Biol,* 12:1071–75.

23. Wei, S. H. Y., & Forbes, W. C. (1968). X-ray diffraction and analysis of the reactions between intact and powdered enamel and several fluoride solutions. *J Dent Res,* 47:471–77.

24. Mellberg, J. R., Laakso, P. V., & Nicholson, C. R. (1966). The acquisition and loss of fluoride by topically fluoridated human tooth enamel. *Arch Oral Biol,* 11:1213–20.

25. Bruun, C. (1973). Uptake and retention of fluoride by intact enamel in vivo after application of neutral sodium fluoride. *Scand J Dent Res,* 81:92–100.

26. Lovelock, D. J. (1973). The loss of topically applied fluoride from the surface of human enamel in vitro using 18F. *Arch Oral Biol,* 18:27–29.

27. Mellberg, J. R. (1973). Topical fluoride controversy symposium. Enamel fluoride uptake from topical fluoride agents and its relationship to caries inhibition. *J Am Soc Prev Dent,* 3:53–54.

28. Rinderer, L., Schait, A., & Muhlemann, H. R. (1965). Loss of fluoride from dental enamel after topical fluoridation. Preliminary report. *Helv Odont Acta,* 9:148–50.

29. Ahrens, G. (1976). Effect of fluoride tablets on uptake and loss of fluoride in superficial enamel in vivo. *Caries Res,* 10:85–95.

30. Wei, S. H. Y., & Schulz, E. M., Jr. (1975). In vivo microsampling of enamel fluoride concentrations after topical treatments. *Caries Res,* 9:50–58.

31. Kanauya, Y., Spooner, P., Fox, J. L., Higuchi, W. I., & Muhammad, N. A. (1983). Mechanistic studies on the bioavailability of calcium fluoride for re-mineralization of dental enamel. *Int J Pharmacol,* 16:171–79.

32. Chandler, S., Chiao, C. C., & Fuerstenau, D. W. (1982). Transformation of calcium fluoride for caries prevention. *J Dent Res,* 61:403–407.

33. Featherstone, J. D. B. (1999). Prevention and reversal of dental caries: Role of low level fluoride. *Community Dent Oral Epidemiol,* 27:31–40.

34. Rolla, G. (1988). On the role of calcium fluoride in the cariostatic mechanism of fluoride. *Acta Odontol Scand,* 46:341–45.

35. ten Cate, J. M. (1997). Review on fluoride, with special emphasis on calcium fluoride mechanisms in caries prevention. *Eur J Oral Sci,* 105:461–65.

36. Beiswanger, B. B., Mercer, V. H., Billings, R. J., & Stookey, G. K. (1980). A clinical caries evaluation of a stannous fluoride prophylactic paste and topical solution. *J Dent Res,* 59:1386–91.

37. Knutson, J. W. (1948). Sodium fluoride solution: Technique for applications to the teeth. *J Am Dent Assoc,* 36:37–39.

38. Mellberg, J. R. (1977). Enamel fluoride and its anticaries effects. *J Prev Dent,* 4:8–20.

39. Mellberg, J. R., Nicholson, C. R., Miller, B. G., & Englander, H. R. (1970). Acquisition of fluoride in vivo by enamel from repeated topical sodium fluoride applications in a fluoridated area: Final report. *J Dent Res,* 49:1473–77.

40. Puttnam, N. A., & Bradshaw, F. (1964). X-ray fluorescence studies on the effect of stannous fluoride on human teeth. *Adv Fluorine Res Dent Caries Prev (ORCA),* 3:145–50.

41. Hoermann, K. C., Klima, J. E., Birks, L. S., Nagel, D. J., Ludwick, W. E., & Lyon, H. W. (1966). Tin and fluoride uptake in human enamel in situ: Electron probe and chemical microanalysis. *J Am Dent Assoc,* 73:1301–5.

42. McDonald, J. L., Schemehorn, B. R., & Stookey, G. K. (1978). Influence of fluoride upon plaque and gingivitis in the beagle dog. *J Dent Res,* 57:899–902.

43. Beiswanger, B. B., McClanahan, S. F., Bartizek, R. D., Lanzalaco, A. C., Bacca, L. A., & White, D. J. (1997). The comparative efficacy of stabilized stannous fluoride dentifrice, peroxide/baking soda dentifrice and essential oil mouthrinse for the prevention of gingivitis. *J Clin Dent,* 8:46–53.

44. Institute of Medicine. (2011). *Advancing oral health in America.* Washington, DC: The National Academies Press.

45. Seppä L., Leppanen, T, Hausen H. (1995). Fluoride varnish versus acidulated phosphate fluoride gel: a 3-year clinical trial. Caries Res 1995;29:327–30.

46. Marinho, V. C., Higgins, J. P., Logan, S., & Sheiham, A. (2002). Fluoride gels for preventing dental caries in children and adolescents. *Cochrane Datab Syst Rev* (Iss 2. Art. No. CD002280.)

47. Azarpazhooh, A., and P. A. Main. (2008). Fluoride varnish in the prevention of dental caries in children and adolescents: A systematic review. *J of Can Dent Assoc,* 74:73–79.

48. Beltran-Aguilar, E. D., Goldstein, J. W., & Lockwood, S. A. (2000). Fluoride varnishes—A review of their clinical use, cariostatic mechanism, efficacy and safety. *J Am Dent Assoc,* 131:589–96.

49. Weintraub, J., Ramos-Gomez, F., Jue, B., et al. (2006). Fluoride varnish efficacy in preventing early childhood caries. *J Dent Res,* 85:172–76.

50. Gibson, G., Jurasic. M. M., Wehler, C. J., & Jones, J. A. (2011). Supplemental fluoride use for moderate and high caries risk adults: A systematic review. *J Public Health Dent,* 71:171–84.

51. Tagliaferro, E. P., Pardi, V., Ambrosano, G. M., Meneghim, Mde C, da Silva, S. R., & Pereira, A. C. (2011, April). Occlusal caries prevention in high and low risk schoolchildren. A clinical trial. *Am J Dent,* 24:109–14.

52. Milsom, K. M., Blinkhorn, A. S., Walsh, T., Worthington, H. V., Kearney-Mitchell, P., Whitehead, H., & Tickle, M. (2011, November). A cluster-randomized controlled trial: Fluoride varnish in school children. *J Dent Res,* 90:1306–11.

53. Pessan J. P., Toumba, K. J., & Buzalaf, M. A. (2011). Topical use of fluorides for caries control. *Monogr Oral Sci,* 22:115–32.

54. Garcia-Godoy, F., Hicks, J., & Flaitz, C. (2002). APF foam application: Caries initiation and progression in vitro. *J Dent Res,* 81(Spec Iss): Abstract 3541.

55. Pimlott, J. F. L. (1999). Professionally applied topical fluorides: Providing optimal patient care using an evidence-based approach. *Probe Sci J,* 33:175–79.

56. Cobb, H. B., Rozier, R. G., & Bawden, J. W. (1980). A clinical study of the caries preventive effects of an APF solution and an APF thixotropic gel. *Pediatr Dent,* 2:263–66.

57. Jiang, H., Tai, B., Du, M., & Peng, B. (2005). Effect of professional application of APF foam on caries reduction in permanent first molars in 6–7-year-old children: 24-month clinical trial. *J Dent,* 33469–73.

58. Whitford, G. M., Adair, S. M., Hanes, C. M., Perdue, E. C., & Russel, C. M. (1995). Enamel uptake and patient exposure to fluoride: comparison of APF gel and foam. *Pediatr Dent,* 17:199–203.

59. Pimlott, J. F. L. (1999). Professionally applied topical fluorides: Providing optimal patient care using an evidence-based approach. *Probe Sci J,* 33:175–79.

60. Knutson, J. W., Armstrong, W. D., & Feldman, F. M. (1947). Effect of topically applied sodium fluoride on dental caries experience. IV. Report of findings with two, four, and six applications. *Public Health Rep,* 62:425–30.

61. Houpt, M., Koenigsberg, S., & Shey, Z. (1983). The effect of prior toothcleaning on the efficacy of topical fluoride treatment. Two-year results. *Clin Prev Dent,* 5:8–10.

62. Katz, R. V., Meskin, L. H., Jensen, M. E., & Keller, D. (1984). Topical fluoride and prophylaxis: A 30-month clinical trial. *J Dent Res,* 63: Abstract 771.

63. Ripa, L. W., Leske, G. S., Sposato, A., & Varma, A. (1983). Effect of prior toothcleaning on biannual professional APF topical fluoride gel-tray treatments. Results after two years. *Clin Prev Dent,* 5:3–7.

64. Bijella, M. F., Bijella, V. T., Lopes, E. S., & Bostos, J. R. (1985). Comparison of dental prophylaxis and toothbrushing prior to topical APF applications. *Community Dent Oral Epidemiol,* 13:208–11.

65. Ekstrand, J., & Koch, G. (1980). Systemic fluoride absorption following fluoride gel application. *J Dent Res,* 59:1067.

66. Ekstrand, J., Koch, G., Lindgren, L. E., & Petersson, L. G. (1981). Pharmacokinetics of fluoride gels in children and adults. *Caries Res,* 15:213–20.

67. LeCompte, E. J., & Whitford, G. M. (1982). Pharmacokinetics of fluoride from APF gel and fluoride tablets in children. *J Dent Res,* 61:469–72.

68. LeCompte, E. J., & Doyle, T. E. (1982). Oral fluoride retention following various topical application techniques in children. *J Dent Res,* 61:1397–1400.

69. LeCompte, E. J., & Rubenstein, L. K. (1984). Oral fluoride retention with thixotropic and APF gels and foam-lined and unlined trays. *J Dent Res,* 63:69–70.

70. McCall, D. R., Watkins, T. R., Stephan, K. W., Collins, W. J., & Smalls, M. J. (1983). Fluoride ingestion following APF gel application. *Br Dent J,* 155:333–36.

71. Pourbaix, S., & Desager, J. P. (1983). Fluoride absorption: A comparative study of 1% and 2% fluoride gels. *J Biol Buccale,* 11:103–8.

72. LeCompte, E. J., & Doyle, T. E. (1985). Effects of suctioning devices on oral fluoride retention. *J Am Dent Assoc,* 110:357.

73. Stookey, G. K., Schemehorn, B. R., Drook, C. A., & Cheetham, B. L. (1986). The effect of rinsing with water immediately after a professional fluoride gel application on fluoride uptake in demineralized enamel: An in vivo study. *Pediatr Dent,* 8:153–57.

74. Jiang, H., Bian, Z., Tai, B. J., Du, M. A., & Peng, B. (2005). The effect of a bi-annual professional application of APF foam on dental caries increment in primary teeth: 24 month clinical trial. *J Dent Res,* 84:265–68.

75. Jiang, H., Tai, B., Du, M., & Peng, B. (2005). Effect of professional application of APF foam on caries reduction in permanent first molars in 6–7 year old children: 24 month clinical trial. *J Dent,* 33:469–73.

76. American Dental Association Council on Scientific Affairs. (2006). Professionally applied topical fluoride, evidence-based clinical recommendations. *J Am Dent Assoc,* 137:1151–59.

77. Lavigne, S. (2000). Not all trays are created equal: An analysis of fluoride tray fit. *Probe Scientific J,* 6:217–24.

78. Averill, H. M., Averill, J. E., & Ritz, A. G. (1967). A two-year comparison of three topical fluoride agents. *J Am Dent Assoc,* 74:996–1001.

79. Galagan, D. F., & Knutson, J. W. (1948). Effect of topically applied sodium fluoride on dental caries experience. VI. Experiments with sodium fluoride and calcium chloride. Widely spaced applications. Use of different solution concentrations. *Public Health Rep,* 63:1215–21.

80. Scheifele, E., Studen-Pavlovich, D., & Markovic, N. (2002). Practitioner's guide to fluoride. *Dent Clin North Am,* 46:831–46.

81. Featherstone, J. D. B. (2001). Elements of a successful adult caries preventive program. *Compend Cont Educ Oral Hygiene,* 8:3–9.

82. Berger, E. K. (2006). Review of professional and take-home fluorides. *Contemp Oral Hyg,* 6:8–9.

83. Horowitz, H. S., & Heifetz, S. B. (1969). Evaluation of topical fluoride applications of stannous fluoride to teeth of children born and reared in a fluoridated community: Final report. *J Dent Child,* 36:355–61.

84. Muhler, J. C. (1960). The anticariogenic effectiveness of a single application of stannous fluoride in children residing in an optimal communal fluoride area. II. Results at the end of 30 months. *J Am Dent Assoc,* 61:431–38.

85. Szwejda, L. F. (1972). Fluorides in community programs: A study of four years of various fluorides applied topically to the teeth of children in fluoridated communities. *J Public Health Dent,* 32:25–33.

86. Brudevold, F., & Nanjoks, R. (1978). Caries preventive fluoride treatment of the individual. *Caries Res,* 12 (Suppl 1): 52–64.

87. Forrester, D. J. (1971). A review of currently available topical fluoride agents. *J Dent Child,* 38:52–58.

88. Horowitz, H. S., & Heifetz, S. B. (1970). The current status of topical fluorides in preventive dentistry. *J Am Dent Assoc,* 81:166–77.

89. Forrester, D. J., & Shulz, E. M., Eds. (1974). *International workshop of fluorides and dental caries reductions.* Baltimore: University of Maryland.

90. Stookey, G. K. (1970). Fluoride therapy. In Bernier, J. L., & Muhler, J. C., Eds. *Improving dental practice through preventive measures* (2nd ed.). St. Louis, MO: Mosby, 92–156.

91. Ripa, L. W. (1981). Professionally (operator) applied topical fluoride therapy: A critique. *Int Dent J,* 31:105–20.

92. Mellberg, J. R., & Ripa, L. W. (1983). Professionally applied topical fluoride. In *Fluoride in preventive dentistry. Theory and clinical applications.* Chicago, IL: Quintessence, 181–214.

93. Katz, S., McDonald, J. L., & Stookey, G. K. (1979). *Preventive dentistry in action* (3rd ed.). Upper Montclair, NJ: DCP Publishing Company.

94. Ripa, L. W. (1989). Review of the anticaries effectiveness of professionally applied and self-applied topical fluoride gels. *J Public Health Dent,* 49:297–309.

95. Ripa, L. W. (1990). An evaluation of the use of professional (operator-applied) topical fluorides. *J Dent Res,* 69:786–96.

96. Wei, S. H. Y., & Yiu, C. K. Y. (1993). Evaluation of the use of topical fluoride gel. *Caries Res,* 27 (Suppl 1):29–34.

97. Johnston, D. W. (1994). Current status of professionally applied topical fluorides. *Community Dent Oral Epidemiol,* 22:159–63.

98. Horowitz, H. S., & Ismail, A. I. (1966). Topical fluorides in caries prevention. In Fejerskov, O., Ekstrand, J., & Burt, B. A., Eds. *Fluoride in dentistry* (2nd ed.). Copenhagen, Denmark: Munksgaard, 311–27.

99. Featherstone, J. D. (2006). Delivery challenges for fluoride, chlorhexidine and xylitol. *BMC Oral Health,* 6 (Suppl 1):S8.

100. Adair, S. M. (2006). Evidence-based use of fluoride in contemporary pediatric dental practice. *Pediatr Dent,* 28:133–42.

101. Fine, S. D. (1974). Topical fluoride preparations for reducing incidence of dental caries. Notice of status. *Fed Reg,* 39:17245.

102. Ripa, L. W. (1981). Professionally (operator) applied topical fluoride therapy: A critique. *Int Dent J,* 31:105–20.

103. Mellberg, J. R., & Ripa, L. W. (1983). Professionally applied topical fluoride. In *Fluoride in preventive dentistry. Theory and clinical applications.* Chicago: Quintessence, 181–214.

104. Katz, S., McDonald, J. L., & Stookey, G. K. (1979). *Preventive dentistry in action* (3rd ed.). Upper Montclair, NJ: DCP Publishing Company.

105. Clark, D. C., Hanley, J. A., Stamm, J. W., Weinstein, D. L. (1985). An empirically based system to estimate the effectiveness of caries-preventive agents. A comparison of the effectiveness estimates of APF gels and solutions, and fluoride varnishes. *Caries Res,* 19:83–95.

106. Arnold, F. A., Jr., Dean, H. T., & Singleton, D. C., Jr. (1944). The effect on carie incidence of a single topical application of a fluoride solution to the teeth of young adult males of a military population. *J Dent Res,* 23:155–62.

107. Frank, R. (1950). Research and clinical evaluation of local applications of sodium fluoride. *Schweiz Mschr Zahnh,* 60: 283–87.

108. Klinkenberg, E., & Bibby, B. G. (1950). Effect of topical applications of fluorides on dental caries in young adults. *J Dent Res,* 29:4–8.

109. Rickles, N. H., & Becks, H. (1951). The effects of an acid and a neutral solution of sodium fluoride on the incidence of dental caries in young adults. *J Dent Res,* 30:757–65.

110. Kutler, B., & Ireland, R. L. (1953). The effect of sodium fluoride application on dental caries experience in adults. *J Dent Res,* 32:458–62.

111. Carter, W. J., Jay, P., Shklair, I. L., & Daniel, L. H. (1955). The effect of topical fluoride on dental caries experience in adult females of a military population. *J Dent Res,* 34:73–76.

112. Muhler, J. C. (1957). Effect on gingiva and occurrence of pigmentation on teeth following the topical application of stannous fluoride or stannous chlorofluoride. *J Periodont,* 28:281–86.

113. Muhler, J. C. (1958). The effect of a single topical application of stannous fluoride on the incidence of dental caries in adults. *J Dent Res,* 37:415–16.

114. Protheroe, D. H. (1961). A study to determine the effect of topical application of stannous fluoride on dental caries in young adults. *Roy Can Dent Corps Q,* 3:18–23.

115. Harris, N. O., Hester, W. R., Muhler, J. C., & Allen, J. F. (1964). *Stannous fluoride topically applied in aqueous solution in caries prevention in a military population* (SAM-TDR-64-26). Brooks Air Force Base, TX: U.S. Air Force School of Aerospace Medicine.

116. Obersztyn, A., Kolwinski, K., Trykowski, J., & Starosciak, S. (1979). Effects of stannous fluoride and amine fluorides on caries incidence and enamel solubility in adults. *Aust Dent J,* 24: 395–97.

117. Viegas, Y. (1970). The caries inhibiting effect of a single topical application of an acidic phosphate solution in young adults. A one year experience. *Rev Saude Publica,* 4:55–60.

118. Curson, I. (1973). The effect on caries increments in dental students of topically applied acidulated phosphate fluoride (APF). *J Dent,* 1:216–18.

119. Mercer, V. H., & Muhler, J. C. (1972). Comparison of single topical application of sodium fluoride and stannous fluoride. *J Dent Res,* 51:1325–30.

120. Ingraham, R. Q., & Williams, J. E. (1970). An evaluation of the utility of application and cariostatic effectiveness of phosphate-fluorides in solution and gel states. *J Tenn Dent Assoc,* 50:5–12.

121. Cons, N. C., Janerich, D. T., & Senning, R. S. (1970). Albany topical fluoride study. *J Am Dent Assoc,* 80:777–81.

122. Horowitz, H. S., & Doyle, J. (1971). The effect on dental caries of topically applied acidulated phosphate-fluoride: Results after three years. *J Am Dent Assoc,* 82:359–65.

123. U.S. Public Health Service. (1987, August). *Oral health of United States adults. The national survey of oral health in U.S. employed adults and seniors: 1985–1986. National findings.* (NIH Publication No. 87–2868). Bethesda, MD: National Institutes of Health.

124. Beltrán-Aguilar, E. D., Barker, L. K., Canto, M. T., et al. (2005). Surveillance for dental caries, dental sealants, tooth retention, edentulism, and enamel fluorosis—United States, 1988–1994 and 1999–2002. *MMWR Surveill,* 5:1–43. Available at www.cdc.gov/mmwr/preview/mmwrhtml/ss5403a1.htm.

125. Hand, J. S., Hunt, R. S., & Beck, J. D. (1988). Incidence of coronal and root surface caries in an older adult population. *J Pub Health Dent,* 48:14–19.

126. Hamasha, A. A., Warren, J. J., Hand, J. S., & Levy, S. M. (2005). Coronal and root caries in the older Iowans: 9-11 year incidence. *Spec Care Dent,* 25:106–10.

127. Garcia, A. L. (1989). Caries incidence and costs of prevention programs. J *Public Health Dent,* 49(5 Spec No):259–71.

128. Griffin, S. O., Regnier, E., Griffin, P. M., & Huntley, V. N. Effectiveness of fluoride in preventing caries in adults. (2007). *J Dent Res,* 86:410–14.

129. Burt, B. A., Ismail, A. I., & Eklund, S. A. (1986). Root caries in an optimally fluoridated and a high-fluoride community. *J Dent Res,* 65:1154–58.

130. Brustman, B. A. (1986). Impact of exposure to fluoride-adequate water on root surface caries in elderly. *Gerodontics,* 2:203–207.

131. Hunt, R. J., Eldredge, J. B., & Beck, J. D. (1989). Effect of residence in a fluoridated community on the incidence of coronal and root caries in an older adult population. *J Pub Health Dent,* 49:138–41.

132. Stamm, J. W., Banting, D. W., & Imrey, P. B. (1990). Adult root caries survey of two similar communities with contrasting natural water fluoride levels. *J Am Dent Assoc,* 120:143–49.

133. Jones, S., Burt, B. A., Petersen, P. E., & Lennon, M. A. (2005). The effective use of fluorides in public health. *Bull World Health Org,* 83:670–76.

134. Jensen, M. E., & Kohout, F. J. (1988). The effect of a fluoridated dentifrice on root and coronal caries in an older adult population. *J Am Dent Assoc,* 117:829–32.

135. Nyvad, B., & Fejerskov, O. (1986). Active root surface caries converted into inactive caries as a response to oral hygiene. *Scand J Dent Res,* 94:281–84.

136. Wallace, M. C., Retief, D. H., & Bradley, E. L. (1993). The 48-month increment of root caries in an urban population of older adults participating in a preventive dental program. *J Pub Health Dent,* 53:133–37.

137. Stookey, G. K. (1990). Critical evaluation of the composition and use of topical fluorides. *J Dent Res,* 69:805–12.

138. Stookey, G. K., Rodlun, C. A., Warrick, J. M., & Miller, C. H. (1989). Professional topical fluoride systems vs root caries in hamsters. *J Dent Res,* 68:372.

139. Hong, L., Watkins, C. A., Ettinger, R. L., & Wefel, J. S. (2005). Effect of topical fluoride and fluoride varnish on in vitro root surface lesions. *Am J. Dent,* 18:182–87.

140. Berger, E. K. (2006). Fluoride varnish treatment for reducing caries: A brief review of the literature. *Contemp Oral Hyg,* 6:8, 9.

141. Semler, S. (2006). Evidence-based solutions to clinical challenges: Prevention-based dentistry—Fluoride varnish. *Journal of Practical Hygiene,* 15:23, 25.

142. Petersson, L. G. (1993). Fluoride mouthrinses and fluoride varnishes. *Caries Res,* 27 (Suppl 1):35–42.

143. Petersson, L. G., Arthursson, L., Ostberg, C., Jonsson, G., & Gleerup, A. (1991). Carries-inhibiting effects of different modes of Duraphat varnish reapplication: A 3-year radiographic study. *Caries Res,* 25:70–73.

144. Association of State and Territorial Dental Directors. Fluorides Committee. Fluoride Varnish: An Evidence-Based Approach. Research Brief. September 2007. Accessed at http://www.astdd.org/docs/Sept2007FINALFlvarnishpaper.pdf.

145. American Public Health Association. (2010). Fluoride varnish for caries prevention. Policy No, 201010. Retrieved from http://www.apha.org/advocacy/policysearch/default.htm?id-1402.

146. American Public Health Association. (2008). Community water fluoridation in the United States. Policy No. 20087. Retrieved from http://www.apha.org/advocacy/policysearch/default.htm?id-1373.

147. Topical fluoride recommendations for high-risk children: Development of Decision Support Matrix. 2007. Retrieved from http://www.mcoralhealth.org/PDFs/TopicalFluorideRpt.pdf.

148. Shobha, T., Nandlal, B., Prabhakar, A. R., & Sudha, P. (1987). Fluoride varnish versus acidulated phosphate fluoride for school children in Manipal. *J Ind Dent Assoc, 59*:157–60.

149. Divaris, K., Preisser, J. S., Slade, G.D. (2012, November). Surface-Specific Efficacy of Fluoride Varnish in Caries Prevention in the Primary Dentition: Results of a Community Randomized Clinical Trial. *Caries Res, 27;47*(1):78–87.

150. Marinho, V. C. C., Higgins, J. P. T., Sheiham, A., Logan, S. (2004) One topical fluoride (toothpastes, or mouthrinses, or gels, or varnishes) versus another for preventing dental caries in children and adolescents. *Cochrane Database of Systematic Reviews 2004*, Issue 1. Art. No.: CD002780. DOI: 10.1002/14651858. CD002780.pub2. Accessed at http://www2.cochrane.org/reviews/en/ab002780.html.

151. Weintraub, J. A., Ramos-Gomez, F., Jue, B., Shain, S., Hoover, C. I., Featherstone, J. D., & Gansky, S. A. (2006). Fluoride varnish efficacy in preventing early childhood caries. *J Dent Res, 85*: 172–76.

152. Association of State and Territorial Dental Directors, Fluorides Committee. 2010. Fluoride Varnish Policy Statement. New Bern, NC: Association of State and Territorial Dental Directors. 5 pp. Rretrieved on October 10, 2012 from http://www.mchoralhealth.org/highlights/flvarnish.html.

153. American Academy of Pediatric Dentistry. Definition of Early Childhood Caries (ECC) revised 2008. http://www.aapd.org/media/Policies_Guidelines/D_ECC.pdf)

154. Fontana, M., & Zero, D. T. (2006). Assessing patients' caries risk. *J Am Dent Assoc, 137*:1231–39.

155. Biller, I. R., Hunter, E. L., Featherstone, M. J., & Silverstone, L. M. (1980). Enamel loss during a prophylaxis polish in vitro. *J Int Assoc Dent Child, 11*:7–12.

156. Stookey, G. K. (1978). In vitro estimates of enamel and dentin abrasion associated with a prophylaxis. *J Dent Res, 57*:36.

157. Vrbic, V., Brudevold, F., & McCann, H. G. (1967). Acquisition of fluoride by enamel from fluoride pumice pastes. *Helv Odont Acta, 11*:21–26.

158. Vrbic, V., & Brudevold, F. (1970). Fluoride uptake from treatment with different fluoride prophylaxis pastes and from the use of pastes containing a soluble aluminum salt followed by topical application. *Caries Res, 4*:158–67.

159. Bixler, D., & Muhler, J. C. (1966). Effect on dental caries in children in a nonfluoride area of combined use of three agents containing stannous fluoride: A prophylactic paste, a solution, and a dentifrice. II. Results at the end of 24 and 36 months. *J Am Dent Assoc, 72*:392–96.

160. Gish, C. W., & Muhler, J. C. (1965). Effect on dental caries in children in a natural fluoride area of combined use of three agents containing stannous fluoride: A prophylactic paste, a solution, and a dentifrice. *J Am Dent Assoc, 70*:914–20.

161. Muhler, J. C., Spear, L. B., Jr., Bixler, D., & Stookey, G. K. (1967). The arrestment of incipient dental caries in adults after the use of three different forms of SnF_2 therapy: Results after 30 months. *J Am Dent Assoc, 75*:1402–406.

162. Obersztyn, A., Piotrowski, Z., Kowinski, K., & Ekler, B. (1973). Stannous fluoride in the prophylaxis of caries in adults. *Czas Stomat, 26*:1181–87.

163. Scola, F. P., & Ostrom, C. A. (1968). Clinical evaluation of stannous fluoride when used as a constituent of a compatible prophylactic paste, as a topical solution, and in a dentifrice in naval personnel. II. Report of findings after two years. *J Am Dent Assoc, 77*:594–97.

164. Scola, F. P. (1970). Self-preparation stannous fluoride prophylactic technique in preventive dentistry: Report after two years. *J Am Dent Assoc, 81*:1369–72.

165. Beiswanger, B. B., Billings, R. J., Sturzenberger, O. P., & Bollmer, B. W. (1978). Effect of an $SnF_2Ca_2P_2O_7$ dentifrice and APF topical applications. *J Dent Child, 45*:137–41.

166. Downer, M. C., Holloway, P. J., & Davies, T. G. H. (1976). Clinical testing of a topical fluoride caries prevention program. *Br Dent J, 141*:242–47.

167. Mainwaring, P. J., & Naylor, N. M. (1978). A three-year clinical study to determine the separate and combined caries-inhibitory effects of sodium monofluorophosphate toothpaste and an acidulated phosphate fluoride gel. *Caries Res, 12*:202–12.

168. Marinho, V. C., Higgins, J. P., Sheiham, A., & Logan, S. (2004). Combinations of topical fluoride (toothpastes, mouthrinses, gels, varnishes) versus single topical fluoride for preventing dental caries in children and adolescents. *Evid Based Dent, 5*:38.

169. Birkeland, J. M., Broch, L., & Jorkjend, J. (1977). Benefits and prognoses following 10 years of a fluoride mouthrinsing program. *Scand J Dent Res, 85*:31–37.

170. Birkeland, J. M., & Torell, P. (1978). Caries-preventive fluoride mouthrinses. *Caries Res, 12* (Suppl 1):38–51.

171. Reports on Councils and Bureaus, Council on Dental Therapeutics, American Dental Association. (1975). Council classifies fluoride mouthrinses. *J Am Dent Assoc, 91*:1250–52.

172. Torell, P., & Ericsson, Y. (1974). The potential benefits to be derived from fluoride mouth-rinses. In Forrester, D. J., & Schulz, E. M., Jr., Eds. *International workshop on fluorides and dental caries reductions.* Baltimore: University of Maryland, 113–76.

173. Heifetz, S. B., Franchi, G. J., Mosley, G. W., MacDougall, O., & Brunelle, J. (1979). Combined anticariogenic effect of fluoride gel-trays and fluoride mouthrinsing in an optimally fluoridated community. *J Clinic Prevent Dent, 6*:21–23.

174. Radike, A. W., Gish, C. W., Peterson, J. K., King, J. D., & Zegreto, V. A. (1973). Clinical evaluation of stannous fluoride as an anticaries mouthrinse. *J Am Dent Assoc, 86*:404–408.

175. Driscoll, W. S., Swango, P. A., Horowitz, A. M., & Kingman, A. (1981). Caries-preventive effects of daily and weekly fluoride mouthrinsing in an optimally fluoridated community: Findings after 18 months. *Pediatr Dent, 3*:316–20.

176. Jones, J. C., Murphy, R. F., & Edd, P. A. (1979). Using health education in a fluoride mouthrinse program: The public health hygienist's role. *Dent Hyg, 53*:469–73.

177. Kawall, K., Lewis, D. W., & Hargreaves, J. A. (1981). The effect of a fluoride mouthrinse in an optimally fluoridated community—Final two year results. *J Dent Res, 60* (Spec Iss A):471. Abstract 646.

178. Ashley, F. P., Mainwaring, P. F., Emslie, R. D., & Naylor, M. N. (1977). Clinical testing of a mouthrinse and a dentifrice containing fluoride. A two-year supervised study in school children. *Br Dent J, 143*:333–38.

179. Triol, C. W., Franz, S. M., Volpe, A. R., Frankl, N., Alman, J. E., & Allard, R. L. (1980). Anticaries effect of a sodium fluoride rinse

and an MFP dentifrice in a nonfluoridated water area. A thirty-month study. *Clin Prev Dent,* 2:13–15.

180. Blinkhorn, A. S., Holloway, P. J., & Davies, T. G. H. (1977). The combined effect of a fluoride mouthrinse and dentifrice in the control of dental caries. *J Dent Res,* 56 (Spec Iss D):D111.

181. Ringelberg, M. L., Webster, D. B., Dixon, D. O., & Lezotte, D. C. (1979). The caries-preventive effect of amine fluorides and inorganic fluorides in a mouthrinse or dentifrice after 30 months of use. *J Am Dent Assoc,* 98:202–208.

182. Horowitz, H. S., Heifetz, S. B., Meyers, R. J., Driscoll, W. S., & Korts, D. C. (1979). Evaluation of a combination of self-administered fluoride procedures for the control of dental caries in a nonfluoride area: Findings after four years. *J Am Dent Assoc,* 98:219–23.

183. Rozier R. G., Adair S., Graham F., Iafolla T., Kingman A., Kohn W., Krol D., Levy S., Pollick H., Whitford G., Strock S., Frantsve Hawley J., Aravamudhan K., & Meyer D. M. (2010, December). Evidence-based clinical recommendations on the prescription of dietary fluoride supplements for caries prevention: a report of the American Dental Association Council on Scientific Affairs. *J Am Dent Assoc,* 141(12):1480–9.

184. Skartveit, L., Wefel, J. S., & Ekstrand, J. (1991). Effect of fluoride amalgams on artificial recurrent enamel and root caries. *Scand J Dent Res,* 99:287–94.

185. Donly, K. J. (1995). Enamel and dentin demineralization inhibition of fluoride-releasing materials. *Am J Dent,* 7:275–78.

186. Erickson, R. L., & Glasspoole, E. A. (1995). Model investigations of caries inhibition by fluoride-releasing dental materials. *Adv Dent Res,* 9:315–23.

187. ten Cate, J. M., & van Duinen, R. N. B. (1995). Hyper-mineralization of dentinal lesions adjacent to glass-ionomer cement restorations. *J Dent Res,* 74:1266–71.

188. Donly, K. J., Segura, A., Kanellis, M., & Erickson, R. L. (1999). Clinical performance and caries inhibition of resin-modified glass ionomer cement and amalgam restorations. *J Am Dent Assoc,* 130:1459–66.

189. Rawls, H. R. (1991). Preventive dental materials: Sustained delivery of fluoride and other therapeutic agents. *Adv Dent Res,* 5:50–56.

190. Vatanatham, K., Trairatvorakul, C., & Tantbironjn, D. (2006). Effect of fluoride- and nonfluoride-containing resin sealants on mineral loss of incipient artificial carious lesion. *J Clin Pediatr Dent,* 30:320–24.

191. Jones, D. W., Jackson, G., Suttow, E. J., Hall, A. C., & Johnson, J. (1988). Fluoride release and fluoride uptake by glass ionomer materials. *J Dent Res,* 67(A):197. Abstract 672.

192. Marinelli, C. B., Donly, K. J., Wefel, J. S., Jakobsen, J. R., & Denehy, G. E. (1997). An in vitro comparison of three fluoride regimens on enamel remineralization. *Caries Res,* 31:418–22.

193. Bynum, A. M., & Donly, K. J. (1999). Enamel deremineralization on teeth adjacent to fluoride releasing materials without dentifrice exposure. *ASDC J Dent Child,* 66:89–92.

194. Donly, K. J., Segura, A., Wefel, J. S., & Hogan, M. M. (1999). Evaluating the effects of fluoride-releasing dental materials on adjacent interproximal caries. *J Am Dent Assoc,* 130:817–25.

195. Bayless, J. M., & Tinanoff, N. (1985). Diagnosis and treatment of acute fluoride toxicity. *J Am Dent Assoc,* 110:209–11.

196. Heifetz, S. B., & Horowitz, H. S. (1986). The amounts of fluoride in current fluoride therapies; safety considerations for children. *J Dent Child,* 77:876–82.

197. McIvor, M. E. (1987). Delayed fatal hyperkalemia in a patient with acute fluoride intoxication. *Ann Emerg Med,* 16:1165–67.

198. Department of Health and Human Services. (1991). U.S. Public Health Service. *Report of the ad hoc subcommittee to coordinate environmental health and related programs. Review of fluoride benefits and risks.* Washington, DC: U.S. Department of Health and Human Services.

199. Whitford, G. M. (1987). Fluoride in dental products: Safety considerations. *J Dent Res,* 66:1056–60.

200. Newbrun, E. (1992). Current regulations and recommendations concerning water fluoridation, fluoride supplements, and topical fluoride agents. *J Dent Res,* 67:1255–65.

201. Keels, M. A., Osterhout, S., & Vann, W. F., Jr. (1988). Incidence and nature of accidental fluoride ingestions. *J Dent Res,* 67 (Spec Iss):335. Abstract 1778.

202. Nochimson, G. Toxicity, fluoride. Retrieved February 29, 2008, from http://www.emedicine.com/emerg/topic181.htm.

203. Szweida, L. F. (1972). Fluorides in community programs: A study of four years of various fluorides applied topically to the teeth of children in fluoridated communities. *J Public Health Dent,* 32:25–33.

myhealthprofessionskit

Visit www.myhealthprofessionskit.com to access the interactive Companion Website for this textbook. Simply select "Dental Hygiene" from the choice of disciplines. Find this book and log in by using your user name and password to access additional learning tools.

Dental Sealants

Christine N. Nathe

OBJECTIVES

After studying this chapter, the student should be able to:

1. Describe how sealants prevent dental caries.
2. Describe the history of sealant development.
3. List the criteria for selecting teeth for sealant placement.
4. Describe the essentials in attaining maximum retention of sealants.
5. Describe the placement of a sealant.
6. Compare the advantages and disadvantages of light-cured and self-cured sealants.
7. List reasons given for the underuse of sealants by practitioners, and analyze the validity of the reasons.

KEY TERMS

Alternative restorative technique (ART), 276
Autopolymerization, 275
Chemical activation, 275
Chemical-cured sealants, 276
Enameloplasty, 274
Etchants, 279
Interim therapeutic restoration (ITM) , 276
Light activation, 275
Photoactivation, 275
Photocure, 275
Polymerization, 275
Prophylactic odontotomy, 274
Tags, 277

INTRODUCTION

Fluorides are highly effective in reducing the number of carious lesions that occur on the smooth surfaces of enamel and cementum. Unfortunately, fluorides are not equally effective in protecting the occlusal pits and fissures, where the majority of carious lesions occur.[1] The placement of sealants is a highly effective means of preventing carious lesions in the pits and fissures in both primary and permanent teeth.[2–4] A Cochrane systematic review examined the effectiveness of second-generation resins compared with no treatment; the resin-based sealants were highly effective in preventing caries in permanent first molars in individuals under 20 years of age and in children 5 to 10 years of age.[5] Another systematic review examined the efficacy of professional measures for caries prevention in high-risk individuals; sealants presented an 88% reduction in caries in that population.[6] Sealants present great preventive value when placed correctly and monitored regularly. A sealant is indicated if an occlusal fissure, fossa, or incisal lingual pit is present. When in doubt, the preferred course of action is to seal and monitor.

A liquid resin, more commonly called a *dental sealant,* is placed over the occlusal surface of the tooth where it penetrates the deep fissures to fill areas that cannot be cleaned with the toothbrush (Figure 16–1 ■). The resin then solidifies, and the hardened sealant subsequently presents a barrier between the tooth and the hostile oral environment. Concurrently, there is a significant reduction of *Streptococcus mutans* on the treated tooth surface.[7] Pits and fissures serve as reservoirs for mutans streptococci; therefore, sealing the niche reduces their oral count.

HISTORICAL PERSPECTIVE

Historically, several agents have been tried to protect deep pits and fissures on occlusal surfaces. In 1895, Wilson reported the placement of dental cement in pits and fissures to prevent caries.[1] In 1929, Bödecker suggested that deep fissures could be

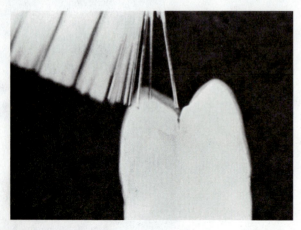

FIGURE ■ 16–1 One reason that 50% of the carious lesions occur on the occlusal surface is that the toothbrush bristle has a larger diameter than the width of the fissure.

(*Source:* Courtesy of Dr. J. McCune, Johnson & Johnson.)

broadened with a large round bur to make the occlusal areas more self-cleansing, a procedure that is called **enameloplasty**.[8,9] Two major disadvantages, however, accompany enameloplasty. First, it requires a dentist, which immediately limits its use. Second, in modifying a deep fissure by this method, it is often necessary to remove more sound tooth structure than would be required to insert a small restoration.

In 1923 and again in 1936, Hyatt advocated the early insertion of small restorations in deep pits and fissures before carious lesions had the opportunity to develop.[10] He termed this procedure **prophylactic odontotomy**. Again, this operation is more of a treatment procedure than a preventive approach because it removes sound tooth structure.

DID YOU KNOW

These early approaches to prevent dental decay were the impetus to the now common routine preventive modality known as *dental sealants.*

Several materials have been unsuccessfully used in an attempt to either seal or make the fissures more resistant to caries. These attempts have included the use of topically applied zinc chloride, potassium ferrocyanide, and ammoniacal silver nitrate; copper amalgam has also been packed into the fissures.[11–13]

A final course of action to manage a deep pit and fissure is one that is often used: Do nothing; wait and watch. This option avoids the need to cut good tooth structure until a definite carious lesion is identified. It also results in many teeth being lost when individuals do not return for periodic examinations. This approach, although used, is a violation of the ethical principle of nonmaleficence which means to do no harm, whereas providing sealants would be promoting the principle of beneficence, which would be providing a benefit.

SEALANT USE IN DENTAL CARE

In the late 1960s and early 1970s, another option, the use of pit-and-fissure sealants became available.[14] Buonocore first described placing sealants using a method to bond polymethylmethacrylate (PMMA) to human enamel conditioned with phosphoric acid.[14] Practical use of this concept, however, was not realized until the development of bisphenol A–glycidyl methylacrylate (Bis-GMA), urethane dimethacrylate (UDMA), and triethylene glycol dimethacrylate (TEGDMA) resins, which possessed better physical properties than PMMA. Buonocore reported the first successful use of resin sealants in the 1960s.[14]

DID YOU KNOW

Nuva-Seal, the first successful commercial sealant, was placed on the market in 1972. Since then, more effective sealants have become available.

Currently, bisphenol A–glycidyl methylacrylate is the most frequently applied sealant. It is a mixture of Bis-GMA and methyl methacrylate. The first sealant clinical trials used cyanoacrylate-based materials, which were later replaced by dimethacrylate-based products. The primary difference between sealants is the method of polymerization; these methods are discussed in the following section.

Bisphenol A (BPA), a plastic found in many products, has generated much press for its estrogenic properties and subsequent safety concerns. Studies have suggested that Bisphenol A can mimic or disrupt estrogenic cell responses.[15] Exposure to BPA from sources other than dental resins contributes to salivary baseline concentration levels and indicates environmental exposure and use of products containing BPA. On the basis of the proven benefits of resin-based dental materials and the brevity of BPA exposure, one review suggested continued use with strict adherence to precautionary application techniques.[16] Use of these materials should be minimized during pregnancy whenever possible.[16] Further research is needed to examine the cumulative estrogenic effects of BPA from dental sealants.[17]

Some sealants contain fillers, which makes classifying the commercial products into filled and unfilled sealants desirable. The filled sealants contain microscopic glass beads, quartz particles, and other fillers used in composite resins. The fillers are coated with products such as silane to facilitate their combination with the Bis-GMA resin. The fillers make the sealant more resistant to abrasion and wear. Because filled sealants are more resistant to abrasion, the occlusion should be checked, and the sealant height might need to be adjusted after placement. In contrast, unfilled sealants wear more quickly but usually do not need occlusal adjustment.

POLYMERIZATION OF SEALANTS

The common sealant is a liquid resin called a *monomer* (a molecule that can be bound to similar molecules to form a polymer, which contains two or more monomers). When the catalyst acts on the monomer, repeating chemical bonds begin to form, increasing in number and complexity as the hardening process, **polymerization**, proceeds (Figure 16–2 ■). Finally, the resultant hard product is known as a *polymer.*

Two methods have been used to catalyze polymerization. The first method is light curing with the use of a visible blue light; synonyms for this method are **photocure, photoactivation**, and **light activation**. Some light-cured sealants contain a catalyst, such as camphoroquinone, which is placed in the monomer at the time of manufacture. The catalyst is sensitive to visible blue-light frequencies. When the monomer is exposed to the visible blue light, polymerization is initiated. The second method is self-curing in which a monomer and a catalyst are mixed together to induce polymerization without the use of a light source; synonyms for this process are *cold cure*, **autopolymerization**, and **chemical activation**. Self-curing sealants are used less frequently in practice.

Polymerization in first-generation sealants was initiated by ultraviolet light; these sealants were replaced by other light-cured sealants that instead required visible blue light. Second-generation sealants were autopolymerized, and third-generation sealants used visible blue light. Fourth- and fifth-generation sealants added a step in which dental-bonding agents were used as a primer before the sealants were placed. Sixth-generation sealants use a self-etching process. Less frequently, glass ionomer cement is used as a dental sealant.

FIGURE ■ 16–2 Polymerization diagram.

Light-Cured Sealants

The main advantage of the light-cured sealant is that the operator can initiate polymerization at any suitable time. Polymerization time is shorter with the light-cured products than with the self-curing sealants. The light-cured process does require purchase of a light source, but this light is also used for polymerization of composite restorations and is available in all dental offices. Light-cured sealants have become the product of choice in most offices. Light-cured sealants should be stored away from bright office lighting, which can sometimes initiate polymerization. The light-cured sealants have a greater compressive strength and a smoother surface, probably because air is introduced into the self-cure resins during mixing.

The light-emitting device consists of a high-intensity white light, a blue filter to produce the desired blue color, usually between 400 to 500 nm, and a light-conducting rod. Some other systems consist of a blue light produced by light-emitting diodes (LED) (Figure 16–3 ■). Most systems have timers for automatically switching off the lights after a predetermined time interval. In use, the end of the rod is held only a few millimeters above the sealant during the first 10 seconds, after which time the rod can be rested on the hardened surface of the partially polymerized sealant. The time required for polymerization is set by the manufacturer and is usually around 20 to 30 seconds. The depth of cure is influenced by the intensity of the light, which can differ greatly with different products and length of exposure. Often it is desirable to set the automatic light timer

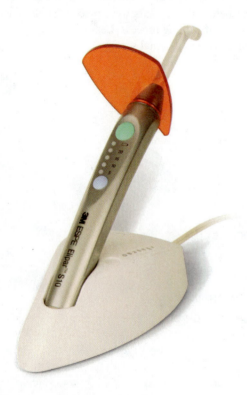

FIGURE ■ 16–3 Light-emitting diode (LED) curing unit for direct, intraoral exposure.

(*Source:* Courtesy of 3M ESPE.)

for longer than the manufacturer's instructions. Even after cessation of light exposure, a final, slow polymerization can continue over a 24-hour period.[18]

Long-term exposure to the intense light can cause damage to the eyes. Staring at the lighted operating field is uncomfortable and does produce afterimages. A filtering device can be used to reduce the effects and filters out the intense blue light. The disk filters out the intense blue light in the 400- to 500-nm range and is sufficiently dark to subdue other light frequencies.

Self-Cured Sealants

Autopolymerizing sealants, sometimes referred to as **chemical-cured sealants**, incorporate a catalyst with the monomer; in addition, another bottle contains an initiator, usually benzoyl peroxide. When the monomer and the initiator are mixed, polymerization begins.

The self-curing resins do not require an expensive light source. However, a great disadvantage is that once mixing has started, if some minor problem is experienced in the operating field, the operator must either continue mixing or stop and make a new mix. For the autopolymerizing resin, the time allowed for sealant manipulation and placement must not be exceeded, even though the material might still appear liquid. Once the hardening begins, it occurs very rapidly, and any manipulation of the material during this critical time jeopardizes retention and surface smoothness. In addition, the operating field must remain completely dry for a longer amount of time, which is obviously a disadvantage. Despite these differences, retention in both the light-cured and the self-cured products appears to be equal.[19,20]

TYPES OF SEALANTS

Glass Ionomer Cement Sealants

Glass ionomer cements have been used as dental sealants. Studies have indicated that they do have the same effective retention rates as those of conventional sealants.[21] Glass ionomer cement is most frequently used when providing the **alternative restorative technique (ART)**, formerly referred to as the *atraumatic restorative technique*. This technique is defined as the nondefinitive restorative treatment procedure for caries prevention that involves removal of soft/demineralized tooth tissue using a hand instrument alone, followed by restoration of the tooth with an adhesive restorative material, such as a glass ionomer cement.[22] ART is used extensively throughout the world as a method to alleviate pain and infection.[23]

Interim therapeutic restoration (ITM) more accurately describes the procedure used in contemporary dental practice in the United States, which can restore and prevent further decalcification and caries in young patients, uncooperative patients, or patients with special health care needs or when traditional cavity preparation and/or placement of traditional dental restorations are not feasible and need to be postponed.[22] This technique is especially valuable in areas of the country where there are shortages of dentists and where dental hygienists are available to place sealants.

Sealants with Bonding Agents

Recently, bonding agents or primers have been added to dental sealant systems. A clinical study conducted over 5 years reported a 50% reduction in occlusal sealant failure and a 66% reduction in buccal–lingual sealant failure when bonding agents were used.[24] One study indicated that in the presence of contamination with saliva, use of bonding under the fissure sealant can reduce microleakage.[25] Another study reported that using a bonding agent or fluoridated sealant did not influence microleakage significantly, either on sound or on questionable fissured surfaces.[26] The use of a bonding agent also increases the time necessary for sealant placement and cost of sealant materials.

Self-Etching Light-Cured Sealants

A new sealant has been introduced; it contains a self-etching additive, which allows placement of the sealant material after a tooth surface is cleaned by oil-free pumice and dried. After waiting for the etching to occur, the light is placed on the sealant. This procedure is much faster than previous methods, and these sealants also include fluoride. One clinical study suggested that self-etched sealants had a significantly higher-bonding strength than a traditional etch and than seal material.[27] However, another study indicated that a self-etch sealant material provided lower bond strength and more marginal leakage than the control.[28]

Fluoride-Releasing Sealants

The addition of fluoride to sealants was considered about 20 years ago based on the finding that the incidence and severity of secondary caries were reduced around fluoride-releasing materials such as the silicate cements used for anterior restorations. Use of a fluoridated resin-based sealant was thought to possibly provide an additional anticariogenic effect if the fluoride released from its matrix was incorporated into the adjacent enamel because fluoride uptake would increase the enamel's resistance to the caries effect.[29]

Fluoride is added to sealants by two methods. The first method involves adding a soluble fluoride to the unpolymerized resin. The second method involves adding an organic fluoride compound that will bind chemically to the resin to form an ion exchange resin. Fluoride-releasing sealants have shown antibacterial properties as well as greater artificial caries resistance compared with a nonfluoridated sealant.[30–34] Fluoridated sealants have also demonstrated a caries-inhibiting effect with a significant reduction in lesion depth in adjacent surface enamel and a reduction in the frequency of wall lesions.[34] Moreover, the fluoridated sealant's laboratory bond strength to enamel is similar to that of nonfluoridated sealants.[35]

However, recent reviews have revealed that, compared with resin-based sealants, fluoride-containing sealants have a poor retention rate after 48 months; they also have not proven to act as a fluoride reservoir with long-term release of fluoride into the oral environment.[20,34,36]

Moisture-Resistant Sealants

A moisture-resistant sealant material, that is not composed of glass ionomer cement is available. This material is composed of acrylic resin and does not contain BPA.[37] At present, no studies can be accessed to assess this sealant material.

Colored versus Clear Sealants

Both clear and colored sealants are available. Colored sealants vary from translucent (clear) to white, yellow, and pink. Some manufacturers sell both clear and colored sealants in either the light-curing or autopolymerizing form. The selection of a colored versus a clear sealant is a matter of individual preference. The colored products permit a more precise placement of the sealant with the visual assurance that the periphery extends halfway up the inclined planes. Both the patient and the operator placing the sealant can more accurately monitor retention. A clear sealant, however, could be considered more acceptable.

Some clinicians prefer the clear sealants because they are more discrete than white sealants. Others prefer the white sealants because they are easier to monitor at recall appointments. On the other hand, some clinicians seem to prefer the clear sealants because it is possible to see under the sealant to detect whether a carious lesion is active or advancing. However, no clinical study has comprehensively compared these issues. Some pit-and-fissure sealants actually change color as they become light polymerized. Color change has not been fully investigated and seems to have only a relative advantage to the dental provider.

SEALANT RETENTION

Resin sealants are retained better on recently erupted teeth than on teeth with a more mature surface. Moreover, they are retained better on first molars than on second molars and on mandibular than on maxillary teeth. This latter finding is possibly caused by the fact that the mandibular teeth being more accessible and easier to see; also, gravity aids the flow of the sealant into the fissures. Sealants appear to be equally retained on occlusal surfaces in primary and permanent teeth.[3] One-year retention rates on primary teeth sealed with a flowable resin material were significantly higher than nonflowable materials.[38]

Sealed teeth from which the dental sealants were later lost still had fewer lesions than control teeth.[39] This finding is possibly due to the presence of tags that are retained in the enamel after the bulk of the sealant has been sheared from the tooth surface. When the resin sealant flows over the prepared surface, it penetrates the fingerlike depressions created by the etching solution. These projections of resin into the etched areas are called **tags** (Figure 16–4 ■). The tags are essential for retention. Scanning electron microscope examination of sealants that were not retained has demonstrated large areas devoid of tags or incomplete tags, usually caused by saliva contamination during the sealing process. If a sealant is forcefully separated from the

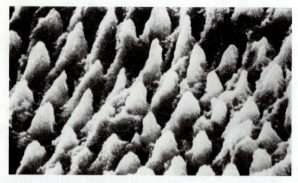

FIGURE ■ 16–4 Tags, 30 micron. Sealant was flowed over etched surface and allowed to polymerize. The tooth surface subsequently dissolved away in acid, leaving tags.

(*Source:* Courtesy Wiley-Blackwell Publishing LTD.)

tooth by masticatory pressures, many of these tags are retained in the etched depressions.

The number of retained sealants decreases at a curvilinear rate. Over the first 3 months, the rapid loss of sealants is probably caused by faulty technique in placement. The fallout rate then begins to plateau with the ensuing sealant losses probably caused by abnormal masticatory stresses. After a year or so, the sealants become very difficult to see or to discern tactilely, especially if they are abraded to the point that they fill only the fissures. In research studies, this lack of visibility often leads to underestimating the effectiveness of the sealants that remain but cannot be identified. Because the most rapid falloff of sealants occurs in the early stages, an initial 3-month appointment recall after placement to determine whether sealants have been lost should be routine, although the recall is not generally done. If sealants are lost, the teeth should be resealed. Teeth successfully sealed for 6 to 7 years are likely to remain sealed.[40]

DID YOU KNOW **?**

Approximately 30% of children have at least one sealed tooth.

Long-term studies reported that, at the 20-year follow-up examination of the first molars, 65% showed complete retention of sealants and 27% partial retention without caries. At a 15-year follow-up of the same sealants, the second molars demonstrated corresponding retention rates of 65% and 30%, respectively.[41,42] Mertz-Fairhurst cited studies in which 90% to 100% of the original sealants were retained over a 1-year period.[40] One review reported 82% of the sealants placed are retained for 5 years.[43] When resealing is accomplished as needed at recall appointments, a higher and more continuous level of protection is achieved. Pit-and-fissure sealants applied during childhood have a long-lasting, caries-preventive effect.[41,42]

CRITERIA FOR SELECTING TEETH FOR SEALANT PLACEMENT

A sealant is indicated under these circumstances:

- The *fossa* (shallow depression) selected for sealant placement is well isolated from another fossa with a restoration.
- The area selected is confined to a fully erupted fossa even though the distal fossa is impossible to seal because of inadequate eruption.
- The selected tooth has an intact occlusal surface when the contralateral tooth surface (surface of tooth in opposite arch) is carious or restored; teeth on opposite sides of the arches usually are equally prone to caries.
- An incipient lesion exists in the pit-and-fissure area.
- Sealant material can be flowed over a conservative class I composite or amalgam to improve the marginal integrity and into the remaining pits and fissures to prevent further recurrent decay.

All teeth meeting these criteria should be sealed and resealed as needed. Sealants should be placed on the teeth of adults if there is evidence of existing or impending caries susceptibility, as would occur following excessive intake of sugar, methamphetamine use, or xerostomia induced by drugs or radiation therapy. Sealants should also be used in communities where fluoride level in the water supply is optimized, as well as in nonfluoridated communities.[43] The following cases are two good illustrations of this philosophy. After a 3-year study, Ripa and colleagues concluded that the time the teeth had been in the mouth (some for 7 to 10 years) had no effect on the vulnerability of occlusal surfaces to caries attack.[44] Also, the incidence of occlusal caries in young Air Force recruits, who were usually in their late teens or early twenties, is relatively high.[45]

DID YOU KNOW

The *Healthy People 2020* document has several objectives that address the need to increase the proportion of children receiving dental sealants.

When priorities, such as in many public health programs, must be based on economic factors, ages 3 and 4 years (preschool) are the most important times for sealing the eligible deciduous teeth; ages 6 to 7 years (second grade) for the first permanent molars; and ages 11 to 13 years (sixth grade) for the second permanent molars and premolars.[46] Currently, 77% of the 12- to 17-year-old children in the United States have dental caries in their permanent teeth.[47] Combining sealant placement and regular fluoride exposure would save many school days, and school dental health clinics or mobile dental health programs would achieve better dental health.[48] If a primary factor in treatment planning is limited resources, the disease susceptibility of the tooth should be considered when selecting teeth for sealants as opposed to the age of the individual.

A sealant is contraindicated under these circumstances:

- Patient behavior does not permit use of adequate dry-field techniques throughout the procedure.
- An open, frank, carious lesion exists on the same tooth.
- Caries exist on other surfaces of the same tooth in which restoration will disrupt an intact sealant.
- A large occlusal restoration is already present.

SEALANT PLACEMENT

For sealant retention, the surface of the tooth must (1) have a maximum surface area, (2) have deep, irregular pits and fissures, (3) be clean, and (4) for most sealant materials, be absolutely dry at the time of sealant placement and uncontaminated with saliva residue. These are the four commandments for successful sealant placement, and they cannot be violated.

Increasing the Surface Area

Sealants do not bond directly to the teeth. Instead, adhesive forces mainly retain them. Increasing the surface area, which in turn increases the adhesive potential, requires the use of tooth conditioners (also called **etchants**), which are composed of a 30% to 50% concentration of phosphoric acid; the etchants are placed on the occlusal surface prior to placement of the sealant.[49] The etchant can be in liquid or gel form; both are equal in abetting retention.[50] Once a tooth is etched, it appears chalky white (see Figure 16–5 ■). If any etched areas on the tooth surface are not covered by the sealant or if the sealant is not retained, the normal appearance of the enamel returns within 1 hour to a few weeks as a result of the salivary constituents' remineralization of the enamel.[51]

The etchant should be carefully applied to avoid contact with the soft tissues. If not confined to the occlusal surface, the acid can produce a mild inflammatory response. It also produces a sharp acid taste that is often objectionable.

Pit-and-Fissure Depth

Deep, irregular pits and fissures offer a much more favorable surface contour for sealant retention compared with broad, shallow fossae (see Figure 16–1). The deeper fissures protect the resin sealant from the shear forces occurring as a result of masticatory movements. Of parallel importance is the possibility of caries development increasing as the fissure depth and slope of the inclined planes increase.[52] Thus, as the potential for caries increases, so does the potential for sealant retention.

Surface Cleanliness

The need and methods for cleaning the tooth surface prior to sealant placement are controversial. Methods used to clean the tooth surface include air polishing, use of hydrogen peroxide, polishing with pumice, brushing with a nonfluoridated toothpaste, and use of laser.[53–56] Comparison of acid etching with laser alone did not demonstrate any significant difference of sealant retention or microleakage. In light of the expense of laser equipment, using a laser prior to sealant placement provides no advantage.[20] Furthermore, cleaning teeth with the newer prophylaxis pastes with or without fluoride (NuPro, Topex) was not shown to affect the bond strength of sealants.[57] Interestingly, in the most cited studies on sealant longevity, Simonsen accomplished the most effective sealant longevity without use of a prior prophylaxis.[41] However, cleaning the tooth surface with oil-free pumice is recommended for sixth-generation sealant material. Whatever the cleaning preferences, either by acid etching or other methods, all heavy stains, deposits, debris, and plaque should be removed from the occlusal surface before applying the sealant material.

It was once thought that the use of fluoride prior to sealant placement would decrease sealant retention. The literature indicates, however, that this concern is not true and that, if the tooth is treated with fluoride and the sealant is not retained, the tooth will still benefit from the prior fluoride placement.[58,59]

Preparing the Tooth for Sealant Application

The preliminary steps for the light-activated and the autopolymerized resins are similar up to the time of application of the resin to the teeth. After the selected teeth are isolated, they are thoroughly dried. If a liquid etchant is being used, it is dabbed on the tooth with a small resin sponge or cotton pellet held with cotton pliers. More commonly, a gel etchant would be placed directly on the tooth by the supplied syringe/canula delivery system. Following the manufacturer's direction for etch time is important; typically 20 to 30 seconds of enamel-etching time is recommended. The etched tooth is then rinsed and dried (Figure 16–6 ■).

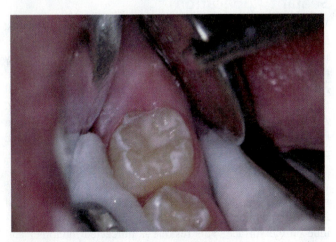

FIGURE ■ 16–5 Tooth after etchant is placed.

(*Source:* University of Kentucky College of Dentistry-OHRI.)

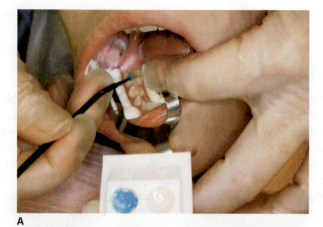

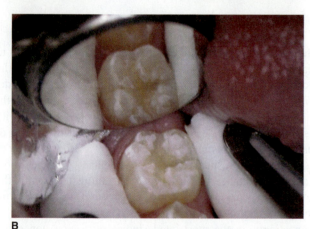

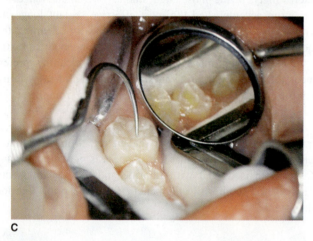

FIGURE ■ 16–6 Sealant placement. A. Gel etchant is applied to teeth, including the lingual cusp on the first molar. B. Etched surface has a "frosty" appearance. C. Application of resin-based sealant.

(*Source:* University of Kentucky College of Dentistry-OHRI.)

The dried tooth surface should have a white, dull, frosty, or chalky appearance because the etching removes approximately 5 to 10 micron of the original surface, although at times inter-rod penetrations of up to 100 micron can occur.[60,61] The etching does not always involve the inter-rod areas; sometimes the

central portion of the rod is etched, and the periphery is unaffected. The pattern on any one tooth is unpredictable.[62] In any event, the surface area is greatly increased by the acid etch.

Drying the Tooth Surface

The teeth must be dry at the time of sealant placement because sealants are hydrophobic. The presence of saliva on the tooth is even more detrimental than water because its organic components interpose a barrier between the tooth and the sealant. When the teeth are dried with an air syringe, the air stream should be checked to ensure that it is not moisture laden. Otherwise, if sufficient moisture is sprayed on the tooth, adhesion of the sealant to the enamel will be prevented. A check for moisture can be accomplished by directing the air stream onto a cool mouth mirror; any fogging indicates the presence of moisture. The omission of this simple step possibly accounts for the interoperator variability in the retention of fissure sealants.

A dry field can be maintained in several ways including use of cotton rolls, and/or the placement of bibulous (absorbent) pads over the opening of the parotid duct. The most successful sealant studies have used cotton rolls for isolation.[41] In one study comparing the retention rate of a rubber dam versus cotton rolls, the sealant retention was approximately equal.[63] Other studies have shown excellent sealant retention after 3 years and after 10 to 20 years.[41,42,64] Another promising dry-field–isolating device for single-operator use, especially when used with cotton rolls, is ejector moisture-control systems, which suction and eject saliva from the mouth.

The use of two operators, such as a dental hygienist or a dentist and a dental assistant, is preferred because it increases the likelihood that a dry field can be maintained. In the event that it becomes necessary to replace a wet cotton roll, it is essential that no saliva contacts the etched tooth surface. If saliva contact is suspected, it is necessary to repeat all procedures up to the time the dry field was compromised, including repeated etching to remove any residual saliva.

Sealant Application

With either the light-cured or autopolymerized sealants, the material should be placed first in the fissures of maximum depth. At times, penetration of the fissure is negated by the presence of debris, air entrapment, narrow orifices, and excessive viscosity of the sealant.[65] The sealant should fill the fissures, but some bulk over the fissure should be present. After the fissures are adequately covered, the material is then brought to a knife-edge approximately halfway up the inclined plane.

Following polymerization, the sealants should be examined carefully before the dry field is discontinued. If any voids are evident, additional sealant can be added without the need for additional etching. The hardened sealant leaves an oil residue on the surface. This residue is unreacted monomer and should be removed with a gauze square. If a sealant requires repair at any time after the dry field is discontinued, repeating the initial etching and drying procedures is prudent. Because all commercial sealants, light-cured and self-cured, are of the same Bis-GMA chemical family, they easily bond to one another.[66]

Occlusal and Interproximal Discrepancies

At times, excess sealant can inadvertently flow into a fossa or the adjoining interproximal spaces. To remedy the first problem, the occlusion should be checked visually or, if indicated, with articulating paper, which has a pigment coating on one or both sides to mark teeth where their occlusal surfaces contact the paper. The marked surfaces indicate the contact points of the teeth. Usually any minor discrepancies in occlusion are rapidly removed by normal chewing action. A large, round cutting bur can be used to rapidly create a broad resin fossa if the premature contact is unacceptable.

The integrity of the interproximal spaces can be checked with the use of dental floss. If any sealant is present, the use of scalers could be required to accomplish removal. If the sealant still cannot be removed, the area should be re-etched to remove the sealant. These corrective actions are rarely needed once proficiency of placement is attained.

Evaluating Retention of Sealants

The finished sealant should be checked for retention without using undue force. If the sealant does not adhere, the placement procedures should be repeated with only about 15 seconds of etching needed to remove the residual saliva before again flushing, drying, and applying the sealant. If two attempts are unsuccessful, the sealant application should be postponed until remineralization occurs and the patient can comply with the procedure.

PLACEMENT OF SEALANTS OVER CARIOUS LESIONS

Sealing over a carious lesion is important because of the professional concern about the possibility of caries progression under the sealant sites. Teeth that were examined in vivo and later subjected to histologic examination after extraction for orthodontic reasons were often found to have areas of incipient or overt caries under many fissures, which the explorer cannot detect. In one study, sealants were purposely placed over small, overt lesions; when compared with control teeth, many of the sealed carious teeth were diagnosed as sound 3 and 5 years later.[67] Handelman has indicated that sealants can be considered a viable modality for arrest of pit-and-fissure caries.[68] The number of bacteria recovered from the area decreased rapidly when the lesion was sealed.[31,67–69] This decrease in bacterial population is probably due to the integrity of the seal between the resin and the etched tooth surface, which does not permit the movement of fluids or tracer isotopes between the sealant and the tooth.[70,71]

Sealants have been placed over more extensive lesions in which carious dentin is involved.[72] Even with these larger lesions, there is a decrease in the bacterial population and arrest of the carious process as a function of time. Clinically detectable lesions in the dentin were covered for 5 years with Nuva-Seal. After that time, the bacterial cultures were essentially negative, and an apparent 83% reversal from a caries-active to a caries-inactive state was achieved.[69] More recently, Mertz-Fairhurst and colleagues demonstrated that sealed lesions became inactive bacteriologically with arrested carious lesions.[73] Researchers found that there were clear efficiencies in sealing incipient surfaces and therefore recommended this practice.[74,75] Sealants that have been placed over incipient lesions should be monitored at subsequent recall/annual dental examination. In addition, there have been reports of sealants being used to achieve penetration of incipient smooth-surface lesions ("white spots") of facial surfaces.

Many times dental providers perform enameloplasty using a bur or an air abrasion to remove demineralized areas and then place a dental sealant. In fact, enameloplasty has no significant differences compared with etching before sealants. Enameloplasty also requires a dentist, which increases the cost of placing sealants.

DENTAL PROVIDERS

The cost of sealant placement increases directly with the operator's level of professional education. In view of cost-effectiveness, a dental hygienist with a dental assistant should be considered the logical providers to place sealants. In most states, dental hygienists are now allowed to place sealants without the presence of a dentist; however, in many states, the dentist is required to examine the tooth to make the decision regarding sealant placement. This requirement increases the time spent in providing sealants and increases the cost of placing the sealants by increasing the number of dental providers required for the procedure.

ECONOMICS

Bear in mind that not every tooth receiving a sealant would necessarily become carious, but the cost of preventing a single carious lesion is higher than the cost of a single sealant application. For instance, calculations have revealed that five sealants would need to be placed on sound teeth to prevent one lesion over a 5-year period, that is, an estimated one tooth for every three sealant applications is prevented from becoming carious.[76] Sealants would be most cost-effective if they could be placed in only those pits and fissures that are destined to become carious. Unfortunately, there is not a caries predictor test of such exactitude, but the use of visual examination plus an economic, portable electronic device that objectively measures conductance (or resistance) would greatly aid in evaluating occlusal risk. Without such a device, it is necessary to rely on professional judgment, which is based on the severity of indicators for caries activity: number of demineralized fissures, level of plaque index, number of incipient and overt lesions, and microbiologic test indications.

In an office setting, treating a tooth is estimated to cost 1.6 times more to than sealing it. A panel of seven experts found that placing sealants, especially on teeth with high caries risk, was a cost-effective measure with positive outcomes.[77] The Task Force on Community Preventive Services, an independent, nonfederal group formed to evaluate oral health interventions, was charged with determining interventions that promote and improve oral health. The Task Force examined the cost of six public health programs for placing pit-and-fissure sealants, revealing a mean cost of $39.10 per person.[78]

DISPARITIES IN DENTAL SEALANT USE

Significant disparities in the number of placed sealants exist. Disparities are found mostly among young children but are also linked to race/ethnicity, income levels, and education.[79] One study reported that white children and children from high-income backgrounds were 60% more likely to have sealants than other racial/ethnic minorities or those from lower incomes. Adults and the elderly generally have lower sealant use even though many of them suffer from xerostomia, which would make them ideal candidates for sealant use.

Barriers that affect the delivery of sealants include (1) legal restrictions on dental hygienists with dental assistants placing sealants without the approval and/or presence of a dentist, (2) lack of consumer knowledge about the effectiveness of sealants and a resultant lack of demand for the product, (3) a shortage of dentists willing to accept patients on Medicaid, and (4) dental providers' concern over the falsely perceived detrimental effect of sealing over a carious lesion.[80]

The safety of dental sealant placement has been demonstrated by many studies showing that, even when placed over incipient and minimally overt caries sites, progression did not occur as long as the sealant remained intact.[81] In addition, several clinical studies have pointed out that dental hygienists and dental assistants could apply sealants, thus providing a more economical workforce for private practice and public health programs.

DID YOU KNOW **?**

Dental sealants can last for up to 10 years and should be assessed at regular intervals.

Dental and public health organizations support the use of dental sealants. The economics and education of the profession and the public are the prime requisites for expanded acceptance of sealants.[80]

SUMMARY

The majority of all carious lesions that occur in the mouth occur on the occlusal surfaces. Which teeth will become carious cannot be predicted; however, if the surface is sealed with a pit-and-fissure sealant, no caries will develop as long as the sealant remains in place. Recent studies indicate an approximate 90% retention rate of sealants 1 year after placement. Even when sealants are eventually lost, most studies indicate that the caries incidence for these teeth is less than that of control surfaces that had never been sealed. Research data also indicate that many incipient and small overt lesions are arrested when sealed. Not one report has shown that caries developed in pits or fissures under an intact sealant.

Sealants are easy to apply, but their application is an extremely sensitive technique. The surfaces that are to receive the sealant must be completely isolated from the saliva during the entire procedure, and etching, flushing, and drying procedures must be timed to ensure adequate preparation of the surface for the sealant. Sealants are comparable to amalgam restorations for longevity but do not require the cutting of tooth structure. Sealants cost less to place than amalgams. Despite their advantages, all dental providers have not embraced the use of sealants even though the American Dental Association, American Dental Hygienists' Association, and the U.S. Public Health Service have endorsed them. Even when small overt pit-and-fissure lesions exist, they can be dealt with conservatively by using ART. What now appears to be required is that the dental and dental hygiene schools teach that sealants are effective interventions, that the dental professional use them, that the dental hygienist and dental assistant be permitted to apply them, and that the public demand them.

PRACTICAL: CONSIDERATIONS

Dental sealants are an excellent means to prevent dental demineralization. The dental provider should promote the use of sealants to all patients, specifically those with high risks. The continued promotion will increase the likelihood that many future adults will live "cavity-free" for a lifetime.

SELF-STUDY QUESTIONS

1. Enamoplasty requires a small cavity preparation before sealant placement and is the preferred method of sealing tooth surfaces.

   a. The first statement is true; the second statement is false.

   b. The first statement is false; the second statement is true.

   c. Both statements are true.

   d. Both statements are false.

   Rationale: First, enamoplasty requires a dentist, which immediately limits its use. Second, in modifying a deep fissure by this method, it is often necessary to remove more sound tooth structure than would be required to insert a small restoration.

2. Fillers are placed in sealants to make them

   a. Able to be placed so that the occusal does not need adjusted

   b. More resistant to abrasion and wear

   c. Classifiable as preventive restoratives

   d. Shorter lasting so that newer materials can be placed.

   Rationale:: The fillers make the sealant more resistant to abrasion and wear. Because filled sealants are more resistant to abrasion, the occlusion should be checked, and the sealant height might need to be adjusted after placement. In contrast, unfilled sealants wear more quickly but usually do not need occlusal adjustment.

3. The most common sealant materials require which type of chemical bonding?

   a. Polymerization

   b. Monomerization

   c. Catalytization

   d. Catalytic monomer chain reaction

   Rationale: The common sealant is a liquid resin called a *monomer* (a molecule that can be bound to similar molecules to form a polymer, which contains two or more monomers). When the catalyst acts on the monomer, repeating chemical bonds begin to form, increasing in number and complexity as the hardening process, polymerization, proceeds. Finally, the resultant hard product is known as a *polymer.*

4. Which providers offer the most cost-effective mechanisms to provide dental sealants to the population?

   a. Dental hygienist and dental assistant

   b. Dentists and dental assistants

   c. Dentists and dental hygienists

   Rationale: The cost of sealant placement increases directly with the level of professional education of the operator. In view of the cost-effectiveness, dental hygienists with dental assistants should be considered the logical providers to place sealants. In most states, dental hygienists are now allowed to place sealants without the presence of a dentist; however, many states require the dentist to examine the tooth to make the decision regarding sealant placement.

5. Dental sealants often are not placed on children who have the highest likelihood of eventual tooth decay. This could be due to lack of resources to obtain care.

   a. The first statement is true; the second statement is false.

   b. The first statement is false; the second statement is true.

   c. Both statements are true.

   d. Both statements are false.

   Rationale: Significant disparities in the number of placed sealants exist, mostly among young children but are also linked to race/ethnicity, income levels, and education

REFERENCES

1. Wilson, I. P. (1985). Preventive dentistry. *Dent Diagn,* 1:70–72.

2. Hotuman, E., Rolling, I., & Poulsen, S. (1998). Fissure sealants in a group of 3–4-year-old children. *Int J Paediatr Dent,* 8:159–60.

3. Garcia-Godoy, F., & Donly, K. J. (2002). Dentin/enamel adhesives in pediatric dentistry. *Pediatr Dent,* 24:462–64.

4. Bletram-Aguilar, E. D., Barker, L. K., Canto, M. T., Dye, B. A., Gooch, B. F., Hyman, J., Jaramillo, F., Kingman, A., Nowjack-Raymer, R., Selwitz, R. H., & Wu, T. (2005). Surveillance for dental caries, dental sealants, tooth retention, edentulism, and enamel fluorosis—US, 1988–1994 and 1999–2002. *Morb Mortality Wkly Rep MMWR,* 54:1–44.

5. Ahovuo-Saloranta, A., Hiiri, A., Nordblad, A., Worthington, H., & Makela, M. (2004). Pit and fissure sealants for preventing dental decay in the permanent teeth of children and adolescents. *Cochrane Datab Syst Rev* (Iss 3. Art. No.: CD001830).

6. Bader, J. D., Shugars, D. A., & Bonito, A. J. (2001). A systematic review of selected caries prevention and management methods. *Community Dent Oral Epidemiol,* 29:399–411.

7. Mass, E., Eli, I., Lev-Dor-Samovici, B., & Weiss, E. I. (1999). Continuous effect of pit and fissure sealing on *S. mutans* presence in situ. *Pediatr Dent,* 21:164–68.

8. Bödecker, C. F. (1929). The eradication of enamel fissures. *Dent Items Int,* 51:859–66.

9. Sturdevant, C. M., Barton, R. E., Sockwell, C. L., & Strickland, W. D. (1985). *The art and science of operative dentistry.* St. Louis, MO: C. V. Mosby.

10. Hyatt, T. P. (1936). Prophylactic odontotomy: The ideal procedure in dentistry for children. *Dent Cosmos,* 78:353–370.

11. Ast, D. B., Bushel, A., & Chase, C. C. (1950). A clinical study of caries prophylaxis and zinc chloride and potassium ferrocyanide. *J Am Dent Assoc,* 41:437–42.

12. Klein, H., & Knutson, J. W. (1942). Studies on dental caries. XIII. Effect of ammoniacal silver nitrate on caries in the first permanent molar. *Am Dent Assoc,* 29:1420–26.

13. Miller, J. (1951). Clinical investigations in preventive dentistry. *Br Dent J,* 91:92–95.

14. Buonocore, M. G. (1971). Caries prevention in pits and fissures sealed with an adhesive resin polymerized by ultraviolet light: A two-year study of a single adhesive application. *J Am Dent Assoc,* 82:1090–93.

15. Söderholm, K. J., & Mariotti, A. (1999, February). BIS-GMA–based resins in dentistry: Are they safe? *J Am Dent Assoc,* 130:201–9.

16. Fleisch A. F., Sheffield P. E., Chinn, C., Edelstein, B. L., & Landrigan, P. J. (2010, October). Bisphenol A and related compounds in dental materials. *Pediatrics,* 126:760–68. Epub.

17. Zimmerman-Downs, J. M., Shuman, D., Stull, S. C., & Ratzlaff, R. E. (2010, [Epub]). Bisphenol A blood and saliva levels prior to and after dental sealant placement in adults. *J Dent Hyg,* 84:145–50.

18. Leung, R. L., Adishian, S. R., & Fan, P. L. (1985). Postirradiation comparison of photoactivated composite resins. *J Prosthet Dent,* 54:645–49.

19. Houpt, M., Fuks, A., Shapira, J., Chosack, A., & Eidelman, E. (1987). Autopolymerized versus light-polymerized fissure sealant. *J Am Dent Assoc,* 115:55–56.

20. Muller-Bolla, M., Lupi-Pegurier, L., Tardieu, C., Velly, A. M., & Antomarchi, C. (2006). Retention of resin-based pit and fissure sealants: A systematic review. *Community Dent Oral Epidemiol,* 34:321–36.

21. Sachin, S. (2011). Glass ionomer cement and resin-based fissure sealants are equally effective in caries prevention. *JADA,* 142: 551–52.

22. American Academy of Pediatric Dentistry. (2008). *Policy on interim therapeutic restorations (ITR).* Chicago, IL: American Academy of Pediatric Dentistry. Retrieved November 10, 2011, from http://www.aapd.org/media/Policies_Guidelines/P_ITR.

23. Frencken, J. E. (2010, January). The ART approach using glass-ionomers in relation to global oral health care. *Dent Mater,* 26:1–6.

24. Feigal, R. J., Musherure, P., Gillespie, B., Levy-Polack, M., Quelhas, I., & Hebling, J. I. (2000). Improved sealant retention with bonding agents: A clinical study of two-bottle and single-bottle systems. *J Dent Res,* 79:1850–56.

25. Askarizadeh, N., Norouzi, N., & Nemati, S. (2008, June). The effect of bonding agents on the microleakage of sealant following contamination with saliva. *J Indian Soc Pedod Prev Den,* 26:64–66.

26. Michalaki, M. G., Oulis, C. J., & Lagouvardos, P. (2010, February). Microleakage of three different sealants on sound and questionable occlusal surfaces of permanent molars: An in vitro study. *Eur Arch Paediatr Dent,* 11:26–31.

27. Gomes-Silva, J. M., Torres, C. P., Contente, M. M., Oliveira, M. A., Palma-Dibb, R. G., & Borsatto, M. C. (2008). Bond strength of a pit-and-fissure sealant associated to etch-and-rinse and self-etching adhesive systems to saliva-contaminated enamel: Individual vs. simultaneous light curing. *Braz Dent J,* 9:341–47.

28. Wadenya, R. O., Yego, C., Blatz, M. B., & Mante, F. (2009 July-August). Bond strength and microleakage of a new self-etch sealant. *Quintessence Int,* 40:559–63.

29. Forsten, L. (1977). Fluoride release from a glass ionomer cement. *Scand J Dent Res,* 85:503–504.

30. Kozai, K., Suzuki, J., Okada, M., & Nagasaka, N. (2000). In vitro study of antibacterial and antiadhesive activities of fluoride-containing light-cured fissure sealants and a glass ionomer liner/base against oral bacteria. *ASDC J Dent Child,* 67:117–22.

31. Carlsson, A., Petersson, M., & Twetman, S. (1997). 2-year clinical performance of a fluoride-containing fissure sealant in young schoolchildren at caries risk. *Am J Dent,* 10:115–19.

32. Loyola-Rodriguez, J. P., & Garcia-Godoy, F. (1996). Antibacterial activity of fluoride release sealants on mutans streptococci. *J Clin Pediatr Dent,* 20:109–11.

33. Jensen, M. E., Wefel, J. S., Triolo, P. T., & Hammesfahr, P. D. (1990). Effects of a fluoride-releasing fissure sealant on artificial enamel caries. *Am J Dent* 3:75–78.

34. Hicks, M. J., Flaitz, C. M., & Garcia-Godoy, F. (2000). Fluoride-releasing sealant and caries-like enamel lesion formation in vitro. *J Clin Pediatr Dent,* 24:215–19.

35. Marcushamer, M., Neuman, E., & Garcia-Godoy, F. (1997). Fluoridated and nonfluoridated unfilled sealants show similar shear strength. *Pediatr Dent,* 19:289–90.

36. Garcia-Godoy, F., Abarzua, I., De Goes, M. F., & Chan, D. C. (1997). Fluoride release from fissure sealants. *J Clin Pediatr Dent,* 22:45–49.

37. Embrace WetBond Pit & Fissure Sealant. Retrieved on November 10, 2011, from http://www.pulpdent.com/products.

38. Corona, S. A., Borsatto, M. C., Garcia, L., Ramos, R. P., & Palma-Dibb, R. G. (2005). Randomized, controlled trial comparing the retention of a flowable restorative system with a conventional resin sealant: One-year follow up. *Int J Paediatr Dent,* 15:44–50.

39. Hinding, J. (1974). Extended cariostasis following loss of pit and fissure sealant from human teeth. *ASDC J Dent Child,* 41:201–203.

40. Mertz-Fairhurst, E. J. (1984). Current status of sealant retention and caries prevention. *J Dent Educ,* 48:18–26.

41. Simonsen, R. J. (1987). Retention and effectiveness of a single application of white sealant after 10 years. *J Am Dent Assoc,* 115:31–36.

42. Wendt, L. K., Koch, G., & Birkhed, D. (2001). On the retention and effectiveness of fissure sealant in permanent molars after 15–20 years: A cohort study. *Community Dent Oral Epidemiol,* 29:302–7.

43. Bohannan, H. M. (1983). Caries distribution and the case for sealants. *J Public Health Dent,* 43:200–4.

44. Ripa, L. W., Leske, G. S., & Varma, A. O. (1988). Longitudinal study of the caries susceptibility of occlusal and proximal surfaces of first permanent molars. *J Public Health Dent,* 48:8–13.

45. Foreman, F. J. (1994). Sealant prevalence and indication in a young military population. *J Am Dent Assoc,* 125:182–84, 186.

46. Simonsen, R. J. (1984). Pit and fissure sealant in individual patient care programs. *J Dent Educ,* 48:42–44.

47. National Institutes of Health. (2001). *Diagnosis and management of dental caries throughout life. NIH consensus statement 2001 March 26–28;* 18:1–24. Retrieved December 4, 2007, from http://consensus.nih.gov/2001/2001DentalCaries115html.htm.

48. U.S. Department of Health and Human Service. (2002, November). Oral health (section 21). In *Healthy People 2010, Vol. 2* (2nd ed.). Washington, DC: U.S. Government Printing Office.

49. Gwinnett, A. J., & Buonocore, M. G. (1965). Adhesives and caries prevention; A preliminary report. *Br Dent J,* 119:77–80.

50. Garcia-Godoy, F., & Gwinnett, A. J. (1987). Penetration of acid solution and gel in occlusal fissures. *J Am Dent Assoc,* 114:809–10.

51. Arana, E. M. (1974). Clinical observations of enamel after acid-etch procedure. *J Am Dent Assoc,* 89:1102–106.

52. König, K. G. (1963). Dental morphology in relation to caries resistance with special reference to fissures as susceptible areas. *J Dent Res,* 2:461–76.

53. Garcia-Godoy, F., & de Araujo, F. B. (1994). Enhancement of fissure sealant penetration and adaptation: The enameloplasty technique. *J Clin Pediatr Dent,* 19:13–18.

54. Kanellis, M. J., Warren, J. J., & Levy, S. M. (2000). A comparison of sealant placement techniques and 12-month retention rates. *J Public Health Dent,* 60:53–56.

55. Chan, D. C., Summitt, J. B., Garcia-Godoy, F., Hilton, T. J., & Chung, K. H. (1999). Evaluation of different methods for cleaning and preparing occlusal fissures. *Oper Dent,* 24:331–36.

56. Sol, E., Espasa, E., Boj, J. R., & Canalda, C. (2000). Effect of different prophylaxis methods on sealant adhesion. *J Clin Pediatr Dent,* 24:211–14.

57. Bogert, T. R., & Garcia-Godoy, F. (1992). Effect of prophylaxis agents on the shear bond strength of a fissure sealant. *Pediatr Dent,* 14:50–51.

58. Warren D. P., Infante, N. B., Rice, H. C., Turner, S. D., & Chan, J. T. (2001). Effect of topical fluoride on retention of pit and fissure sealant. *J Dent Hyg,* 75:21–24.

59. El-Housseiny, A. A., & Sharaf, A. A. (2005). Evaluation of fissure sealant applied to topical fluoride treated teeth. *J Clin Pediatr Dent,* 29:215–19.

60. Pahlavan, A., Dennison, J. B., & Charbeneau, G. T. (1976). Penetration of restorative resins into acid-etched human enamel. *J Am Dent Assoc,* 93:1170–76.

61. Silverstone, L. M. (1974). Fissure sealants. Laboratory studies. *Caries Res,* 8:2–26.

62. Bozalis, W. G., & Marshall, G. W. (1977). Acid etching patterns of primary enamel. *J Dent Res,* 56:185.

63. Straffon, L. H., Dennison, J. B., & More, F. G. (1985). Three-year evaluation of sealant: Effect of isolation on efficacy. *J Am Dent Assoc,* 110:714–17.

64. Wood, A. J., Saravia, M. E., & Farrington, F. H. (1989). Cotton roll isolation versus Vac-Ejector isolation. *ASDC J Dent Child,* 56:438–41.

65. Silverstone, L. M. (1983). Fissure sealants: The enamel-resin interface. *J Public Health Dent,* 43:205–15.

66. Myers, C. L., Rossi, F., & Cartz, L. (1974). Adhesive taglike extensions into acid-etched tooth enamel. *J Dent Res,* 53: 435–41.

67. Mertz-Fairhurst, E. J., Williams, J. E., Pierce, K. L., Smith, C. D., Schuster, G. S., Mackert, J. R., Jr., Sherrer, J. D., Wenner, K. K., Richards, E. E., & Davis, Q. B. (1991). Sealed restorations: 4-year results. *Am J Dent,* 4:43–49.

68. Handelman, S. L., Washburn, F., & Wopperer, P. (1976). Two-year report of sealant effect on bacteria in dental caries. *J Am Dent Assoc,* 93:967–70.

69. Going, R. E., Loesche, W. J., Grainger, D. A., & Syed, S. A. (1978). The viability of microorganisms in carious lesions five years after covering with a fissure sealant. *J Am Dent Assoc,* 97:455–62.

70. Theilade, E., Fejerskov, O., Migasena, K., & Prachyabrued, W. (1977). Effect of fissure sealing on the microflora in occlusal fissures of human teeth. *Arch Oral Biol,* 22:251–59.

71. Jensen, O. E., & Handelman, S. L. (1978). In vitro assessment of marginal leakage of six enamel sealants. *J Prosthet Dent,* 39:304–6.

72. Handelman, S. L. (1982). Effect of sealant placement on occlusal caries progression. *Clin Prev Dent,* 4:11–16.

73. Mertz-Fairhurst, E. J., Schuster, G. S., & Fairhurst, C. W. (1986). Arresting caries by sealants: Results of a clinical study. *J Am Dent Assoc,* 112:194–97.

74. Heller, K. E., Reed, S. G., Bruner, F. W., Eklund, S. A., & Burt, B. A. (1995). Longitudinal evaluation of sealing molars with and without incipient dental caries in a public health program. *J Public Health Dent,* 55:148–53.

75. Oong, E. M., Griffin, S. O., Kohn, W. G., Gooch, B. F., & Caufield, P. W. (2008, March 1). The effect of dental sealants on bacteria levels in caries lesions: A review of the evidence *JADA,* 139: 271–78.

76. Rock, W. P., & Anderson, R. J. (1982). A review of published fissure sealant trials using multiple regression analysis. *J Dent,* 10:39–43.

77. Quinonez, R. B., Downs, S. M., Shugars, D., Christensen, J., & Vann, W. F., Jr. (2005). Assessing cost-effectiveness of sealant placement in children. *J Public Health Dent,* 65:82–89.

78. Truman, B. I., Gooch, B. F., Sulemana, I., Gift, H. C., Horowitz, A. M., Evans, C. A., Griffin, S. O., & Carande-Kulis, V. G. (2002). Task Force on Community Preventive Services. Reviews of evidence on interventions to prevent dental caries, oral and pharyngeal cancers, and sports-related craniofacial injuries. *Am J Prev Med,* 23:21–54.

79. U.S. Department of Health and Human Services. (2000). *Oral health in America: A report of the Surgeon General: Executive summary.* Rockville, MD: U.S. Department of Health and Human Services, National Institute of Dental and Craniofacial Research, National Institutes of Health.

80. Cohen, L., LaBelle, A., & Romberg, E. (1988). The use of pit and fissure sealants in private practice: A national survey. *J Public Health Dent,* 48:26–35.

81. Handelman, S. L. (1991). Therapeutic use of sealants for incipient or early carious lesions in children and young adults. *Proc Finn Dent Soc,* 87:463–75.

Nutrition, Diet, and Associated Oral Conditions

Carole A. Palmer
Linda D. Boyd

KEY TERMS

OBJECTIVES

After studying this chapter, the student should be able to:

1. Describe the rationale for the dietary reference intakes, MyPlate, Dietary Guidelines for Americans, and food labels.

2. Describe the potential oral effects of poor nutrition during organogenesis.

3. Evaluate the effect of dietary patterns and food composition on cariogenic potential.

4. Describe the effects of food on saliva's buffering capacity.

5. Describe the role of nutrition in oral diseases.

6. Explain nutritional factors that place groups with certain medically compromising conditions or special needs at higher risk for oral disease.

INTRODUCTION

Oral health, diet, and nutritional status are closely linked (Figure 17–1 ■). Nutrition is essential for the growth, development, and maintenance of oral structures and tissues. During periods of rapid cellular growth, nutrient deficiencies can have an irreversible effect on the developing oral tissues. Early malnutrition is associated with enamel hypoplasia, salivary gland hypofunction, and changes in saliva composition that increase a child's susceptibility to dental caries in the deciduous teeth.[1,2] Throughout life, nutritional deficiencies or toxicities can affect host resistance, healing, oral function, and oral-tissue integrity. For example, immune response to local irritants and healing of periodontal tissues can be impaired when nutritional status is compromised. Because the oral epithelium has more rapid cell turnover than most other tissues in the body, clinical signs of malnutrition often manifest first in the oral cavity.

After tooth eruption, diet affects the dentition topically rather than systemically. Dietary factors and eating patterns can initiate, exacerbate, or minimize dental decay. Fermentable carbohydrates are essential for the implantation, colonization, and metabolism of bacteria in dental plaque. Factors such as eating frequency and carbohydrate retentiveness on the dentition influence the progression of carious lesions whereas foods containing calcium and phosphorus, such as cheese, enhance remineralization. Frequent intake of acidic foods or beverages can cause enamel erosion. Conversely, impaired dental function can lead to poor nutritional health. Older adults with loose or missing teeth or ill-fitting dentures often reduce their intake of foods that require chewing, such as fresh fruits, vegetables, meats, and breads.[3] When the variety of foods in a diet is reduced, the risk of nutrient inadequacies increases. The patient who undergoes oral or periodontal surgery might require dietary guidance to prevent deleterious changes in the diet. Patients with diabetes mellitus, oral cancer, or depressed immune function can suffer from oral conditions that compromise nutritional status. The dental clinician needs to understand how diet and nutrition can affect oral health and how oral conditions can affect food choices and ultimately nutritional status. This chapter provides an overview of the relationships between

diet, nutrition, and dental practice and offers appropriate suggestions for patient guidance.

DIET ASSESSMENT AND COUNSELING IN DENTAL CARE

The modern dental practitioner not only is concerned with educating patients for the prevention of caries and periodontal disease but also plays an important role in screening patients for other health risks. Just as a medical history and blood pressure evaluation are used to screen for underlying medical conditions, a dietary assessment and screening can help pinpoint potential nutritional problems that can affect or be affected by dental care. Because of the large number of patients seen regularly in a dental practice, the dentist and dental hygienist are in an excellent position to recognize areas of **nutritional risk**. The role of the dental provider should be to screen patients for nutritional risk, provide dietary guidance related to oral health, and refer patients to nutrition professionals for treatment of other nutrition-related systemic conditions.[3]

Patients should be carefully screened and/or assessed to determine the level of prevention and nutrition guidance needed as outlined in the U.S. Preventive Services Task Force guidelines.[4]

Primary Prevention

Primary prevention is fundamental to oral health because it provides guidance on healthy behaviors to help prevent oral diseases before they can occur. This would include guidelines for a healthy diet and information on dietary implications in dental caries and periodontal disease. Ideally, all patients, especially caregivers of young children, should receive oral health/nutrition guidance. At the very least, however, patients and groups at increased risk for developing oral problems should be targeted for preventive guidance. Risk levels can be determined by implementing a structured risk assessment, such as Caries Risk Management by Risk Assessment (CAMBRA), which categorizes patients into level of risk based on a variety of factors. Examples of the types of patients who might be at increase risk include:

- Adolescents at risk of caries because of high intake of soft drinks, sports drinks, and snack foods.
- Caries-prevention counseling for patients with xerostomia or cariogenic diet patterns.
- Proactive diet suggestions for new denture wearers or those having jaw fixation.
- Diet advice before radiation or chemotherapy.
- Healthy diet guidance for people with severe periodontal disease.

Using current diet patterns as a basis for discussion, patients should be taught the role of diet in systemic health and in caries etiology and prevention, examples of cariogenic and noncariogenic eating patterns, and how to adapt one's usual diet

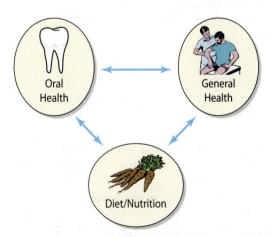

FIGURE ■ 17–1 Relationships between nutrition and health.

to lower the cariogenic risk. The dental team should be encouraged to provide primary preventive education routinely to prevent oral disease rather than waiting until a problem exists to intervene (secondary prevention).

Secondary Prevention

Secondary prevention is intervention to arrest a disease condition that has already occurred and prevent further disease and/or recurrence. This is usually the level at which the dental team intervenes because a problem has already been presented. Examples include:

- Early childhood caries.
- New or recurrent carious lesions in any age group.
- Extensive cervical demineralization.
- Adolescents with cervical decalcification after removal of orthodontic appliances.
- Adults with decalcification due to gastroesophageal reflux disease.
- Severe periodontal disease.
- Xerostomia-related caries/demineralization.

Individuals with these problems need the immediate aforementioned interventions as well as more detailed guidance on how to reduce cariogenicity of their current diet. This guidance would involve determining the factors influencing current habits and working with the patient to develop appropriate and acceptable strategies for improvement.

Tertiary Prevention

This strategy provides supportive and rehabilitative services to maximize the quality of life, especially for[4] adults with a history of caries and many restorations and elderly persons with new prosthetic devices.

This level of prevention might require ongoing dietary counseling to promote long-term change to prevent recurrence of caries. In addition, it could require dietary counseling to discuss methods of preparing foods to facilitate consumption of a healthy diet when chewing can be compromised by tooth loss or new dentures.

THE BASIS FOR A HEALTHY DIET

Dietary Reference Intakes

Daily food intake must meet metabolic requirements for energy (calories) and provide the essential nutrients that the body cannot synthesize in sufficient quantities to meet physiologic needs. Since the 1940s, the **Food and Nutrition Board (FNB)** of the National Academy of Sciences published the **recommended dietary allowances (RDAs)**, which were guides for daily nutrient intake to support growth and maintenance of body tissues and to prevent deficiency diseases.[5]

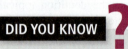

DID YOU KNOW

In the 1940s, deficiency diseases such as pellagra and rickets were very common and led to the development of RDAs.

Beginning in 1997, the FNB refocused the format and purpose of the nutrition recommendations to address nutritional requirements for preventing chronic degenerative diseases and the risk of excess nutrient intake.[5] These **dietary reference intakes (DRIs)** (Table 17–1 ■) are quantitative estimates of nutrient values to be used for planning healthy diets and assessing current ones. The reference values vary according to gender and life stage. The most recently released RDAs also report the upper limit of nutrient intake considered safe, that is, the **tolerable upper intake level (UL)**. This reference value was needed because increased intake of nutrients, primarily as dietary supplements, can have harmful effects.

TABLE ■ 17–1   **Types of Daily Reference Intakes (DRI)**

Estimated average requirement (EAR)

The daily nutrient intake value estimated to meet the needs of half (50%) of all healthy people in a life stage and gender group.

Recommended dietary allowance (RDA)

The average daily nutrient value considered adequate to meet the nutrient needs of nearly all (97%–98%) healthy people in a life stage and gender group.

Adequate intake (AI)

An intake value assumed to be adequate for healthy people in each life stage and gender group when there is not enough data to determine an RDA.

Tolerable upper intake level (UL)

The highest level of daily nutrient intake likely not to pose adverse health risks for almost all individuals in a life stage and gender group. The risk of adverse effects increases with intakes above the UL.

(*Source:* Reprinted with permission from *Dietary Reference Intakes: The Essential Guide to Nutrient Requirements,* 2006 by the National Academy of Sciences, Courtesy of the National Academies Press, Washington, D.C.)

DID YOU KNOW

Food once was the major source of nutrients, but now that supplements are widely available, it has become necessary to set a UL to prevent the harmful effects of excess intake.

Nutrient intakes generally average out over time, and it is unusual for healthy people eating a varied diet to exhibit nutrient deficiencies. If an individual reports an intake of one or more nutrients below the DRIs, more information would be necessary to determine the risk for a nutritional deficiency. A single diet history is never adequate to assess diet risk. A comprehensive nutritional assessment of an individual's status requires several diet histories over time plus clinical, biochemical, and anthropometric assessment.[5]

Dietary Guidelines for Americans

The Dietary Guidelines for Americans were first published in 1980 and are revised every 5 years.[6] The guidelines are designed to complement the DRIs by recommending a pattern of eating to promote health and prevent chronic disease. The 2010 Dietary Guidelines for Americans were redesigned and include two overarching concepts with four key recommendations.[6] Revision of the guidelines recognizes the rising concern over the epidemic of overweight and obesity as well as an increasing number of households unable to acquire adequate food to meet their needs.[6] The focus areas and general recommendations can be found in (Table 17–2 ■).[6]

DID YOU KNOW

ChooseMyPlate helps individuals use the Dietary Guidelines for Americans to choose a healthy diet and encourage physical activity.

In comparison with previous editions, these new guidelines place more emphasis on consuming a nutrient-dense diet, staying physically active, and maintaining calorie balance over time to achieve and maintain a healthy weight. The focus on preventing obesity results from the increased risk that obesity presents for many chronic and degenerative diseases, such as heart disease, stroke, diabetes, arthritis, high blood pressure, and some kinds of cancer. The recommendations emphasize balance, moderation, and variety in food choices; they also promote increased use of whole grains, fruits, and vegetables and decreased use of saturated fat, added sugars, cholesterol, and salt. In particular, the guidelines for sodium are to reduce intake to 1,500 mg. in those over age 51 and in African Americans and those who have hypertension, diabetes, or chronic kidney disease.[6] In addition, the guidelines address food safety in an effort to combat food-borne illness, an important public health concern.[6]

The 2010 Dietary Guidelines for Americans focus on a healthy weight according to the **body mass index (BMI)** and waist circumference. The BMI is a medical standard for defining obesity that not only is highly correlated with independent measures of body fat but also is used to determine whether a person is at increased health risk because of excess weight[7] (Table 17–3 ■).

DID YOU KNOW

BMI does not account for weight from muscle and might not be an accurate measure of overweight and obesity in athletes and muscular individuals.

A healthy BMI of 19 to 24.9 is associated with the lowest statistical health risk.[8]

MyPlate

MyPlate (Figure 17–2 ■) is a useful planning tool based on the 2010 Dietary Guidelines for Americans. ChooseMyPlate focuses on balancing calories, identifies foods to increase as well as foods to decrease.[9] The symbol used for MyPlate is a plate that illustrates the five food groups to be included as well as an estimate of portions (i.e. half the plate should be fruits and vegetables).

As in previous nutrition guidelines, MyPlate foods are grouped according to similar nutrient composition. The food categories are grains, vegetables, fruits, dairy, and protein. Variety is essential to ensure adequate nutrition because each group provides some, but not all, essential nutrients. The size of food group portion on MyPlate is meant to indicate proportionality, which refers to how much food a person should choose from each food group. MyPlate recommends that people eat more of some foods (fruits, vegetables, whole grains, and fat-free or low-fat milk products) and less of other foods (saturated and trans fats, added sugars, cholesterol, salt, and alcohol).[9] Rather than providing specific numbers of servings, MyPlate directs people to the ChooseMyPlate.gov Web site for personalized recommendations (Figure 17–2 ■, Figure 17–3 ■, Table 17–4 ■).[10]

Food Labels

The Nutrition Facts panel found on most processed food packages helps the consumer select foods that meet nutritional recommendations (Figure 17–4 ■). The National Labeling and Education Act of 1990 requires that comprehensive nutrition information must appear on the labels of most processed foods, processed meats, and poultry products. In addition, nutrition information at point of purchase is voluntary for fresh fruits, vegetables, and raw fish. In accordance with the most recent mandatory food labeling regulations published by the Food and

TABLE ■ 17–2   2010 Dietary Guidelines for Americans

Balancing calories to manage weight

- Prevent and/or reduce overweight and obesity through improved eating and physical activity behaviors.
- Control total calorie intake to manage body weight. For people who are overweight or obese, this means consuming fewer calories from foods and beverages.
- Increase physical activity and reduce time spent in sedentary behaviors.
- Maintain appropriate calorie balance during each stage of life—childhood, adolescence, adulthood, pregnancy and breastfeeding, and older age.

Food and food components to reduce

- Reduce daily sodium intake to less than 2,300 milligrams (mg) and further reduce intake to 1,500 mg for persons who are 51 and older and those of any age who are African American or have hypertension, diabetes, or chronic kidney disease. The 1,500 mg recommendation applies to about half of the U.S. population including children and the majority of adults.
- Consume less than 10 percent of calories from saturated fatty acids by replacing them with monounsaturated and polyunsaturated fatty acids.
- Consume less than 300 mg per day of dietary cholesterol.
- Keep *trans* fatty acid consumption as low as possible by limiting foods that contain synthetic sources of *trans* fats, such as partially hydrogenated oils, and by limiting other solid fats.
- Reduce the intake of calories from solid fats and added sugars.
- Limit the consumption of foods containing refined grains, especially refined grain foods containing solid fats, added sugars, and sodium.
- Alcohol consumption should be in moderation—up to one drink per day for women and two drinks per day for men—and only by adults of legal drinking age.

Foods and nutrients to increase

Individuals should meet the following recommendations as part of a healthy eating pattern while staying within their calorie needs.

- Increase vegetable and fruit intake.
- Eat a variety of vegetables, especially dark green and red and orange vegetables and beans and peas.
- Consume at least half of all grains as whole grains. Increase whole-grain intake by replacing refined grains with whole grains.
- Increase intake of fat-free or low-fat milk and milk products, such as milk, yogurt, cheese, or fortified soy beverages.
- Choose a variety of protein foods, which include seafood, lean meat and poultry, eggs, beans and peas, soy products, and unsalted nuts and seeds.
- Increase the amount and variety of seafood consumed by choosing seafood in place of some meat and poultry.
- Replace protein foods that are high in solid fats with choices that are low in solid fats and calories and/or are sources of oils.
- Use oils to replace solid fats where possible.
- Choose foods that provide more potassium, dietary fiber, calcium, and vitamin D, which are nutrients of concern in American diets. These foods include vegetables, fruits, whole grains, and milk and milk products.

Recommendations for specific population groups

Women capable of becoming pregnant

- Choose foods that supply heme iron, which is derived from hemoglobin such as iron in red meats, fish and poultry; nonheme iron is found in plants such as beans and lentils. Non-heme iron is poorly absorbed and can be enhanced by consumption of vitamin C rich foods. Heme iron is more readily absorbed by the body than non-heme iron.
- Consume 400 micrograms (mcg) per day of synthetic folic acid (from fortified foods and/or supplements) in addition to food forms of folate from a varied diet.

Women who are pregnant or breastfeeding

- Consume 8 to 12 ounces of seafood per week from a variety of seafood types.
- Due to their high methyl mercury content, limit white (albacore) tuna to 6 ounces per week and do not eat the following four types of fish: tilefish, shark, swordfish, and king mackerel.
- If pregnant, take an iron supplement as recommended by an obstetrician or other health care provider.

Individuals ages 50 years and older

- Consume foods fortified with vitamin B_{12}, such as fortified cereals, or with dietary supplements.

Building Healthy Eating Patterns

- Select an eating pattern that meets nutrient needs over time at an appropriate calorie level.
- Account for all foods and beverages consumed and assess how they fit within a total healthy eating pattern.
- Follow food safety recommendations when preparing and eating foods to reduce the risk of food-borne illnesses.

(*Source:* U.S. Department of Agriculture and U.S. Department of Health and Human Services. *Dietary Guidelines for Americans, 2010.* 7th Edition, Washington, DC: U.S. Government Printing Office, December 2010.)

TABLE ■ 17–3 Body Mass Index (BMI)

BMI	19	20	21	22	23	24	25	26	27	28	29	30	31	32	33	34	35
Height (Inches)	Body Weight (Pounds)																
58	91	96	100	105	110	115	119	124	129	134	138	143	148	153	158	162	167
59	94	99	104	109	114	119	124	128	133	138	143	148	153	158	163	168	173
60	97	102	107	112	118	123	128	133	138	143	148	153	158	163	168	174	179
61	100	106	111	116	122	127	132	137	143	148	153	158	164	169	174	180	185
62	104	109	115	120	126	131	136	142	147	153	158	164	169	175	180	186	191
63	107	113	118	124	130	135	141	146	152	158	163	169	175	180	186	191	197
64	110	116	122	128	134	140	145	151	157	163	169	174	180	186	192	197	204
65	114	120	126	132	138	144	150	156	162	168	174	180	186	192	198	204	210
66	118	124	130	136	142	148	155	161	167	173	179	186	192	198	204	210	216
67	121	127	134	140	146	153	159	166	172	178	185	191	198	204	211	217	223
68	125	131	138	144	151	158	164	171	177	184	190	197	203	210	216	223	230
69	128	135	142	149	155	162	169	176	182	189	196	203	209	216	223	230	236
70	132	139	146	153	160	167	174	181	188	195	202	209	216	222	229	236	243
71	136	143	150	157	165	172	179	186	193	200	208	215	222	229	236	243	250
72	140	147	154	162	169	177	184	191	199	206	213	221	228	235	242	250	258
73	144	151	159	166	174	182	189	197	204	212	219	227	235	242	250	257	265
74	148	155	163	171	179	186	194	202	210	218	225	233	241	249	256	264	272
75	152	160	168	176	184	192	200	208	216	224	232	240	248	256	264	272	279
76	156	164	172	180	189	197	205	213	221	230	238	246	254	263	271	279	287

(*Source:* U.S. Department of Health and Human Services. (2000, October). *The practical guide: Identification, evaluation and treatment of overweight and obesity in adults.* (NIH Publication No. 00-4084). Bethesda, MD: U.S. Department of Health and Human Services, National Institutes of Health, National Heart, Lung, and Blood Institute.)

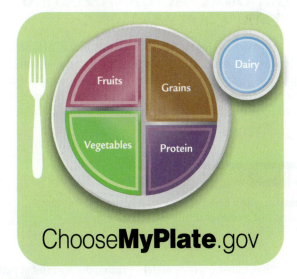

FIGURE ■ 17–2 MyPlate.

(*Source:* U.S. Department of Agriculture, Center for Nutrition Policy and Promotion. (2011, August). ChooseMyPlate. Retrieved September 5, 2011, from http://www.choosemyplate.gov/index.html.)

Drug Administration (FDA) on April 1, 2008,[10] the nutrition panel on processed foods must include the following:

• A standardized serving size (designed to make nutritional comparisons of similar products easier and reflecting the serving sizes that people actually eat).

• The number of servings per container.

• The amounts of total calories and calories from fat per serving.

• The number of grams per serving of total fat, saturated fat, trans fat, cholesterol, sodium, total carbohydrates, dietary fiber, sugars, and protein.

In addition, the nutritional contribution of one serving of the product must be stated as a percentage of the **daily values**, which are based on the RDA for adult males for macronutrients (protein, fat, carbohydrates), vitamins, minerals, and other food components such as dietary fiber. The recommended daily values are based on a 2,000-calorie diet. Depending on age, gender, and activity level, a person might need more or less than 100% of a daily value. It also helps consumers see how a food fits into an overall daily diet.

Other information, such as the amounts of polyunsaturated or monounsaturated fats or other vitamins and minerals, is optional. In addition, descriptors such as "free," "low," "high," "light," "lean," or "reduced" might be used on the label as long as a standard portion meets defined criteria. For example, to be labeled "low-calorie," a serving must have no more than 40 calories. To be labeled "low-fat," no more than 3 grams of fat per serving is allowed.

A health claim, by definition, demonstrates scientific evidence about a substance that can include a food, food

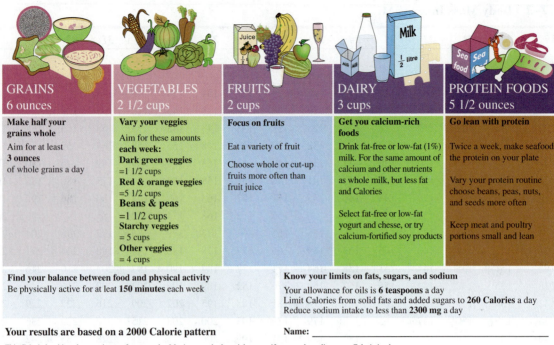

GRAINS 6 ounces	VEGETABLES 2 1/2 cups	FRUITS 2 cups	DAIRY 3 cups	PROTEIN FOODS 5 1/2 ounces
Make half your grains whole Aim for at least **3 ounces** of whole grains a day	**Vary your veggies** Aim for these amounts each week: **Dark green veggies** =1 1/2 cups **Red & orange veggies** =5 1/2 cups **Beans & peas** =1 1/2 cups **Starchy veggies** = 5 cups **Other veggies** = 4 cups	**Focus on fruits** Eat a variety of fruit Choose whole or cut-up fruits more often than fruit juice	**Get you calcium-rich foods** Drink fat-free or low-fat (1%) milk. For the same amount of calcium and other nutrients as whole milk, but less fat and Calories Select fat-free or low-fat yogurt and chesse, or try calcium-fortified soy products	**Go lean with protein** Twice a week, make seafood the protein on your plate Vary your protein routine choose beans, peas, nuts, and seeds more often Keep meat and poultry portions small and lean

Find your balance between food and physical activity
Be physically active for at leat **150 minutes** each week

Know your limits on fats, sugars, and sodium
Your allowance for oils is **6 teaspoons** a day
Limit Calories from solid fats and added sugars to **260 Calories** a day
Reduce sodium intake to less than **2300 mg** a day

Your results are based on a 2000 Calorie pattern   Name: _____
This Calorie level is only an estimate of your needs. Monitor your body weight to see if you need to adjust your Calorie intake

FIGURE ■ 17–3 Sample MyPlate recommendations.

(*Source:* U.S. Department of Agriculture, Center for Nutrition Policy and Promotion. (Aug. 26 2011). ChooseMyPlate. Retrieved 9/5/11 from http://www.choosemyplate.gov/index.html).

TABLE ■ 17–4   Tips to Get Started Using MyPlate

- Make half your grains whole
- Vary your veggies
- Focus on fruit
- Get your calcium-rich foods
- Go lean with protein
- Find your balance between food and physical activity

(*Source:* U.S. Department of Agriculture and U.S. Department of Health and Human Services. Dietary Guidelines for Americans, 2010. 7th Edition, Washington, DC: U.S. Government Printing Office, December 2010.)

component, or dietary ingredient and a disease or health-related condition. There are currently two categories of health claims: those with **significant scientific agreement (SSA)** and those with **qualified health claims**. SSAs are supported by significant scientific evidence with widespread agreement among different studies and researchers.[11] These claims undergo rigorous review and are approved by the FDA. The qualified health claims also rely on scientific evidence, but the evidence does not have to be as strong as that required for SSAs. Qualified health claims differ from SSAs in that they must be accompanied by a disclaimer.[11] See Table 17–5 ■ for current health claims with SSA that are allowed to be placed on food labels.[11] In October 2006, a health claim for the use of fluoridated water to reduce the risk of dental caries was approved.

NUTRITIONAL FACTORS AFFECTING THE ORAL CAVITY

Nutrition plays an important role in the initial growth and development of oral tissues and in their continuous integrity through the lifespan. Optimal nutrition during periods of hard and soft tissue development allow these tissues to reach their optimal potential for growth and resistance to disease. also

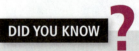

DID YOU KNOW

Nutrition and diet impact not only the risk for dental caries but also overall tissue and healing.

Malnutrition, either over- or undernutrition, during critical periods of organogenesis can have irreversible effects on developing tissues. Examples of this effect can be seen in the tetracycline staining of teeth, dental fluorosis, enamel defects in children born prematurely, and the fever-induced enamel hypoplasia seen in the primary teeth.[12,13] During early childhood, protein-energy malnutrition (PEM) can result in an increased caries risk.[14–16] Malnutrition after initial organ and tissue development is usually reversible but can compromise tissue regeneration and healing and increase susceptibility to oral diseases. Nutrients for which deficiencies or excesses have been directly associated with oral conditions are calories; protein; calcium; phosphorus;

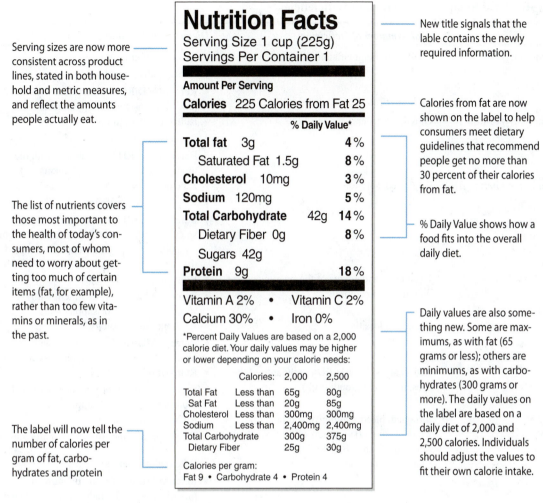

Serving sizes are now more consistent across product lines, stated in both household and metric measures, and reflect the amounts people actually eat.

The list of nutrients covers those most important to the health of today's consumers, most of whom need to worry about getting too much of certain items (fat, for example), rather than too few vitamins or minerals, as in the past.

The label will now tell the number of calories per gram of fat, carbohydrates and protein

New title signals that the lable contains the newly required information.

Calories from fat are now shown on the label to help consumers meet dietary guidelines that recommend people get no more than 30 percent of their calories from fat.

% Daily Value shows how a food fits into the overall daily diet.

Daily values are also something new. Some are maximums, as with fat (65 grams or less); others are minimums, as with carbohydrates (300 grams or more). The daily values on the label are based on a daily diet of 2,000 and 2,500 calories. Individuals should adjust the values to fit their own calorie intake.

*This label is only a sample. Exact specifications are in the final rules.
Source: Food and Drug Administration 1992.

FIGURE ■ 17–4 Food label.

(*Source:* Food and Drug Administration, Center for Food Safety and Applied Nutrition, http://www.fda.gov/food/labelingnutrition/consumerinformation/ucm078889.htm).

TABLE ■ 17–5   Health Claims Allowed on Food Labels

1. Calcium, vitamin D and osteoporosis
2. Dietary lipids (fat) and cancer
3. Dietary saturated fat, cholesterol, and risk of coronary heart disease (CHD)
4. Dietary noncariogenic carbohydrate sweeteners and dental caries
5. Fiber-containing grain products, fruits, and vegetables and cancer
6. Folic acid and neural tube defects
7. Fruits and vegetables and cancer
8. Fruits, vegetables, and grain products that contain fiber, particularly soluble fiber and CHD
9. Sodium and hypertension
10. Soluble fiber from certain foods and CHD
11. Soy protein and CHD
12. Sterols and plant stanol esters and CHD
13. Fluoridated water and reduced dental caries

vitamins C, A, and D; iodine; and fluoride. See Table 17–6 ■ for a summary of the oral symptoms of nutrient deficiencies.

Protein Energy Malnutrition (PEM)

Protein energy malnutrition represents a multinutrient deficiency with inadequate intake of protein, calories and micronutrients. PEM impacts nearly 30% of children worldwide and is reported to impact 3 to 21% of children under 5 years old in various regions and populations of the United States.[17]

Protein, the most abundant organic compound in the body, is required for the synthesis of virtually all body tissues and structures. Protein is necessary for DNA and RNA synthesis, and tensile strength of collagen as well as the viscous, microbial, and buffering properties of saliva. Thus, aberrations in protein nutrition can have far-reaching oral and systemic effects.

The normal turnover of epithelial tissue in the oral cavity requires a continual supply of nutrients. For example, every 3 to 6 days, the basal epithelium of the gingiva undergoes renewal.[15] Thus, any severe deficiency of protein/calorie intake will result

TABLE ■ 17–6   Oral Symptoms of Nutrient Deficiencies

Nutrient	Oral Symptom of Deficiency	Dietary Considerations
Riboflavin (vitamin B_2) or iron	Cheilosis or angular stomatitis	• Rule out other etiology • Use palliative treatment • Refer to MD/RD for treatment with diet modifications and/or supplements
Riboflavin (vitamin B_2) or iron	Glossitis (magenta tongue)	• Rule out other etiology • Palliative treatment • Refer to MD/RD for treatment with diet modifications and/or supplements
Niacin (vitamin B_3) or vitamin B_{12}	Bright red, sore tongue	• Rule out other etiology • Use palliative treatment • Refer to MD/RD for diet modifications: avoiding spicy or acidic foods, eating foods at room temperature, eating nutrient and energy-dense foods that are soft and moist
Riboflavin	Hyperemia and edema of the pharyngeal and oral mucous membranes	• Rule out other etiology • Refer to MD/RD for treatment with diet modifications and/or supplements
Folate	Atrophic glossitis	• Rule out other etiology • Refer to MD/RD for treatment with diet modifications and/or supplements
Biotin	Red, scaly, skin rash, frequently around the eyes, nose, and mouth (rare)	• Rule out other etiology • Refer to MD/RD for treatment with diet modifications and/or supplements
Vitamin C	Inflamed, bleeding gingiva and impaired wound healing (symptoms of scurvy, which is rare in the United States)	• Rule out other etiology • Treat with diet modifications and/or supplements
Vitamin A	Changes in taste	• Rule out other etiology • Refer to MD/RD for treatment with diet modifications to include nutrient and energy-dense foods and/or supplements • Avoid foods that can cause aversion
Iron	Esophageal webs, thin membranes in the esophagus, that can result in dysphagia	• Rule out other etiology • Use palliative treatment • Refer to MD/RD for treatment with diet modifications to include iron-rich foods and/or supplements

MD, physician; RD, registered dietitian.
(*Source:* Food and Nutrition Board. (2006). *Dietary reference intakes: The essential guide to nutrient requirements*. Washington, DC: Food and Nutrition Board. (2006). *Dietary reference intakes: The essential guide to nutrient requirements*. Washington, DC: National Institute of Medicine. Reprinted with permission from the National Academies Press, Copyright 2006, National Academy of Sciences.)

in a decrease in mitotic activity in the crevicular epithelium and elsewhere throughout the body.[16] Recent research has shown higher risk for dental caries and periodontitis in adolescents who have experienced PEM during the early childhood.[17] In animals, protein malnutrition during the developmental stage results in impaired protein synthesis.[18]

Animal models also demonstrated a 40% reduction in collagen production following a short-term (4-day) fast.[19] These findings suggest even short-term states of undernutrition can impact collagen synthesis.

In children malnourished during early childhood, delays in tooth eruption, enamel structural defects, decreased saliva flow, reduced salivary buffering capacity, and impaired salivary antimicrobial activity occur leading to increased caries susceptibility.[20–23]

With the exception of the cleansing and diluting effects of saliva, oral defense mechanisms depend on an adequate supply of proteins. The glycoproteins that result in aggregation of bacteria arise from the salivary glands. Lysozyme, salivary peroxidase, and lactoferrin are also glycoproteins. Secretory

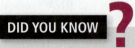

DID YOU KNOW

It is difficult and many times a violation of ethical principles to perform nutrition deficiency studies because of the protection of human subjects from excessive risk in research.

immunoglobulin A (sIgA) arises mainly from the labial and buccal glands.[24] The cell types involved in cellular immunity, polymorphonuclear lymphocytes and macrophages as well as the enzymes used in phagocytosis, also require protein for their production.[25]

Probably one of the most deleterious effects of protein/calorie deficiency is the *depletion of the cellular and immunocellular defenses* of both the oral and the connective sides of the barrier epithelial cells lining the gingival crevice. In general, the severity of the impaired immunologic response parallels the severity of the protein or calorie deficiency.[25] Chronic undernutrition can also compromise cytokine response and affect immune cell function. In other words, undernutrition can impact immune response tissue regeneration and response to insult or infection.[25]

Minerals

Calcium, vitamin D, and phosphorus are essential for proper development and maintenance of mineralized tissues, especially teeth and alveolar bone. A deficiency of these nutrients during critical phases of tooth development in children can result in hypomineralization of developing teeth and possible delayed eruption patterns.[26] The rate of enamel hypoplasia in primary teeth in children born prematurely is more than threefold that of children born at term.[26] In addition, the rate of enamel hypoplasia in permanent teeth in these children is more than twofold that of controls.[26] Preterm infants miss the intrauterine period when 80% of the body calcium, phosphorus, and magnesium are accumulated. As a result, these infants have much higher requirements for calcium and phosphorus.[27,28] In addition, very low birthweight infants have immature kidneys and cannot metabolize adequate levels of vitamin D, further impairing tooth development.[28]

Iron deficiency is the most common nutrient deficiency in the United States. The primary clinical manifestation of iron deficiency in the oral cavity is pallor of the oral tissues and tongue.

DID YOU KNOW ?

Iron deficiency anemia is most common in pregnant women and young children.

The tongue can appear shiny with blunted filiform papillae. The effects of iron deficiency on mineralized tissues are less clear. In rats, even a marginal deficiency of iron in the diet predisposes the rats to caries.[29] Conversely, supplementing a caries-promoting diet with iron produced a major reduction in caries with the greatest effect shown in the neonatal period.[29] In addition, iron serves as a cofactor with ascorbic acid in collagen synthesis as does copper.[30]

Zinc regulates function in inflammation by inhibiting the release of lysosomal enzymes and histamines. A zinc deficiency can inhibit collagen formation, retard osteogenesis and bone matrix mineralization, and reduce cell-mediated immunity.[30] Zinc deficiency can also result in delayed wound healing, defective keratinization of epithelial cells, epithelial thickening, atrophic oral mucosa, and xerostomia. In addition, zinc is essential for taste and odor sensitivity. Declines in taste experienced by many elders can be a result of zinc deficiency.

Vitamins

Vitamin A is essential for the development and continued integrity of all body organs and tissues, including the epithelial mucosa of the oral cavity. Vitamin A deficiency impairs cell differentiation. The result is defective tissue formation and impaired healing. Vitamin A deficiency also results in impairment of both specific and nonspecific immunoprotective mechanisms. Deficiency can affect tissue response to bacterial infection, mucosal immunity, parasitic and viral infection, activity of natural killer cells, and phagocytosis.[31] Vitamin A toxicity can show similar effects with impaired healing response being the most direct affect in the oral cavity.[32] Other effects include proliferation of oral epithelium, reduction of the keratin layer, thickening of the basal membrane, and increase in the granular layer.

In a case report, a patient who took 200,000 IU of vitamin A daily for over 6 months presented with painful gingival lesions, nausea, vomiting, xerostomia, and headaches. Clinical examination revealed gingival erosions, ulcerations, bleeding, swelling, loss of keratinization, color changes, and desquamation of the lips.[32] All pathologic manifestations disappeared within 2 months of the elimination of the vitamin A supplements without a change in oral hygiene habits.

In addition to the effects of high levels of vitamin A intake on soft tissue, a review of 20 studies demonstrated high doses of vitamin A resulted in an increased risk for hip fracture.[33] Whether this effect can impact alveolar bone health is unclear, but it is an area requiring further research.

Vitamin C, ascorbic acid, is essential to oral health. Synthesis of hydroxyproline, an essential component of collagen, requires ascorbic acid. Defects in collagen synthesis are responsible for the many manifestations of vitamin C deficiency called *scurvy*. Its signs in the oral cavity include spontaneous bleeding, infusions of blood into interdental papillae, loosening and exfoliation of teeth, detachment of oral epithelial tissue, and impaired wound healing (Figure 17–5 ■).

The effects of vitamin C deficiency are best studied in animal models in which all factors can be controlled.[34] Acute scurvy was produced by placing monkeys on a vitamin C–deficient diet for 12 weeks. The hydroxyproline content of the gingiva started to decline in the first four weeks and occurred at a faster rate than in skin. By the end of the eighth week, the synthesis of hydroxyproline was totally impaired. The results were extensive gingival pocket formation and tooth mobility due to degradation of the collagen making up periodontal ligament fibers.

Although frank scurvy is rare, even marginal deficiencies can result in alterations in collagen synthesis (Figure 17–5 ■).

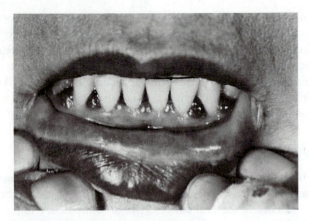

FIGURE ■ 17–5 Scurvy.
(*Source:* Pearson Education.)

Thus, deficient or marginal ascorbic acid intakes might be a conditioning factor in the development of gingivitis and one of the early manifestations of vitamin C deficiency.[35] The most recent epidemiologic data from the Third National Health and Nutrition Examination Survey (NHANES III) suggest that the odds of having periodontal disease are 1.2 times higher in those with low dietary vitamin C intakes.[36] In the same study, smokers and former smokers with low vitamin C intake were at 1.6 times higher risk of having periodontal disease.[36] In a recent clinical study, patients with periodontitis were found to have lower plasma vitamin C levels than healthy controls. After grapefruit consumption by patients with periodontitis, plasma vitamin C levels rose and bleeding scores improved.[37] Research findings suggest people with marginal vitamin C deficiency supplemented with ascorbic acid have a statistically significant increase in hydroxyproline in periodontal tissues.[38]

Ascorbic acid is essential to immune-related functions, such as resistance to oral infection, via its role in leukocyte formation and subsequent phagocytosis. In addition, vitamin C protects the integrity of cells from damage during the oxidative stress that occurs during the inflammatory response. Therefore, during infections and stress, vitamin C levels in the plasma and leukocytes decline rapidly.[39]

Conversely, chronic vitamin C excess can precipitate a scurvylike condition (rebound scurvy) upon cessation of the vitamin. Because the impact of deficient levels of vitamin C is first observed in gingival tissues, dentists and dental hygienists in clinical practice could be the first to diagnose the phenomenon.[40]

The B-complex vitamins primarily function as coenzymes in energy metabolism. B-complex vitamins are found widely in foods and are usually found together. With the exception of B_{12} in the elderly and folic acid in pregnant women, deficiencies of single B vitamins are uncommon (except in alcoholics). The Dietary Guidelines for Americans 2010 provides specific recommendations for people older than 50 years to consume vitamin B_{12} in its crystalline form (i.e., fortified foods or supplements) because of a reduced ability to absorb naturally occurring vitamin B_{12}.[6]

Oral signs and symptoms of B-complex vitamin deficiencies include cracks in the corners of the mouth referred to as *cheilosis,* and inflammation, burning, redness, pain, and swelling of the tongue.[41-42]

DIET AND ENAMEL DEMINERALIZATION

Dental demineralization can result from excessive toothbrushing, regurgitation of stomach acid (as in the eating disorder bulimia), gastro-esophageal reflux disease, or excessive consumption of acid-containing foods or beverages. The demineralizing effect of acid from the diet is magnified in the presence of xerostomia because saliva helps to neutralize acids and help flush them from the oral cavity.

Dietary sources of acid include citrus fruits and juices, acidogenic sports drinks, snacks containing citrus acid, carbonated beverages, chewable vitamin C tablets, or excessive regurgitation of gastric contents into the mouth.[43] Recently, attention has been focused on the increased frequency of consumption of carbonated beverages, both regular and diet, which contain acids and are possible contributors to an increase in enamel demineralization.[43] It is important to differentiate this type of erosion or demineralization from the caries process in which acid produced from plaque bacteria causes enamel demineralization.

DIET AND DENTAL CARIES

Role of Carbohydrates

Dental caries is a diet-related, infectious, and transmissible disease that is strongly affected by diet. *Streptococcus mutans* are the predominant oral bacteria that initiate the caries process. Development of clinical caries is contingent upon the interaction of three local factors in the mouth: *a susceptible tooth, cariogenic bacteria,* and *fermentable carbohydrate.* Newly erupted teeth with a thin enamel layer, such as those found in many children born prematurely, are very susceptible to caries. Tooth morphology, especially the presence of deep pits and fissures, influences the likelihood mutans streptococci will attach to and colonize the tooth's surface. Plaque bacteria ferment starches and sugars, producing organic acids. These acids demineralize dental enamel.

Other dietary factors counteract the damaging effects of carbohydrates. The presence of protective minerals and ions, such as fluoride, calcium, and phosphorus in plaque and saliva, promote remineralization of incipient lesions. In addition to transporting minerals, saliva contains buffering agents, bicarbonates, and phosphates, which neutralize organic acids. Thus, the amount and composition of saliva affect the caries process. Other host factors influencing caries risk include genetic predisposition, immune status, malnutrition during tooth formation, education level, and income status.

The most recent NHANES III 1999–2002 reported that 92% of adults showed evidence of coronal caries and 18% of adults had root caries.[44] In the same survey, children and teens aged 5 to 17 years had 59% evidence of dental caries in the permanent teeth.[44] For these caries-prone children and adults, nutrition counseling about the damaging effects of fermentable carbohydrates on teeth is essential.

Through epidemiologic and clinical studies, the causal relationship between sugar consumption and dental caries has been established. Animal studies suggest that an increase in the concentration of sucrose in the diet enhances dental plaque formation and caries risk.[45,46] Sucrose plays a more dominant role than other sugars in the development of smooth-surface caries because it can be fermented by oral bacteria but, unlike the other simple sugars, it is a substrate for mutans streptococcus synthesis of intracellular and extracellular polysaccharides.[45,46] Extracellular dextran, a storage form of sugar, allows for continued acid formation even when eating and drinking are not occurring. One of these extracellular polysaccharides called *glucan* enables the *Streptococcus mutans* to adhere to the smooth enamel surfaces and contributes to the structural integrity of plaque biofilm.[46] It also appears that the plaque biofilm formed in relation to sucrose intake contains low concentrations of calcium, phosphorus, and fluoride, which are critical elements in the demineralization and remineralization of the tooth surface, and might further increase sucrose's cariogenic potential.[46]

In 1996 in the United States, average caloric sweetener intake was 103 pounds per capita with middle income households having the highest consumption.[47,49] Consumption varies by age and is even higher in 12- to 19-year-olds who consume 137.2 pounds per capita. A systematic review of 77 studies meeting inclusion criteria identified 106 factors related to prevalence/incidence of dental caries.[48] The categories of factors included sociodemographics, diet, oral hygiene, breast/bottle feeding, and oral bacterial flora. The evidence points most consistently to infection with *Streptococcus mutans,* a cariogenic diet, and poor plaque biofilm removal as significant risk factors for dental caries in young children.[48] Caries has declined in Western countries in recent years except in children 2–5 years old which increased from 24% in 1988–1994 to 28% in 1999–2004.[44] Factors thought to contribute to this decline include fluoride intake from water, the use of fluoridated dentifrices, improved biofilm (plaque) control, use of dental sealants, and more frequent visits to a dental provider.

The use of sugar alcohols and alternative sweeteners in foods has played a role in reducing caries. Perhaps one of the most promising sugar substitutes to be studied is xylitol, a sugar alcohol that has been demonstrated to be noncariogenic as well as a promotor of remineralization.[49] Xylitol's ability to inhibit metabolic acid production by mutans streptococci results in minimal depression of plaque pH.[50] Maintenance of the plaque pH close to the saliva pH also fosters remineralization of teeth. In addition, the substitution of xylitol for fermentable sugars in the diet results in a less cariogenic bacterial flora. The importance of other nonfermentable sweeteners in caries control is detailed in Chapter 18.

In addition to simple sugars, cooked starch–sugar combinations as in doughnuts, cookies, potato chips, and some ready-to-eat breakfast cereals produce a prolonged acidogenic response when retained in interproximal spaces.[51] When starches are cooked, they are partially degraded, which allows the salivary alpha-amylase to convert starch particles retained on the tongue, oral mucosa, and teeth to maltose. Making maltose available to plaque bacteria extends the length of time that plaque pH will remain low and permit enamel demineralization to occur. Thus, retentive high-starch foods might be more acidogenic than high-sugar, low-starch foods that are rapidly eliminated from the mouth.[51–52]

Effects of Eating Patterns and Physical Form of Foods

Other dietary factors that affect might minimize or increase risk of caries development include the frequency of eating, physical form of the carbohydrate (liquid versus solid), retentiveness of a food on the tooth surface, sequence in which foods are consumed (e.g., cheese eaten before a sweet food limits the pH drop), and presence of minerals in a food.

Frequent between-meal snacking on sugar or processed starch-containing foods increases plaque formation and keeps the pH low, extending the time for demineralization to occur. When total daily sugar intake was held constant, increasing the frequency of sugar intake for groups of rats resulted in increased number of *Streptococcus mutans* in plaque and the amount of caries experienced.[53] The positive relationship between frequency of sugar intake and caries in humans was first demonstrated in the Vipeholm study, and a recent systematic review continues to support a moderately significant relationship.[48,54] Subjects who consumed candies between meals developed more caries than those who were fed equal amounts of sugars with meals. Because bacterial fermentation can continue as long as carbohydrate adheres to the enamel and exposed dentinal tooth surfaces, the physical consistency of food can affect caries risk. Starchy foods, such as soft bread and potato chips, which are retained on tooth surfaces for prolonged periods of time, result in a low pH that might last up to 60 minutes with each eating exposure.[51,54] The sequence in which foods are eaten also affects how low the plaque pH falls and how long it remains depressed. Sugared coffee consumed at the end of a meal will cause the plaque pH to remain low longer than when an unsweetened food is eaten following sugared coffee.[55–57] If peanuts are eaten before or after sugar-containing foods, the plaque pH is less depressed.[57]

Caries-Protective Foods and Nutrients

Some components of foods are protective against dental caries. Protein, fat, phosphorus, and calcium inhibit caries in rats.[56] Aged natural cheeses have been shown to be cariostatic.[59] When cheese is eaten after a sucrose rinse, the plaque pH remains higher and enamel demineralization is lower than when no cheese follows a sucrose rinse. The protective effect of cheeses is attributed to their texture, which stimulates salivary flow, and their protein, calcium, and phosphate content, which neutralizes plaque acids. Many dairy products such as some yogurts are now fortified with live probiotic *Lactobacillus rhamnosus GG,* which also has been shown to have an inhibitory affect on a wide range of bacteria including *Streptococcus* species.[60] Studies have demonstrated a 37% to 56% reduction in caries risk with short- and long-term exposure, respectively, to these probiotic dairy products.[60,61] Fluoride found in drinking water, foods, and dentifrices increase a tooth's resistance to demineralization and enhance remineralization of carious lesions.

Lipids seem to accelerate oral clearance of food particles. Some fatty acids, linoleic and oleic, in low concentration inhibit growth of mutans streptococcus. Lectins, proteins found in plants, appear to interfere with microbial colonization and might affect salivary function.[62]

Measurement of Foods' Cariogenic Potential

Because it is unethical to conduct human experiments to measure the true cariogenic potential of foods, other indirect tests have been developed. These tests enable researchers to classify foods into at least three categories: protective, low, and high cariogenic potential. Currently, the cariogenic potential or the ability to induce caries in humans might be assessed indirectly by measuring the ability of a test food to cause caries formation in animals, acid production in dental plaque, or demineralization of enamel.[1]

Animal studies have been conducted using a programmed feeding machine. In one study, 20 common snack foods were presented to rats at specified intervals during the day.[63] After sulcal and smooth-surface caries were scored in the animals, **cariogenic potential indices (CPIs)** were computed for each food. The sucrose group had a CPI value of 1 (Table 17–7 ■). A food with a CPI of 0.4 had low cariogenic potential. Those snack foods with high cariogenic potential had 1% or more hydrolyzable starch in combination with sucrose or other sugars.

Acid production in the mouth during bacterial fermentation of a food is predictive of the contribution of that food to the caries process. Measurement of plaque acidogenicity can be measured by determining the pH of a plaque sample taken from the mouth or in situ. Foods that cause the plaque pH

TABLE ■ 17–7   Diet Suggestions for Caries Prevention

Food Group	Suggestions
General	• Limit number of meals/snacks • Avoid sticky or retentive foods
Grains/cereals (3–8 ounce equivalents/day[a])	• Have whole grains • Have popcorn for snacks • Avoid crackers, donuts, potato chips between meals
Fruits (1–2 cups/day)	• All fruits are fine: fresh, frozen, canned, juices • Have fruits for dessert/snacks • Avoid dried fruits or fruit roll-ups • Do not sip slowly or often on fruit juices • Avoid fruit drinks
Vegetables (1–3 cups/day)	• All vegetables are fine: fresh, frozen, canned, juices, potatoes • Limit sweetened salad dressings • Have raw vegetables for snacks
Protein (2–6 ounces/day)	• All proteins are fine: meat, fish, poultry, eggs, beans (lentils, etc.), tofu, nuts • Have nuts for snacks
Dairy[b] (2–3 cups/day)	• Have milk in coffee, soup • Have cheese in sandwiches, casseroles, etc. • Have cheese for snacks
Oils and sweets	• Avoid slowly dissolving candies • Have sweets as dessert with a meal, not between meals • Avoid constant sipping on sweet beverages (soda, sports drinks)
Other	• Have flavored club soda or diet soda • Use sugar-free gum, preferably one containing xylitol • Have water between meals and with snacks

[a] ounce equivalent = one slice of bread, 1 cup of cereal, or 1/2 cup cooked rice, pasta, or cereal.
[b] Aim for fat-free or low-fat products unless increased calories are indicated.
(*Source:* Based on Hallett, K. B., O'Rourke, P. K. (2006). Pattern and severity of early childhood caries. Community Dent Oral Epidemiol, 34(1):25–35.)

to fall below the critical demineralization level (pH 5.5–5.0) are considered acidogenic. Measurement of oral plaque pH requires placement of a wire-telemetric appliance containing a pH microelectrode in the space where a tooth is missing in the mouth. As the test food is chewed, the pH under undisturbed plaque at the site of the indwelling electrode is continually transmitted to an external receiver. The rate of the fall and rise of the pH at an interproximal site can be recorded continuously by plaque telemetry. Foods found to have low acidogenic potential using this method include aged cheeses and some vegetables, meats, fish, and nuts.[64] To assess the ability of a food to demineralize dental enamel, investigators developed an intraoral cariogenicity. Bovine or human dental enamel slabs are imbedded in a prosthesis and placed in the mouth where a tooth is missing. After ingesting a test food, changes in surface microhardness or enamel porosity are determined.[65] Because each test measures a different aspect of cariogenicity, foods are ranked differently. It is recommended that two testing methods be used to determine food acidogenicity and cariogenicity potential.[66,67] See Table 17–7 ■ for diet suggestions for caries prevention.

NUTRITION AND PERIODONTAL DISEASES

Like caries, periodontal disease is infectious and multifactorial in etiology and occurs when virulence of the bacterial challenge is greater than the host defense and repair capability. The course of periodontal disease involves periods of progression and remission. Unlike the direct causative relationship between carbohydrates and caries, nutritional factors seem to play a much more subtle role in periodontal status. Nutritional factors can alter host susceptibility to periodontal disease and/or modulate its progress.[68] The nutritional factors related to preventing infection and enhancing wound healing in general applies to the prevention and management of periodontal disease as well.[69] If both the challenge to and the defense and repair capabilities of the periodontal tissues are in balance, nutrition could be the deciding factor in whether health or disease results. Even when the periodontium is healthy, there is continual need for nutrients to maintain the tissues. Once inflammation is established, the need for nutrients increases.

Host defense in the gingival crevice and connective tissue requires an adequate intake of all nutrients to ensure adequate production and function of defense and supporting cells.[70–73] With the increased needs of cellular immunity and the additional demands by the tissue cells attempting to maintain and repair damaged areas, a high supply of all nutrients is needed. This phenomenon has led to evidence showing that nutrient requirements might be higher at local sites of increased stress than in the rest of the body. Such localized challenges might result in end-organ nutrient deficiencies.[74,75]

Nutrients being investigated for their role in downregulating the inflammatory response in periodontal disease includes vitamin D, omega-3 fatty acids, and antioxidants.[76–77] Studies

TABLE ■ 17–8   Dietary Suggestions for Patients with Periodontal Disease

- Eat a *nutritionally adequate diet* following **MyPyramid** and the USDA Dietary Guidelines for Americans.
- Increase the use of saliva-stimulating fibrous foods.
- Take multivitamin/mineral supplements in doses *no higher* than 1–2 times RDA levels.
- *Avoid fad diets:* They could be deficient in nutrients.
- Avoid *single-vitamin* supplements.

RDA, recommended dietary allowance

suggest the metabolites of vitamin D alter the inflammatory response through its role in signaling keratinocytes of the epidermis to respond to disruption of the barrier function.[78] A recent study of patients undergoing periodontal maintenance therapy compared those taking calcium and vitamin D supplements and found fewer markers of inflammation in those using supplements.[81] Omega-3 fatty acids are another nutrient group that have been shown to modulate the inflammatory response, but more studies are needed to determine the effect on periodontal inflammation in humans.[81] Just as some nutrients might downregulate the inflammatory response, other nutrients might upregulate it. Nutrients that enhance markers of inflammation include refined carbohydrates and saturated fats.[81] The "takehome" message from the ongoing research is that to maintain a healthy weight to prevent obesity associated with upregulation of the inflammatory response, patients should consume a diet rich in whole grains, fruits, and vegetables and low in saturated fat.

When routine scaling, prophylaxis, and oral plaque-control procedures fail to reverse gingivitis and before any treatment for periodontitis is attempted, a thorough diet evaluation and counseling are indicated. The patient should be informed about the importance of systemic nutrition in the defense and repair of oral tissues. Recommendations should be made to help ensure optimal nutrition for patients with periodontal disease (see Table 17–8 ■).

LIFESTYLE DIET AND ORAL HEALTH ISSUES

Early Childhood Caries

Early childhood caries (ECC), which was formerly referred to as "baby bottle tooth decay" or "nursing caries" is defined as one or more decayed, missing (due to caries), or filled tooth surfaces in any primary tooth in a preschool age child between birth and 71 months of age. Severe early childhood caries (S-ECC) refers to a more severe pattern of progressive or rampant caries in children under 3 years of age.[79] The NHANES, 1999–2002 estimated the overall prevalence of ECC to be 27.9%.[80] This value is an increase from 24.2% prevalence reported in the NHANES, 1988–1994.[80] However, a much higher prevalence has been seen among Alaskan and Oklahoma Native American (53%), Navajo (72%), and Cherokee (55%) children attending Head Start programs.[81,82]

Dietary risk factors for ECC include putting a child to sleep at naptime or bedtime with a bottle containing a sugar-containing liquid, allowing an infant to breast-feed at-will, extended use of the nursing bottle or sippy cup beyond 1 year of age, and frequent snacking or sipping on sugar-containing beverages throughout the day.[83] Results of the 1991 National Health Interview Survey show that 16.7% or 3.5 million children between 6 months and 5 years of age are put to sleep with a liquid in the bottle other than plain water.[84] Recent research suggests high risk for ECC was associated with the following: parent or guardian with <12 years of education, family with a poverty income ratio (PIR) <1.3, no dental visit within the preceding year, no daily intake for breakfast, failure to discontinue bottle feeding by age 1, and bottle feeding.[85] Children with healthy eating habits as measured by the Healthy Eating Index (HEI) were 44% less likely to exhibit ECC.[85]

Other risk factors for ECC include childhood illness and the use of liquid prescription medications with high sucrose content, such as amoxicillin, for extended lengths of time.[86]

Children who develop maxillary anterior caries are at increased risk of developing posterior caries in the future.[87] To prevent early childhood caries, dentists, dental hygienists, pediatricians, and other health care professionals should ask parents about their infant-feeding practices. Those parents who report inappropriate feeding practices should receive counseling. Programs serving low-income families, such as the Special Supplemental Food Program for Women, Infants, and Children (WIC), can play a major role in providing education to parents at higher risk for using inappropriate feeding practices. Refer to Table 17–9 ■ for dietary recommendations to reduce the risk of EEC.

Eating Disorders

Eating disorders are often first diagnosed in the dental office because of the pain and discomfort caused by dental complications.[88] There are a number of types of eating disorders, but the primary types include **anorexia nervosa**, bulimia nervosa, and binge-eating disorder. Lifetime prevalence of anorexia nervosa, bulimia nervosa (BN), and binge eating disorder (BED) are estimated to be 0.9%, 1.5%, and 3.5% in women and 0.3%, .05% and 2.0% in men.[89] Less than half of those with BN or BED ever seek treatment.[89] Changes in the oral tissues are often one of the first signs of an eating disorder. Dental professionals should recognize the oral effects of eating disorders (Table 17–10 ■) and talk with the patient about these concerns.

Anorexia nervosa is typified by self-starvation and excessive weight loss. Bulimia nervosa usually consists of secretive cycles of binge eating extremely large quantities of food followed by purging through vomiting, laxative use, or overexercising. In contrast, **binge-eating disorder (BED)** involves periods of uncontrolled, continuous eating much like bulimia nervosa, but no purging is involved. BED is strongly associated with severe obesity.[89]

All eating disorders require a multidisciplinary approach to care including physicians, psychiatrists, psychologists, nutritionists, and social workers. Initially, patients often deny having an eating disorder. The dental professional's approach to the discussion must be empathetic and nonjudgmental to elicit the information necessary to lead into the discussion of eating disorders and their potential impact on oral and general health. Studies have demonstrated that dental practitioners are uncomfortable in discussing concerns and/or suspicions about eating disorders with patients. In response to this issue, the National Eating Disorders Association in cooperation with the

TABLE ■ 17–9 Diet Suggestions to Reduce the Risk of Early Childhood Caries

- Do not allow babies to sleep with a bottle containing anything other than water.
- Do not allow infants to constantly drink from a sippy cup if it contains juice, milk, or a sweet beverage.
- Do not allow older children to use slowly dissolving hard candies, lollipops, or the like on a regular basis.
- Do not allow children to snack frequently throughout the day.
- Do clean an infant's teeth daily as soon as they erupt into the mouth.
- Do provide nutritious snacks such as fruits and vegetables rather than sweets between meals.
- Do have regular meal and snack times, and minimize the number of between-meal snacks.
- Do give children sweets at dessert time when they can brush teeth immediately afterwards.

(*Source:* Based on Hallett, K. B., & O'Rourke, P. K. (2006). Pattern and severity of early childhood caries. *Community Dent Oral Epidemiol,* 34:25–35.)

TABLE ■ 17–10 Signs and Symptoms of Eating Disorders

- Mucosal lesions: mucosal atrophy, glossitis (erythema and atrophy), erythematous lesions (palatal and pharyngeal from inducing vomiting)
- Dental erosion: lesions on the lingual (*perimolysis*) and occlusal surfaces of teeth resulting from the effects of vomiting; teeth might become brittle and translucent, and erosion can occur as early as 6 months from the start of the condition
- Increased dentin hypersensitivity. In extreme cases, the pulp might be exposed, leading to periapical infection or pulpal necrosis
- Salivary manifestations: enlargement of the parotid salivary glands and hyposalivation (xerostomia)
- Dental caries
- Oral burning sensation
- Gingivitis
- Unprovoked, spontaneous tooth pain

(*Source:* Based on Rosso, L., Campisi, G., DiFede, O., Di Liberto, C., Panzarella, V., & Lo Mazio, L. (2010). Oral manifestations of eating disorders: A critical review. *Oral Diseases,* 14: 479–84.)

TABLE ■ 17–11   Script for Discussing Eating Disorders with the Dental Patient

Introduce the issue . . .	• I am noticing (name the conditions) on your teeth, gums, tongue, throat, etc.
	• This is something I have seen in individuals who engage in (name the behavior: e.g. vomiting, consuming excessive soda, gastroesophageal reflux, etc.)
Ask for information . . .	• How do you think this condition might have occurred in your mouth?
Provide resources . . .	• Are you seeing a professional about these behaviors/condition(s)?
	• Because eating disorders impact your oral, mental, and physical health, it is very important to seek professional help from a counselor, medical doctor, nutritionist, support group, or some combination of these. For eating disorders information and treatment referrals, contact the National Eating Disorders Association at 800-931-2237 or visit www.NationalEatingDisorders.org.
Discuss next steps . . .	• While you are getting help for these behaviors and establishing healthier eating habits, I would like to suggest some options for improving your oral health (i.e., mouthguards, avoid brushing immediately after vomiting, the use of fluorides, etc.)

(*Source:* National Eating Disorders Association. (2002). Dental complications of eating disorders: Information for dental practitioners. Retrieved November 26, 2006, from http://www.nationaleatingdisorders.org.)

Washington Dental Service Foundation developed a script for a suggested approach to this discussion (Table 17–11 ■).

The diagnosis of this disorder by the dental provider and the realization of the dental destruction caused by the disorder often convince patients to agree to treatment. The patient must be cautioned that, for dental rehabilitation to be successful, the underlying problem (the eating disorder and its causes) must be resolved.

Aging Issues

The aging patient often faces a variety of challenges that can undermine both oral health and nutritional status. A study among community dwelling elders found depression, satisfaction with social support, functional status, and oral health were all significant factors in nutritional health.[90] A multinational study indicated a high prevalence of malnutrition among elders in a variety of settings including rehabilitation centers (50.5%), hospitals (38.7%), and nursing homes (13.8%).[91] Compared with younger individuals, elders have a significantly decreased ability to respond to physiologic challenges. This impairment is particularly true of infectious disease because of the immunosenescence that occurs with aging. Sensory function decreases, leading to impaired taste and smell, which can have an impact on the enjoyment of food and impact nutritional status.[92] Changes in the gastrointestinal system can affect the ability to digest, absorb, and use food properly. Functional problems, such as arthritis or vision difficulties, can affect the ability to prepare and eat food. Psychosocial problems such as loneliness, depression, lack of money, and poor access to food all can undermine good eating habits.

Problems in the oral cavity, such as xerostomia and loose teeth, have been considered major contributors to the poor eating habits of the elderly and might be a major contributor to malnutrition.[92-94] Several studies have shown that dentate status can affect eating ability and subsequent diet quality.[95-98] Individuals with one or two complete dentures had a 20% decline in diet quality compared with those with

at least partial dentition in one or both arches.[99] Another study showed that, compared with those with 25 or more teeth, edentulous individuals consumed less fiber and carotene, and fewer vegetables but more cholesterol, saturated fat, and calories.[100] Dentures can affect taste and swallowing ability, especially if they are maxillary dentures. The denture covers taste buds found on the upper palate. When the upper palate is covered, it becomes difficult to detect the location of food in the mouth and might predispose individuals to choking. For this reason, dentures might be a cause of choking in adults.[101]

Xerostomia is common in the older population, in part because of xerostomic medications commonly taken. Xerostomia makes eating more difficult and increases the cariogenic potential of the diet.[102] It has also been associated with burning mouth syndrome and inadequate diet.[102]

Conversely, nutrition is an important factor in oral status. In a sample population of 843 elderly people, there was a significant association between low levels of ascorbic acid and the prevalence of oral mucosal lesions.[103] Low calcium intake throughout life has been shown to contribute to osteoporosis. In turn, osteoporosis in alveolar bone is thought to be a contributing factor to the resorption of alveolar bone that ultimately results in tooth loss.[104] The alveolar process is composed primarily of trabecular bone, which is more labile to calcium imbalances than is cortical bone. Thus, the alveolar bone provides a potential labile source of calcium available to meet other tissue needs. Because the alveolar process is thought to undergo resorption before other bones, it is projected that changes detected in the alveolar process might eventually be used for early detection of osteoporosis and risk for bone fracture.[105] Mandibular bone mass was correlated with total body calcium and bone mass of the radius and vertebrae in dentate and edentulous postmenopausal women with osteoporosis with the highest correlation between total body and mandibular bone mass.[106] Thus, the mandible reflects the mineral status of the entire skeleton. Calcium intake in postmenopausal osteoporotic women was also correlated with mandibular density, supporting the hypothesis that low calcium intake might contribute to

TABLE ■ 17–12 Dietary Suggestions to Assist in Dental Concerns of Older People

Food Group	Difficulty Chewing or Swallowing	Impaired Taste or Appetite	Dry Mouth
Dairy products	Have cottage cheese, yogurt instead of hard cheeses	Use flavored milk and yogurt; add powdered milk to foods to increase protein and calorie intakes	Add milk or yogurt to moisten dry foods
Meats and proteins	Substitute fish, eggs, peanut butter, tofu for hard-to-chew meats	Chew thoroughly	Add broths, gravies, and sauces
	Cut into small pieces	Add herbs and spices instead of salt	
Fruits and vegetables	Use cooked, canned	Have ripe fruits and raw vegetables with skins	Use soups and stews with high water content
	Cut into small pieces or puree		
Grains	Avoid breads with hard crusts; use pasta, rice, cooked cereals	Use whole grains such as rye and pumpernickel	Moisten breads, cereals with milk or broths
Other	Avoid seeds and nuts that tend to slip under dentures	Wine before a meal might stimulate the appetite when used in moderation.	Use candy or gum with non-nutritive sweeteners instead of sucrose-containing products. Drink plenty of fluids.

(*Source:* American Academy of Family Physicians, American Dietetic Association, and National Council on Aging. (1992). *Nutrition interventions manual for professionals caring for older Americans.* Washington, DC: Nutrition Screening Initiative.)

reduced bone density.[107–108] In a study of 329 healthy post-menopausal women, an inverse relationship was shown between bone mineral density and number of existing teeth with those women who received dentures after the age of 40 having the lowest bone mineral density.[109]

Older patients should be carefully screened for nutritional risk factors and should be educated about the importance of good nutrition to general and oral health. MyPlate provides guidelines for healthy food choices and can be used as a tool against which to evaluate individual diets. If major nutritional problems are suspected, the patient should be referred to a registered dietitian.[110] When new dentures are provided, patients should be counseled on how to adapt their usual diet to a softer consistency for the first few days after denture insertion. See Table 17–12 ■ for dietary suggestions for older dental patients.

DENTAL AND NUTRITIONAL IMPLICATIONS OF COMMON CHRONIC CONDITIONS

Diabetes Mellitus

The dental patient with poorly controlled diabetes is at greater risk for developing oral infections and periodontal disease than the patient without diabetes.[111] Conversely, epidemiologic evidence suggests that periodontal disease is an independent predictor of diabetes.[112]

Recommendations for individuals with diabetes are much the same as those found in the 2010 Dietary Guidelines for Americans. Medical nutrition therapy is a standard of care for those with prediabetes or diabetes, and the focus is on achieving and maintaining a healthy weight by reducing the intake of

saturated and trans fat and monitoring carbohydrate intake to achieve glycemic control.[113] The nutrition care plan generally requires that patients have meals and snacks of specific nutrient composition at regularly scheduled intervals, coordinated with medications, insulin or oral agents, and exercise. Dietary management has changed from the high-fat, low-carbohydrate diets of past decades to the more liberal use of complex carbohydrates and the changes in fat intake known to be associated with a healthy diet in general.[114] Frequent use of hard candies or other foods taken to counteract hypoglycemia are an indication that the diabetes is not well controlled. Patients with uncontrolled diabetes should be referred to their physician for further management. In the dental office, quickly assimilated carbohydrate sources, such as juices, cake frosting, soda, or glucose tablets, should be kept readily available in the event that a diabetic patient develops symptoms of hypoglycemia. Table 17–13 ■ provides diet guidelines for the patient with diabetes mellitus.

Immunocompromising Conditions

Immunocompromised patients, such as those with cancer or HIV/AIDS, often have increased requirements for nutrients while having major physiologic and psychosocial impediments to eating.[115] A recent cross-sectional study found that HIV-positive subjects had low ascorbate levels, suggesting that vitamin C requirements in those with HIV infection might be significantly higher than the RDA.[116]

Even though HIV is now considered a chronic disease by many because of the success of highly active antiretroviral therapy (HAART), people who have it still exhibit oral lesions, xerostomia, increased periodontal pocket depths, and orofacial pain that can all impact adequate nutritional intake.[117] Thirty-five percent of all head and neck cancer patients are nutritionally

TABLE ■ 17–13   Diet Guidelines for the Patient with Diabetes Mellitus

- Have regular physician appointments to monitor health status and medications
- See a registered dietitian for personalized medical nutrition therapy
- Have regular meal and snack times; do not skip meals, snacks, or medications
- Have a balance of whole grains, proteins, fruits, vegetables, and dairy products in your meals and snacks
- Have concentrated sweets (candy, cakes, cookies, etc.) only occasionally because they contribute to rapid rises in blood sugar (consult a registered dietitian)
- Avoid the use of slowly dissolving hard candies, mints, breath mints, and the like because they can raise blood sugar and contribute to dental caries

(*Source:* U.S. Department of Health and Human Services. (October 2000). *The practical guide: Identification, evaluation and treatment of overweight and obesity in adults* (NIH Publication No. 00-4084). Bethesda, MD: U.S. Department of Health and Human Services, National Institutes of Health, National Heart, Lung, and Blood Institute.)

compromised at initial diagnosis.[118] The consequences of poor nutrition increases eating difficulty by causing painful oral mucositis, candidiasis, dysphagia, and severe xerostomia.[119]

Cancer often sets up a syndrome of weight loss and wasting in which both metabolism and nutrient losses increase. The cancer often causes severe anorexia, taste changes, and early satiety. The pain and discomfort of oral infections, such as the herpes simplex and oral candidiasis found in AIDS and chemotherapy patients, can also impair the desire and ability to eat.[118]

When providing dental treatment to patients suffering from cancer or AIDS, dental providers need to understand the nutrition principles underlying the care, so that dental services provided can be coordinated effectively with total care. The nutrition care plan initially focuses on providing high-caloric intake in frequent small meals. Liquid supplements might be used if optimal nutrition cannot be achieved via food alone. In more serious cases, patients might need enteral (tube) feedings or more advanced nutritional support.[120] A high-calorie, high-protein diet has high total calories, fat, and possibly simple carbohydrates.[120] In these cases, the dental provider should not caution patients to reduce the frequency of eating because this directive will contradict nutritional management goals. Rather, thorough cleaning after each eating event and the use of fluoride and xylitol-containing products should be stressed. Patients with cancer should be cautioned, however, about the potential oral sequelae of an increased frequency of eating. Patients should also be cautioned to avoid the use of slowly dissolving hard candy, which is often used to mitigate the discomfort caused by the xerostomia. The most important monitoring tool for these patients is weight status. The patient should be queried at each visit about how their weight is being maintained. Involuntary weight loss of 10 pounds or more is a warning for the need for more intensive care. See Table 17–14 ■ for general diet guidelines for immunocompromised dental patients.

ORAL SURGERY AND INTERMAXILLARY FIXATION

Patients who have had oral surgery, whether therapeutic or as a result of trauma, need special nutritional consideration.[121] An adequate diet before surgery is needed to support adequate postsurgical response. If food consumption will be impaired for a short period of time, the risk of nutritional deficiency is low. The risk of deficiency increases with length of eating impairment. The surgery itself can result in anorexia, inability to

TABLE ■ 17–14   General Diet Guidelines for Patients Needing Soft or Liquid Diet or Increased Calories

Food Group (Daily Amount)	Liquid Choices	Soft Choices	To Increase Calories
Dairy products and other calcium sources (at least 3 servings/day; a serving is 1 cup)	All forms of milk, milk shakes, instant breakfast drinks, soft custards, ice cream, yogurt, pudding	All forms of milk, milk shakes, instant breakfast drinks, soft custards, ice cream, yogurt, pudding Soft cheeses such as cottage cheese	Double-strength milk mix: 1 cup nonfat dry milk powder and 1 quart whole milk Provides twice the protein, vitamins, and minerals, and 1.5 times the calories
Proteins (at least 5 ounces/day; one slice of meat is about 1 ounce; a usual serving of protein is 4–5 ounces)	Broth, strained cream soups, eggs in custard, strained or pureed meat or poultry in soups, plain yogurt, pudding	Eggs, cheese, milk and milk shakes, pea and bean soups, soups with tender meat, fish, poultry, chowders, tender meat in gravy	Hearty meat, fish, poultry, beans, tofu, peanut butter, stews, soups, chowders, meat, sauces, pot roasts Gravies and sauces added to most fish and poultry Eggs added to soups, sauces, and hot cereal

(continued)

TABLE ■ 17–14 (Continued)

Food Group (Daily Amount)	Liquid Choices	Soft Choices	To Increase Calories
Fruits (at least 3 servings/day; a serving is 1/2 cup)	Fruit juices, nectars, ices, popsicles, applesauce, strained fruits	Fruit juices, ices, nectars, popsicles, applesauce, pureed or strained cooked fruits, canned fruits, fruit gelatins	Soft
Vegetables (at least 4 servings/day; a serving is 1/2 cup)	Vegetable juices, strained or pureed vegetables mixed with broth	Vegetable juices, strained or pureed vegetables mixed with broth	Soft, cooked vegetables, vegetable soups, stews, juices, sauces, and gravies
		Pureed, soft, canned, cooked vegetables	Starchy vegetables such as potatoes, winter squash, creamed corn
Grains (at least 3 servings/day; a serving is one slice)	Soft bread with crusts removed softened in soup or milk; diluted cereals	Cooked cereals, soft breads, mashed potatoes, pasta, rice, crackers in soup	Creamy, hot cereals, noodles, pasta, bread
			Dry cereals added to soups and sauces
			Wheat germ added to cereals
			Breakfast drinks, custards, frappes, yogurt, etc.
			French toast, pancakes, bread pudding
			Avoid dry toast and hard crusty bread unless soaked in beverage or soup

chew, and increased metabolic requirements.[122] After surgery, a patient might need a liquid diet for 1 or 2 days but should progress as soon as possible to a soft diet of high nutritional quality until a normal diet can be resumed. In some cases, nutritionally complete liquid supplements might be appropriate and should be prescribed in consultation with the patient's dietitian and physician. Often patients prefer purees of normal foods over commercial liquid supplements.[122] Multivitamin and mineral supplements might be appropriate as well. Table 17–15 also provides examples of dietary suggestions for oral surgery patients.

SUMMARY

Nutritional status and dietary habits can affect and be affected by specific oral conditions. Comprehensive patient care requires that nutritional factors be considered in the etiology, progression, and sequelae of oral problems.

Dental providers should routinely screen patients for nutritional issues, provide dentally oriented counseling, and refer patients to dietitians for further care. The nutritional implications in dental conditions are many and complex. No longer can dental professionals take the stance that nutrition is outside their scope of practice.

PRACTICAL CONSIDERATIONS

Dental professionals have an important role in supporting the overall health and wellness of their patients, including encouraging good nutrition. The first step in the process is assessment of dietary habits and intake as part of risk assessment for caries and periodontal disease. Once assessment is complete, national evidence-based guidelines, such as the 2010 Dietary Guidelines for Americans, Dietary Reference Intakes (DRIs), and MyPyramid, should be utilized to develop nutrition recommendations. When patients have special needs, medical nutrition therapy often becomes necessary because of the complex issues involved, and these patients need to be referred to their primary care provider and a registered dietitian.

SELF-STUDY QUESTIONS

1. Which of the following is *not* a dietary factor that might increase risk of dental caries?

   a. Frequency of eating meals and snacks containing simple or retentive carbohydrates

   b. Oral retentiveness of foods

   c. Amount of fermentable carbohydrate consumed

   d. Amount of protein eaten for breakfast

   Rationale: Protein is not cariogenic because it is made up of amino acids and is not broken down by salivary amylase in the mouth, so it cannot be used as energy by caries promotion bacteria. The other possible answers have all been shown by evidence to increase the risk for dental caries.

2. All of the following place a child at high risk for early childhood caries (ECC) *except* one of the following. Which one is the exception?

   a. Family with a poverty income ratio < 1.3

   b. No dental visit within the preceding year

   c. Children with healthy eating habits as measured by the Healthy Eating Index

   d. Failed to discontinue bottle feeding by age 1

   Rationale: Children with healthy eating habits were 44% less likely to have ECC. Evidence shows that children of parents or guardians with lower levels of education and SES are more likely to experience ECC. All children should have a dental home by age 1 and regular anticipatory guidance and preventive care to reduce the risk of ECC. Inappropriate feeding practices such as bottle feeding after age 1 increase a child's risk for ECC.

3. Based on the Caries Potential Index, which of the following is the *best* choice for an anticariogenic snack for a patient at high risk for dental caries?

   a. Cola flavored soda

   b. Cheese

   c. Raisins

   d. Soda crackers

   Rationale: Cheese is composed of protein and fat and has an anticariogenic effect because of its high calcium and phosphorus content. The calcium and phosphorus raise the pH of saliva and buffer the acids produced by bacteria. Soda, raisins, cookies, and crackers are either refined or retentive carbohydrates capable of being metabolized in the mouth by cariogenic bacteria to lower salivary pH.

4. A protein deficiency might result in all of the following *except* one. Which one is the exception?

   a. Enhanced DNA and RNA synthesis

   b. Changes in viscosity or quality of saliva

   c. Loss of tensile strength of collagen

   d. Changes in buffering properties of saliva

   Rationale: Protein functions include DNA and RNA synthesis, which also impact development of immune cells, collagen, and immune function. A protein deficiency would impair DNA and RNA synthesis.

5. You do not have time in your office to provide the patient all the nutrition education she needs. If you were to choose one overall goal for change, what is the most important area to address at this time to reduce her caries risk?

   a. Reduce the frequency of sugary and retentive snacks

   b. Add more fruits and vegetables to the daily diet

   c. Reduce fat intake

   d. Add more dairy to the diet

   Rationale: Although all these recommendations would assist the patient in developing a healthy diet, the recommendation that would most impact caries risk is reducing the frequency of sugary and retentive snacks. Sugary and retentive snacks have the greatest caries potential and the more frequently they are eaten, the longer the teeth are bathed in acids produced by cariogenic bacteria.

REFERENCES

1. Psoter, W. J., Reid, B. C., & Katz, R. V. (2005). Malnutrition and dental caries: A review of the literature. *Caries Res,* 39(6):441–47.

2. Psoter, W., Gebrian, B., Prophete, S., Reid, B., & Katz, R. (2008). Effect of early childhood malnutrition on tooth eruption in Haitian adolescents. *Community Dent Oral Epidemiol,* 36:179–89.

3. Papas, A. S., Palmer, C. A., Rounds, M. C., Herman, J., McGandy, R. B., Hartz, S. C., Russell, R. M., & DePaola, P. (1989). Longitudinal relationship between nutrition and oral health. *Ann NY Acad Sci,* 561:124–42.

4. U.S. Preventive Services Task Force. (1996). *Guide to clinical preventive services* (2nd ed.). Baltimore: Williams & Wilkins.

5. Food and Nutrition Board. (2006). *Dietary reference intakes: The essential guide to nutrient requirements.* Washington, DC: National Institute of Medicine.

6. U.S. Department of Agriculture and U.S. Department of Health and Human Services. (2010, December). *Dietary Guidelines for Americans,* 2010. (7th ed). Washington, DC: U.S. Government Printing Office.

7. American Dietetic Association. (1997). Weight management—position of ADA. *J Am Diet Assoc,* 97:71–74.

8. Meisler, J. G., & St. Jeor, S. (1996). Summary and recommendations from the American Health Foundation's Expert Panel on Healthy Weight. *Am J Clin Nutr,* 63(Suppl 1): 474S–77S.

9. U.S. Department of Agriculture, Center for Nutrition Policy and Promotion. (2011, August). ChooseMyPlate. Retrieved September 5, 2011, from http://www.choosemyplate.gov/index.html.

10. Food and Drug Administration, Center for Food Safety and Applied Nutrition. (2008, April). Food labeling: Nutrition labeling of food. Retrieved January 22, 2011, from http://frwebgate1.access.gpo.gov/cgi-bin/GPOgate.cgi?WAISdocID=cUsC2S/20/3/0&WAISaction=retrieve.

11. Food and Drug Administration, Center for Food Safety and Applied Nutrition. (1999, December). Health claims meeting significant scientific agreement (SSA). Retrieved January 22, 2011, from http://www.fda.gov/Food/LabelingNutrition/LabelClaims/HealthClaimsMeetingSignificantScientificAgreementSSA/default.htm#Approved_Health_Claims.

12. Den Besten, P. K. (1999). Mechanism and timing of fluoride effects on developing enamel. *J Public Health Dent,* 59(4):2226–30.

13. Seow, W. K., Young, W. G., Tsang, A. K., & Daley, T. (2005). A study of primary dental enamel from preterm and full-term children using light and scanning electron microscopy. *Pediatr Dent,* 27:37409.

14. Navia, J. M. (1970). Evaluation of nutritional and dietary factors that modify animal caries. *J Dent Res,* 49:1213–28.

15. Enwonwu, C. (1974). Role of biochemistry and nutrition in preventive dentistry. *J Am Soc Prev Dent,* 4:6–17.

16. DePaola, D. P., & Kuftinec, M. M. (1976). Nutrition in growth and development of oral tissues. *Dent Clin North Am,* 20:441–59.

17. Russell, S. L, Psoter, W. J., Jean-Charles, G., Prophte, S., & Gebrian, B. (2010). Protein-energy malnutrition during early childhood and periodontal disease in the permanent dentition of Haitian adolescents aged 12–19 years: A retrospective cohort study. *Int J Paediatr Dent,* 29(3):222–29.

18. Menaker, L., & Navia, J. M. (1974). Effect of undernutrition during the perinatal period on caries development in the rat: Changes in whole saliva volume and protein content. *J Dent Res,* 53:592–97.

19. Spanheimer, R., Zlatev, T., Umpierrez, G., & Digitolamo, R. (1991). Collagen production in fasted and food-restricted rats: Response to duration and severity of food deprivation. *J Nutr,* 121:518–24.

20. Alvarez, J. O., Caceda, J., Woolley, T. W., Carley, K. W., Baiocchi, N., Caravedo, L., & Navia, J. M. (1993). A longitudinal study of dental caries in the primary teeth of children who suffered from infant malnutrition. *J Dent Res,* 72:1573–76.

21. Alvarez, J. O., Eguren, J. C., Caceda, J., & Navia J. (1990). The effect of nutritional status on the age distribution of dental caries in the primary teeth. *J Dent Res,* 69:1564–66.

22. Johansson, I., Saellstrom, A. K., Rajan, B. P., & Parameswaran, A. (1992). Salivary flow and dental caries in Indian children suffering from chronic malnutrition. *Caries Res,* 26:38–43.

23. Alvarez, J. O., Lewis, C. A., Saman, C., Caceda, J., Montalvo, J., Figueroa, M. L., Izquierdo, J., Caravedo, L., & Navia, J. M. (1988). Chronic malnutrition, dental caries, and tooth exfoliation in Peruvian children aged 3–9 years. *Am J Clin Nutr,* 48:368–72.

24. Vogel, R. (1985). Oral fluids: Saliva and gingival fluid. In Pollack, R. L., & Kravitz, E., Eds. Nutrition in oral health and disease. Philadelphia, PA: Lea & Febiger, 84–107.

25. Watson, R. R., & McMurray, D. M. (1979). Effects of malnutrition on secretory and cellular immunity. In Furia, T. E., Ed. *CRS—Critical reviews of food and nutrition.* Cleveland, OH: CRS Press.

26. Aine, L., Backstron, M. C., Maki, R., Kuusela, A. L., Koivisto, A. M., Ikonen, R. S., & Maki, M. (2000). Enamel defects in primary and permanent teeth of children born prematurely. *J Oral Pathol Med,* 29:403–409.

27. Demarini, S. (2005). Calcium and phosphorus nutrition in preterm infants. *Acta Paediatr Suppl,* 94:87–92.

28. Seow, W. K., Masel, J. P., Weir, C., & Tudehope, D. I. (1989). Mineral deficiency in the pathogenesis of enamel hypoplasia in prematurely born, very low birthweight children. *Pediatr Dent,* 11:297–302.

29. Sintes, J., & Miller, S. (1983). Influence of dietary iron on the dental caries experience and growth of rats fed an experimental diet. *Arch Latinoam Nutr,* 33:322–28.

30. Kwun, I. S., Cho, Y. E., Lomeda, R. A., Shin, H. I., Choi, J. Y., Kang, Y. H., & Beattie, J. H. (2010). Zinc deficiency suppresses matrix mineralization and retards osteogenesis transiently with catch-up possibly through Runx 2 modulation. *Bone,* 46:732–41.

31. DePaola, D., Faine, M., & Palmer, C. (1999). Nutrition in relation to dental medicine. In Shils, M., Olson, J, Shike, M, & Ross, A. C., Eds. Modern nutrition in health and disease (9th ed.). Philadelphia, PA: Lea & Febiger.

32. deMenzes, A. C., Costa, I. M., & El-Guindy, M. M. (1984). Clinical manifestations of hypervitaminosis A in human gingiva: A case report. *J Periodontol,* 8:474–76.

33. Crandall, C. (2004). Vitamin A intake and osteoporosis: A clinical review. *J Womens Health,* 12:939–53.

34. Ostergaard, E., & Löe, H. (1975). The collagen content of skin and gingival tissues in ascorbic acid deficient monkeys. *J Period Res,* 10:103–14.

35. Nakamoto, T., McCroskey, M., & Mallek, H. M. (1984). The role of ascorbic acid deficiency in human gingivitis—A new hypothesis. *J Theor Biol,* 108:163–71.

36. Nishida, M., Grossi, S. G., Dunford, R. G., Ho, A. W., Trevisan, M., & Genco, R. J. (2000). Dietary vitamin C and the risk for periodontal disease. *J Periodontol,* 71:1215–23.

37. Staudte, H., Sigusch, B. W., & Glockmann, E. (2005). Grapefruit consumption improves vitamin C status in periodontitis patients. *Br Dent J,* 199:213–17.

38. Buzina, R. Aurer-Kozelj, J., Srdak-Jorgić, K., Bühler, E. & Gey, K. F. (1986). Increase of gingival hydroxyproline and proline by improvement of ascorbic acid status in man. *Int J Vitam Nutr Res,* 56: 367–72.

39. Wintergerst, E. S., Maggini, S., Hornig, D. H. (2006). Immune-enhancing role of vitamin C and zinc and effect on clinical conditions. *Ann Nutr Metab,* 50:85–94.

40. Charbeneau, T. D., & Hurt, W. C. (1983). Gingival findings in spontaneous scurvy. A case report. *J Periodontol,* 54:694–97.

41. DePaola, D., Faine, M., & Palmer, C. (1999). Nutrition in relation to dental medicine. In Shils, M., Olson, J., Shike, M., & Ross, A. C., Eds. Modern nutrition in health and disease (9th ed.). Philadelphia, PA: Lea & Febiger.

42. Institute of Medicine. (1998). *Dietary reference intakes for thiamin, riboflavin, niacin, vitamin B_6, folate, vitamin B_{12}, pantothenic acid, biotin, and choline.* Washington, DC: National Academy Press.

43. Lussi, A., & Jaeggi, T. (2008). Erosion-diagnosis and risk factors. *Clin Oral Invest,* 12(Suppl 1):S5–13.

44. Dye, B. A., Tan, S., Smith, V., Lewis, B. G., Barker, L. K., Thornton-Evans, G., et al. (2007). Trends in oral health status: United States, 1988–1994 and 1999–2004. National Center for Health Statistics. *Vital Health Stat,* 11.

45. Klein, M. L., DeBaz, L., Agidi, S., Lee, H., Xie, G., Lin, A., et al. (2010). Dynamics of *Streptococcus mutans* transcriptome in response to starch and sucrose during biofilm development.

46. Anderson, C. A., Curzon, M. E., Van Loveren, C., Tatsi, C., & Duggal, M. S. (2009). Sucrose and dental caries: A review of the evidence. Obes Rev, 10(Suppl 1):41–54.

47. USDA, Economic Research Service. (2005). Sweetener consumption in the US: Distribution by demographics and product characteristics. Retrieved January 23, 2011, from http://www.ers.usda.gov/Publications/SSS/aug05/sss24301/sss24301.pdf.

48. Harris, R., Nicoll, A. D., Adair, P. M., & Pine, C. M. (2004). Risk factors for dental caries in young children: A systematic review of the literature. *Community Dental Health,* 21(Suppl):71–85.

49. Deshpande, A., & Jadad, A. R. (2008). The impact of polyol-containing chewing gums on dental caries: A systematic review of original randomized controlled trials and observational studies. *J Am Dent Assoc,*139:1602–14.

50. Duane, B. (2010). Xylitol gum, plaque pH and mutans streptococci. *Evid Based Dent,* 1:109–10.

51. Pollard, M. A., Imfeld, T., Higham, S. M., Agalamanyi, E. A., Corzon, M. E., Edgar, W. M., & Borgia, M. (1996). Acidogenic potential and total salivary carbohydrate content of expectorants following the consumption of some cereal-based foods and fruits. *Caries Res,* 30:132–37.

52. Kashket, S., Zhang, J., & Van Houte, J. (1996). Accumulation of fermentable sugars and metabolic acids in food particles that become entrapped on the dentition. *J Dent Res,* 75:1885–91.

53. König, K. G., & Schmid, P. (1968). An analysis of frequency-controlled feeding of small rodents and its use in dental caries experiments. *Arch Oral Biol,* 13:13–26.

54. Gustafson, B., Quensel, E., & Lanke, L. (1954). The Vipeholm dental caries study: The effect of different carbohydrate intake on caries activity in 436 individuals observed for five years. *Acta Odontol Scand,* 11:232–64.

55. Lingstrom, P., Birkhed, D., Ruben, J., & Arends, J. (1994). Effect of frequent consumption of starchy food items on enamel and dentin demineralization and on plaque pH in situ. *J Dent Res,* 73:652–60.

56. Mundorff-Shrestha, S. A., Featherstone, J. D. B., & Eisenberg, A. D. (1994). Cariogenic potential of foods, II. Relationship of food composition, plaque microbial counts, and salivary parameters to caries in the rat model. *Caries Res,* 28:106–15.

57. Rugg-Gunn, W., Edgar, M., & Jenkins, G. N. (1981). The effect of altering the position of a sugary food in a meal upon plaque pH in human subjects. *J Dent Res,* 60:867–72.

58. Edgar, W. M., & Bowen, W. H. (1982). Effects of different eating patterns on dental caries in the rat. *Caries Res,* 16:384–88.

59. Jensen, M. E., Harlander, S. K., & Schachtele, C. F. (1984). Evaluation of the acidogenic and antacid properties of cheeses by telemetric recording of dental plaque. In Hefferen, J. J., Koehler, H. M., & Osborn, J. C., Eds. Food, nutrition and dental health (vol. 5). Park Forest South, IL: Pathotox.

60. Nase, L., Hatakka, K., Savilahti, E., Saxelin, M., Ponka, A., Poussa, T., Korpela, R., & Meurman, J. H. (2001). Effect of long-term consumption of a probiotic bacterium, *Lactobacillus rhamnosus GG,* in milk on dental caries and caries risk in children. *Caries Res,* 35:412–20.

61. Ahola, A. J., Yli-Knuuttila, H., Suomalainen, T., Poussa, T., Ahlstrom, A., Meurman, J. H., & Korpela, R. (2002). Short term consumption of probiotic-containing cheese and its effect on dental caries risk factors. *Arch Oral Biol,* 47(11):799–804.

62. Bowen, W. H. (1994). Food components and caries. *Adv Dent Res,* 8:215–20.

63. Mundorff, S. A., Featherstone, J. D. B., & Bibby, B. G. (1990). Cariogenic potential of foods, I. Caries in the rat model. *Caries Res,* 24:344–55.

64. Jensen, M. E. (1985). Dental caries: A diet-related disease. *Curr Q,* 1:18–20.

65. Koulourides, T., & Chien, M. C. (1992). The ICT in situ experimental model in dental research. *J Dent Res,* 71:822–27.

66. DePaola, D. (1986). Executive summary: Scientific consensus conference on methods for assessment of the cariogenic potential of foods. *J Dent Res,* 65(Spec Iss):1540–43.

67. Curzon, M. E. J., & Pollard, M. A. (1996). Integration of methods for determining the acid/cariogenic potential of foods: A comparison of several different methods. *Caries Res,* 30:126–31.

68. Vogel, R., & Alvares, O. F. (1985). Nutrition and periodontal disease. In Pollack, R. L., & Kravitz, E., Eds. Nutrition in oral health and disease. Philadelphia PA: Lea & Febiger, 136–50.

69. Navia, J. M., & Menaker, L. (1976). Nutritional implications in wound healing. *Dent Clin North Am,* 20:549–67.

70. Alfano, M. C., Miller, S. A., & Drummond, J. F. (1975). Effect of ascorbic acid deficiency on the permeability and collagen biosynthesis of oral mucosal epithelium. *Ann NY Acad Sci,* 258:253–63.

71. Alfano, M. C., & Masi, C. W. (1978). Effect of acute folic acid deficiency on the oral mucosal permeability. *J Dent Res,* 57:312.

72. Joseph, C. E., Ashrafi, S. H., Steinberg, A. D., & Waterhouse, J. P. (1982). Zinc deficiency changes in the permeability of rabbit periodontium to 14-C-phenytoin and 14C-albumin. *J Periodont,* 53:251–56.

73. Alfano, M. C. (1976). Controversies, perspectives and clinical implications of nutrition in periodontal disease. *Dent Clin North Am,* 20:519–48.

74. Malleck, H. M. (1978). An investigation of the role of ascorbic acid and iron in the etiology of gingivitis in humans. (Doctoral thesis). Cambridge, MA: Institute Archives, Massachusetts Institute of Technology.

75. Whitehead, N., Ryner, F., & Lindenbaum, J. (1973). Megaloblastic changes in the cervical epithelium. Association with oral contraceptive therapy and reversal with folic acid. *JAMA,* 226:1421–24.

76. Merchant, A. T., Pitiphat, W., Franz, M., & Joshipura, K. J. (2006). Whole grain and fiber intakes and periodontitis risk in men. *Am J Clin Nutr,* 83:1395–1400.

77. Miley D. D., Garcia, M. N., Hildebolt, C. F., Shannon, W. D., Couture, R. A., Anderson Spearie, C. L., Dixon, D. A., et al. (2009). Cross-sectional study of vitamin D and calcium supplementation effects on chronic periodontitis. *J Perio,* 80:1433–39.

78. Bikle. D. D. (2008). Vitamin D and the immune system: Role in protection against bacterial infection. *Current Opin Nephro & Hypertension,* 17:348–52.

79. American Academy of Pediatric Dentistry, American Academy of Pediatrics. (2008). Policy on Early Childhood Caries (ECC): Classifications, consequences, and preventive strategies. http://www.aapd.org/media/policies_guidelines/p_eccclassifications.pdf.

80. Beltran-Aguilar, E. D., Barker, L. K, Canto, B. A., Gooch, B. F., Griffin, S. O., Hyman, J., Jaramillo, F., Kingman, A., Nowjack-Raymer, R., Selwitz, R. H., & Wu, T. (2005). Surveillance for dental caries, dental sealants, tooth retention, edentulism, and enamel flourosis—United States, 1988–1994 and 1999–2002. *MMWR Morb Mortal Wkly Rep,* 54: 1–44.

81. Kelly, M., & Bruerd, B. (1987). The prevalence of baby bottle tooth decay among two Native American populations. *J Pub Health Dent,* 47:94–97.

82. Broderick, E., Mabry, J., Robertson, D., & Thompson, J. (1989). Baby bottle tooth decay in Native American children in Head Start Centers. *Pub Health Rep,* 104:50–54.

83. Palmer, C. A, Kent, R., Loo, C. V., Hughes, E., Stutius, N., Pradhan, M., Dahlan, E., et al. (2010). Diet and caries-associated bacteria in severe early childhood caries. *J Dent Res,* 89:1224–29.

84. Kaste, L. M., & Gift, H. C. (1995). Inappropriate infant bottle feeding. *Arch Pediatr Adolesc Med,* 149:786–91.

85. Nunn, M. E., Braunstein, N. S., Krall Kayce, E. A., Dietrich, T., Garcia, R. I. , & Henshaw, M. M. (2009). Healthy Eating Index is a predictor of early childhood caries. *J Dent Res,* 88:361–66.

86. Hallett, K. B., & O'Rourke, P. K. (2006). Pattern and severity of early childhood caries. *Community Dent Oral Epidemiol,* 34:25–35.

87. O'Sullivan, D. M., & Tinanoff, N. (1993). Maxillary anterior caries associated with increased caries risk in other primary teeth. *J Dent Res,* 72:1577–80.

88. National Eating Disorders Association. (2002). Dental complications of eating disorders: Information for dental practitioners. Retrieved November 26, 2006, from http://www.nationaleating-disorders.org.

89. Hudson J. I., Hiripi, E., Pope, H. G., & Kessler, R. C. (2007). The prevalence and correlates of eating disorders in the National Comorbidity Survey replication. *Biol Psychiatry,* 2007,61: 348–58.

90. Chen, C. C. (2005). A framework for studying the nutritional health of community-dwelling elders. *Nurs Res,* 54:13–21.

91. Kaiser, M. J., Bauer, J. M., Ramsch, C., Uter, W., Guigoz, Y., Cederholm, et al. (2010). Frequency of malnutrition in older adults: A multinational perspective using the mini nutritional assessment. *J Am Geriatr Soc,* 58:1734–48.

92. Schiffman, S. S. (1991). Taste and smell losses with age. *Contemporary Nutrition,* General Mills Nutrition Department: 16:6–8.

93. Brodeur, J. M., Laurin, D., Vallee, R., & Lachapelle, D. (1993, November). Nutrient intake and gastrointestinal disorders related to masticatory performance in the edentulous elderly. *J Prosthet Dent,* 70:468–73.

94. Position of the American Dietetic Association. (2007). Oral health and nutrition (2007). *J Am Diet Assoc,* 107:1418–28.

95. Slagter, A. P., Olthoff, L. W., Bosman, F., & Steen, W. H. (1992). Masticatory ability, denture quality, and oral conditions in edentulous subjects. *J Prosthet Dent,* 68:299–307.

96. Touger-Decker, R., Schaefer, M., Flinton, R., & Steinberg, L. (1996). Effect of tooth loss and dentures on diet habits. *J Prosthet Dent,* 75:831.

97. Sebring, N. G., Guckes, A. D., Li, S., & McCarthy, G. R. (1995). Nutritional adequacy of reported intake of edentulous subjects treated with new conventional or implant-supported mandibular dentures. *J Prosthet Dent,* 74:358–63.

98. Greksa, L. P., Parraga, I. M., & Clark, C. A. (1995). The dietary adequacy of edentulous older adults. *J Prosthet Dent,* 73:142–45.

99. Papas, A., Palmer, C., McGandy, R., Hartz, S. C., & Russell, R. M. (1987). Dietary and nutritional factors in relation to dental caries in elderly subjects. *Gerodontics,* 3:30–37.

100. Joshipura, K., Willett, W., & Douglass, C. (1996). The impact of edentulousness on food and nutrient intake. *J Am Dent Assoc,* 127:459–67.

101. Anderson, D. L. (1977). Death from improper mastication. *Int Dent J,* 27:349.

102. Gueiros, L. A., Soares, M. S. M., & Laeo, J. C. (2009). Impact of ageing and drug consumption on oral health. *Gerodontology,* 26:297–301.

103. Vaanen, M. K., Markkanen, H. A., Tuovinen, V. J., Kullaa, A. M., Karinpau, A. M., & Kumpusalo, E. A. (1993). Periodontal health related to plasma ascorbic acid. *Proc Finn Dent Soc,* 89:51–59.

104. Paganini-Hill, A. (1995). The benefits of estrogen replacement therapy on oral health. The Leisure World cohort. *Arch Intern Med,* 155:2325–29.

105. Jonasson, G., Alstad, T., Vahedi, F., Boseaus, I., Lisnner, L., & Hakeberg, M. (2009). Trabecular pattern in the mandible as bone fracture predictor. *Oral Surg, Oral Med, Oral Path, Oral Rad, Endo,* 108:42–51.

106. Kribbs, P. J., Chestnut, C. H., Ott, S., & Kilcoyne, R. F. (1990). Relationships between mandibular and skeletal bone in a population of normal women. *J Prosthet Dent,* 63:86–89.

107. Kribbs, P. J. (1990). Comparison of mandibular bone in normal and osteoporotic women. *J Prosthet Dent,* 63:218–22.

108. Houki, K., DiMuzio, M. T., & Fattore, L. (1994). Mandibular bone density and systemic osteoporosis in elderly edentulous women. *J Bone Miner Res,* 9 (Suppl):S211.

109. Krall, E. A., Dawson-Hughes, B., Papas, A., & Garcia, R. I. (1994). Tooth loss and skeletal bone density in healthy postmenopausal women. *Osteoporos Int,* 4:104–109.

110. American Academy of Family Physicians, American Dietetic Association, and National Council on Aging. (1992). *Nutrition interventions manual for professionals caring for older Americans.* Washington, DC: Nutrition Screening Initiative.

111. Pla, G. W. (1994). Oral health and nutrition. *Prim Care Clin Off Pract,* 21:121–23.

112. Simpson, T. C., Needleman, I., Wild, S. H., Moles, D. R., & Mills, E .J. (2010). Treatment of periodontal disease for glycemic control in people with diabetes. *Cochrane Datab Syst Rev,* 5:1–65.

113. Demmer, R. T., Jacobs, D. R., & Desvarieux, M. (2008). Periodontal disease and incident Type 2 diabetes. *Diabetes Care,* 31:1373–79.

114. American Diabetes Association. (2011). Standards of medical care in diabetes–2011. *Diabetes Care,* 34(Suppl 1):S11–S61.

115. U.S. Department of Veteran's Affairs. (2010). Diet and nutrition in HIV. http://www.hiv.va.gov/patient/diet/single-page.asp.

116. Stephensen, C. B., Marquis, G. S., Jacob, R. A., Kruzich, L. A., Douglas, S. D., & Wilson, C. M. (2006). Vitamin C and E in adolescents and young adults in HIV infection. *Am J Clin Nutr,* 83:870–79.

117. Nittayananta, W., Talungchit, S., Jaruratanasirikul, S., Silpapojakul, K., Chayakul, P., Nilmanat, A., et al. (2010). Effects of long-term use of HAART on oral health status in HIV-infected subjects. *J Oral Path Med,* 39:397–406.

118. Capuano, G., Gentile, P. C., Bianciardi, F., Tosti, M., Palladino, A., & DiPalma, M. (2010). Prevalence and influence of malnutrition on quality of life and performance status in patients with locally advanced head and neck cancer before treatment. *Support Care Cancer,* 18:433–37.

119. National Cancer Institute. Nutrition in cancer care (PDQ): Health professional version. Retrieved February 1, 2011, from http://www.cancer.gov/cancertopics/pdq/supportivecare/nutrition/healthprofessional.

120. Dwyer, J. T., Efstathion, M. S., Palmer, C., & Papas, A. (1991). Nutritional support in treatment of oral carcinomas. *Nutr Rev,* 49:332–37.

121. Kendall, B. D., Fonseca, R. J., & Lee, M. (1982). Postoperative nutritional supplementation for the orthognathic surgery patient. *J Oral Maxillofac Surg,* 40:205–13.

122. Soliah, K. (1987). Clinical effects of jaw surgery and wiring on body composition: A case study. In *Dietetic currents* (vol. 14). Columbus, OH: Ross Laboratories, 13–16.

Sugar and Other Sweeteners

Michelle L. Sensat
Jill L. Stoltenberg

KEY TERMS

OBJECTIVES

After studying this chapter, the student should be able to:

1. Define *sugars, sweeteners,* and *sugar substitutes.*
2. Identify the three sugars that are composed of glucose, fructose, or galactose.
3. Differentiate between cariogenic sugars and noncariogenic sweeteners.
4. Describe the potential impact that excessive sugar intake has on dental and systemic health.
5. Explain the role of sugar in the caries process.
6. Suggest alternative sweetener options that are noncariogenic on the basis of a working knowledge of comparative sweetness to sucrose.
7. Identify contraindications that can preclude someone from using a specific sugar substitute.
8. Describe the role of xylitol in the prevention of dental caries.
9. Describe preventive strategies to halt or decrease caries frequency in the high-risk or at-risk patient.

INTRODUCTION

Sweeteners are sugars or substances added to foods and beverages that provide a pleasurable taste and, in some cases, added energy. Those that provide energy are termed "nutritive" or **caloric sweeteners** (i.e., sucrose, fructose, and sugar alcohols). Those that do not provide energy are called *non-nutritive* or **noncaloric sweeteners**, as well as *sugar substitutes* (i.e., acesulfame-K, aspartame, neotame, saccharin, and sucralose). A list of nutritive sweeteners used in the food supply is in Table 18–1 ■.

Sweetness is a stimulus that can be imparted by a wide variety of molecules. Sugars, amino acids, peptides, proteins, olefinic alcohols, nitroanilines, saccharin, chloroform, and many other organic compounds are capable of imparting a sweet taste.[1]

To most people, the word *sugar* refers to the common crystalline, granular table sugar, or sucrose. However, sucrose is only one of many naturally occurring sugars found in the human diet. Chemically, sugars are a group of compounds composed of carbon (C), hydrogen (H), and oxygen (O) atoms, also known as carbohydrates.[2]

Naturally occurring sugars can be divided into two classifications of carbohydrates: simple sugars, or monosaccharides, and disaccharides. **Monosaccharides** contain 3 to 7 carbon atoms per monomer and include the following primary simple sugars in the human diet: glucose, fructose, and galactose. Mannose, another monosaccharide, also plays a minor role in the human diet.[2] Figure 18–1 ■ shows examples of structural formulas for several naturally occurring sugars. These simple sugars are readily absorbed.[3] **Disaccharides** are two monosaccharides, or two monomers, that are joined together. Primary disaccharides (Figure 18–2 ■) in the human diet include sucrose (one glucose and one fructose), lactose (one galactose and one glucose), trehalose (two molecules of α-glucose, 1Ø 1 linkage), and maltose (two molecules of α-glucose, 1Ø 4 linkage).[2]

This chapter will discuss both nutritive and non-nutritive sweeteners, comparing contributions of each to commercial food products, their effects on the dental caries process, and their place in caries prevention.

TASTE PERCEPTION AND SENSATION

Total perception of food is complex. Multiple senses are at work: taste; olfaction (which includes smells, or aromas); touch, also called *mouth feel,* from texture of food and fat content; and thermoreception and nociception caused by strong spices and irritants.[4] There are generally four categories of primary stimuli with regard to taste: sweet, sour, salty, and bitter. One other primary taste, savory, also termed *umami,* is controversial.[4] Mixtures of these primary stimuli are found in complex foods.

TABLE ■ **18–1** Nutritive Sweeteners in the Food Supply

Sweeteners (Other Names)[a]	Description
Monosaccharides	
Glucose/dextrose (dextrin, corn sugar)	Used in food processing and canned foods
Fructose (fruit sugar, levulose)	Produces laxative effect at intake of 20 grams or more
Disaccharides	
Sucrose (granulated, powdered, brown, turbinado [raw], invert sugar)	Sweetens and tenderizes baked goods
High-fructose corn syrup (HFCS)	Used in soft drinks
Corn syrup (corn sugar, corn syrup solids)	Used in candy, snack foods, ice cream, fruit drinks, nondairy creamers
Maltose (malt sugar or syrup)	Made from barley; used in malt flavored foods and alcoholic beverages
Molasses/sorghum/maple syrup	Used in breads and on pancakes, waffles
Honey (raw, comb, creamed)	Harvested from bees; not safe for infants
Lactose (milk sugar)	Used in whipped toppings and commercial baked goods

[a]All provide 4 kcal/g.

FIGURE ■ **18–1** Primary monosaccharides in foods.

(*Source:* Sigman-Grant, M., & Morita, J. (2003). Defining and interpreting intakes of sugars[1,2,3,4]. *American Journal of Clinical Nutrition,* 78 (4 Suppl):815S–26S.)

FIGURE ■ 18–2 Primary disaccharides in foods.

(*Source:* Sigman-Grant, M., & Morita, J. (2003). Defining and interpreting intakes of sugars[1,2,3,4]. *American Journal of Clinical Nutrition*, 78 (4 Suppl):815S–26S.)

The chemical detection of taste agents occurs in specialized epithelial cells called **taste receptor cells**; they are present in vertebrates as ovoid clusters or taste buds. Each taste bud contains 50 to 100 cells. These buds are found embedded within the nonsensory lingual epithelium and are found within specialized connective tissues called *papillae,* including fungiform, foliate, and circumvallate papillae. Taste buds are also found in the palate, pharynx, and upper portion of the esophagus.[4]

Taste sensation is initiated by the arrival of a stimulus at the taste buds. Recognition of the taste agent or agents occurs when receptor sites of the taste bud cells carry, by cranial nerves VII, IX, and X, messages to the brain that are then processed and recognized as either sweet, sour, salty, bitter, or some combination of these primary stimuli.[4]

HISTORY OF SWEETENERS

The first recorded sweetener was honey used in the ancient cultures of Greece and China.[5] Honey later was replaced by **saccharose**, or common sugar, originally made from sugar cane. A large industry for sugar cane production in the Western Hemisphere was in place by the 17th century and supplied sweeteners to Europe. Napoleon's scientists developed sugar extraction from sugar beets when France was isolated from major shipping early in the 19th century.

DID YOU KNOW ?

Early human cultures valued sweetness and considered it rare enough that they kept naturally available sweeteners from their regions for special religious or celebratory events.

During the world wars, saccharose production largely came from sugar beets rather than sugar cane because of the ease of production. The search for other sweeteners led to new chemical developments. During World Wars I and II, **saccharin**, the first artificial sweetener and first manufactured in 1879 by Remsen and Fahlberg, became used widely because of its low production costs and the shortage of regular sugar.[5] As the economy recovered after the wars, sugar became more plentiful and affordable. Unfortunately, with the growing candy and fast-food industry, obesity soon increased in Western societies. Since the 1950s, a push to use saccharin shifted from cost concerns to calorie reduction and weight control. Profitable market demand soon followed for reduced-calorie diet products, which contained reduced sugar or substitution of sugar with artificial sweeteners. Saccharin, however, was known for not only its sweetness but also its bitter aftertaste, so there was an interest to create new, better-tasting reduced-calorie sweeteners.[5]

In the 1950s, a breakthrough was achieved with the development of **cyclamate**. It tasted better than saccharin and blended very well with it. Cyclamate, saccharin, and other additives were then mixed together and sold under the name Sweet'N Low, which became widely used in the United States. Cyclamate was used in tablet or liquid form as a tabletop sweetener and as a sweetener in soft drinks.

In 1970, the U.S. Food and Drug Administration (FDA) banned cyclamate from all diet foods and fruits because of suspicion of induced cancer in laboratory animals.[6] In all other countries, however, it is still used today, particularly in combination with other sweeteners.

In 1981, **aspartame** was approved and marketed as NutraSweet. This allowed dairy products such as yogurt, to be sold as "diet" or "light" reduced-calorie foods for the first time.[7]

Saccharin, cyclamate, and aspartame were known as the "first-generation sweeteners." Second-generation sweeteners soon followed, including acesulfame-K, sucralose, alitame, and neotame, which differ widely in their key markets throughout the globe. These second-generation sweeteners, unfortunately, had limitations similar to those of the first-generation sweeteners. Their taste was often bitter with a metallic aftertaste, and they provided an unreal feeling in the mouth compared with regular sugar. Many synergic artificial sweeteners, that is, sweeteners that enhance each others' flavor, are now combined to improve the overall quality of sweetened products (i.e., a combination of acesulfame-K, aspartame, and others in soft drinks).[5]

Today consumers' feelings are mixed concerning use of artificial sweeteners, largely because of earlier reports of cancer risks with these substances. In the 1980s, when many sweeteners were new to the market, there were several published reports of carcinogenic effects associated with use of artificial sweeteners. Their publication was unfortunate because many of the reports lacked a sound scientific background or were poorly investigated.[5] Some scientific publications of that time also were not well researched and possessed erroneous statistical analyses of findings. In the last decade, the cancer and artificial sweetener link has not been discussed as frequently as earlier, although some long-term studies with saccharin and cyclamate have been conducted and published.[5] There appears to be no resurgence in concern with regard to saccharin use, and popularity of new products has shifted demand to the newer, sweeter, and better tasting artificial sweeteners.

SUCROSE AND CONSTITUENTS

Sucrose is a nutritive sweetener and the most commonly used tabletop sweetener. It is a disaccharide (one glucose and one fructose) and provides 4 kilocalories/gram (kcal/g; approximately 16 kcal per teaspoon) when consumed. Sucrose is manufactured from the processing of sugar cane or sugar beets, and through refinement, yellow-brown pigments are removed to produce the white crystalline form of common table sugar. Molasses is sucrose in its least refined state.[8] Sucrose, cane, or beet sugar is used in the following food items in descending order of frequency: bakery and cereal products; candy and other confectionary items; ice cream and dairy products; beverages; canned, bottled, and frozen foods; and other miscellaneous foods.[9]

Fructose, a component of sucrose, is also often added to foods to synergize the sweetness potential of sucrose and some non-nutritive sweeteners.[10] As a monosaccharide, fructose provides 4 kcal/g when consumed. Fructose makes up 50% of a sucrose molecule, and the other 50% is glucose which is present in fruit, also known as *fruit sugar* or *levulose*, and is added to foods and beverages as high-fructose corn syrup (HFCS; 42%–55% fructose) or in a crystallized form.[8] Fructose has replaced sucrose in many foods and beverages because of its intense sweetness, reduced cost, and properties that enhance flavor, color, and product stability.[10] Corn syrups can be found in beverages, processed foods, cereal and baked goods, dairy products, candy, and other confectionary goods.[9]

Exact data on sugar consumption is difficult to obtain because of limitations of data gathering. Two major surveys that are used to estimate a person's intake of food are the Continuing Survey of Food Intakes by Individuals and the National Health and Nutrition Examination Survey.[11] For the intake of sugars, the 24-hour dietary recall method is used most often. The major limitation with the data gathered is that these surveys rely on self-reported, retrospective, recall of dietary intake.[12] Furthermore, the data are cross-sectional and provide no information regarding previous or subsequent consumption beyond the days of the dietary intake recall or what an individual person might do if presented with alternative food choices.[2] Accuracy of self-reported food intake is also a problem.[13,14]

In an article published in 2003, the reported mean population intake of added sugars was approximately 80 grams, which equals a mean of 15.8% of total energy intake.[15,16] Average intake for children younger than 12 years was less than 19% of total energy, approximately 20% of total energy for adolescents, and then decreased throughout adulthood.

Uses of Sucrose

Sucrose has, in addition to its sensory qualities, functional properties that make it desirable for use in the food industry. It is ideal in the following roles:

- *Sweetening agent:* The character of the sweetness of a product can be varied according to the pH and temperature used to manufacture it as well as by its interaction with other ingredients. Level of sweetness is important to the acceptance of certain foods.[17]
- *Flavor blender and modifier:* In some foods, sucrose assists in blending flavors; in other foods (i.e., pickles), it reduces the acidic and/or sour taste.
- *Texture and bodying agent:* Sucrose imparts a texture that is highly acceptable to consumers. It gives fullness and a distinctive mouth feel to foods and beverages.
- *Dispersing/lubricating agent:* In dry packaged mixes, sucrose keeps other ingredients from packing too closely. This permits a better blending of the ingredients during food preparation.
- *Caramelization/color agent:* Caramelization during cooking and baking produces a brown color, which provides a desirable, characteristic flavor and aroma to the food product.
- *Bulking agent:* When sucrose is replaced by a noncaloric sweetener that can be hundreds of times sweeter, other ingredients must be added to replace the lost sucrose "bulk" to maintain the food's normal appearance and consistency.[18]

Evaluation of the Health Aspects of Sucrose

In the United States, sucrose (along with several other sweeteners) is a generally recognized to be safe (GRAS) ingredient, and other artificial sweeteners are categorized as food additives.

These distinctions are defined by the 1958 Food Additives Amendment to the Federal Food, Drug, and Cosmetic Act.[8] The FDA must approve the safety of all food additives. The *Code of Federal Regulations* (21 CFR 171), revised in 2002, defines food additives and procedures necessary for evaluating the safety of these substances. When reviewing potential sweeteners as food additives, the FDA asks the following questions: (1) How is it made? (2) What are its properties in foods and beverages (i.e., product specifications)? (3) How much of the sweetener will be consumed, and will certain groups be particularly susceptible to the food additive?[4] Is the sweetener safe, and does it cause adverse effects, including cancer, or chronic toxicity, to the individual or offspring?[8]

In recent years, intake of sugars was suggested to be associated with a variety of health issues, namely obesity, diabetes and glycemic response, hyperlipidemias, behavioral disorders, and dental caries.[8,19] After intense scrutiny, many supposed adverse health effects of sugars were found to lack a scientific foundation.[20] Sugars alone were not associated with obesity, hyperactivity in children, diabetes, and coronary heart disease.[21] A position statement by the American Dietetic Association clarifies this issue: "Consumers can safely enjoy a range of nutritive and nonnutritive sweeteners when consumed in a diet that is guided by current federal nutrition recommendations, such as the Dietary Guidelines for Americans and the Dietary References Intakes, as well as individual health goals."[8] Furthermore, the Institutes of Medicine suggest a maximum intake level of nutritive sweeteners to be less than 25% of total energy; otherwise, dietary quality suffers.[8]

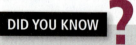

DID YOU KNOW ?

Oxygenated beverages, as opposed to carbonated beverages, are effective against oral halitosis.

SUGARS AND DENTAL CARIES FORMATION

Substantial research implicates sugars (i.e., sucrose, glucose, fructose, maltose) and all fermentable carbohydrates as principal dietary substances that promote caries formation.[22–26] Although the connection between sweet carbohydrates and dental decay has been observed for hundreds of years, two landmark animal studies and three human clinical studies have

contributed to the understanding of the importance of sugar, along with bacterial biofilms, in the development of caries.

In 1955, the first animal study was conducted with laboratory rats in a gnotobiotic (germ-free) environment.[27] One group of rats was fed a cariogenic diet containing large amounts of sugar. The second group was fed the same diet; however, at the same time, specific microorganisms were introduced to the otherwise germ-free environment. Rats receiving the cariogenic diet alone did not develop caries; those with the cariogenic diet in the presence of bacteria did develop carious lesions. Observations at that time and since have clearly demonstrated that certain strains of microorganisms (i.e., *Streptococci mutans* and lactobacilli) are more caries productive than others.

Another study using rats as subjects fed them a caries-producing diet by means of a stomach tube with no food actually coming in contact with the teeth.[28] No caries resulted. When the same diet was fed orally and contacted the teeth, caries did occur. These two studies conclusively demonstrated that (1) bacteria are essential for caries development, regardless of diet, and (2) the action of sugar in the caries process is local, not systemic (Table 18–2 ■).

Several human studies have further clarified the animal studies. Two of the most often cited studies occurred at Hopewood House[29] in Australia and at Vipeholm in Sweden.[30]

Hopewood House was an orphanage in Australia that housed up to 82 children. From its beginning, sugar and other refined carbohydrates were excluded from the children's diet. Carbohydrates were served in the form of whole meal bread, soybeans, wheat germ, oats, rice, potatoes, and some molasses. Dairy products, fruits, raw vegetables, and nuts were prominently featured in the typical menu. Dental surveys of these children from the ages of 5 to 11 years revealed a greatly reduced caries incidence compared with the state school population in that age group even though the orphaned children's oral hygiene was poor with about 75% suffering from gingivitis. When the children became old enough to earn wages in the outside economy, they deviated from the orphanage diet. A steep increase of decayed, missing, and filled teeth (DMFT) after the age of 11 years indicated that the teeth did not acquire any permanent resistance to caries.

The Vipeholm study was conducted at a mental institution in the southern city of Vipeholm, Sweden. Adult patients on a nutritionally adequate diet were observed for several years and found to have a slow caries rate. The patients were then divided into different groups to compare the cariogenicity accompanying various changes in frequency and consistency of carbohydrate

TABLE ■ 18–2   Caries in Rats Fed a Decay-Producing Diet via Normal and Stomach Tube Routes

Group	Methods of Feeding	No. of Rats	Avg. No. of Carious Molars	Avg. No. of Carious Lesions
A	Normal	13	5.0	6.7
B	Stomach tube	13	0	0

(*Source:* Kite, O., Shaw, J., & Sognnaes, R. (1950). The prevention of experimental tooth decay by tube-feeding. The American Society for Nutrition Sciences, *Journal of Nutrition*, 42:89–103. Reprinted with permission.)

intake. Sucrose was included in the diet as toffee, chocolate, or caramel, in bread, or in liquid form. Caries increased significantly when foods containing sucrose were ingested between meals. In addition to the frequency of eating, the consistency of the sugar-containing food was very important. Sticky or adherent forms of food that maintained high sugar levels in the mouth for longer periods of time were much more cariogenic than forms that were rapidly cleared.

The Vipeholm study also demonstrated that it was possible to increase the average consumption of sugar from about 30 to 330 grams with little increase in caries when the additional sugar was consumed at mealtime and in solution form.[30] Two important points about the design of the Vipeholm study are the use of excessive quantities and abnormal presentations of food, and by today's standards, it would not have received ethical clearance.

Additional evidence of sugar's link to dental caries comes from a genetic disease. Some people have a lowered caries incidence attributable to a condition known as **hereditary fructose intolerance (HFI)**. After the intake of fructose, these persons experience nausea, vomiting, and excessive sweating; they can also develop malaise, tremor, coma, and convulsions. As a result, these individuals carefully avoid foods with fructose or sucrose that has fructose as one of the metabolic products. Those HFI individuals who have survived this disorder by successfully avoiding fructose or sucrose from any source are either caries free or have very few caries.[31] The low prevalence of caries in HFI persons is an indication that starchy foods alone do not produce decay whereas foods with sugar do produce decay.

What annual level of sugar consumption makes a diet highly cariogenic? A truly safe level has not been established, although animal and human studies that have examined the drop and recovery of plaque pH after consumption of specific foods have suggested an annual intake between 10 and 15 kg per person per year.[32]

Two similar epidemiologic studies of the caries prevalence in 12-year-olds and the per-capita sugar use have been done. The first, conducted in 47 countries, showed a statistically significant relationship between the availability of sugar and the number of DMFT.[33] When the daily per capita supply of sugar was less than 50 grams, the DMFT index was less than 3.0 (Table 18–3 ■). More recently, a study in 90 countries showed a statistically significant relationship between the logarithm of DMFT and sugar consumption at a slope of 0.021 per kilogram per person per year.[34] It is interesting to note that this association disappeared when the data from only 29 industrialized countries were analyzed. This finding indicates that factors other than sugar consumption (i.e., oral hygiene, professional care, fluoride use) should be considered when explaining variations in caries prevalence.

It is erroneous to think that oral hygiene and optimum fluoride exposure alone will protect teeth from deleterious dietary practices. It is also an oversimplification to believe that simply removing "sugar" from the diet is an adequate approach to preventing caries progression. The caries-promoting activity of carbohydrates and sweeteners varies according to frequency of

TABLE ■ 18–3 Sugar Supply and Caries Prevalence in 12-Year-Old Children from 47 Countries

	Sugar Supply (gram/person/day)		
DMFT Index	**50**	**50–120**	**120**
3.0	21 countries	9 countries	
3.0–5.0		9 countries	1 country
5.0		1 country	6 countries

DMFT, decayed, missing, filled teeth.
(*Source:* Reprinted by permission from Sreebny, L. M. (1982). *Community Dent Oral Epidemiol,* 10:1–17.33.)

intake and combined intake with other foods that can vary in protein or fat content.

Processed, high-starch snacks, whether gelatinized, baked, or fried, produce as much acid in dental plaque as sucrose alone but at a slower rate.[35,36] Foods containing both cooked starch and sucrose have been shown to enhance caries potential,[37] which is enhanced because the starch brings the sucrose into closer contact with the tooth surface.[38] It is important to emphasize that added sugars can be part of a total diet when recommended intake guidelines are followed and when the sugars are eaten with meals while avoiding food and beverage intake that contains sugars or starches between meals for caries prevention.[8,39]

DID YOU KNOW ?

Cranberry extract prevents adhesion of *Streptococcus mutans* bacteria to teeth.

The modern understanding of the dental caries process, called the *chemoparasitic theory,* was described by W. D. Miller in 1890.[40] Caries is caused by dissolution of teeth by acid produced during the metabolism of dietary carbohydrates by oral bacteria. The resultant lowered pH favors the growth of *S. mutans* and other acidogenic bacteria. The two primary bacteria involved in caries formation are *S. mutans* and lactobacilli.[41]

Plaque composition studies have established that persons who regularly consume dietary components with a high fermentable sugar content have increased proportions of *S. mutans* and lactobacilli in their dental plaque, tipping the delicate balance of the oral environment to a more acidic, demineralizing role.[42] Significant factors regulating homeostasis in the mouth include the integrity of the host defenses (i.e., salivary flow) and the composition of the diet.[43] Stimulation of salivary flow or suppression of sugar catabolism and acid production by the use of metabolic inhibitors and nonfermentable artificial sweeteners in snacks could assist in the maintenance of microbial homeostasis in plaque and thus a reduction in caries incidence.[42] For instance, the use of fluorides, consumption of foods and beverages that contain nonfermentable sugar substitutes such as aspartame or polyols, stimulation of salivary flow after main meals by chewing sugar-free gum, and selection of a diet that favors remineralization (i.e., content high in calcium, phosphate, and protein) are all ways to prevent the lowered pH and breakdown of microbial homeostasis in dental plaque biofilms.[41,42]

DID YOU KNOW?

Casein phosphopeptide-amorphous calcium phosphate (CPP-ACP), one trade name known as Recaldent, prevents enamel demineralization and promotes remineralization of enamel subsurface lesions in animal and human in situ caries models.

POLYOLS AS SWEETENERS

Because of their sweet taste, several **polyols** are currently used as sugar substitutes. They are not sugars but are **sugar alcohols**. Each molecule resembles a sugar with the exception that an alcohol grouping (-OH) is attached to each carbon atom of the polyol (Figure 18–3 ■). Polyols can have a chemical structure that is derived from monosaccharides (e.g., sorbitol, mannitol, xylitol, erythritol), disaccharides (e.g., isomalt, lactitol, maltitol), or polysaccharide-derived mixtures (e.g., maltitol syrup, hydrogenated starch hydrolysates [HSH][8]. The sweetness of polyols varies considerably, and only a few of them suffice as sugar substitutes.

Polyols have 40% of the caloric content of sucrose,[44] which is an advantage to those limiting caloric intake for weight control. Another advantage is that polyols have physical characteristics similar to sucrose, so their substitution in products does not alter the overall quality, size, and weight of the products to which they are added. However, one disadvantage to using polyols in baked goods is that browning (i.e., caramelization) does not occur.

FIGURE ■ 18–3 Comparison of the structural formula of a polyol and common sugar.

Sorbitol

Sorbitol is a sugar alcohol (polyol) that occurs naturally in many fruits and berries. It is produced commercially from glucose and is on the GRAS list as a "bulk" sweetener for use in chewing gum, chocolates, jams and jellies, frozen confections, and other confectionaries.[8] It is only half as sweet as sucrose. Although considered noncariogenic, in solution it is slowly fermented by *S. mutans*.[45] In patients with reduced salivary gland function, it has been shown to be cariogenic with prolonged use.[46] Sorbitol is not easily metabolized or absorbed by the gastrointestinal (GI) tract and can cause diarrhea if large quantities are ingested.[45]

DID YOU KNOW?

Grape seed extract has shown a positive effect in the in vitro demineralization and/or remineralization of artificial root caries lesions. Oleanolic acid in raisins suppresses in vitro adherence of cariogenic *Streptococcus mutans* biofilm.

Mannitol

Mannitol is a naturally occurring polyol found in seaweed, but is also commercially obtained from the sugar mannose. Oral microorganisms metabolize this sweetener very slowly, so there is virtually no cariogenic activity with its use.[47] Mannitol is used as a dusting agent for chewing gum and as a bulking agent in powdered foods.[8]

Xylitol

Xylitol is the polyol that has received the greatest amount of attention by the dental profession for its anticaries benefits. Xylitol is a naturally occurring caloric 5-carbon sugar alcohol. It is nonfermentable by oral bacteria and exhibits antibacterial properties.[48] Discovered in wood chips in 1890 and in wheat and oat straw in 1891, xylitol is produced commercially from birch trees and other hardwoods that contain xylan. Recently, in an effort to reduce production costs, biotechnology has been used to produce xylitol from corncobs and from the waste of sugar cane and other fibers.[49–55] Xylitol's sweetness approximates that of sucrose; however, it is about 10 times more costly to produce than sucrose.

Xylitol is used primarily in chewing gum, although it can also be found in mints, mouthrinses, some dentifrices, slow-melting tablets, syrup, and candy.[56] The growing use of xylitol as a sweetener in low concentrations in foods and other consumables is increasing the public's exposure to xylitol and can have an additive benefit aside from therapeutic dose exposure.[57]

Xylitol can influence oral ecology through a chain of different antibacterial events. It

- Decreases bacterial metabolism and produces a less dramatic drop in dental plaque pH. Metabolic by-products produced by oral bacteria include xylitol-5-phosphate, which is a toxic end point. Very few oral species can use this substance for energy production.

- Reduces the volume and amount of supragingival plaque due to a reduced production of extracellular polysaccharides and biofilm matrix.

- Promotes the selection of xylitol-resistant mutans streptococci, which are thought to be less virulent and adhesive than xylitol-susceptible strains.

- Stimulates salivary secretion.[56]

These properties are suggestive of xylitol's ability to decrease the acid challenge on the pathologic side and promotion of remineralization through stimulation of saliva on the protective side of the delicate caries balance.[56]

Many studies have shown that xylitol creates a protective effect and reduces tooth decay in part by reducing levels of *S. mutans* found in plaque and saliva and by reducing the level of lactic acid produced by the bacteria.[45,50,58–62] In a double-blind cohort study in Belize, 1,277 schoolchildren were randomly assigned to nine treatment groups, consisting of four xylitol groups of differing doses, two xylitol–sorbitol groups of differing doses, two sucrose groups of differing doses, and one sorbitol group. When four blinded and calibrated dentist examiners carried out dental examinations at baseline, 16, 28, and 40 months applying World Health Organization (WHO) criteria for caries detection, the most significant caries reduction was found in the group assigned to the highest xylitol concentration.[58] In a more recent study by Hildebrandt and colleagues, xylitol chewing gum was compared with a xylitol mouthrinse, and both were found to cause a similar reduction in oral *S. mutans* levels.[63]

Evidence is sufficient for clinicians to consider including xylitol-containing products for the prevention of dental caries in high-risk populations (Figure 18–4 ■). However, sufficient dose and frequency of use must be followed to obtain the desired result. The following are guidelines for patient-based caries management with xylitol-containing products:

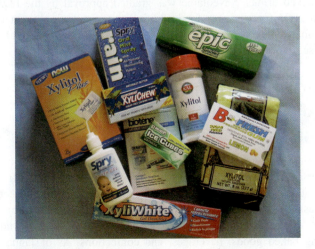

FIGURE ■ 18–4 Selected xylitol-containing products.
(*Source:* Courtesy of Jill Stoltenberg.)

- Patients at risk for dental caries could be recommended to use xylitol-containing products in addition to daily fluoride exposure.

- At least 5g of xylitol per day is needed to achieve an optimum therapeutic effect on S. mutans.

- Daily intake should be divided into three to four doses. Exposure time should be at least 5 to 10 minutes with each dose.

- Xylitol products that actively stimulate salivary flow should be recommended for use.

- Recommended products should contain as much xylitol per unit as possible and ideally with xylitol as the single sweetener.[56]

Furthermore, several dental associations, including the American Academy of Pediatric Dentistry, recommend clinical use of xylitol in children more than 4 years of age.[56]

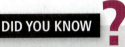

DID YOU KNOW

Xylitol has also been found to decrease ear infections in children.

Xylitol's effectiveness increases at a higher frequency of consumption as well as a higher dose. The main side effect associated with consumption of polyols, including xylitol, is osmotic diarrhea but only when consumed in very large quantities.[50] Nevertheless, those persons with preexisting gastrointestinal disorders should consider this potential problem before starting a dosing regimen.

INTENSE SWEETENERS

With regard to primary preventive dental practices, noncariogenic sweeteners and sugar substitutes used in foods, beverages, oral medications, mouthrinses, dentifrices, and candy are highly desirable for preventing dental caries and some adverse health effects. For these reasons, dental providers advocate their use.

Because of their intense sweetness compared with sucrose, noncariogenic sweeteners and sugar substitutes are used in very small quantities and thus, in the long term, are economical. The following section describes the most popular intense sweeteners currently used in the United States, ones currently being introduced into the market, and those used elsewhere in the world but not yet approved for use in the United States.

Saccharin

Saccharin is approximately 200 to 700 times sweeter than sucrose. It is nonnutritive and noncariogenic. It is the oldest of the artificial sweeteners used in the United States and is marketed under the brand name of Sweet 'N Low. Each year,

8 million pounds of saccharin are used in food: 2 to 3 million pounds as tabletop sweetener, 1 to 2 million pounds in beverages, and 3 million pounds in personal care products. Despite a decline in usage since a peak in 1982, saccharin remains the largest volume, lowest-cost intense sweetener used in the world today.[8,64]

Saccharin is approved for use as a food additive in foods and beverages, tabletop sugar substitutes, and gum. It can also be used in cosmetics and pharmaceuticals. Since 2001, products that contain saccharin no longer need to carry a warning about saccharin's association with cancer in laboratory animals. In 1977, the FDA proposed a ban on the use of saccharin because it was reported to cause bladder cancer in laboratory rats. In 2000, the National Toxicology Program of the National Institutes of Health concluded that saccharin should be removed from the list of potential carcinogens, and in 2001 federal legislation allowed the warning label placed on products to be removed.[65] The FDA has approved saccharin in the following forms: ammonium saccharin, calcium saccharin, and sodium saccharin. In beverages, amounts cannot exceed 12 mg per fluid ounce, as a sugar substitute it cannot exceed the sweetening power of 1 teaspoon of sucrose (20 mg) for use in cooking or at the table, and in processed foods amounts it cannot exceed 30 mg per serving.[8] The product label must list saccharin as an ingredient and state the amount contained per serving as indicated above.[66]

Aspartame

Aspartame, a dipeptide, is 160 to 220 times sweeter than sucrose. It is sold under the brand names Nutrasweet and Equal. Upon digestion, intestinal esterases hydrolyze aspartame to aspartic acid, methanol, and phenylalanine, which are components found naturally in fruits, vegetables, meats, and milk.[67] Metabolized aspartame provides 4 kcal/g, but because of its intense sweetness, only very small amounts are needed, so the amount of caloric intake is negligible.[8]

In 1981, the FDA approved aspartame as a sweetener in dry goods (i.e., tabletop sweetener, cold breakfast cereals, gelatins, and puddings) and in chewing gum. In 1983, the approval was expanded to include carbonated beverages. In 1996, the FDA further approved aspartame as a "general purpose sweetener" for use in all foods and beverages. More than 100 nations have also approved aspartame for use as a sweetener.[8]

Aspartame is available in liquid, granular, encapsulated, and powder forms. Soft drinks account for more than 70% of aspartame consumption, but it also is added to more than 6,000 foods, personal care products, and pharmaceuticals. The United States accounts for up to 75% of sales, leading the world in aspartame demand. One disadvantage of aspartame is that excessive heating causes decomposition and lessens its sweetening ability.[8] Another serious consideration is its ingestion by persons with phenylketonuria. Phenylketonuria is a homozygous recessive inborn error of metabolism in which individuals affected cannot metabolize phenylalanine. In persons with this rare condition, excessive intake of aspartame can cause higher plasma phenylalanine levels and many adverse effects.[68] The FDA requires that foods containing aspartame have the following label with prominent wording: PHENYLKETONURICS: CONTAINS PHENYLALANINE.[69]

Acesulfame-K

Acesulfame-K (acesulfame potassium) is a non-nutritive sweetener approximately 200 times sweeter than sucrose.[8,45] It was approved by the FDA in 1988 for use in dry food products. In 1994, approval was expanded for use in yogurt, refrigerated desserts, syrups, and baked goods. Acesulfame-K is currently approved for use in foods, beverages, pharmaceuticals, and cosmetics in more than 30 countries.[45] Interestingly, 95% of the consumed sweetener is excreted unchanged in the urine, so consumption does not affect intake of potassium.[70] It can withstand high temperatures, making it ideal for cooking and baking, and is available in granular forms to blend with other nutritive and non-nutritive sweeteners.[8]

Sucralose

Sucralose, sold under the brand name Splenda, is a noncariogenic and non-nutritive sweetener that is 600 times sweeter than sucrose. It is poorly absorbed (approximately 11%–27%) and is largely excreted in the feces and urine unchanged. Sucralose was first approved in 1998 for use as a tabletop sweetener and in a number of desserts, confections, and nonalcoholic beverages. In 1999, sucralose was approved as a general-purpose sweetener. In a review of more than 110 studies in humans and animals, this sweetener did not pose carcinogenic, reproductive, or neurologic risk to humans.[71]

Neotame

Neotame is a new product developed by the manufacturers of NutraSweet. It is very similar in structure to aspartame and has a highly intense sweetness with a clean taste. It is 7,000 to 13,000 times sweeter than sucrose and is heat stable for baking. It has been reported to be stable for use in carbonated soft drinks, powdered soft drinks, yellow cake, yogurt, and hot-packed drinks.[72] Neotame was granted approval by the FDA in 2002 for use as a food additive and sweetening agent to enhance flavor in several food categories. It is not approved for use in meat and poultry.[8,73,74]

NONNUTRITIVE SWEETENERS NOT APPROVED IN THE UNITED STATES

Alitame

Alitame is 2,000 times sweeter than sucrose without the bitter or metallic taste of most high-intensity sweeteners.[75] It is blended with other sweeteners to enhance the quality of sweetness. In 1986, a petition was submitted to the FDA for approval of alitame as a tabletop sweetener and use in products including baked goods, beverages, and confections. As of January 2003, this petition was in the abeyance category (i.e., deficiencies were found, a new petition must be submitted, and another review is necessary).[8] Currently, alitame is approved for use in foods and beverages in Australia, New Zealand, Mexico, People's Republic of China, and Columbia.[8]

Cyclamate

Cyclamate is more than 30 times sweeter than sucrose. It is currently in use by more than 50 countries worldwide; however, the FDA banned cyclamates in 1969 by as a food ingredient when the saccharin/cyclamate mixture was shown to cause cancer in laboratory rats.[76] The concern was that it could be toxic in some individuals who metabolize cyclamate to cyclohexylamine.[77] In 1982, the Cancer Assessment Committee of the FDA determined that cyclamate was not carcinogenic. Although this conclusion was reaffirmed later in 1985 by the National Academy of Sciences, the petition to reapprove cyclamate is still under review by the FDA.

Neohesperidin

Neohesperidin dihydrochalcone is 1,500 times sweeter than sucrose. It imparts a licorice flavor to foods and beverages and can enhance the mouth feel of beverages. In the United States, it is GRAS as a flavor ingredient but not as a sweetener.[8]

Stevia (Steveoside)

Stevioside is a natural sweetener extracted from leaves of *Stevia rebaudiana* Bertoni, a shrub in South America, also known as *honey leaf of sweet chrysanthemum* or *sweet herb of Paraguay*.[78,79] Extracts from these leaves are used in many countries for sweetening the following products: pickled vegetables, sea foods, soft drinks, soy sauce, and confectionary products. Stevioside is used extensively in Japan, China, Russia, Korea, Paraguay, Argentina, Indonesia, Malaysia, Australia, New Zealand, South America, and others, mainly as a sweetener in local teas, medicines, food, and beverages.[80] Collectively, these extracts are known as *steviol glycosides*.

A white crystalline compound, Stevioside is a natural herbal sweetener that is noncaloric and is more than 100 to 300 times sweeter than table sugar. Its sweetness is superior in quality to that of sugar in mildness and refreshment.[81] It is heat stable to 198°C, nonfermentable, and a flavor enhancer and possesses antiplaque and anticaries qualities. Stevioside must be kept in an airtight container to prevent moisture absorption.[82]

This phytochemical not only has been established as a noncaloric sweetener but also exhibits other pharmacological activities. Stevia leaves are also used for their medicinal properties in those with hypertension, obesity, topically applied as a dressing for wounds, and other skin disorders.[83] Other documented properties of Stevia are that it is antibacterial, antifungal, antiinflammatory, antimicrobial, antiviral, antiyeast, cariotonic, diuretic, hypoglycemic, hypotensive, and vasodilating. It does not possess neurological or renal side effects as do other artificial sweeteners. Mild stevia leaf used for tea has also been shown to offer excellent relief for an upset stomach. It is suitable for diabetics and phenylketonuria (PKU) patients as well

as for those intending to lose weight. No allergic reactions to it seem to exist.[82]

DID YOU KNOW?

Tea polyphenols can inhibit the sucrose-dependent adherence of oral cariogenic bacterium to the tooth surface.

Stevioside also supports the prevention of dental caries. *Streptococcus mutans* experiences growth suppression and secretes less acid when grown on media containing stevioside when compared to media containing sucrose, glucose, or fructose. It is also safe and nontoxic.[84,85–87] The routine daily consumption of 5 to 6 ml of stevia leaf extract per kilogram of body weight as a dietary sweetener is safe.[88]

Steviol glycosides have not been approved as food ingredients in the United States or the European Union; however, the leaves of Stevia or their extracts are sold in the United States as dietary supplements. In 2007, the Joint FAO/WHO Expert Committee on Food Additives (JECFA) declared that steviol glycoside sweeteners must be composed of at least 95% of the known steviol glycosides.[89]

Thaumatin

Thaumatin acts as a flavor enhancer and is a protein mixture that imparts an intensely sweet taste.[8] In the United States, thaumatin is GRAS as a flavor adjunct in a number of categories of foodstuffs.[8]

HEALTH CONSIDERATIONS

Obesity

Non-nutritive sweeteners have the potential to promote weight loss in those persons who are overweight and/or obese. Originally, the goal during development of the sweeteners was to provide a sweet taste to foods and beverages without providing energy (i.e., high caloric content) to persons wanting to control energy intake.[8]

Diabetes and Glycemic Response

Sweeteners do not cause diabetes, but high intake of nutritive sweeteners in a susceptible individual should be avoided because it has been determined that high intake of fructose can lead to high blood lipid levels for persons with diabetes. A safer alternative is to use non-nutritive sweeteners whenever possible.[8]

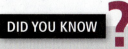

DID YOU KNOW?

Compounds isolated from licorice root can help prevent cavities.

Hyperlipidemias

Diets high in nutritive sweeteners have been shown to increase serum triacylglycerol and low-density lipoprotein cholesterol levels in short-term studies. Fructose has been found to be more hyperlipidemic than sucrose. For those controlling cholesterol levels, intake of this nutritive sweetener should be decreased whenever feasible.

Behavioral Disorders

Although once believed to be associated with excessive sugar consumption, hyperactivity is not the result of sugar intake in children.[8] It is important to note, too, that when the FDA approved use of non-nutritive sweeteners and accepted levels for consumption in children, no adverse effects were found if intake remained within the recommended guidelines.[8]

SUMMARY

A wide variety of chemicals can add to the sweetness of the human diet. Each sweetener has its benefits and its disadvantages. Nutritive sweeteners, which humans have used the longest, impart calories with their use, and they support dental decay with frequent oral contact. Nonetheless, sweetness is highly sought and highly valued by humans. It is no wonder that the market demand for both nutritive and non-nutritive sweeteners is so high. Humans' affinity for sweet taste is established in utero and continues throughout one's lifetime.

With the current push to prevent weight gain and dental caries and to control glycemic response in those who have diabetes, market demand will continue to drive the development of improved, sweeter, and more cost-effective non-nutritive alternatives to sucrose. Particularly with regard to xylitol as a phenomenon in the effort to prevent dental caries, consumers will see a push to develop more xylitol products for decay prevention as well as further efforts to cut costs associated with its manufacture.

PRACTICAL CONSIDERATIONS

Prevention and control of dental caries is one of the primary responsibilities of the dental health professional. Helping patients expand their knowledge of the strong evidence-based link between "nutritive" or caloric sweeteners and caries is a positive first step in reinforcing healthy behavior or planting the seed for behavior modification. In the United States, it is particularly important to also address the role of non-nutritive sweeteners and sugar alcohols in the prevention of systemic conditions such as obesity, diabetes, and other metabolic disorders.

Today's care is based on assessing each person's level of risk for contracting disease. Therefore, caries risk assessment tools are essential for establishing a plan for care. These tools most often include protective, risk, and clinical factors.

Dietary habits, frequency of eating, and use of xylitol are critical components. A patient/professional relationship based on good communication skills, trust, and respect can help transform patient behavior. For patients at risk for caries, elimination of caloric sweeteners is not the goal. Sensible reduction of intake and/or alteration of when caloric sweeteners are ingested (i.e., with a meal rather than between meals) should be the take-home message for patients. Non-nutritive sweeteners should also be encouraged. Recommending products with xylitol, however, have the potential to transform the oral flora and, therefore, have the greatest impact in reducing risk for patients. Dispensing such products from the dental practice, medical practice, or community clinic will increase the likelihood of use.

ACKNOWLEDGMENT

The authors extend their gratitude to the late Robert J. Feigal, D.D.S., Ph.D., Professor, Division of Pediatric Dentistry, School of Dentistry, University of Minnesota, for his thoughtful review and helpful comments during the preparation of this chapter.

SELF-STUDY QUESTIONS

1. The first recorded sweetener was

    a. Sugar cane

    b. Glycerin

    c. Xylitol

    d. Honey

Rationale: The first recorded sweetener was honey used in the ancient cultures of Greece and China and later replaced by saccharose, or common sugar.

2. The Institutes of Medicine suggest a maximum intake level of nutritive sweeteners to be less than what percentage of total energy?

a. 15%

b. 20%

c. 25%

d. 30%

Rationale: The Institutes of Medicine suggest no more than 25% of total energy provided by the intake of nutritive sweeteners; otherwise dietary quality suffers.

3. Processed, high-starch snacks produce _____ acid in dental plaque as sucrose alone, _____ .

   a. as much, but at a slower rate

   b. as much, and at the same rate

   c. less, and at a slower rate

   d. less, but at a faster rate

Rationale: Processed, high-starch snacks, whether gelatinized, baked, or fried, produce as much acid in dental plaque as sucrose alone but at a slower rate. Caries potential is enhanced because the starch brings the sucrose in closer contact with the tooth surface.

4. Xylitol creates a protective effect and reduces tooth decay in part by reducing the level of what acid that can be produced by cariogenic bacteria?

   a. phosphoric acid

   b. lactic acid

   c. malic acid

   d. sulfuric acid

Rationale: Bacteria cannot metabolize xylitol into lactic acid as occurs in metabolic pathways when refined or fermentable carbohydrates are consumed.

5. Sucrose is a nutritive sweetener that provides how many kcal/g when consumed?

   a. 0

   b. 4

   c. 8

   d. 12

Rationale: Sucrose, a disaccharide (one glucose and one fructose) provides 4 kilocalories/gram (kcal/g; approximately 16 kcal per teaspoon) when consumed.

REFERENCES

1. Tamussi, P. (2006). The history of sweet taste: Not exactly a piece of cake. *J Mol Recognit,* 19:188–99.

2. Sigman-Grant, M., & Morita, J. (2003). Defining and interpreting intakes of sugars[1,2,3,4]. *Am J Clin Nutr,* 78 (Suppl 4):815S–26S.

3. Mc Murry, J. (1998). *Fundamentals of organic chemistry* (4th ed.). Pacific Grove, CA: Brooks/Cole Publishing Company.

4. American Society for Neurochemistry. (1999). Neural processing and behavior 48. Molecular biology of olfaction and taste (part 7). In Siegel, G. J., Albers, R. W., & Price, D. L., Eds. *Basic neurochemistry. Molecular, cellular and medical aspects* (6th ed.). Baltimore: Lippincott Williams & Wilkins, 1–7.

5. Bright, G. (1999). Low-calorie sweeteners—From molecules to mass markets. *World Rev Nutr Diet,* 85:3–9.

6. Cohen, S. M., Anderson, T. A., de Oliveira, L. M., & Arnold, L. L. (1998). Tumorigenicity of sodium ascorbate in male rats. *Cancer Res,* 58:2557–61.

7. Lindley, M. G. (1999). New developments in low-calorie sweeteners. *World Rev Nutr Diet,* 85:44–51.

8. American Dietetic Association. (2004). Position of the American Dietetic Association: Use of nutritive and nonnutritive sweeteners. *J Am Diet Assoc,* 104:255–75.

9. U.S. Department of Agriculture. Economic Research Service. (2000). *Sugar and sweetener situation and outlook yearbook.* Beltsville, MD: U.S. Department of Agriculture.

10. Hanover, L., & White, J. (1993). Manufacturing, composition, and applications of fructose. *Am J Clin Nutr,* 5 (Suppl):724S–32S.

11. Briefel, R. (2001). Nutrition monitoring in the United States. In Bowman, B., & Russell, R. M., Eds. *Present knowledge in nutrition* (8th ed.). Washington, DC: ILSI Press, 617–35.

12. van Staveren, W., & Ocke, M. C. (2001). Estimation of dietary intake. In Bowman, B., & Russell, R. M., Eds. *Present knowledge in nutrition* (8th ed.). Washington, DC: ILSI Press, 605–16.

13. Macdiarmid, J., & Blundell, J. E. (1997). Dietary under-reporting: What people say about recording their food intake. *Eur J Clin Nutr,* 51:199–200.

14. Hirvonen, T., Mannisto, S., Roos, E., & Pietinen, P. (1997). Increasing prevalence of underreporting does not necessarily distort dietary surveys. *Eur J Clin Nutr,* 51:297–301.

15. U.S. Department of Agriculture. Products from the CSFII/DHKS 1994–96, 1998, 2002. Retrieved December 23, 2006, from http://www.barc.usda.gov/bhnrc/foodsurvey/Products9496.html.

16. Murphy, S., & Johnson, R. K. (2003). The scientific basis of recent US guidance on sugars intake. *Am J Clin Nutr,* 78:827S–33S.

17. Schiffman, S. S., Sattely-Miller, E. A., Graham, B. G., Bennett, J. L., Booth, B. J., Desai, N., & Bishay, I. (2000, February). Effect of temperature, pH, and ions on sweet taste. *Physiol Behav,* 68:469–81.

18. Davis, E. (1995). Functionality of sugars. Physicochemical interactions in foods. *Am J Clin Nutr,* 62 (Suppl):170S–77S.

19. Guthrie, J., & Morton, J. (2000). Food sources of added sweeteners in the diets of Americans. *J Am Diet Assoc,* 100:43–48, 51.

20. Schneeman, B. (1995). Summary of the proceedings of a workshop: Nutritional and health aspects of sugars. *Am J Clin Nutr,* 62 (Suppl):294S–96S.

21. Mardis, A. (2001). Current knowledge of the health effects of sugar intake. *Fam Econ Nutr Rev,* 13:87–91.

22. Rugg-Gunn, A. J. (1989). Diet and dental caries. In Murray, J. J., Ed. *The prevention of dental diseases* (2nd ed.). Oxford: Oxford University Press, 4–114.

23. Scheinin, A., & Makinen, K. K. (1975). Turku sugar studies I–XXI. *Acta Odontol Scand,* 33 (Suppl 70):1–349.

24. Koulourides, T., Bodden, R., Keller, S., Manson-Hing, L., Lastra, J., & Housch, T. (1976). Cariogenicity of nine sugars tested with an intraoral device in man. *Caries Res,* 10:427–41.

25. Kandelman, D. (1997). Sugar, alternative sweeteners and meal frequency in relation to caries prevention: New perspectives. *Br J Nutr,* 77 (Suppl 1):S121–S28.

26. Sreebny, L. (1982). Sugar and human dental caries. *World Rev Nutr Diet,* 40:19–65.

27. Orland, F., Blayney, J., Harrison, R., Reyniers, J., Trexler, P., Ervin, R., Gordon, H., & Wagner, M. (1955). Experimental caries in germ-free rats inoculated with enterococci. *J Am Dent Assoc,* 50:259–72.

28. Kite, O., Shaw, J., & Sognnaes, R. (1950). The prevention of experimental tooth decay by tube-feeding. *J Nutr,* 42:89–103.

29. Marthaler, T. M. (1967). Epidemiological and clinical dental findings in relation to intake of carbohydrates. *Caries Res,* 1:222–38.

30. Gustafsson, B. E., Quensel, C. E., Lanke, L. S., Lundqvist, C., Grahnen, H., Bonow, B. E., & Krasse, B. (1954). The Vipeholm dental caries study. The effect of different levels of carbohydrate intake on caries activity in 436 individuals observed for five years. *Acta Odont Scand,* 11:232–64.

31. Newbrun, E., Hoover, C., Mattraux, G., & Graf, H. (1980). Comparison of dietary habits and dental health of subjects with hereditary fructose intolerance and control subjects. *J Am Dent Assoc,* 101:619–26.

32. Sheiham, A. (1991). Why free sugar consumption should be below 15 kg. per person per year in industrialized countries: The dental evidence. *Br Dent J,* 171:63–65.

33. Sreebny, L. M. (1982). Sugar availability, sugar consumption and dental caries. *Community Dent Oral Epidemiol,* 10:1–17.

34. Woodward, M., & Walker, A. R. P. (1994). Sugar consumption and dental caries: Evidence from 90 countries. *Br Dent J,* 176:297–302.

35. Grenby, T. H. (1991). Snack foods and dental caries. Investigations using laboratory animals. *Brit Dent J,* 171:353–61.

36. Mörmann, J. E., & Mühlemann, H. R. (1981). Oral starch degradation and its influence on acid production in human dental plaque. *Caries Res,* 15:166–75.

37. Mundorff, S. A., Featherstone, J. D. B., Bibby, B. G., Curzon, M. E. J., Eisenberg, A. D., & Espeland, M. A. (1990). Cariogenic potential of foods. 1. Caries in the rat model. *Caries Res,* 24:344–55.

38. Sgan-Cohen, H. D., Newbrun, E., Huber, R., Tenenbaum, G., & Sela, M. N. (1988). The effect of previous diet on plaque pH response to different foods. *J Dent Res,* 67:1434–37.

39. U.S. Department of Health and Human Services. (2000). *Nutrition and your health: Dietary guidelines for Americans* (5th ed.). (Home and Garden Bulletin No. 232). Washington, DC: U.S. Government Printing Office.

40. Miller, W. D. (1973). *The microorganisms of the human mouth.* In König, K. G., Ed. Basel, Switzerland: S. Karger.

41. Touger-Decker, R., & van Loveren, C. (2003). Sugar and dental caries. *Am J Clin Nutr,* 78 (Suppl):881S–92S.

42. Marsh, P. D. (2006). Dental plaque as a biofilm and a microbial community—Implications for health and disease. *BMC Oral Health,* 6 (Suppl 1):S14.

43. Marsh, P. D. (1989). Host defenses and microbial homeostasis: Role of microbial interactions. *J Dent Res,* 68:1567–75.

44. Lindley, M. G., Birch, G. G., & Khan, R. (1976). Sweetness of sucrose and xylitol. Structural considerations. *J Sci Food Agric,* 27:140–44.

45. Roberts, M. W., & Wright, J. T. (2002). Food sugar substitutes: A brief review for dental clinicians. *J Clin Pediatr Dent,* 27 (1):1–4.

46. Wennerhoim, K., Arends, J., Birkhed, D., Ruben, J., Emilson, C. G., & Dijkman A. G. (1994). Effect of xylitol and sorbitol in chewing-gums on mutans streptococci, plaque pH and mineral loss of enamel. *Caries Res,* 28:48–54.

47. Imfeld, T. (1993). Efficacy of sweetness and sugar substitutes in caries prevention. *Caries Res,* 27 (Suppl 1):50–55.

48. Söderling, E. M. (2009). Xylitol, mutans streptococci, and dental plaque. *Adv Dent Res,* 21: 74-78.

49. Bertrand, M. G. (1891). Rechercheszur quelques derives du xylose. *Bull Soc Chim Paris,* 5:554–57.

50. Ly, K. A., Milgrom, P., & Rothen, M. (2006). Xylitol, sweeteners, and dental caries. *Pediatr Dent,* 28:154–63.

51. Tada, K., Horiuchi, J., Kanno, T., & Kobayashi, M. (2004). Microbial xylitol production from corn cobs using *Candida magnoliae. J Biosci Bioeng,* 98:228–30.

52. Latif, F., & Rajoka, M. I. (2001). Production of ethanol and xylitol from corn cobs by yeasts. *Bioresour Technol,* 77:57–63.

53. Buhner, J., & Agblevor, F. A. (2004). Effect of detoxification of dilute-acid corn fiber hydrolysate on xylitol production. *Appl Biochem Biotechnol,* 119:13–30.

54. Dominguez, J. M., Gong, C. S., & Tsao, G. T. (1996). Pretreatment of sugar cane bagasse hemicellulose hydrolysate for xylitol production by yeast. *Appl Biochem Biotechnol,* 57–58:49–56.

55. Santos, J. C., Pinto, I. R., Carvalho, W., Mancilha, I. M., Felipe, M. G., & Silva, S. S. (2005). Sugarcane bagasse as raw material and immobilization support for xylitol production. *Appl Biochem Biotechnol,* 121–124:673–83.

56. Twetman, S. (2010). Treatment protocols: Nonfluoride management of the caries disease process and available diagnostics. *Dent Clin N Am,* 54:527-40.

57. Milgrom, P., Ly, K. A., & Rothen, M. (2009). Xylitol and its vehicles for public health needs. *Adv Dent Res,* 21: 44–47.

58. Hayes, C. (2001). The effect of non-cariogenic sweeteners on the prevention of dental caries: A review of the evidence. *J Dent Educ,* 65:1106–109.

59. Ashley, D., & Barbieri, S. (2005, December). The use of xylitol in caries prevention. *Access Mag,* 24–27.

60. Peldyak, J., & Mäkinen, K. K. (2002). Xylitol for caries prevention. *J Dent Hyg,* 76:276–83.

61. Hansen, A. (2006, August). Xylitol: A dental phenomenon. *Access Mag,* 24–26.

62. Hildebrandt, G. H., & Sparks, B. S. (2000). Maintaining mutans streptococci suppression with xylitol chewing gum. *J Am Dent Assoc,* 131:909–16.

63. Hildebrandt, G. H., Lee, I., & Hodges, J. S. (2006, March). Reducing oral mutans streptococci levels with xylitol mouth rinse. *J Dent Res,* 85 (Spec Iss A). Abstract 1542.

64. Bizzari, S., Jackel, M., & Yoshida, Y. (1996). High intensity sweeteners. In *Chemical Economics Handbook.* Menlo Park, CA: SRI Consulting.

65. Department of Health and Human Services: Public Health Service. National Toxicology Program. (2001, May). Announces the availability of the *Report on Carcinogens* (9th ed.). *Fed Reg,* 66:29340–42.

66. Food and Drug Administration. (2002). Food additives permitted in food or in contact with food on an interim basis pending additional study. 66(104). Saccharin, ammonium saccharin, calcium saccharin, and sodium saccharin. 21 CFR 180.37

67. Ranney, R., Oppermann, J., Muldoon, E., & McMahon, F. (1976). Comparative metabolism of aspartame in experimental animals and humans. *J Toxicol Environ Health,* 2:441–51.

68. Wolf-Novak, L. C., Steginck, L. D., Brummel, M. C., Persoon, T. J., Filer, L. J., Jr., Bell, E. F., Ziegler, E. E., & Krause, W. L. (1990). Aspartame ingestion with and without carbohydrate in phenylketonuric and normal subjects. Effect on plasma concentrations of amino acids, glucose, and insulin. *Metabolism,* 39:391–96.

69. Food and Drug Administration. (2002). Food additives permitted for direct addition to food for human consumption: Aspartame. 21 CFR 172.804.

70. Walker, R. Acesulfame potassium: WHO food additives (Series 28). Retrieved December 6, 2007, from http://www.inchem.org/documents/jecfa/jecmono/v28je13.htm.

71. Food and Drug Administration. Food additives permitted for direct addition to food for human consumption: Sucralose. 21 CFR 172.64 (1998).

72. Witt, J. (1999). Discovery and development of neotame. *World Rev Nutr Diet,* 85:52–57.

73. Garbow, J. R., Likos, J. J., & Schroeder, S. A. (2001). Structure, dynamics, and stability of β-cyclodextrin inclusion complexes of aspartame and neotame. *J Agric Food Chem,* 49:2053–60.

74. Neotame. (2002). Retrieved January 17, 2007, from http://www.neotame.com.

75. Auerbach, M., Locke, G., & Hendrick, M. (2001). Alitame. In Nabors, L., Ed. *Alternative sweeteners* (3rd ed.). New York: Marcel Dekker, 31–40.

76. Price, J., Biava, C., Oser, B., Vogin, E., Steinfeld, J., & Ley, H. (1967). Bladder tumors in rats fed cyclohexylamine or high doses of a mixture of cyclamate and saccharin. *Science,* 167:1131–32.

77. Kojima, S., & Ichibagase, H. (1966). Cyclohexylamine, a metabolite of sodium cyclamate. *Chem Pharm Bull,* 14:971.

78. Geuns, J. M. C. (2003). Phytochemistry: Stevioside. *Science Direct,* 64:913–21.

79. Brahmachari, G., Mandal, L. C., Roy, R., Mondal, S., & Brahmachari, A. K. (2011). Stevioside and related compounds-molecules of pharmacological promise: A critical overview. *Arch Pharm Chem Life Sci,* 1:5–19.

80. Elkins, R. (1997). *Nature's sweetener.* Pleasant Grove, UT: Woodland Publishing.

81. Kinghorn, A. D., & Soejarto. D. D. (1989). *Med Res Rev,* 9:91–115.

82. Goyal, S. K., Samsher, & Goyal, R. K. (2010). Stevia (Stevia rebaudiana) a bio-sweetener: A review. *Int J Food Sci Nutr,* 61:1–10.

83. Kinghorn, A. D., Soejarto, D. D., Nanayakkara, N. P. D., Compadre, C. M., Makapugay, H. C., Hovanec-Brown, J. M., Medon, P. J., & Kamath, S. K. (1984). *J Nat Prod,* 47:439–44.

84. Thomas, J. E., & Glade, M. J. (2010). Stevia: It's not just about calories. *Open Obes J,* 2:101–9.

85. Grenby, T. H. (1991). Update on low-calorie sweeteners to benefit dental health. *Int Dent J,* 41:217–24.

86. Grenby, T. H. (1997). Dental aspects of the use of sweeteners. *Pure Appl Chem,* 69: 709–14.

87. Phillips, K. C. (1987). In T. H. Grenby, ed. *Developments in Sweeteners.* London: Elsevier Applied Science, 1–43.

88. Carakostas, M. C., Curry L. L., Boileau A. C., & Brusick, D. J. (2008). Overview: The history, technical function, and safety of rebaudioside A, a naturally occurring steviol glycoside, for use in food and beverages. *Food Chem Toxicol,* 46 (Suppl 7): S1-S10.

89. Joint FAO/WHO Expert Committee on Food Additives (JECFA). (2008). Steviol glycosides in combined compendium of food additive specifications, 68th Meeting of the Joint FAO/WHO Expert Committee on Food Additives (Online Edition). FAO/JECFA Monograph 4, Rome: Food and Agriculture Organization of the United Nations (FAO), Rome, Italy x, 61–64.

PEARSON myhealthprofessionskit

Visit www.myhealthprofessionskit.com to access the interactive Companion Website for this textbook. Simply select "Dental Hygiene" from the choice of disciplines. Find this book and log in by using your user name and password to access additional learning tools.

Health Education and Promotion Theories

Mary Catherine Hollister

KEY TERMS

OBJECTIVES

After studying this chapter, the student should be able to:

1. Define *patient autonomy*.

2. Explain the elements of the major health education theories.

3. Apply appropriate health education models to cases.

4. Identify principles of adult learning.

5. Use motivational interviewing techniques to devise a patient education strategy.

INTRODUCTION

In U.S. society today, health information abounds. Anyone with exposure to media has heard about the dangers of smoking, methods to control weight, and bad effects of high cholesterol levels; the individual also knows that every healthy diet should contain whole grains and lots of fruits and vegetables. If information alone changed health behaviors, our society would be full of fit, nonsmoking individuals with normal blood pressure and cholesterol levels.

Because the most common oral diseases, dental caries and periodontal diseases, are preventable, an informed, motivated patient, practicing basic preventive techniques is likely to have good oral health for life. Other risk factors, such as medical condition, history of disease, and access to dental care, can contribute to dental diseases, but lifestyle choices such as tobacco use, dietary choices, and oral hygiene practices play a significant role in oral health. Unlike family history, use of medications, and other factors that can affect oral health, lifestyle choices are under the patient's control. Therefore, it is the dental professional's responsibility to assist the patient in adopting healthy lifestyle choices that will promote good oral health. The most common method of assisting a patient with lifestyle choices is through health education.

Health education, also called *patient education,* too often consists of information only. The dental professional provides the patient information orally and in writing through pamphlets, Web sites, or other printed materials. The dental professional then considers the "job done." The obligation of patient education has been fulfilled. It is the patient's responsibility to take that information and change behaviors. This approach can be effective with a very small number of patients, but most nod and smile and go back to business as usual. Patients do indeed need accurate information to make a behavior change, but information alone is usually not sufficient to bring about a behavior change.[1]

HISTORY OF HEALTH EDUCATION

Early health educators often took a paternalistic approach to their work. Providers focused on a prescribed regimen and dictated behaviors to patients. The provider was considered the expert who imparted knowledge to the patients. Patients were expected to absorb that knowledge and change behaviors accordingly. Those patients who did not follow provider recommendations were often considered noncompliant and were subject to more "expert-to-patient" education.[1]

DID YOU KNOW ?

Patient education involves much more than the provider just imparting knowledge to the patient.

Over the years, the understanding of patient education has changed. Current health education theories recognize the importance of **patient autonomy**, which has been defined as the capability and right of patients to control the course of their own medical treatment and participate in the treatment decision-making process.[2] Patient autonomy is of prime consideration in giving informed consent for clinical procedures. In addition to consent for clinical procedures, however, the provider must involve the patient in the entire decision-making process. This means recognizing patient autonomy in providing patient education.

In recognizing patient autonomy, the provider allows the patient to decide the most relevant health issues to be addressed and encourages the patient to take an active part in both health behaviors and health management.[1,3] Enlisting the patient as an active participant, allowing the patient to have autonomy in deciding the best course of action to take, and helping the patient achieve those goals have proven to be much more successful in bringing about healthy lifestyle choices than the previous method of expert-to-patient information exchange.[1,3]

DID YOU KNOW ?

A little personal attention goes a very long way. Practitioners who took time to get to know their patients and tailored a personal health message found that their patients were much more successful at changing health behaviors.

It might seem obvious that all patients want good oral health, so decisions about healthy practices and treatments will be similar in most patients. Upon closer examination, this might not be as clear cut as it seems. Consider two patients with slightly yellow anterior teeth and one carious lesion on an upper first molar requiring a two-surface restoration. The first patient is a sales representative who is very concerned about the appearance of his smile. Therefore, less aesthetic amalgam posterior restorations and anterior veneers can be his treatment of choice. The second patient is very environmentally conscious and is unwilling to accept mercury-containing amalgam restorations. She might accept less aesthetic anterior teeth and request no treatment for them and a resin posterior restoration.

The following theories differ in approach and basic philosophies, but all theories currently being embraced in health education recognize the importance of patient autonomy and self-determination. It is important to note that each of the theories discussed has strengths and weaknesses. Each can be appropriate in certain situations; no single theory will be useful in every circumstance.

HEALTH BELIEF MODEL

First proposed in the 1950s by Hockbaum and adopted in the 1970s by the U.S. Public Health Service, the **health belief model** (HBM) was one of the first attempts to view health in a social context (Figure 19–1 ■). The theory was a milestone in health education because it placed a high value on the attitudes of the learner and recognized the importance of the learner's readiness to enact meaningful behavior change.

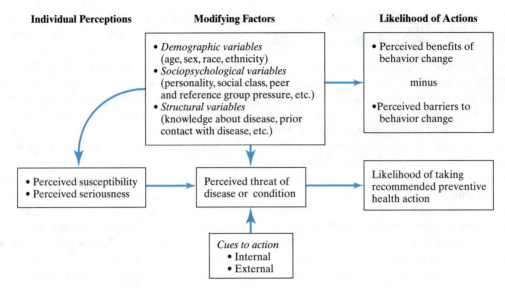

FIGURE ■ 19–1 Health belief model.

(*Source:* From Nathe, C. (2010). *Dental Public Health and Research: Contemporary Practice for the Dental Hygienist* (3rd ed.). Upper Saddle River, NJ: Pearson.)

The underlying principle of the HBM implies that individuals with better information make better health decisions. Hochbaum eloquently stated that "you will find it worthwhile to keep an open mind. If you are prepared to accept new concepts, you will understand yourself much better; with a better understanding of how and why you make your choices, you will be much better able to make them intelligently, independently, and maturely."[4]

The HBM is a staged theory; each step in the decision process depends on the previous decision or belief. Briefly, individuals must first believe they are susceptible to a condition; second, they must believe the condition is serious; third, they must believe there is a successful intervention for the condition; and last, they must overcome all barriers to using the intervention. Each step is contingent on the previous belief.

Oral Health Applications

Studies have shown good correlation between current actions and beliefs and correlating stages in the model. Cross-sectional research has found reliable correlations between oral hygiene behaviors and appropriate HBM stages.[5,6] However, research has not supported the HBM as a model that will produce predictable changes.[7–9] One possible explanation for the apparent contradiction is that, in cross-sectional studies, behavior is measured *after* the change has occurred. After a change occurs, individuals are likely to report that, as their beliefs changed, so did their behaviors. However, changing beliefs, as with only giving increased information, might not be sufficient for behavior change. That can explain why research has not confirmed the predictive value of the HBM.

The strength of the HBM is that it acknowledges the patient's values and attitudes toward health behaviors. Limitations are that increased information and changing beliefs might not be sufficient to cause behavior change and that behavior changes rarely follow a logical, stepwise progression.[3]

TRANSTHEORETICAL MODEL AND STAGES OF CHANGE

The **transtheoretical model and stages of change** developed by Prochaska, Norcross, and DiClemente is based on an individual's readiness to adopt a new health behavior (Figure 19–2 ■).[10] Like HBM, stages of change represent distinct beliefs and levels of readiness, but unlike HBM, stages of change include methods for assessing stages and helping patients progress through those stages. The transtheoretical theory states that, as individuals move through a series of readiness stage, certain behaviors and attitudes characterize each staged. Assessing an individual's stage allows health care workers and educators to tailor the intervention appropriate to the person's stage of readiness.[10] Key to applying the theory in a health education setting is accurately identifying an individual's stage of readiness to learn and to make behavior changes. Individuals might skip over stages or lapse to previous stages, but an awareness of the patient's current stage of readiness allows the practitioner to provide appropriate assistance in moving toward healthier lifestyle choices.

The six stages of change are precontemplation, contemplation, preparation, action, maintenance, and termination. In the precontemplation stage, an individual has little or no interest and no intention of changing a behavior. In the contemplation stage, the individual is considering making a change within the next 6 months. The individual will examine the pros and cons of making a change, carefully weighing the benefits of changing versus the costs of changing. In the next stage, preparation, the individual is ready to make the change and actively makes plans to enact the change. In the **action stage**, the change has been adopted, and in the maintenance stage, the change has been continuous for at least 6 months. The termination stage, often not attained, represents a stage in which the change is permanent to the extent that it is as if the previous behavior never

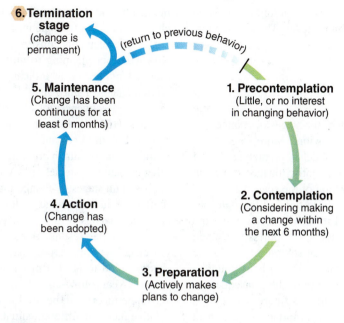

6. Termination stage (change is permanent)

(return to previous behavior)

5. Maintenance (Change has been continuous for at least 6 months)

1. Precontemplation (Little, or no interest in changing behavior)

4. Action (Change has been adopted)

2. Contemplation (Considering making a change within the next 6 months)

3. Preparation (Actively makes plans to change)

FIGURE ■ 19–2 Transtheoretical model.

(*Source:* Based on Transtheoretical model. (From the Ministry of Children and Family Development. Retrieved from http://www.mcf.gov.bc.ca/publications/privacy_charter/stages.gif.)

existed. Those in true termination are unlikely to return to the previous behavior.[10,11]

Individuals move through the stages using a process of decisional balance. They can weigh the benefits and costs, or pros and cons, of the change. Benefits can include health, emotional, or social gains. Costs can be represented by obstacles such as social pressures, addiction that creates a physical dependence on the habit, or merely a desire to continue the behavior. As the scale tips more toward the benefit end of change, the individual can move to the next step. Self-efficacy (explained more fully in the following social cognitive theory section) develops as individuals begin to believe a change in behavior is likely to affect an outcome. Because the individuals believe that a change is possible, that they have the ability to enact the change, and that their actions will affect health outcomes, a move to a more advanced stage is likely.[10,11]

The strength of the theory is that it allows the provider or counselor to provide the precise intervention for which the participant is ready. At each stage, the goal of the counselor is to assist the learner to identify benefits in the behavior change

and overcome obstacles that would prevent the change. In this way, the practitioner helps tip the decisional balance in favor of the change. The practitioner does not dictate behavior change, but the practitioner and the learner identify relevant, immediate areas of concern, negotiate goals, and agree on short-term behaviors.[10,11]

Health care providers can help learners move through the stages using multiple mechanisms. Consciousness raising, vicarious learning, self-efficacy, self-evaluation, and environmental evaluation are useful in the precontemplation, contemplation, or preparation stage. Raising consciousness can alert the individual to a severe health problem and possible outcomes. Media campaigns, television programs, or celebrity illnesses may have a great impact on the public's consciousness of a disease or condition and could affect a person's willingness to advance to a higher stage of readiness.[11] Vicarious learning can occur when individuals observe poor outcomes in others, thereby learning without actually experiencing that poor outcome. Self-efficacy is gained as the learner gains confidence that personal actions have an effect on outcomes. Self-evaluation and environmental evaluation assess personal habits and social environments that could affect a personal habit. Each of these strategies promotes autonomy in the learner and promotes a partnership between the practitioner and the learner in health behavior modification.[11]

In the action and maintenance stages, strategies such as counterconditioning and contingency management can be useful. By substituting one habit for another, counterconditioning can empower an individual to develop a healthy alternative for an unhealthy habit. Contingency management such as preplanning strategies for managing high-stress circumstances and rewarding positive changes can be most useful for helping individuals who have reached these higher stages. Those in the termination stage might provide assistance or counseling to others trying to change the behavior.[11]

Oral Health Applications

Research has recorded the validity of the stages of change and decisional balance in oral care behaviors. More research is needed to test the accuracy of the model in predicting altered behaviors for oral health care.[12] Currently, tobacco cessation is the most frequently used application of the stages of change with regard to oral health and has been verified through longitudinal research.[13,14] When used in tobacco counseling, the clinician must first establish the patient's readiness to change stage. A person who has no intention of stopping tobacco use would be a precontemplator. For this patient, a brief counseling session offering information on the health consequences of using tobacco and offering support at a future date should the patient decide to quit would be appropriate. A person in this stage might not be willing to set a quit date or develop quitting strategies. A patient in the contemplation stage would be considering quitting and might be willing to set a quit date. Offering support through counseling, providing information and quit aides through identifying quitting resources such as classes or support groups would be appropriate for someone at this stage. This patient is moving toward making a change, so frequent encouragement and information about the benefits of the change might help tip the decisional balance in favor of proceeding to the next stage.

The patient in the preparation stage is ready to make the change. This person could enroll in a cessation class or purchase nicotine gum or patches and should be willing to set a quit date and develop contingency plans to overcome cravings or trigger behaviors. Assistance for this patient can be writing the quit date in the oral health record, identifying plans for replenishing gum or patches, helping develop plans to overcome stressful situations that can trigger the desire for tobacco, and offering verbal encouragement.

A person in the action stage could be enrolled in a cessation class or using a pharmaceutical resource and would have stopped using tobacco products for 1 to 2 months. For this patient, frequent contacting to encourage continued abstinence, providing additional quit aides, completing a dental examination and prophylaxis, or taking other measures to support the current change is the most beneficial. Patients in maintenance who have continued the behavior change for more than 6 months might be willing to help others overcome tobacco addiction through peer counseling. This would also be appropriate for individuals in termination, although many tobacco users never reach this stage.

Prochaska, Redding, and Evers,[13] primary proponents of these stages of change, tested a staged intervention against a standard self-help cessation program by following participants for 18 months. Results were similar at 12 months. At 18 months, the staged group moved ahead. Behaviors and attitudes about smoking and readiness often match the appropriate stage in cross-sectional studies. A program evaluation at a clinic for the medically underserved asked smokers to assess their stage of change. Smokers who planned to quit within 6 months scored higher on statements consistent with quitting than did smokers who were not planning to quit. Decisional balance scores of those planning to quit indicated more concerns over negative consequences of smoking.[14,15]

The effectiveness of changes in health behavior that are based on HBM theory as the sole basis of interventions has been mixed. Longitudinal analysis of smoking cessation programs found similar results in programs based on stages of change and other cessation strategies.[15,16] A systematic review of clinical trials based on stages of change interventions found the approach ineffective in school-age children.[17] Cross-sectional and prospective analysis of a workplace smoking cessation program showed similar results. Behaviors and attitudes significantly correlated with the appropriate stage of change. However, the theory failed to predict progression through the stages at the 1- and 2-year follow-up.[18] These mixed results demonstrate that no single theory can be used in all situations. Each theory has relative merits in different situations. The challenge is to apply the appropriate theory in appropriate situations.

Stages of change is an important theory because it encourages the learner to consider pros and cons of making a change, and it encourages counselors to meet individuals at their particular state of readiness. Identification of the appropriate readiness to learn stage forms the foundation of motivational interviewing, which is discussed in the following chapter on tobacco cessation.

THEORY OF REASONED ACTION

The **theory of reasoned action** stresses the importance of attitudes and intentions to change a behavior (Figure 19–3 ■). According to this theory, the most important determinant of behavior is intention. Very few actions that produce a healthy outcome happen without ample knowledge and full intention to practice the healthy behavior. Two cognitive processes are at work to develop healthy behaviors: (1) belief about what

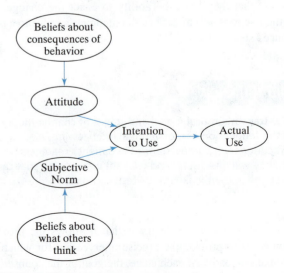

FIGURE ■ 19–3 Theory of reasoned action.

significant others think is important and (2) personal motivation to comply with those significant people. Other external variables that will influence attitudes and, thus, behaviors are internally processed within the context of significance.[19]

This theory is also called *planned behavior* because people make rational decisions based on knowledge, values, and attitudes. Therefore, a person's *intent* to perform a certain action is the most immediate and relevant predictor of carrying out that action. The two kinds of beliefs that shape intentions are behavioral beliefs and normative beliefs.[19]

Behavioral beliefs are those attitudes held by the individual alone. A person forms attitudes based on relative risks, benefits, and possible outcomes. Therefore, personal knowledge and perception of importance to personal health influence behavioral beliefs. **Normative beliefs** are those held by other people who influence the individual. If a certain behavior is expected or is the social norm or is expected by someone important to the individual, those expectations will have a bearing on an individual's intentions and, therefore, behavior.[19] Social norms might be formed in families, local communities, or larger societal communities. Celebrities' actions or experiences might influence social norms and, thus, health behaviors. When President Ronald Reagan was diagnosed with colon cancer, there was a sharp increase in tests for that disease. However, the effect was not sustained, and testing returned to previous levels within 6 months after the media attention dropped.

If the dental professional takes time to determine the social norms of a particular patient, the provider can use positive societal norms to assist a patient in adopting those positive behaviors as seen in the following example.

A 21-year-old woman who is 6 months pregnant with her first child presents for routine dental care. She has little knowledge of oral care for infants. She has a friend who gave her child a nighttime bottle with no ill effects, so she plans to do the same. However, she saw a television show on early infancy and learned that the mother's oral status, as well as nighttime bottle-feeding, could cause severe tooth decay. She wants her baby to have a beautiful smile, and wants her friends and family to think she is a good mother.

This woman's desire to be a good mother and please her friends and family are powerful motivators to learn how to care for her child. The television show on baby care might set social norms for her to follow. Knowing that she values her family and friends' opinions, the dental provider can ask about other oral health practices among her family members or friends. If she describes a person who followed healthy practices, the provider can suggest she consult that person for advice. Because she has indicated that she gathers health information from television, the provider can also suggest other reputable media sources of information and advice.

A limitation of this theory is the reliance on intentions, which might not accurately predict actual behavior change. Intentions will predict behavior only if they are stable and consistent. When faced with an unexpected obstacle, individuals might change their intentions and therefore not carry out the intended behavior. Another limitation of this theory is that intentions must be matched very closely to the behavior to have predictive power.[19]

Social norms and community expectations are powerful predictors of individual behavior, according to this theory. Used in a community intervention, the theory might be better able to predict the behavior of the collective community than of one individual. Social norms do not change as readily as individual choices. Therefore, social norms are more stable and provide strong normative beliefs to those in a close community.[19]

This theory helps explain an individual's perceptions of normal and expected behavior. The theory seems to be most successful in predicting behaviors that are completely within the individual's control and in which intentions remain stable, such as daily oral hygiene practices. Extraneous factors outside the individual's control, such as fatigue or change of environment, might quickly change intentions and therefore change behavior and outcome.

Oral Health Applications

The theory of reasoned action has been shown to explain behavior changes and predict planned behavior among a wide range of people.[20] Applying this concept to patient education, a teenager might consistently practice oral hygiene at home, but a change in environment such as moving to student housing at college can change intentions and behavior. Changes in the social norms or expectations of peers, change in routine, or fatigue associated with student life might affect oral hygiene routines.[21]

Community or cultural expectations can play a large role in affecting oral health behaviors. In communities where large numbers of children have early childhood caries, seeing children with crowned anterior teeth, extracted anterior teeth, or active decay can be regarded as a normal part of childhood. Changing the populations' expectations of acceptable oral health can make a noticeable impact on oral health and dietary behaviors.

DID YOU KNOW ?

The 6-month checkup recommendation came from a radio advertisement for toothpaste. Sometimes even professionals follow a practice because it has become an accepted social (or professional) norm even if the reason for that practice is unknown.

If severe caries (Figure 19–4 ■) is accepted as a normal part of childhood, caregivers cannot attribute personal actions to oral diseases. The clinician must assess the patient's/caregiver's dental knowledge and values to devise an effective health education plan. This approach could be applied to a local Head Start daily toothbrushing program. This program is mandated by the Head Start performance standards and is a consistent resource for Head Start students and parents. Dental professionals involved in these programs can apply the theory of reasoned action to encourage daily brushing, thereby creating a behavioral norm for the family. Social norms of daily brushing and use of fluoridated toothpaste that become firmly established within a family can have lasting effects, long after the children leave the Head Start program.

SOCIAL LEARNING THEORY

Social learning theory (SLT) states individuals do not learn or change behavior in a linear fashion. Rather changes take place bidirectionally; environment, information, and behavior all affect one another (Figure 19–5 ■).

As an individual learns more, behaviors and environment can change, causing more knowledge to be gained, which, in turn, reinforces behavior and healthy environments. This reciprocal determinism is key to understanding the theory. Behaviors do not move along a predictable continuum. Each element reinforces another as behavior is learned, practiced, reinforced in certain environments, and refined.[21]

Social learning theory was a product of behavioralists such as B. F. Skinner and others who believed behavior was a direct result of conditioning.[22] Psychologist Albert Bandura agreed with the basic tenets of the theory but placed a focus on personal agency and actions rather than pure conditioning. To refocus the theory from a pure behavioralist view, Bandura renamed the theory **social cognitive theory (SCT)**.[23] Self-efficacy, the main construct of the SCT, is the belief that one's personal actions will have an impact on outcome. Individuals with high self-efficacy practice forethought and planning, develop contingency plans, and put effort into overcoming obstacles. Self-efficacy is gained as information, behavior, and environment interact in a reciprocal manner. Lapses are a part of the learning process as the individual uses personal choices to develop behaviors consistent with individual choice and lifestyle.[24,25]

Self-efficacy is gained through several mechanisms. Enactive attainment, or experiencing success, is the most powerful method. As an individual gains new knowledge and puts that knowledge to use, the individual can personally experience

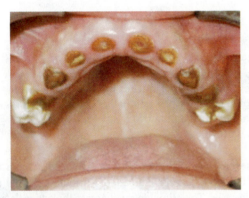

FIGURE ■ 19–4 Early childhood caries.

(*Source:* Courtesy of Sharon Peterson.)

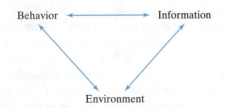

FIGURE ■ 19–5 Social learning theory.

the outcome resulting from the actions. Vicarious learning is another method of gaining self-efficacy. Individuals do not have to experience the effects of poor health choices if they can learn from others' experiences. The third method is through verbal persuasion. Affective states such as pain or fatigue will deter self-efficacy.

Enactive attainment, or performance accomplishment, allows the learner to experience the results of actions. Providers can assist this experience by encouraging the learner to model behaviors (participant modeling) or suggesting a trial period. Learners might not only experience a successful outcome but also might develop coping skills for stressful situations, or times when the desired behavior is difficult to continue. During a trial period, the learner can also develop unique methods of implementing suggested behaviors.[26]

Vicarious learning through modeled behavior allows the patient to develop expectations based on others' experiences. It also allows patients to learn of poor outcomes without actually experiencing them. A patient who has lost a tooth because of severe caries can be motivated to change behaviors to prevent losing more teeth. A patient who has not actually experienced tooth loss can adopt healthy practices to prevent tooth loss by hearing of someone else's behaviors and resulting outcome.[27]

Modeled behavior is not as powerful at changing behavior as is personal experience, so repeated encounters with the patient to encourage changes can be needed. Successes gained through repeated efforts by the model can be more influential than behaviors changed with ease. This concerted effort demonstrates the possibility of overcoming obstacles through planning and forethought, even in stressful situations. Modeling can be more successful if the model has similar characteristics to the patient, thus increasing the relevance of the model to the patient.[27]

Verbal persuasion is a necessary follow-up for those attempting to sustain a changed behavior. Persuasion will include assisting the patient to develop goals, determine expectations of outcomes, and formulate strategies for coping with challenging situations. Simply telling a patient what to expect is much less powerful than actual experience or personal testimonies. But verbal persuasion is an important component for tailoring a program to a particular patient and encouraging successful changes.[27]

One example is seen in the following situation. A 42-year-old male presents with severe generalized gingivitis and isolated 4 mm pockets. The patient has a family history of type 2 diabetes and hypertension, although the patient has neither condition. Upon questioning, the provider learns that the patient's father experienced loose teeth, resulting in the need for full dentures at an early age. The patient wants to keep his teeth.

The dental provider can use vicarious learning to explain to the patient how periodontal disease could have been the reason for his father's tooth loss. The provider can teach proper oral hygiene techniques to control gingivitis and schedule subsequent appointments to treat the early periodontitis. At a subsequent appointment, the patient experienced improved gingival health because of his oral hygiene efforts. Verbal persuasion will attribute the improved oral status to the patient's practices. Thus, the provider has allowed the patient to experience success through his own efforts (enactive attainment), allowed him to learn of poor outcomes through his father's experience (vicarious learning), and pointed out that the results are a direct result of his efforts (verbal persuasion).

Health behaviors will change as individuals gain knowledge, practice new skills, and experience changing environments. For example, a person might learn about nutrition from a medical provider or dietitian. The individual can then try a new recipe or food. The person can also attend a nutrition class, which in turn provides exposure to others who can share knowledge and experiences. Altered behaviors can produce desired results of overall well-being or weight loss. Frequently contacting the dietitian or attending nutrition classes provides opportunities for verbal persuasion to continue encouragement of new behaviors. Personal testimonies provide vicarious learning for class members. A continuous process of knowledge, experiences, and environment slowly changes the individual's understanding and behaviors. This process can be very slow, requiring frequent reinforcement of positive changes. Over time, self-efficacy is gained as the individual finds that changed behaviors can produce desired results.

Oral Health Applications

Self-efficacy has been an accurate predictor of oral health in both cross-sectional and longitudinal studies.[27–30] It has been shown to be a significant predictor of behavior in conditions such as managing diabetes and oral health.[28,29] Research using both quantitative and qualitative methods indicated that cognitive experiences and supportive and emotional dimensions, as well as childhood experiences, influence dental attitudes and behaviors.[27,28] Dental self-efficacy was found to be a determinant in oral health and oral hygiene among diabetes patients and for general oral health in adults and adloescents.[28,29] Self-efficacy has been shown to be consistent with improvements in oral hygiene over time, but the benefit can be short term only. Periodontal patients showed improvements in oral hygiene and dental self-efficacy 6 months after the initial intervention, but differences were lost over time.[28] Researchers have proposed that self-efficacy can be a useful part of a multidimensional model to predict early childhood caries (ECC).[30]

DID YOU KNOW?

Adults tend to continue healthy practices that began in childhood. Children who receive regular dental care are more likely to have routine dental exams and treatment as adults.[28]

A limitation of self-efficacy is that it tends to be domain specific, and similar domains can influence one another. For example, as a person gains knowledge about plaque control, self-efficacy can increase in the areas of personal hygiene in general. However, that self-efficacy cannot extend to other health domains. An individual can have high expectations that oral health is attainable through personal oral hygiene but low expectations in other health

areas.[28] Therefore, a patient can be confident in his or her ability to practice daily oral hygiene but has little confidence in having regular dental professional care. Such a patient can brush and floss daily but seek only emergency dental care.

LOCUS OF CONTROL

Like social cognitive theory, locus of control is an extension of SLT. As with SLT, environment, knowledge, and behavior interact to affect lifestyle choices. Developed by Wallston, Wallston, and Kaplan in the mid-1970s, **locus of control (LOC)** deals with perception of personal control over those elements and pertinent health issues. Internal LOC occurs when individuals think their personal actions determine health status. External LOC means individuals perceive others as being in control of health decisions and health status. External sources can be fate, chance, luck, God, or powerful others.[31] Unlike self-efficacy, which is domain specific, LOC tends to be more global. As such, a person with internal LOC would perceive control over health status regardless of the health condition, and an individual with external LOC would consider outside forces as influential in any health issue.

The theory has been refined since its introduction. As originally presented and in much subsequent research, LOC has been considered a global orientation to health behavior. Scales to measure LOC were designed to be mid-level in specificity so they could be used to predict behaviors or outcomes for any condition. Validation of the theory, however, has found this approach to be problematic because healthy people respond differently to the questions on the scales than do chronically ill individuals.[32] Several researchers have used the basic scales, but they found that they needed to be modified to measure specific diseases or conditions such as diabetes[32] and headaches.[33] Oral health research commonly uses the Multidimensional Oral Health Locus of Control Scale with items specific to oral health behaviors and influences.[34,35]

Oral Health Applications

Locus of control has been found to be predictive for personal health behaviors. Researchers found that individuals with higher internal beliefs practiced better oral hygiene and received more dental services than individuals with chance beliefs (external LOC). Those individuals were more likely to have lower oral hygiene scores and use dental services only as needed for emergency care.[35] Researchers measured psychological factors in a group of university students and then provided standard oral hygiene instructions. Clinical measures taken before the education and repeated 10 weeks later showed that LOC and strong dental health values were associated with oral hygiene scores.[36] This theory continues to be refined for use in various populations and conditions.

SENSE OF COHERENCE

Antonovsky took a very different tack in health promotion and disease prevention. Antonovsky's central premise is that it is more useful to study health than to study disease. He referred to this method of study as "salutogenesis," the beginnings of health. *Salutogenesis* defines health in terms of a continuum of ease to disease and the conditions surrounding the individual that provide coping resources. Antonovsky's objection to the study of pathogenesis is that it tends to dichotomize people into either a "healthy" or "ill" state. He contends there is a continuum of "ease" or perfect health with no limitations to "dis-ease" or severe disease or disability resulting in severe limitations of daily life. Most individuals exist somewhere in between these two extremes.[37]

The salutogenesis model closely examines the role of stressors and tension as contributing factors for health and disease. A **stressor** is defined as a source of disturbance that upsets a sense of equilibrium. This disturbance can come from external or internal sources such as illness, hereditary factors, job stress, or lack of personal control. Many sources of stimuli are handled routinely by an individual and are not stressors. Stressors produce tension, and it is the perception of stress and the tension response that has an effect on an individual.[37]

To deal with and possibly use stressors to enhance the life experience, people build a network of generalized resistance resources (GRRs). A GRR is more than a specific coping skill for a particular event. Rather, GRRs include all available resources at an individual, community, and cosmic level that enable people to manage daily stressors as well as cataclysmic events. A network of GRRs can contain a person's heredity, education, knowledge, finances, physical resources, values, attitudes, or faith.

Generalized resistance resources can help an individual avoid stressors as in practicing good health habits or avoiding dangerous situations. They can also enable a person to effectively manage a stressor and avoid psychologic, emotional, or physical impairment. An examination of the list of GRRs shows that they encompass a broad range of elements. Included are biologic elements such as the immune system, cognitive elements such as knowledge, material resources such as personal income or medical insurance, social factors such as support and social norms, and macrosocial support such as a belief in divine purpose.[37]

A GRR has an element of farsightedness. This quality allows an individual to envision coping strategies and anticipate the response of the environment. The coping strategy is not the actual behavior but the planned behavior. This strategy can give an individual a measure of personal control, but the actual response or behavior can be limited by circumstances such as physical ability or material resources.[37]

Sense of coherence is the main construct of salutogenesis and is central to a salutogenic orientation to health and disease. **Sense of coherence** (SOC) is a method of seeing the world and one's place in it. It is cognitive, perceptual, and social. Individuals who have a strong network of GRRs will develop an overall SOC that is global in perspective, that is, SOC can be used in any situation to deal with a number of various stressors. Individuals with strong SOC find problems manageable, comprehensible, and meaningful. Stressors are manageable if the individual has sufficient resources to handle the situation and the means to use those resources. Stressors are comprehensible if they are predictable or make sense and meaningful if the individual is willing to expend time and energy to deal with those stressors.[37]

Oral Health Applications

Researchers have found that a mother's SOC significantly associated with several oral health indicators in adolescents.[38] Strong maternal SOC was associated with gingival health, overall number of caries, number of anterior caries, and professional dental visits. No longitudinal studies have been conducted to measure the long-term impact of SOC on oral health. From a pathogenic perspective, a clinician diagnoses a condition and works to cure it. From a salutogenic perspective, a clinician can work with a patient on goal-oriented behavior that will strengthen the SOC, thereby moving the patient toward the "ease" end of the ease/dis-ease continuum. Sense of coherence will move a person toward consistency and stability.[38] The following case is a perfect example.

A 35-year-old female patient presents with multiple carious lesions. She says her family has "soft teeth," so she thinks her decay rate is completely out of her control. She also has difficulty controlling her weight and attributes her body size to her family history. Upon questioning, the dental provider discovers the patient has very good oral hygiene skills but lacks knowledge about nutrition related to oral health. She has been trying to lose weight and has been slowly sipping on a sugar-sweetened soft drink throughout the day.

The dental provider can increase the patient's SOC by identifying resources available to her for improved health through the dental office, Internet, and printed resources. She has dental insurance, so she is able to receive all needed restorations and regular preventive visits thereafter. She has established a trusting relationship with the dental provider, so she is willing to accept advice. By identifying resources, the provider has helped make oral health manageable. When the patient understands that decay is the result of personal behavior, the oral health becomes comprehensible. Through conversations with the patient, the provider has learned that oral health is very important to the patient, but she felt that tooth loss was inevitable. She now believes that she can save her teeth; therefore, she now feels her oral health is meaningful and is willing to expend time and effort needed to ensure good oral health.

Each theory has its strengths and limitations (Table 19–1 ■). No single theory will apply to all situations. Often combining pertinent elements of several theories will produce the best results. Researchers have suggested that multidimensional models can prove to be the most effective, particularly for conditions with multiple risk factors such as early childhood caries.[39]

Before deciding on a course of behavior modification for an individual, the dental professional must consider the patient's values and beliefs, readiness to change, perception of control, perception of the effectiveness of personal actions, and behavioral and social norms as well as available resources. If the dental professional is considering proposing a change of policy for a community, school, or other group of people, the primary

TABLE ■ 19–1   Summary of Health Behavior Models

Theory	Major Elements
Health belief model (HBM)	1. Perceived susceptibility
	2. Perceived seriousness
	3. Perceived effectiveness of the intervention
	4. Perceived ability to overcome obstacles
Transtheoretical stages of change	Behavior changes move through a predictable set of stages including:
	1. Precontemplation
	2. Contemplation
	3. Preparation
	4. Action
	5. Maintenance
	6. Termination
Theory of reasoned action	1. People make rational decisions based on knowledge, values, and attitudes.
	2. Intentions and behavior changes are affected by behavioral beliefs and normative beliefs.
Social learning theory (SLT)	Change is effected through knowledge, environment, and behavior.
Social cognitive theory (SCT) (self-efficacy)	1. Extension of SLT places an emphasis on personal actions.
	2. Self-efficacy is the belief that personal actions will affect outcomes.
	3. Self-efficacy is gained through enactive attainment, vicarious learning, and verbal persuasion.
	4. As self-efficacy increases, individuals plan for contingencies, and persevere through difficulties.
Locus of control (LOC)	1. Extension of SLT places an emphasis on perception of personal control.
	2. Internal LOC: Personal actions determine health status.
	3. External LOC: Other people or factors strongly influence health status.
Sense of coherence (SOC)	1. Health lies on a continuum of ease to dis-ease.
	2. Stressors move an individual to the dis-ease end of the continuum.
	3. Individuals develop a network of general resistance resources that reduce stressors.
	4. Individuals with high SOC find stressors manageable (they have the resources to cope), comprehensible (stressors make sense), and meaningful (willing to spend resources to deal with the stressor).

considerations can be social norms, community resources, and level of knowledge.

IMPLEMENTATION OF HEALTH EDUCATION MODELS

Once the dental professional has mastered the concepts of health education theories, the challenge is to effectively implement those theories for various target audiences. Implementation will be very different for children, teens, adults, communities, or other groups. The intervention's setting can also affect the implementation scheme. For example, different strategies can be needed in changing behaviors of independently living seniors as opposed to seniors with similar abilities who reside in an assisted-living facility or a nursing home. The following section addresses implementation of learning theories for various target audiences.

ADULT HEALTH EDUCATION

Adults have unique learning needs influenced by a wealth of experience and established practices that work. The goals of this section are to introduce some concepts about adult learning and to give some suggestions for using the previously discussed health education models for adult patient education.

Adults come to health providers with well-established habits and preexisting knowledge. Adults have achieved a concept of self-direction gained by knowledge and experience accumulated throughout their lives from various sources. As such, adults must be considered autonomous and self-directed. In a situation in which a self-directing adult is not perceived as autonomous, tension and resentment can develop and education might not be effective.[40]

Adults have been taught in school, had education from health care providers, and practiced health behaviors. Their current practices are a result of incorporating knowledge into practices that work for them. Adults will seldom change a behavior just from gaining new knowledge. When participating in an educational activity, adults know what goals they want to achieve. Therefore, information should be presented in a results-oriented manner so that adults will have a valid reason to change behaviors. Even with expanded knowledge, adults will need some help putting new knowledge into practice.[41]

A key point of adult learning is *relevance*. This concept applied here means that adults must understand why new information or a changed behavior is needed before true learning can take place. Self-directing adults must be considered partners in learning; successful clinicians will consider the adult's values, preferences, and biases of previous knowledge and experience. Adults must be ready to learn and might learn only those things that they perceive to be a benefit to daily life. The second key point is that information must be practical, which means the information presented meets the patient's readiness to learn and can be put to immediate use.[41]

Putting these concepts to work in a health education situation, the provider must, through talking with and observing the patient, determine the patient's interests, attitudes, and current knowledge. The provider must also assess what the patient is ready to learn and what information can be put to immediate use. Determining appropriate topics of education at any point in time might be tricky because the provider must first determine what those topics are. The counselor will have to interview the patient to determine current level of knowledge, interests, and needs. The provider must also refrain from giving the patient *everything*! If information is relevant and practical, it is more likely that the patient will try out the knowledge, observe success, and gain self-efficacy. Using these techniques empowers the patient, honors her or his autonomy, and allows her or him to gain self-efficacy. An example could be that a patient presents for emergency dental care to relieve pain. The dental provider provides the emergency treatment, proceeds to counsel the patient on additional oral health needs, and recommends a comprehensive dental examination. The provider can make the counseling relevant by linking oral health to other patient concerns such as possible diabetes or cardiovascular complications.

The provider makes the counseling practical by ensuring the patient has the means necessary to use the information immediately. Questions regarding insurance status, previous use of the dental health care system, and previous dental health experiences can allow the provider to help the patient act immediately on the recommendation.

How could adult education techniques be used in oral health? Providers should empower patients to be partners in care. To accomplish this, providers must concentrate on individual assessments of knowledge and interest. Discussing past dental experiences, oral health expectations, and previous successes can help the patient and provider identify treatment goals. This process will not be the same for every patient! Understanding that all education for adults must meet their immediate needs (relevance) and be put to immediate use (practical) will encourage patients to be an active participant in their health care.

Providers could be reluctant to allow patients to dictate treatment planning. Patients might not understand the need for certain treatments or sequences of planned procedures. The provider and the patient must negotiate goals. Patient education can be more successful if the following principles of adult education are used: the patient's need to know, the patient as decision maker, the patient's acknowledgment of previous experiences, and the provider's meeting patients at their level of readiness to learn and providing relevant and practical information. This approach allows providers and patients to work together in achieving healthy choices for better oral health.

One example could be a patient with type 2 diabetes who presents with a draining abscess, but the tooth is not causing any pain. Because of the lack of pain or interference with daily activities, the patient does not want to have the tooth treated. The provider can make education *relevant* by advising the patient on the impact of chronic infection on blood sugar. The provider can make the education *practical* by addressing other issues of concern to the patient such as anxiety, cost of treatment, or other perceived barriers to care. The patient then becomes a full partner in setting treatment goals. The patient can make fully informed decisions and is more likely to follow comprehensive treatment recommendations.

MOTIVATING PATIENTS

Learning is a dynamic process that involves *motivation* to learn and knowledge retention, reinforcement, and transference. All learners must have a motivation to accept new information or skills. Once the learner has a degree of incentive to learn or change behavior, the information or skills must be presented in a manner that will allow the learner to retain the knowledge and reinforce skills. *Positive reinforcement* occurs with a positive outcome and can lead to increased self-efficacy. *Negative reinforcement* occurs with a bad outcome and can come from the instructor or from natural results of behavior. For example, a dental provider can instruct a patient to floss daily. If the patient does not adopt that behavior and the gum tissue continues to bleed, that is a negative consequence of the patient's behavior. It is then the provider's responsibility to persuade the patient to continue daily flossing so that positive results can be achieved.[41]

Transference occurs when new knowledge or skills are applied to a different setting. It can be evident if a young mother learns about brushing and flossing and then teaches her children similar practices.

As in presenting education to adults, motivating the adult learner requires certain considerations. Six sources of adult motivation are as follows:

- *Social relationships:* Changing behavior to meet people or improve social activities.
- *External expectations:* Desire to please someone in authority.
- *Social welfare:* Desire to improve society.
- *Personal advancement:* Improvement on the job or achievement of a personal goal.

- *Escape stimulation:* Avoidance of boredom.
- *Cognitive interest:* Learning for the sake of learning.

Adults also have many barriers to learning. These barriers can include lack of time, interest, money, confidence, or failure to see the need to change. The challenge of the health educator is to minimize barriers and increase the reason for learning. A specific method of achieving this goal is through the use of motivational interviewing.

MOTIVATIONAL INTERVIEWING

As discussed in the previous section, learners and providers must be partners. This is a departure from the counseling style in which the provider is seen as expert and the patient as novice. The patient is the expert on identifying needs and concerns as well as his or her state of readiness to learn and change behaviors. The provider is an expert on the health condition and effective interventions. The provider must meet the patient at an appropriate level to assist behavior changes. A technique known as *motivational interviewing* has successfully used the principles of adult education, readiness to learn, and self-efficacy to empower patients to adopt healthy lifestyle changes.[42,43] Motivational interviewing focuses on patients' readiness to learn and change and helps engage patients to motivate them to progress along the stages of change model.

DID YOU KNOW ?

Understanding your patient's personal goals will greatly increase the chance of behavior change. Letting the patient set the behavior change schedule is empowering and allows the practitioner and patient to become a team working toward a shared goal.

Motivational interviewing (MI) is defined as patient-centered counseling that helps the patient resolve conflicts and ambivalence. Behavior changes are encouraged by encouraging patients to set personal goals as negotiated with the health care provider.[43] To effectively use MI, the provider needs to understand its spirit. Techniques, length of interviews, and number of encounters can vary, but the essence of MI is described in the key points outlined here:

1. Motivation to change is initiated by the patient, not the provider.
2. It is the patient's responsibility to determine conflict or ambivalence between different courses of action.
3. Direct persuasion is not effective in changing behavior.
4. Counseling style is quiet and encourages patient participation.
5. The provider must assist the patient in examining conflict or ambivalence.
6. Readiness to change is not stagnant or an innate trait but constantly fluctuates.
7. The counseling relationship is a partnership.[42]

Through interviews and observations, the learner and counselor work together to decide topics of immediate concern. The counselor must avoid the temptation to overload the patient with information. The patient will have more than one encounter with medical professionals. These multiple encounters offer the opportunity to expand education and improve health behaviors.

How do you determine the patient's current needs? Questions to the patient can reveal much about her or his current level of knowledge and interest. Some possible questions to pose regarding dental needs and oral hygiene practices include the following:

- What concerns do you have about your mouth?
- Tell me about your past experiences with dental treatment.
- What methods have you used in the past to clean between your teeth?
- What do you know about how to prevent gum (periodontal) disease?

Frequently, individuals with severe dental disease report no dental problems. If a brief look in the patient's mouth reveals obvious dental disease and the patient reports no problems, the clinician should stop after the first two questions and focus on the need for good oral health, possibly touching on the association between chronic oral infections and diabetes mellitus or cardiovascular complications. That would be an example of giving only relevant information. For a better understanding of MI, it can be useful to recognize characteristics of counseling that are *not* MI. Motivational interviewing has not taken place if the counselor:

1. Argues that the patient has a problem in need of change.
2. Offers direct advice without determining the patient's interest in change.
3. Adopts a superior attitude to the patient.
4. Does most of the talking.
5. Labels the patient.
6. Uses coercion.[42]

ORAL HEALTH APPLICATION

The benefits of MI have been demonstrated for conditions as diverse as early childhood caries and adult periodontitis.[44,45] Mothers of young children at high risk for developing caries were counseled using MI techniques; a control group received written information and viewed a videotape. Mothers in the experimental group received one session of MI and six follow-up calls within the first year. There were no clinical interventions for either group in the first year. After 2 years, the children in the experimental group had significantly fewer new caries than children in the control group. The researcher concluded that the MI techniques had a protective effect for early childhood caries.[43] Similar results were obtained by counseling adults with moderate periodontal disease. The MI group showed more improvement regarding bleeding on probing and oral hygiene scores than the control group.[45]

SUMMARY

Health education is complex and challenging. Providers must assess the learner's knowledge, interest, and values, must then identify the appropriate learning approach, and then design a personal oral health plan for the patient. This can seem overwhelming and not realistic within the available patient treatment time. However, after the provider has become comfortable with the various learning theories, determining patient needs and designing patient education becomes a natural part of the oral health appointment.

PRACTICAL CONSIDERATIONS

Have you ever made a big change in your life, particularly in a health-related area? Have you lost weight, started an exercise routine, stopped smoking, started wearing seat belts, or engaged in any other healthy lifestyle change? If yes, consider what helped you make those changes. You probably had access to accurate information. Was that enough to make a major change? Did you join a support group, journal your progress, or share your experiences with friends?

As you enjoyed some success, did you reflect on changes in your appearance or how you felt? Were you influenced by your surroundings or expectations of people you respect? As you think about your personal successes, compare your experiences with the health theories described in this chapter. You might find that at least one, perhaps more than one, theory could help explain how or why you were able to make better choices.

SELF-STUDY QUESTIONS

1. If a patient considering a lifestyle change is contemplating the benefits of the change, what stage will he or she move to as he or she makes plans to act on the decision?
   a. Preparation
   b. Action
   c. Contemplation
   d. Termination

   Rationale: Understanding the flow of decision making is critical to effectively use the stages of change model. This is true when presenting information and when engaged in motivational interviewing.

2. Adopting a style or action popularized by celebrities can be a motivating factor for behavior change according to which theory?
   a. Health belief model
   b. Theory of reasoned action
   c. Locus of control
   d. Stages of change

   Rationale: A clear understanding of social norms, such as peer pressure, is necessary to use this theory to develop a patient education plan.

3. Self-efficacy, the main concept of social learning theory, is an example of
   a. A global learning theory-skill in which opinions apply equally to all areas of health
   b. Domain-specific theory, which states that skills and opinions apply only to a specific health condition or behavior
   c. Mixed theory, which has features of both global and domain-specific theories
   d. None of the above

   Rationale: Self-efficacy is domain specific; therefore, individuals can believe that actions taken in one area such as nutrition can affect other health outcomes but that actions taken in another area, such as oral hygiene, can have little impact on health. Domains can overlap, but very distinct domains can have different levels of self-efficacy.

4. Sense of coherence is an example of
   a. A global learning theory-skill in which opinions apply equally to all areas of health
   b. Domain-specific theory, which states that skills and opinions apply only to a specific health condition or behavior
   c. Mixed theory, which has features of both global and domain-specific theories
   d. None of the above

   Rationale: Individuals with a high sense of coherence have a network of resources that address physical, emotional, and social needs. Such a network is comprehensive by nature and therefore applies globally to expected and unexpected health needs.

5. Encouraging a patient to set individual oral hygiene goals is an example of what patient education technique?
   a. Determining the patient's locus of control
   b. Counseling through stages of change
   c. Identification of the health belief model stage
   d. Motivational interviewing

   Rationale: Motivational interviewing is an education technique that uses many of the health models to assist a patient in determining his or her health priorities and treatment goals.

REFERENCES

1. Radely, A. (1994). *Making sense of illness: The social psychology of health and disease.* London, UK: Sage Publications.

2. Ascension Health. (2006). Healthcare ethics. Autonomy. Retrieved November 3, 2006, from http://www.ascensionhealth.org/ethics/public/isssues/autonomy.asp.

3. Wanyonyi, K. L., Themessl-Huber, M., Humphris, G., & Freeman, R. (2011). A systematic review and meta-analysis of face-to-face communication of tailored health messages: Implications for practice. *Patient Educ Couns.*

4. Hochbaum, G. (1970). *Health behavior.* Belmont, CA: Wadsworth Publishing, 70.

5. Pine, C. M., McGoldrick, P. M., Burnside, G., Curnow, N. M., Chesters, R. K., Nicholson, J., & Huntington, E. (2000). An intervention programme to establish regular toothbrushing: Understanding parents' beliefs and motivating children. *Int Dent J* (Suppl):312–23.

6. Nakazono, T. T., Davidson, P. L., & Anderson, P. M. (1997). Oral health beliefs in diverse populations. *Adv Dent Res,* 11:235–44.

7. McCall, K. D., Glasgow, R. E., & Gustafson, C. (1985). Predicting levels of dental behaviors. *J Am Dent Assoc,* 111:601–5.

8. Weisenburg, N., Kegeles, S. S., & Lund, A. K. (1980). Children's health beliefs and acceptance of dental preventive activity. *J Health Soc Behav* 21:59–74.

9. Groner, J. A., Ahijevych, K., Grossman, L. K., Rich, L. N. (2000). The impact of a brief intervention on maternal smoking behavior. *Pediatrics,* 105:267–71.

10. Prochaska, J. O., Norcross, J. C., & DiClemente, C. C. (1994). *Changing for good.* New York: Avon Books.

11. Prochaska, J. O., Redding, C. A., & Evers, K. E. (1997). *Health behavior and education.* San Francisco, CA: Jossey-Bass.

12. Bertrand, J. T., & Anhang, R. (2006). The effectiveness of mass media in changing HIV/AIDS-related behaviour among young people in developing countries. *World Health Organ Tech Rep Ser,* 938:205–41.

13. Tillis, T. S., Stoch, D. J., Cross-Poline, G. N., Annan, S. D., Astroth, D. B., & Wolfe, P. (2003). The transtheoretical model applied to an oral self-care behavior change: Development and testing of instruments for stages of change and decisional balance. *J Dent Hyg,* 77:16–25.

14. Amomori, M., Korhonen, T., Kinnunen, T., Michie, S., & Murtoma, H. (2011). Enhancing implementation of tobacco use prevention and cessation counseling guideline among dental providers: A cluster randomized controlled trial. *Implement Sci.*

15. Lawrence, T., Aveyard, P., Evans, O., & Cheng, K. K. (2003). A cluster randomised controlled trial of smoking cessation in pregnant women comparing interventions based on the transtheoretical (stages of change) model to standard care. *Tob Control,* 12:168–77.

16. Carlson, L. E., Taezner, P., Koopmans, J., & Casebeer, A. (2003). Predictive value of aspects of the Transtheoretical Model on smoking cessation in a community-based, large-group cognitive behavioral program. *Addic Behav,* 28:725–40.

17. Aveyard, P., Cheng, K. K., Almond, J., Sherratt, E., Lancashire, R., Lawrence, T., Griffin, C., & Evans, O. (1993). Cluster randomised controlled trial of expert system based on the transtheoretical ("stages of change") model for smoking prevention and cessation in schools. *British Med J,* 319:948–53.

18. Herzog, T. A., Abrams, D. B., Emmons, K. M., Linnan, L. A., & Schadel, W. G. (1999). Do processes of change predict smoking stage movements: A prospective analysis of the transtheoretical model. *Health Psychol,* 18:369–75.

19. Ajzen, I., & Fishbein, M. (1980). *Understanding attitudes and predicting social behavior.* Englewood Cliffs, NJ: Prentice Hall.

20. Buunk-Werkhoven, Y. A., Dijkstra, A., & Van Der Schans, C. P. (2010). Determinants of oral hygiene behavior: A study based on the theory of planned behavior. *Community Dent Oral Epidemiol.*

21. Hollander, E. P., & Hunt, R. G., Eds. (1976). *Current perspectives in social psychology* (4th ed.). London, UK: University Press.

22. Collier, G., Minton, H. L., & Reynolds, G., Eds. (1991). *Currents of thought in American social psychology.* New York, NY: Oxford Press.

23. Bandura, A. (1986). *Social foundation of thought and action: A social cognitive theory.* Englewood Cliffs, NJ: Prentice Hall.

24. Bandura, A. (2001). Social cognitive theory: An agentic perspective. *Annu Rev Psychol,* 52:1–26.

25. Bandura, A. (1997). *Self efficacy: The exercise of control.* New York, NY: Freeman.

26. Bandura, A. (1977). Self-efficacy: Toward a unifying theory of behavioral change. *Psycholog Rev,* 84:191–215.

27. Lee, K. Y, Wong, M. C. M., Lam, K. F., & Schwartz, E. (2011). Age, period, and cohort analysis of regular dental care behavior and edentulism: A marginal approach. *BMC Oral Health.*

28. Syrjala, A. M., Kneckt, M. C., & Knuuttila, M. L. (1999). Dental self-efficacy as a determinant to oral health behaviour, oral hygiene and HbA1c level among diabetic patients. *J Clin Periodontol,* 26:616–21.

29. Vakili, M., Zohreh, R., Haidar, N., & Parastoo, Y. (2011). Determinants of oral health behaviors among high school students in Shahrekord, Iran based on Health Promotion Model. *J Dent Hyg,* 85:39–48.

30. Litt, M. D., Reisine, S., & Tinanoff, N. (1995). Multidimensional causal model of dental caries development in low-income preschool children. *Pub Health Rep,* 11: 607–17.

31. Wallston, K. A., Stein, M. A., & Smith, C. A. (1994). Form C of the MCHL scales: A condition specific measurement of locus of control. *J Pers Assess,* 63:534–53.

32. Ferraro, L. A., Price, J. H., Desmond, S. M., & Roberts, S. M. (1987). Development of a diabetes locus of control scale. *Psychol Rep,* 61:763–70.

33. Vandecreek, L., & Odonnell, F. (1992). Psychometric characteristics of the headache-specific locus of control scale. *Headache,* 32:239–41.

34. Baker, S. R., Mat, A., & Robinson, P. G. (2010). What psychosocial factors influence adolescents' oral health? *J Dent Res,* 89:1230–35.

35. Peker, K., & Bermek, G. (2010). Oral health: Locus of control, health behavior, self-rated oral health and socio-demographic factors in Istanbul adults. *Acta Odontol Scand,* 69:54–64.

36. Stenstrom, U., Einarson, S., Jacobsson, B., Lindmark, U., Wenander, A., & Hugoson, A. (2009). The importance of psychological factors in the maintenance of oral health: A study of Swedish university students. *Oral Health Prev Dent,* 7: 225–33.

37. Antonovsky, A. (1979). *Health stress and coping.* San Francisco, CA: Jossey-Bass.

38. de Silva, A. N, Mendoca, M. H., & Vettore, M. V. (2011) The association between low socioeconomic status mother's Sense of

Coherence and their child's utilization of dental care. *Community Dent Oral Epidemiol,* 39(2):115–26.

39. Atherton, J. S. (2005). Knowles' andragogy: An angle on adult learning. Retrieved October 9, 2006, from http://www.learningandteaching.info/learning/knowlesa.htm.

40. Leib, S. (1991). Principles of adult learning. Retrieved November 27, 2006, from http://honolulu.hawaii.edu/intranet/committees/FacDevCom/guidebk/teachtip/adults-2.htm.

41. Weinstein, P., Harrison, R., & Benton, T. (2006). Motivating mothers to prevent caries: Confirming the beneficial effect of counseling. *J Am Dent Assoc,* 137:789–93.

42. Rollnick, S., & Miller, W. Motivational interviewing: What is it? Retrieved November 27, 2006.

43. Heinz, S. J. (2010). Teaching dental students motivational interviewing techniques: Analysis of a third year class assignment. *J Dent Educ,* 72: 1351–57.

44. Weinstein, P., Harrison, R., & Benton, T. (2006) Motivating mothers to prevent caries: Confirming the beneficial effect of counseling. *J Am Dent Asso,* 137:789–93.

45. Jonsson, B., Ohrn, K., Lindberg, P., & Oscarson, N. (2010). Evaluation of an individually tailored oral health education programme on periodontal health. *J Clin Periodontol,* 37(10): 912–19.

PEARSON
myhealthprofessionskit™

Visit www.myhealthprofessionskit.com to access the interactive Companion Website for this textbook. Simply select "Dental Hygiene" from the choice of disciplines. Find this book and log in by using your user name and password to access additional learning tools.

Tobacco Cessation

Joan M. Davis

OBJECTIVES

After studying this chapter, the student should be able to:

1. Describe population characteristics of tobacco users in the United States and the resultant morbidity and mortality.

2. Describe the oral diseases and lesions related to the use of tobacco, both smoked and smokeless.

3. Describe the different types of tobacco and their uses, emphasizing the harmful toxins, carcinogens, and nicotine levels in both smoked and smokeless tobacco.

4. Describe the process of nicotine addiction as a chemical dependence as well as the behavioral and social aspects of the addiction process.

5. Identify the specific FDA-approved pharmacotherapies available for tobacco cessation, including nicotine-replacement therapy and oral medication as well as emphasizing the appropriate assessment of the dependence level to nicotine and the most beneficial use of available medications.

6. Identify the various components of an effective tobacco-dependence intervention using the Public Health Service Guideline, stages of change model, and motivation for behavior change.

7. Describe the specific components of a tobacco-dependence intervention in the dental office setting, emphasizing the specific roles of the dental team for a comprehensive program.

8. Identify the elements of successful tobacco-prevention strategies in the office and community settings.

KEY TERMS

Bidis, 344
Clove cigarettes, 345
Dose response, 343
Fagerstrom Test for Nicotine Dependence (FTND), 349
Kreteks, 345
Main-stream smoke, 344
Reverse-smoking, 346
Second-hand smoke, 341
Side-stream smoke, 344
Smokeless (spit) tobacco, 342
Substance dependence, 347
Water pipes, 345

INTRODUCTION

Dental providers have a unique opportunity to see basically healthy individuals, often throughout their entire lives. This regular, long-term contact provides the clinician the opportunity to identify tobacco use and provide appropriate tobacco intervention based on both clinical findings and a supportive, patient-centered relationship. For those patients who have not initiated tobacco use or quit using tobacco, the clinician has the opportunity to encourage a tobacco-free life.

TOBACCO USE: MORBIDITY, MORTALITY, AND U.S. POPULATION TRENDS

Tobacco use continues to be the primary cause of preventable death and disease in the United States; approximately 443,000 premature deaths are attributed to smoking annually.[1] Of these estimated premature deaths of adults 35 year or older, 41% were attributed to lung cancer, 33% to cardiovascular disease, and 26% to respiratory disease. Lung cancer, chronic obstructive pulmonary disease (COPD), and ischemic heart disease are the top three causes of death due to smoking.[1] In the *Surgeon General's How Tobacco Smoke Causes Disease: The Biology and Behavioral Basis for Smoking-Attributable Disease,* Department of Health and Human Services Secretary Sebelis stated that smoking continues to be the leading cause of preventable death in the United States and that it is the time to use the evidence-based knowledge and tools to make a profound difference in the lives of generations to come. This report provided definitive evidence that smoking was a causative factor for numerous diseases in addition to lung cancer (Figure 20–1 ■), including but not limited to the following cancers: laryngeal, oral, pharynx, esophageal, pancreatic, bladder and kidney, cervical, endometrial, stomach, and acute leukemia.[2]

Fortunately, tobacco use in the United States fell from 42% of adult smokers 18 years and older (51.9% males, 33.9 % females) in 1965 to 20.6% of adult smokers (23.5% males, 17.9% females) in 2009[3]; 3.5% Americans over 18 years old reported using smokeless tobacco in 2007.[4] It is estimated that the decline in smoking over the past 50 years has resulted in the reduction of approximately 40% of deaths due to lung cancer in males.[5] See Table 20–1 ■ for a breakdown of characteristics of the estimated 45.1 million people 18 years or older who report smoking every day. Unfortunately, the decline in adult smoking has stalled over the past several years. Much needs to be done to meet the objectives of *Healthy People 2020* of reducing adult smoking levels to 12.0% and smokeless levels to 0.3%.[6] Focused public health efforts are needed to prevent initiation of tobacco use; a need also exists for expanded cessation and policy measures focused on the populations with the highest percentage of smoking, those with a general education diploma at 43.2%, those below the poverty level at 29.9%, and Native American/Alaska Indian native populations.[3]

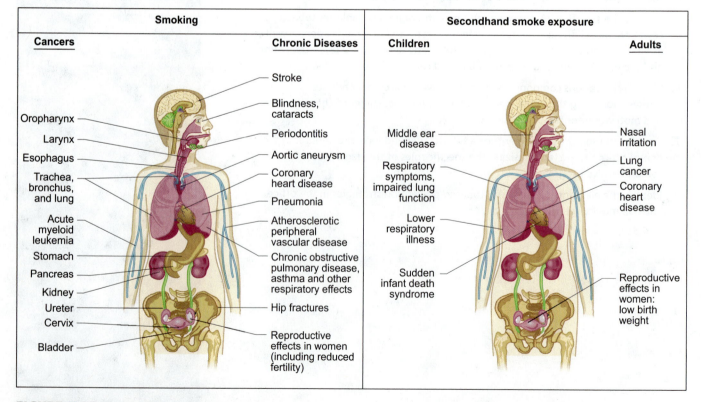

FIGURE ■ 20–1 How tobacco smoke causes disease.

(*Source:* U.S. Department of Health and Human Services. (2010). *How tobacco smoke causes disease: The biology and behavioral basis for smoking-attributable disease.* Rockville, MD: Public Health Service, Office of Surgeon General.)

TABLE ■ 20–1 Characteristics of Adults over 18 Years Who Are Current Smokers from the National Health Interview Survey, United States, 2009

Race/Ethnicity	Percentage
White	22.1%
Black	21.3
Hispanic	14.5
Native American/ Alaskan Native	23.2
Asian	12.0
Education	
0–12 yrs (no diploma)	26.4
9–11 yrs	33.6
GED diploma	49.0
High school grad.	25.0
Assoc. degree	19.7
Some college	22.3
Undergrad degree	5.6
Graduate degree	7.1
Age	
18–24	21.8
25–44	24.0
45–64	21.9
> 65	9.5
Poverty status	
At or above	19.4
Below	31.1
TOTAL	20.6% (46.6 million)

(*Source:* Centers for Disease Control and Prevention. (2010). Adult Tobacco Survey – 19 states, 2003–2007. *MMWR Morb Mortal Wkly Rep*, 59(SS-3):1–25.)

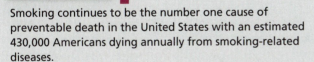

DID YOU KNOW

Smoking continues to be the number one cause of preventable death in the United States with an estimated 430,000 Americans dying annually from smoking-related diseases.

Initiation of tobacco use continues to occur primarily before the age of 18 years with 46.3% of students in grades 9 through 12 reporting having tried cigarette smoking sometime in their lives.[7] Although youth rarely encounter the known chronic health effects as a result of smoking, this risk behavior can lead to the establishment of a life-long use of tobacco and a much higher risk of developing smoking-related diseases. A total of 19.5% of high school students reported current cigarette use and 8.9% reported using smokeless (15.0% males, 2.2% females) in the past 30 days.[7,8] As with the tobacco-use trend reported in adult data, reported youth tobacco use has also declined, but much needs to be done to reach the *Healthy People 2020* goal of less than 16%.[6]

The harm of tobacco smoke is not limited to those who are actually lighting up and smoking. **Second-hand smoke** is responsible for premature death and disease for nonsmokers who are exposed to it. Between 2007 and 2008, it is estimated that 88 million nonsmokers were exposed to second-hand smoke. Of those, 32 million children were exposed to the hundreds of toxins found in second-hand smoke.[4] This exposure can lead to an increased risk of acute respiratory infection, ear infections, and more severe asthma in children as well as coronary heart disease and lung cancer in nonsmoking adults exposed to second-hand smoke.[9] Indoor air laws are designed to protect the health and welfare of both workers and patrons, not to limit the rights of others. Smoke-free initiatives are evidence-based health and safety initiatives and need to be supported.

DID YOU KNOW

As of January 2011, a total of 35 states and territories had laws in effect that require 100% smoke-free workplaces. See www.no-smoke.org for an update of smoke-free laws.

TOBACCO-RELATED ORAL DISEASES AND LESIONS

The Directors for the National Cancer Institute and the National Institute for Dental Research emphasized that helping patients to stop using tobacco can be the single most important service dental professionals can provide for their patients' health. The physical consequences of using smoked and/or **smokeless (spit) tobacco** on the oral cavity are numerous and potentially life threatening (Table 20–2 ■).[10] Although the oral effects of smoked and smokeless tobacco are sometimes presented together, the actual tissue changes, damage, or disease caused by each type of tobacco are often unique to the specific form of tobacco used. All forms of tobacco contain the addictive drug nicotine as well as cancer-causing nitrosamines; however, when tobacco is burned, more than an additional 4,000 chemicals are generated and inhaled with each puff, causing a higher level of harm. The vast majority of reported health consequences of tobacco use are referring to smoked, not smokeless, tobacco.[2] For example, tobacco that is smoked has been clearly shown to be a causative factor in the development of periodontitis[11] whereas smokeless tobacco has not. It is important to remember, though, that there is no safe or harmless tobacco product. All forms of tobacco are harmful and can lead to chemical dependence; therefore, one form should never be substituted for another.

TABLE ■ 20–2   Oral Lesions and Conditions Related to Tobacco Use

Oral cancer (smoked & smokeless)
Leukoplakia (smoked)
    Homogeneous leukoplakia
    Nonhomogeneous leukoplakia (precancer)
        Verrucous leukoplakia
        Nodular leukoplakia
        Erythroleukoplakia
Other tobacco-induced oral mucosal conditions
    Snuff dipper's lesions (smokeless only)
    Smoker's palate (nicotine stomatitis; smoked only)
    Smoker's melanosis
Tobacco-associated effects on the teeth and supporting tissues
    Tooth loss (premature mortality)
    Staining
    Abrasion
    Periodontal diseases
        Periodontitis (smoked)
        Focal recession (smokeless)
        Necrotizing ulcerative gingivitis (smoked)
Other tobacco-associated oral conditions
    Gingival bleeding
    Calculus
    Halitosis/Malodor
    Leukoedema
    Chronic hyperplastic candidiasis (candidal leukoplakia)
    Median rhomboid glossitis
    Hairy tongue
Possible association with tobacco
    Oral clefts
    Dental caries
    Lichen planus
    Salivary changes
    Taste and smell

(*Source:* Mecklenburg, R. E., Greenspan, D., Kleinman, D. V., Manley, M. W., Niessen, L. C., Robert-son, P. B., & Winn, D. E. (1996). *Tobacco effects in the mouth* (NIH Publication No. 96-3330). Bethesda, MD: U.S. Department of Health and Human Services, Public Health Service, National Institutes of Health.)

Oral Cancer/Precancerous Lesions

In 2010, 36,540 new cases of oral (tongue, mouth, pharynx, other oral cavity) and pharyngeal cancers with approximately 7,880 deaths resulting were estimated to occur in the United States.[12] The primary risk factors for the development of which account for more than 75% of oral cancers.[13,14] Rodriguez reviewed various risk factors in 137 cases of oral cancer in patients below the age of 46 and found that smoking accounted for 77% of all reported oral and pharyngeal cancers, alcohol consumption for 52%, and the combined effect of heavy smoking and drinking for 83% of the cancers in the study.[15] Smokers are more likely to develop leukoplakia than nonsmokers.[16] A clear dose response also exists; the more a person smokes or uses any type of tobacco product, the more likely a form of leukoplakia, which is a premalignant lesion, will develop. Fortunately, most leukoplakias will resolve if smoking is discontinued.[2,16]

DID YOU KNOW ?

Smoked tobacco and alcohol use account for approximately 70% of oral cancers each year in the United States.

Smokeless tobacco poses an oral cancer risk because of the presence of tobacco-specific nitrosamines found in all tobacco products and is able to cause smokeless tobacco-specific leukoplakia called *snuff dipper's pouch*.[10,17] Although early research reported smokeless tobacco greatly increased the risk of oral cancer with long-term use,[18] later research introduced the idea that smokeless tobacco poses a lower risk than smoked tobacco.[19,20] The level of risk from using smokeless tobacco depends a great deal on how much and how long it is used as well as on the specific type of smokeless tobacco, which contains a range of nitrosamines depending on the product.[19] As stated previously, there is no safe form of tobacco, and it should never be suggested that someone replace one form of tobacco with another as a harm-reduction strategy: *tobacco kills*. Dental health care providers are ethically bound to screen for oral cancer on every adult patient on a regular basis and to provide appropriate tobacco interventions to help all tobacco-using patients to quit, no matter what form they use.[19]

Periodontal Diseases

The majority of adults in the United States suffer from some level of mild-to-moderate periodontitis; 4.2% suffer from a severe form.[21] Of those adults with periodontitis, it is estimated

that 42% (6.4 million) of the cases can be attributed to cigarette smoking and 11% (1.7 million) to smokers who had already quit but show past damage. For those periodontal patients who continue to smoke, it is estimated that 75% of their periodontitis is attributed to smoked tobacco.[22] Even when gender, age, and plaque index was controlled for, smoking remained the primary contributing factor for the presence of established periodontal disease.[23] As with the risk of oral cancer, the level of periodontal destruction is exposure dependent. The number of cigarettes plus the number of years smoked, known as **dose response**, often is an indicator for the level of periodontal destruction.[23,24] In addition, smokers have deeper probing depths, gingival recession, loss of attachment, and bone loss than nonsmokers.[23–25] Cigarette smoking is a potential contributing factor in necrotizing ulcerative gingivitis,[26] possibly doubles the risk of root canal therapy,[27] and can increase healing complications after placement of endosseous dental implants.[28]

DID YOU KNOW ?

Approximately 75% of periodontitis cases are attributed to smoked tobacco.

The exact mechanism of tobacco smoke and the impact on periodontal health are not known, but research is pointing to the chemicals in tobacco smoke altering the host inflammatory and immune response (Table 20–3 ■).[29–38] A strong host response is essential for the body to fight the bacterial assault and prevent or fight the breakdown of the immune response, resulting in gingivitis and progression to periodontitis. Smoking alters the body's ability to mount a host response at both the local and systemic levels by changes in vasculature[29]; these changes manifest as reduction of bleeding upon probing, potentially causing misinterpretation of periodontal health[30]; reduction of oxygen in the periodontal pocket, which can alter subgingival flora[31]; interference with production of cytokines, thus inhibiting the systemic immune response[32]; an increase in proteolytic enzymes, resulting in periodontal destruction[33–35]; compromised periodontal ligament attachment to the root surface after root planing[36]; and a decrease in lymphocyte production.[37,38] Patients who smoke not only are more likely to present with moderate or advanced periodontitis but also often respond poorly to nonsurgical periodontal therapy[39] and periodontal re-care therapy[38] compared with nonsmokers or smokers who have quit. Fortunately, many of the soft-tissue changes associated with smoking, such as an increase of blood flow and gingival crevicular fluid, return to the status of a nonsmoker over

TABLE ■ 20–3 *Potential* Negative Impact on Periodontal Tissues from Smoked Tobacco

- Change in vasculature—reducing immune response
- Reduction of oxygen in the periodontal pocket—affecting composition of subgingival flora
- Increase in proteolytic enzymes—leading to periodontal destruction
- Compromised PDL attachment to root surface—poor healing following periodontal therapy

time.[40] Bone loss, on the other hand, remains as a historical marker of past tobacco use. Patients should be asked not only whether they currently use tobacco but also whether they have ever used it in order to better understand the current level of periodontitis and to provide relapse-prevention information. The research is clear: Cigarette smoking is a major risk factor for periodontitis and is considered to have a strong causal association to the development of this chronic disease.[11,22–39]

Smokeless Tobacco and Periodontal Disease

The use of smokeless tobacco directly affects the oral tissue where the snuff or chew tobacco directly touches the mouth. The consequences of the gingival and mucosal tissue being covered with tobacco, which releases nicotine, cancer-causing nitrosamines, and a high level of sweetening agents, results in a significantly larger amount of recession and attachment loss, possibly resulting from chemical injury rather than bacterial assault. It is believed that there exists no clear demonstrated association between use of smokeless tobacco and generalized severe periodontitis.[41–43] In one study, Fisher reviewed population-based records of 12,932 adults in the National Health and Nutrition Examination Survey III study and found that the smokeless-tobacco users were twice as likely as nontobacco users to have evidence of severe active periodontal disease than the control group smokers.[44] More research is needed to examine the relationship between smokeless tobacco and generalized periodontal disease to clarify this point. Regardless of the type of tobacco use, the American Academy of Periodontology strongly recommends inclusion of tobacco cessation in periodontal therapy.[45]

TOBACCO TYPES, TOXINS, AND CARCINOGENS

Understanding the cause of the numerous systemic and oral consequences of tobacco use requires the ability to identify the types of tobacco on the market, how they are used, and what toxic components each contains. Although all forms of tobacco

are harmful, the tobacco type, amount used, and duration of use can have a great impact on the risk for disease.[2]

The most common form of tobacco used by adults in the United States is cigarette smoking at 20.6%, cigar smoking at 5.4%, and pipe smoking at 0.08%.[46] Smoked tobacco inhaled by the consumer (**main-stream smoke**) contains an estimated more than 4,000 compounds and more than 60 carcinogens, including tobacco-specific nitrosamines (Table 20–4 ■),[47–49] whereas **side-stream smoke** (also known as *involuntary exposure to tobacco smoke, environmental tobacco smoke,* or *second-hand smoke*) has most of the same toxins (ammonia, nitrogen oxides, and chemical carcinogens). However, that exposure can be up to 100 times higher than mainstream smoke.[50] Second-hand smoke not only poses significant health risks[9] but also can result in an increase in periodontitis.[51] The chemically complex mixture of toxins, carcinogens, and inert substances is a result of the combination of the tobacco leaf, pesticides used to grow the plant, the curing or fermenting process, additives, and the burning process. Even with the introduction of low-tar, filtered cigarettes in the late 1950s, smoking-related morbidity and mortality did not decrease.[2,52] Although filtered cigarettes deliver lower tar and nicotine as measured by a "smoking machine," smokers compensate for the lower nicotine dose by inhaling more deeply, covering filter vents, and smoking more.[52]

DID YOU KNOW?

Cigarette smoke contains more than 4,000 toxins and over 60 carcinogens.

Newer trends in smoked-tobacco use among high school students include the use of bidis (pronounced "bee-dees") at 2.4%, kreteks (pronounced "cree-teks") at 2.4%,[53] water pipes, and flavored cigarettes. **Bidis** are small, hand-rolled cigarettes imported from India or Southeast Asia. This hand-rolled "poor man's cigarette" is made from flakes and dust of dark tobacco leaves with vanilla, licorice, strawberry, cinnamon, or mango

TABLE ■ 20–4 A Sample of the Carcinogens/Toxins Found in Tobacco Smoke

Nitrogen	Argon	Hydrogen	Ammonia
Nitrogen oxides	Hydrogen cyanide	Hydrogen sulfide	Methane
Isoprene	Butadiene	Acetylene	Benzene
Toluene	Styrene	Formic acid	Acetic acid
Propionic acid	Methyl formate	Formaldehyde	Acetaldehyde
Acrolein	Acetone	Methanol	Furan
Pyridine	Picolines	3-vinylpyridine	Tobacco specific
Nicotine	Anatabine	Naphthalene	N-nitrosamines
Oxygen	Carbon dioxide	Carbon monoxide	

(*Source:* National Cancer Institute, Smoking and Tobacco Control. (1998). *Cigars, health effects and trends.* (Monograph 9, NIH Publication No. 98-4302). Bethesda, MD: U.S. Department of Health and Human Services, National Institutes of Health, National Cancer Institute, 73–97; National Toxicology Program. (2000). *9th report on carcinogens* (11th ed.). Bethesda, MD: U.S. Department of Health and Human Sciences, National Institute of Environmental Health Sciences. Retrieved 11/21/06, from http://www.cdc.gov/tobacco/ETS_Toolkit/PublicPlaces/secondhand-smoke; Johnson G. K., & Guthmiller, J. M. (2007). The impact of cigarette smoking on periodontal disease and treatment. *Periodontol 2000,* 44:178–94.)

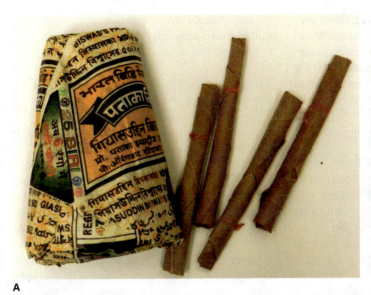

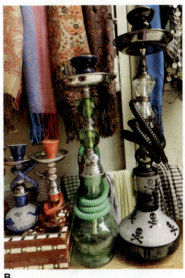

FIGURE ■ 20–2 Alternative tobacco products. A. Kreteks or clove cigarettes B. Hookahs or water pipes.

(*Source:* Courtesy of Joan M. Davis.)

flavoring added to give a sweet taste and mask the strong tobacco smoke. These flavored, unfiltered cigarettes are attractive to youth because they are relatively inexpensive compared with cigarettes. Bidis are sold in tattoo parlors, on the Internet, and at other venues that cannot enforce regulations such as those adhered to by more traditional tobacco retail locations.

Kreteks, or **clove cigarettes**, are imported from Indonesia and contain a mixture of tobacco, cloves, and other additives. Although little research has been conducted on the physical effects of clove cigarettes, people who smoke them have been found to inhale more deeply and therefore are provided basically the same level of nicotine as that from regular cigarettes. Both bidis and kreteks deliver more nicotine, carbon monoxide, and tar than standard cigarettes[54,55] and pose possible health risks. **Water pipes** (hookahs, narghile, shisha, or arghile), originating in Africa and Asia, are becoming popular among college students and others in the United States.[56] The water pipe contains a bowl in which fermented tobacco and flavorings are burned with the use of charcoal. The hookah smoke bubbles through water and is then breathed in via tubes, often by multiple users. Although users feel that the water "filters" out the toxins, hookah smoke has been shown to contain many of the same toxins found in cigarette smoke.[57] Unfortunately, youth and young adults are trying alternative tobacco and herbal products, believing that they are not as harmful as regular cigarettes (Figure 20–2 ■). When these products are formally tested, they often yield higher amounts of tobacco toxins. Therefore, the provider must ask youth and young adults if they are using any tobacco products rather than just asking "Do you smoke?" to better assess their use and become familiar with how tobacco is used in the community.

DID YOU KNOW

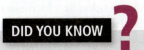

Hookah, or water pipe smoke, has been shown to contain many of the same toxins found in cigarette smoke.

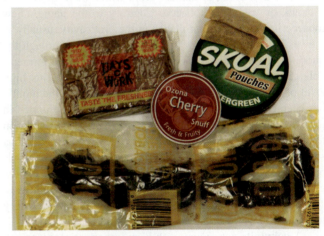

FIGURE ■ 20–3 Types of Smokeless Tobacco: chewing, block and rope, snuff, and pouches.

(*Source:* Courtesy of Joan M. Davis.)

The use of smokeless tobacco has increased slightly (3.5%, men at 7% and women at 0.3%) in the United States among individuals 18 years old and remains high (at 6.1%) in those under the age of 18 years.[46] Alarmingly, data indicate that more than 17% of current tobacco users are utilizing several or multiple types of tobacco for smoking as well as smokeless tobacco. Use of multiple types of tobacco can lead to a more serious nicotine addiction and incidence of disease.[7] In recent years, the tobacco industry has marketed the use of spit tobacco to smokers who are not allowed to smoke and can choose another type of tobacco use. As with smoked tobacco, smokeless comes in many and varied forms (Figure 20–3 ■). All smokeless tobacco contains tobacco-specific cancer-causing nitrosamines[58–60] and nicotine, which are "free" or available for absorption by the body in the presence of base chemicals (sodium carbonate and ammonium carbonate) added by the tobacco companies. The higher the pH, the more nicotine is available (approximately one can of snuff equals four packs of cigarettes) and, therefore, the greater potential effect on the brain. Introductory spit products, such as Bandits (U.S. Tobacco Co.) have a lower pH and more flavoring than Copenhagen (U.S. Tobacco Co.) or Kodiak (Genuine Tobacco Co.), thus allowing youth or novices to experiment on flavored, low-nicotine products to adjust to using them before graduating to more potent and addictive products.[61,62] The two main forms of smokeless tobacco used in this country are snuff and chewing tobacco.

Snuff is finely ground tobacco sold in three forms: moist (fine or long cut), packets or sachets, and dry. Moist snuff comes in round flat tins; the user takes a pinch between two fingers and places the "dip" somewhere in the vestibule area in the buccal mucosal fold. Saliva then bathes the dip, forming tobacco juice, which is swallowed or spit—hence, the term "spit tobacco." Snuff is also sold in packets designed to contain the loose, fine-cut moist snuff to make it more acceptable to users who could be just trying it out or do not want to be seen using loose tobacco.

Chew tobacco comes in loose leaves, in a twist of tobacco leaves, or in a block of tobacco from which the user cuts off a chunk or "plug" of tobacco. Contrary to the name, chew tobacco is not chewed but placed in the oral cavity, usually in the vestibule area, to allow the nicotine to diffuse through the buccal mucosa. Chew tobacco contains 30% to 40% fermentable carbohydrates compared with 2% in snuff.[63] This high level of sugar, repeatedly placed in one location in the mouth, has been shown to lead to 4 times more root caries reported in tobacco chewers than in snuff users or smokers.[64] In addition to the presence of nitrosamines, chew tobacco contains *Bacillus* species, which produce organic toxins and can lead to the development of localized tissue damage in chewers.[65] And finally, cigars, chew, and snuff tobacco products have been shown to contain abrasive particles (silicone dioxide or silica), possibly leading to dental attrition.[66]

A culturally aware approach is an important aspect for all patient care but especially when providing tobacco-dependence interventions for patients from other cultures. Tobacco is commonly used all over the world in pastes and powders, as desserts, in toothpaste, in small packets (Swedish snuff, "snus"), and mixed with slaked lime, spices, ash, and/or fungus, which can be smoked, smoked on the burning end (**reverse smoking**), sucked on, chewed, or wiped on the teeth and gingiva. It is not unusual for women to be regular users of these products, and they can give tobacco to their children to use.[67] One of the more common alternative tobacco practices found in the United States is betel-quid and areca-nut (an Indian import) chewing. An areca-nut paste is mixed with slack lime and tobacco and then wrapped in a betel leaf called a *betel-quid* (numerous other names and ingredients are used in other parts of Southeast Asia). Alone, the use of areca-nut products poses a high risk of developing oral cancer. Combined with tobacco (known as "Gutka") increases the risks of leukoplakia, oral submucous fibrosis, oral cancer, and abnormal reproductive health outcomes are increased.[68,69] Clearly, an open-ended inquiry, such as "Tell me about your tobacco use," will best determine how to customize a tobacco intervention. In addition, all tobacco-related health effects identified in the oral examination should

be incorporated into the cessation message, thus making the quit message personally meaningful.

NICOTINE USE: A BIOCHEMICAL DEPENDENCE

The use of tobacco is a complex, multifactorial human behavior that encompasses biochemical, behavioral, and social components.[70] From a single puff of smoked tobacco or plug of smokeless tobacco, nicotine enters the bloodstream through the lungs or oral mucosa and travels throughout the body. This powerful psychoactive drug (subjectively affecting mood and feelings) binds to the nicotinic acetylcholine receptors in the brain, autonomic ganglia, and the neuromuscular junction and releases a cascade of biochemicals, including acetylcholine, dopamine, serotonin, norepinephrine, β endorphin, glutamate, pituitary hormones, and vasopressin.[71,72] This nicotine-initiated biochemical release affects numerous body systems, including (1) cardiovascular system, increasing heart rate and blood pressure and vasoconstriction in extremities; (2) respiratory system; (3) skeletal motor, causing feelings of relaxation; and (4) gastrointestinal system, through stimulation of the afferent chemical receptors and the autonomic nervous system.[71,72] The steady infusion of nicotine and sodium found in smokeless tobacco has been linked to the possible acceleration of coronary disease and vascular disease.[73] In addition, nicotine suppresses the appetite and increases body metabolism, often leading to an artificially lower weight for tobacco users. Once tobacco use is discontinued, an average of 5 to 10 pounds is gained, thus returning the individual to a non-nicotine or normal weight.[74]

The extent to which nicotine affects the central nervous system is determined by the method and amount of tobacco used. Inhaled tobacco smoke quickly moves from the lungs to the brain in approximately 7 seconds. The 1 to 2 mg of bioavailable nicotine remains in the system for 20 to 30 minutes and then rapidly drops off, cueing the user to replenish the nicotine with another cigarette. This peak-and-valley pattern explains the need for smokers to use tobacco every 1 to 2 hours depending on their level of dependence. Smokeless tobacco slowly diffuses through the mucous membrane and clears the system slowly, giving a more stable infusion of nicotine.[71] Because of the slow diffusion, smokeless tobacco users might smoke when they first wake to rapidly replenish the drug and then use smokeless tobacco to maintain a constant dosing of the drug.

The release of dopamine causes a sense of well-being, relaxation, and stress reduction whereas release of norepinephrine (adrenaline) causes a sense of heightened alertness. These effects reward and reinforce the continued use of the tobacco, leading to nicotine dependence. For the first-time user, this powerful drug can cause dizziness, nausea, vomiting, and headache (toxicity). However, with repetition and increase in the amount used (dosing), these negative effects disappear, and a tolerance or desensitization of the neuroreceptors develops, requiring an increased and steady use of nicotine to obtain the desired effect.[71] In addition, with the continued use and increased dose of nicotine, the brain adapts to this chemical assault by significantly increasing (up-regulating) the number of nicotinic neuroreceptors by 50% within a few weeks.[75,76] Unfortunately, the creation of additional receptors and desensitization of existing nicotinic receptors combined with the memory of positive reinforcement from endorphin release produces a powerful craving, a strong drive to use the substance, and avoidance of withdrawal if not given the needed dose of nicotine. The cravings and avoidance of withdrawal drive a user to sustain or increase the amount and/or frequency of tobacco use, thus establishing chemical and behavioral dependence, even when presented with compelling health consequenses.[77,78]

Now considered a chronic, relapsing, progressive disease, a formal diagnosis of **substance dependence** is made if a user meets three of the six major criteria in the diagnostic criteria from *Diagnostic Statistical Manual of Mental Disorders, Fourth Edition.*[79] Habitual self-administration, the development of tolerance, compulsive drug-taking behavior, and withdrawal are central components for diagnosing substance dependence disorders for alcohol, cocaine, heroin, and nicotine. Nicotine withdrawal symptoms include depressed mood, insomnia, irritability, anxiety, difficulty concentrating, restlessness, decreased heart rate, and increased appetite.[79]

> **DID YOU KNOW ?**
>
> Patients maynot want to quit in order to *avoid withdrawal symptoms,* which include depressed mood, insomnia, irritability, anxiety, difficulty concentrating, restlessness, decreased heart rate, and an increase in appetite.

Not all tobacco users become dependent but might smoke or chew at will, in very small amounts, or only on weekends (the latter called *social smokers* or *chippers,* one to five cigarettes a day.) The National Survey of Drug Abuse and Health reported that approximately 57.7% of those ages 12 year or older who had smoked for a month or more, met the criteria for nicotine dependence.[80] Although a patient can use limited amounts or is not currently dependent, even a small amount of tobacco exposes the individual to carcinogens, toxins, and nicotine; therefore, the user should be encouraged to quit.[81]

Current research points to a genetic basis for tobacco-use behavior and the likelihood of relapse once tobacco use is discontinued. This genetic risk factor can explain why some people can quit seemingly at will and why others cannot seem to quit no matter how hard they try. Knowing whether a patient is genetically predisposed to nicotine use can aid in developing appropriate behavioral and pharmacotherapy interventions for a dependent patient who finds it difficult to quit.[82,83]

TOBACCO USE: A BEHAVIORAL AND SOCIAL ADDICTION

Equally important to the chemical dependence of nicotine is the repetitive, habitual actions connected with each puff or dip and the reinforcing experience of relaxation and sense of well-being. Each cigarette is a drug-delivery system containing approximately 1 to 2 mg of bioavailable nicotine with

inhalation through the lungs being a very effective mechanism to deliver this drug to the brain.[71] Tobacco companies enhanced this deadly delivery system by adding ammonia to cigarettes in the 1970s to raise the pH and increase the available nicotine, creating a better "hit" and subsequent positive reinforcement.[84] With approximately ten puffs taken per cigarette, a one-pack-per-day smoker repeats the administration of nicotine 200 times each day to maintain relatively stable levels of the drug to satisfy cravings or avoid withdrawal symptoms.[85] The repetitions are often connected to specific activities performed each day, such as getting out of bed, having a cup of coffee, driving, spending time with friends or in a favorite activity, and after eating—causing cigarettes to be habitually connected to every aspect of life's activities. The ritual of handling, placing, and using the tobacco is often reported to be as pleasurable as the effects of the nicotine and should be considered when developing a cessation plan. Helping patients overcome this multifactorial addiction by necessity involves behavioral and pharmacologic assistance.

> **DID YOU KNOW ?**
>
> Providing both cessation medications and behavioral therapy can dramatically increase a patient's chance to successfully quit long-term.

Pharmacotherapy for Treatment of Nicotine Dependence

The clinical practice guideline *Treating Tobacco Use and Dependence*[70] of the U.S. Public Health Service (PHS) established the importance of treating nicotine addiction as a disease and recommended the use of appropriate cessation medications and behavioral interventions based on the patient's level of dependence and need. This resource provides an in-depth discussion and reference material on cessation medications and can be found at http://www.surgeongeneral.gov/tobacco/treating_tobacco_use08.pdf.

Dental and medical professionals can have a significant impact on tobacco quit rates and should be actively involved in helping patients quit. Smokers trying to quit on their own succeed approximately only 3% to 5% of the time.[70] The PHS guideline reports that a brief cessation intervention by a health care provider combined with appropriate medication can increase the success of maintaining abstinence to 30%. With approximately 58% of the estimated 45 million smokers in the United States indicating that they would like to quit within the next six months[4] and at least 50% of those smokers visiting their dentist's office each year, the potential impact that dental clinicians could have on tobacco-related oral and general health is immense.

The discussion and recommendation of appropriate pharmacotherapies to help manage withdrawal symptoms for those who are nicotine dependent is an important aspect of a cessation intervention. Tobacco cessation medications are safe and effective and have been shown to double the chances of a quit attempt being successful.[70,86] Although the various cessation medications are effective, they are not equally helpful to all users.[87] For example, women do not respond as well to nicotine-replacement therapy as men.[88] And for the most part, although pharmacotherapy can assist in quit attempts, medications plus behavioral assistance has been shown to be the most effective. Therefore, because tobacco dependence is a multifactorial chronic relapsing disease, the combination of both behavioral and pharmacologic assistance is required to increase the chances of long-term success.[70]

First-Line Medications

The U.S. Food and Drug Administration (FDA) has approved several medications for over-the-counter (OTC) or prescription use in the treatment of nicotine dependence for both smoked and smokeless tobacco. First-line medications are approved for tobacco cessation but second-line medications for tobacco cessation are not FDA approved for that use (i.e., off-label use).

Nicotine replacement therapies (NRT) are medications that provide nicotine in various forms intended to lessen or relieve withdrawal symptoms, but they have not been shown to relieve cravings. Although it seems counterintuitive to treat nicotine addiction with nicotine, the administration of "pure" nicotine removes the exposure to tobacco's nitrosamines and toxins while behavioral changes are being made during the quit process. When used properly, NRT can provide approximately 30% to 80% of the nicotine normally obtained from tobacco use. By self-dosing, the user has control over the amount of nicotine needed for cessation.[71,73,89,90] Studies have shown that whatever the form of NRT used, the chances of quitting increased by 50% to 70%.[91] The patient must be advised to follow the label directions carefully because (1) an excess of nicotine-replacement can cause toxicity and (2) too little nicotine makes insufficient amounts available to ease withdrawal symptoms.[90] In either case, improper use of the medication is common and often leads to a return to tobacco use, called a *relapse*. This "failure" can give the tobacco user a sense that the pharmacotherapy did not work, leaving her or him reluctant to try again.

Pregnant and lactating women should be encouraged to quit tobacco without using cessation medications. However, when the benefits to the mother and child exceed the risks of cessation medications, a medical consult should be obtained for optimal care.[70]

DID YOU KNOW ?

The PHS *Treating Tobacco Use and Dependence Clinical Practice Guideline* recommends that all tobacco dependence interventions include the discussion of cessation medications.

Available NRT Products in the U.S. *OTC Nicotine Gum (Nicotine Polacrilex; 2 or 4 mg).* Nicotine gum was the first

NRT approved for tobacco cessation by the FDA in the 1980s and has been shown to double the odds of a successful cessation attempt.[70] Unfortunately, many users chew this product like regular gum, leading to nicotine toxicity (stomachache, nausea) and is often discontinued. The patient should be instructed to (1) chew the gum a few times until a peppery/mint flavor is tasted, (2) place the gum in the vestibule area until the peppery taste is gone, (3) repeat this cycle approximately every 20 to 30 minutes, and (4) not use more than 20 pieces of 4 mg gum or 30 pieces of 2 mg gum. The level of nicotine peaks in the bloodstream in about 20 to 30 minutes. Patients should be advised to avoid coffee, juices, and soft drinks 15 minutes before and while they use the gum because a low, or acidic, pH will interfere with the nicotine absorption through the mucous membrane. Patients with temporomandibular joint problems or dentures have reported difficulties chewing the gum and can benefit from using the nicotine lozenge.

OTC Nicotine Lozenge (Nicotine Polacrilex with Aspartame; 2 or 4 mg) The nicotine lozenge, much like the gum, is an effective nicotine-replacement delivery system for tobacco users with low or high nicotine dependence.[91] The lozenge delivery system is easy to use (no chewing/parking) and delivers a complete dose of nicotine. As with nicotine gum, acidic beverages can interfere with the absorption of nicotine. Patients should be advised to avoid food, juice, coffee, or soft drinks 15 minutes before or during the use of the lozenge.

Sublingual lozenges are nicotine-containing tablets placed under the tongue; they are available in other countries but not yet in the United States.

OTC Nicotine Transdermal Patch (7, 14, and 21 mg or 15 mg) The nicotine transdermal patch (Nicoderm CQ®, Nicotrol®) has been shown to be a safe and effective form of NRT, which works by diffusing a steady dose of nicotine through the skin.[70,91] The nicotine level peaks in about 4 to 8 hours and is maintained for 15 to 24 hours. Patients might experience mild skin irritation, but this side effect often resolves in a few days, or the patch can be moved to different locations. Insomnia has been reported with the transdermal patch and can indicate that the dose should be lowered.

Prescription Nicotine Inhaler The nicotine inhaler consists of a small cartridge that attaches to a cigarlike mouthpiece; it has been shown to be safe and effective in helping tobacco users quit.[70,91] The nicotine is not actually inhaled but is "puffed" into the mouth where the medication is held and then diffused through the oral mucosa. This system mimics the behavior of smoking and can meet a smoker's emotional need to place something in the mouth. Mouth and throat irritation, coughing, and rhinitis are common but temporary side effects of this NRT.

Prescription Nicotine Nasal Spray Nicotine nasal spray is administered directly into the nasal cavity, delivering a rapid dose of nicotine, which can benefit highly addicted users. The nasal spray has been reported to cause local irritations and congestion in about 94% of the users. Because of the more immediate dose of nicotine, this form of NRT poses a risk of addiction developing in about 15% to 20% of patients using the nicotine nasal spray.[70]

Proper Dosing of Nicotine Replacement

The proper amount and type of NRT to recommend to a patient depends on several factors, including (1) type of tobacco used, (2) amount of tobacco used, (3) level of nicotine dependence, (4) former experience with cessation medications, (5) medical contraindications, and (6) patient preference. Because each cigarette provides the user 1 to 2 mg of available nicotine, a reasonable amount or dose to recommend can be 1 mg of NRT to one cigarette smoked or one plug of smokeless used, which is basically the recommendation for use on NRT package instructions. As with all medications, the dosing should be adjusted for individual differences and needs. For example, if an individual smokes five cigarettes a day, using a 21-mg patch could easily cause nicotine toxicity. If a person smokes two packs a day, then a 7-mg patch would not be an adequate replacement. A smokeless-tobacco user can benefit from using the gum or lozenge to place in the mouth instead of a plug. A smoker might prefer the nicotine inhaler to provide the feel of something in the hands and mouth, and a chipper might prefer a 2-mg lozenge to use as needed. NRT offers the option of using them on a fixed schedule or as needed.

A combination of NRTs can be a beneficial option by providing an ad libitum delivery of nicotine. For example, a nasal spray, gum, lozenge, or inhaler can be used with the patch, which delivers a slower, steady amount of nicotine or with oral medications (bupropion and varenicline). This combination of medications allows for individualizing medications according to the patient's needs and preferences, which can yield higher quit rates.[87] The amount and form of NRT should be carefully considered and reduced at the first sign of toxicity.

Another important factor in determining the level and type of NRT is the degree of nicotine dependence. The **Fagerstrom Test for Nicotine Dependence (FTND)** consists of six basic questions on smoking behavior and has been widely used to assess the level of dependence.[92] The Heaviness of Smoking Index is a two-question survey that was adapted from the FTND and yields a quick indication of the level dependence[93]:

1. How soon after you wake up do you smoke your first cigarette?
   a. Within 5 minutes?
   b. 6–30 minutes?
   c. After 60 minutes?
2. How many cigarettes per day do you smoke?
   a. 10 or less
   b. 11–20
   c. 21–30
   d. 31 or more

A person who smokes within 30 minutes or less after waking and/or smokes 21 or more cigarettes per day is considered highly dependent. Because smokeless tobacco is used differently than smoked tobacco, the FTND was adapted for smokeless-tobacco use.[94] Like the FTND, the Fagerstrom Test for Nicotine Dependence—Smokeless Tobacco reports that the primary indicator of the level of dependence is related to how soon the smokeless tobacco is used when the user wakes and if the tobacco juice is swallowed. Knowing the level of tobacco dependence assists the clinician and patient in developing a cessation plan that includes appropriate behavioral responses and levels of medications necessary to address anticipated cravings and withdrawal symptoms.

Non-NRT Cessation Medications

Prescription bupropion SR (Zyban®), also marketed as an antidepressant (Wellbutrin®), was approved for smoking cessation by the FDA in 1997; it has been shown to be safe and approximately doubles the likelihood of successfully quitting long term.[70,95] Although the exact mechanism is unknown, bupropion is believed to act on the neuroreceptors to mimic the effects of nicotine on dopamine and norepinephrine production and to lessen withdrawal symptoms as well as delay weight gain.[95] This non-nicotine medication is taken in pill form and should be started 1 to 2 weeks before the quit date. Bupropion SR should not be prescribed for patients with a history of alcoholism, eating disorders, or seizure disorders or for those using monoamine oxidative inhibitors.[70]

Prescription varenicline (Chantix®), taken in pill form, was approved in 2006 by the FDA for smoking cessation and was designed specifically as a cessation medication. Varenicline is a partial agonist that binds to nicotinic acetylcholine receptors, which block nicotine from stimulating high levels of dopamine, thus short-circuiting the reward/dependence cycle. As a partial agonist, varenicline stimulates the nicotinic receptor, releasing a moderate level dopamine, thus relieving both cravings and withdrawal symptoms.[96,97] This medication can be used for up to one year, possibly reducing the likelihood of relapse.[70]

Although research has shown both bupropion and varenicline to be relatively safe, nonaddictive, and more effective than a plaebo,[70,97] the FDA (http://www.fda.gov/downloads/Drugs/DrugSafety/DrugSafetyNewsletter/UCM107318.pdf) has received reports of adverse effects of both drugs including suicidal intentions, changes in behavior, agitation, and depressed mood.[98] Other adverse effects when using varenicline include hypersensitivity reactions, serious skin reactions (rare), accidental injury, and nausea (up to 30%). As oral health care professionals, we must carefully screen patients for potential emotional and physical contraindications as we discuss potential cessation medications. However, the benefit of these medications to help patients quit smoking must also be considered as we provide tobacco cessation interventions. For more detailed information on varenicline, see Prescribing Information at http://www.pfizer.com/files/products/uspi_chantix.pdf. Prescription clonidine, nortriptyline, and rimonabant have been used for nicotine-dependence treatment but are not approved by the FDA for smoking cessation. The PHS guideline does not recommend the use of second-line medications for use in normal clinical cessation therapy.[70]

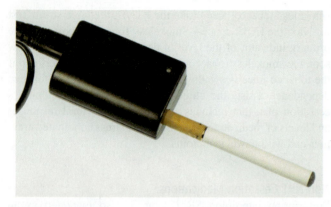

FIGURE ■ 20–4 FDA warns of health risks posed by e-cigarettes.

(*Source:* http://www.fda.gov/downloads/ForConsumers/ConsumerUpdates/UCM173430.pdf.)

Electronic cigarettes (Figure 20–4 ■) have been promoted as an alternative form on tobacco use for those who are in smoke-free locations or for use as a smoking cessation aid. However, they can contain harmful vapors, and the FDA has not approved their use in the United States.

Other Considerations

The *combination of first-line tobacco dependence medications* has been explored with indications of increased cessation effectiveness. Possible combinations include nicotine patch + other NRT (gum, lozenge or nasal spray); nicotine patch + inhaler; Buproprion + nicotine patch,[70,87] and varenicline + bupropion.[99] The use of various combinations allow for a steady dose of medication while giving the patient the option of titrating the dose of nicotine as needed. Because varenicline acts as a partial agonist of the nicotinic receptor, the concurrent use of NRT remains in question and is not advised.

Our role as oral health professionals is to assess the patient for medical and psychological contraindications, discuss various options, and then allow the patient to choose the medication that would best suit her or his needs. Follow-up must be a component of all tobacco cessation treatment plans that include medications, preferably within one week of starting the prescription. This will aid the patient's efforts to quit as well as identify any adverse outcomes from the recommended or prescribed medications.[70]

Another important consideration when providing care to patients who smoke is the potential of prescription medications adversely interacting with the more than 4,000 components found in tobacco smoke.[100] Common drugs that interact with tobacco smoke include theophylline, caffeine, antidepressants, cardiovascular drugs, anticoagulants, steroid hormones, and insulin (Table 20–5 ■). Smokers might require a higher dose of medication to achieve the desired effect. This reduction in action, in part, results from the tobacco smoke's stimulating the action of hepatic enzymes, leading to an increased clearance of drugs and therefore

TABLE ■ 20–5 Drug Interactions with Tobacco Smoking (TS)

Drug	*Tobacco Smoke Effect*
Theophylline	Increased drug clearance
Insulin	Decreases subcutaneous absorption
Beta blockers	Less effective
Oral contraceptives	Increased drug clearance potential

(*Source:* Data from Zevin, S., & Benowitz, N. L. (1999). Drug interactions with tobacco smoking: An update. *Clin Pharmacokinet,* 36:425–38.)

requiring a higher dose of medication. When a person no longer smokes, the body adjusts hepatic enzyme activity leading to the reduction of medication needed to obtain the desired effect. Whether the patient is ready to make a quit attempt or not, awareness of these potential smoking/drug interactions should be evaluated as a part of patient assessment. Patients who smoke should be advised to consult their attending physician when smoking is reduced or stopped.

DID YOU KNOW ?

Tobacco smoke can adversely affect many prescription medications and should be reassessed when smoking is reduced or discontinued.

Acupuncture, herbal remedies, hypnosis, auriculotherapy, and numerous other methods to end tobacco dependence, although popular, are not evidence based. Until these methods have independent supporting research to back their claims, they should not be formally recommended as cessation methods.[70] However, these methods can increase a user's belief that he or she can succeed (self-efficacy) and ultimately can help that individual.

COMPONENTS OF AN EFFECTIVE TOBACCO DEPENDENCE INTERVENTION

Dental health care providers assess risk by taking health histories, using radiographs, and making clinical evaluations, thereby developing treatment plans and providing oral health interventions as a regular and normal part of the oral care appointment. The inclusion of tobacco assessment and cessation is not only appropriate but also an ethical obligation on the part of every clinician. Because tobacco use is the primary cause of oral cancer and periodontitis not to mention the number one cause of preventable death and disease in this country, every effort must be made to make tobacco cessation a normal part of dental care and a component of public health outreach.

Substantial evidence shows that even a brief tobacco-dependence intervention (TDI) provided by a health care provider can be effective in helping a patient successfully quit. The more time oral professionals spend providing a TDI, the greater will be the benefit to the patients, resulting in an increase in successful quit rates.[70] Unfortunately, oral professionals continue to report barriers to offering tobacco interventions such as lack of time, training, and reimbursement, and they continue to offer limited TDIs.[101,102] Conversely, patients have viewed tobacco interventions as a part of overall health care and have expressed satisfaction when TDIs were provided.[103]

It is important to approach any behavioral change with sensitivity and to adapt the message and evidence of tobacco-related oral disease to the patient (Table 20–6 ■).[104] The concept of active listening, adapting the needed behavioral change to the person, and then helping the patient adopt the change is at the core of what is called motivational interviewing.

The gold standard for tobacco interventions worldwide is the PHS guideline *Treating Tobacco Use and Dependence.* The centerpiece of this seminal (original) document is the use of the 5 A's (ask, advise, assess, assist, arrange) and

TABLE ■ 20–6 The "Spirit" of Motivational Intervention in Health Care

- *Collaborative:* Interactions are shared with the clinician facilitating/providing appropriate information.
- *Evocative:* The patient is encouraged to explore the health behavior change from her or his own experience rather than letting the clinician create a solution.
- *Honoring patient autonomy:* Care should be taken to ensure that the patient maintains control of their own health choices and not be told what to do or "educated" into compliance.

(*Source:* Based on Rollnick, S., Miller, W. R., & Butler, C. (2008). *Motivational interviewing in health care.* New York, NY: Guilford Publications.)

the 5 R's (relevance, risks, rewards, roadblocks, repetition) (Figure 20–5 ■).

Ask

Asking whether a patient uses tobacco is the first step in establishing oral health risks when interviewing a patient during an initial appointment or subsequent appointments. Establishing tobacco use can be done with questioning or by adding

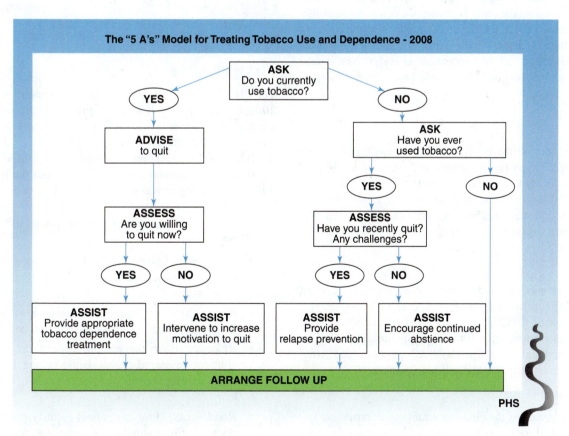

FIGURE ■ 20–5 The PHS Five A's Model

(*Source:* Treating Tobacco Use and Dependence Slide overview at http://www.ahrq.gov/clinic/tobacco/slideoverview/brftobaccosl.htm.)

TABLE ■ 20–7 Example of a Health History of Tobacco Use Assessment

ARE YOU USING TOBACCO?

1. YES or NO

    a. Any tobacco product: cigarettes (# per day_____) / cigar / snuff / pipe / bidi

    b. If YES, how long have you been using tobacco products? _____ years.

    c. How soon do you use tobacco when you wake up in the morning?
Within: __ 5 min __10 min __20 min __ 30 min +

    d. Are you interested in reducing or quitting tobacco use? YES NO

    e. Would you like help in reducing/quitting: _____ now _____ this month _____ later _____
not interested right now

    f. If you have tried to quit, what have you tried or used? _____ (This should
give a fairly good idea of the patient's current *stage*.)

tobacco-use questions on the health history (Table 20–7 ■). A verbal follow-up and clarification can "assess" the behavioral and emotional issues associated with the tobacco use.

Advise

All tobacco users should be encouraged to quit; how the statement is posed can either create resistance or an opportunity for change. One approach is an open-ended question such as "Today is a great day to quit. How do you feel about that?" as opposed to "You need to quit smoking." One approach opens the door for discussion; the other encourages a defensive response. Clearly, with a TDI, 5 A's, the stages model (Figure 20–6 ■), and 5 R's blend together depending on the patient's response. Knowing all aspects of an intervention provides the clinician the understanding and tools to provide an appropriate service without alienating the tobacco user.

Assess

Taking into account the behavioral factors, emotional factors, level of addiction, past quit attempts, and current sense of willingness and ability to quit are all important in providing a TDI. The use of the stages-of-change model can aid in assessing readiness to quit, thus guiding the clinician in what and how much to share with the tobacco user.

Assist

This concept was discussed under the action stage. Briefly, assistance should include pharmacotherapy discussion, recommendation of OTC nicotine replacement therapies, writing of a prescription, referral to the phone quit line or online resources, preparation of a personalized quit plan, and provision of resource materials and self-help pamphlets.

Arrange

This concept involves the clinician arranging or providing follow-up on a TDI for a person who is ready to quit and has set a quit date. A simple follow-up letter, postcard, or call has been shown to boost the success of a quit attempt.[70]

DID YOU KNOW **?**

Asking and *advising* a patient to quit should be offered to all tobacco-using patients at every appointment. If a patient is ready to quit, the clinician should *assess* what the patient has done in the past and *assist* her or him in developing a quit plan. Follow up, or *arrange*, the intervention with a phone call or postcard or at the next dental visit will increase the chances of a successful quit.

PHS's Five R's

The PHS *Treating Tobacco Use and Dependence Guideline: 2008 Update* uses 5 R's at the precontemplation or contemplation stage with the patient who is not ready to quit but has entered into some level of discussion.[70] The use of motivational interviewing techniques can help avoid making the patient defensive when talking about the benefits of quitting. Offering unwanted information should be avoided in order to create a basis of future discussions at recare appointments. The motivational messages of the 5 R's are as follows:

- *Relevance:* Tailor specific health information (periodontal disease, stain, leukoplakia) to the patient's health status.

- *Risks:* Explore whether the patient knows and understands the health risks associated with tobacco use.

- *Rewards:* Have the patient identify the benefits of quitting: improved health, better-tasting food, saving money, fresher breath, and better-smelling clothing and hair.

- *Roadblocks:* Have the patient identify possible barriers to quitting: withdrawal symptoms, fear of failure, depression, weight gain, lack of support, and loss of friends.

Pre-contemplation: Not willing to quit or even think about it.	• Provide a pamphlet and let the patient know you are there to help when the patient is ready to quit. • Use the spirit of motivational interviewing, that is, the PHS 5 R's. • Relate any evidence of tobacco-related disease during patient care to a quit message. • Note intervention in patient chart (intervention takes about 1 to 2 minutes).
Contemplation: Willing to quit in the next 6 months, May be stuck in this stage for years, May have several previous failed quit attempts.	• Give pamphlet, briefly review pharmacotherapy option, provide information about state/federal quitlines (1-800-QUIT-NOW or www.smokefree.gov). • Offer future assistance when patient is ready. • Relate any evidence of tobacco-related disease during patient care. • Note intervention and stage in chart (takes about 1 to 2 minutes).
Preparation: Willing to quit within the next month, ready to set a quit date.	• Provide emotional support, and affirm benefits of not using tobacco stated by patient. • Explore different options to aid the patient to quit. • Explain pharmaceutical options; determine best fit. • Refer patient to a tobacco quitline/online support. • Provide printed resource materials (cessation workbook). • Encourage development of a support system (family, friends). • Help to set a quit date and note date in patient chart for future follow-up. • Allow the patient to select the quit plan—write it out, copy the plan, and place it in the chart (takes approximately 20 minutes).
Action: Has recently quit within the past 6 months.	• Provide emotional support, affirm benefits of not using tobacco stated by patient. • Review pharmaceuticals, if any, being used; support proper use. • Refer patient to a tobacco quitline/online support if patient has not accessed these resources. • Encourage use of the support system (family, friends). • Note quit date and patient's progress in chart. • Provide words of encouragement to continue (takes approximately 2 to 3 minutes).
Maintenance: Has abstained for at least 6 months (relapse prevention).	• Provide verbal support; point out any positive oral-health effects. • Help patient develop strategies to prevent relapse (takes approximately 1 minute).

FIGURE ■ 20–6 Tobacco Dependence Interventions Using the Stages of Change Model.

• *Repetition:* Use the 5 R's and motivational interviewing techniques each time a tobacco user receives dental treatment—keep the intervention short and focused. Actively listen to the patient; reflect his or her feelings, frustrations, and goals back to the patient. Allow the patient to choose a realistic quit plan that will work for him or her. Avoid "educating" the patient. Stress benefits of quitting.

An effective approach can be to say, "Chris, we have found evidence of moderate-to-severe periodontitis in your mouth, which can be a cause of your malodor. Periodontitis is a bacterial infection that your body has been unable to fight, most likely because of the toxins and carbon monoxide found in your tobacco smoke. Without a strong immune system, the ongoing bacterial infection will put you at an increased risk for losing your teeth—even with regular cleanings and good home care." The

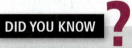

DID YOU KNOW

If a patient is not ready to quit, the PHS *Treating Tobacco Use and Dependence* 5 R's and brief motivational interviewing should be employed with the goal of establishing rapport and trust to build the next TDI on.

patient will need time to consider this information. Motivation to change often comes from very personal reasons and must not be related to the fear of cancer or lung disease. An effective TDI requires a learned and practiced skill that must consider numerous issues not to mention the time and office support needed to accomplish this essential service.

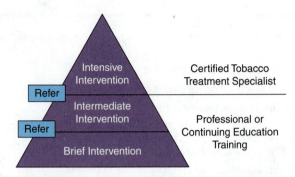

FIGURE ■ 20–7 Levels of tobacco dependence interventions.
(*Source:* Reprinted by permission. Davis et al., (2010), Education of tobacco use prevention and cessation for dental professionals – a paradigm shift. International Dental Journal, 60: 60–72. doi: 10.1922/IDJ_2535Davis13.)

LEVELS OF A TDI

Over the last 20 years, numerous strategies have been presented to aid clinicians in consistently and effectively providing TDI. The PHS guideline suggests using a brief (a few minutes) or an intensive (more than 20 minutes) intervention with repeated visits and reports that with all levels of intervention, the success of a cessation attempt increases when more time is spent.[70] The dental setting offers clinicians flexibility to offer varying levels of intervention ranging from a brief to moderate to an intensive intervention (Figure 20–7 ■), depending on the time and level of training the clinician has.

Brief Intervention (1+ minute)

Both the American Dental Hygienists' Association's Ask, Advise, Refer program (www.askadviserefer.org) and the American Dental Association's smoking and tobacco cessation program (www.ada.org/2615.aspx) encourage clinicians to offer at least a brief tobacco intervention at each visit. The clinician is directed to ask about tobacco use, advise the patient to quit, and then give resource information, emphasizing the use of the state or federal quitline (1-800-QUIT-NOW or www.smokefree.gov). The advantage to this system is that it provides a clear plan of action for use in a limited period of time. An adaptation to this model can be to ask and quickly assess the patient's stage via the health history and then advise the person to quit and offer help when he or she is ready to quit.

The clinician could place quitline information and an informational pamphlet in a bag with toothbrush and paste. This is an effective TDI strategy if the patient is not interested in setting a quit date and leaves open the possibility for continued discussion at future recare appointments.

Moderate Intervention (5 to 10 minutes)

A moderate intervention can be necessary for those individuals who have thought about previous conversations with the clinician, want more information on medications, resources, want more detail on how tobacco is affecting them, and are interested in moving forward toward a future quit attempt. Cessation is a process as is helping a patient quit. If trust and a sense of support are cultivated, the clinician will have numerous opportunities to offer the information and support that the patient is ready to hear. This process can require several years before the patient is ready to set a quit date. Success is a successful quit, but success also encompasses the process of moving the patient toward that goal. Dental professionals are well placed to spend the extra time needed during a recare appointment while still staying on time.

Intensive Intervention (20 or more minutes)

For those individuals who are ready to quit, need help creating a quit plan, or are highly addicted and have tried everything and failed, an intensive intervention could be indicated. The more time the provider spends with the patient, the more successful the quit attempt will be.[70] The intensive intervention should focus on past quit attempts, assessment of the patient's belief in being able to succeed, medications, barriers, establishing a support system, and a patient-developed quit plan. Few clinicians are able to create 20 minutes in an already tight schedule. Options to assist the patient could be to run over into the next appointment or to schedule another appointment for that specific purpose although dental insurance at this time does not cover that service. Another option is to refer the patient to a tobacco-counseling program or support group. Several institutions now offer tobacco-dependence specialist certification. Dental health professionals can pursue this specialty to better serve the community and the patients in their practices.

SUMMARY

Every dental patient who uses tobacco is at an increased risk for general and oral diseases including cardiovascular disease, oral cancer, and periodontitis. Tobacco-dependence interventions by dental clinicians can and do make a difference. The combination of behavioral therapy, pharmacotherapy, and follow-up has been shown to increase a tobacco user's ability to successfully quit from 3% to 5% on his or her own to 30% or more with clinician assistance. Dental health care professionals have the knowledge, opportunity, and ethical responsibility to offer an appropriate, patient-centered tobacco-dependence intervention as normal patient care.

PRACTICAL CONSIDERATIONS

Establishing a TDI In-Office Program

The dental office is composed of numerous individuals in different roles with all members working together as a team to provide quality patient care. This is especially true for the integration of TDIs.[105,106]

A successful TDI program consists of several basic components that need to be put in place: (1) acquiring information, (2) providing tobacco-dependence training/orientation to the office staff, (3) establishing a clear working relationship concerning the level of TDI to be offered and learning how to recommend medications and determine the level of follow-up, and (4) maintaining and evaluating the effectiveness of the TDI program by reviewing patient's and staff's verbal reaction.

Step 1

The collection of tobacco-dependence resources and services is very important when offering cessation interventions. The PHS guideline *Treating Tobacco Use and Dependence: 2008 Update*[70] is an important resource available to guide dental clinicians when recommending and/or prescribing pharmacotherapies.

Excellent sources for low- or no-cost tobacco-dependence materials include the local health department, the American Cancer Association, and the American Lung Association. The Centers for Disease Control and Prevention (CDC) also offers extensive educational and patient-cessation pamphlets, videos, and posters that can be ordered at http://www.cdc.gov/tobacco.

Another important cessation resource is the tobacco quitline, which has been proven to be effective in helping tobacco users quit[107] and can be a time-saving tool for a busy office. State quitlines offer two basic types of services: *reactive* (the tobacco user takes the initiative to call the quitline for counseling and information) and *proactive*: the clinician faxes a signed permission form to the quitline then the quitline makes *proactive* calls to the tobacco user to aid in their quit attempt..

In preparation for offering a TDI, the patient's health history should include data on tobacco use, level of dependence, and readiness to quit and then be evaluated and revised at each visit. This review will save the clinician a substantial amount of time and greatly aid with assessment. For example, (1) a hygienist offers a TDI, (2) the patient agrees to be contacted by a nicotine-dependence specialist from the state's quitline and signs the form requesting the service and giving permission for the dental office to fax the request, (3) the receptionist faxes the request, and (4) a trained specialist calls the patient over the next several weeks. This service greatly enhances and expands the TDI provided by the dental staff.

Another component of a new service is the insurance code for reimbursement. Although the American Dental Association has a code for tobacco cessation (D1320 – CDT-10, 2011; see www.ada.org), insurance does not pay for that service at this time.

Step 2

As with anything new, starting or enhancing a TDI program must include all dental team members' commitment to and support of it. Unfortunately, many providers still believe that they lack the training or experience to provide cessation services. Dental team members are able to increase their sense of self-efficacy and clinical ability by taking one or more of the many excellent continuing education courses or in-service, reading journal articles, and learning from self-instruction materials.[101,106–108]

Step 3

The scope of the office TDI protocol should be established before offering patients cessation services. Patients are not served well if the dental hygienist provides an effective TDI during the recare appointment that interests the patient in quitting by using bupropion, but the attending dentist feels uncomfortable prescribing an antidepressant (bupropion SR) for cessation and discusses only needed restorations with the patient. The roles and scope of services need to be established for each dental team member according to the following sample distribution of responsibilities:

- *Dentist:* Diagnose, conduct TDI, and prescribe medications.
- *Dental hygienist:* Perform comprehensive oral assessment, diagnose (depending on state law), conduct TDI, make referrals, recommend OTC medications, make chart notations, and follow-up at recare appointments.
- *Dental assistant:* Provide resource materials and make chart notation of TDI.
- *Receptionist:* Send referral/fax request to quitline, make formal follow-up, and schedule time for TDI.

Step 4

As with any services, the TDI program should be evaluated for staff and patient acceptance and effectiveness. Staff meetings and patient comments as well as self-reports of quit attempts and successful quits can all aid in evaluation. This evaluation could be done informally or during staff meetings.

Tobacco-Use Prevention

Ideally, the most effective way to avoid tobacco-related disease and death is by preventing its use in the first place. In the dental office/clinic, several positive steps can be taken to send a tobacco-free message, such as providing only magazines that do not contain tobacco advertising, posting a sign that invites patients to ask about smoking-cessation assistance, making informational material on the benefits of quitting and quitlines available in the waiting room, and asking youth (10 years and older) whether they have tried any tobacco products and providing support for their decision to not use them. These actions send a message that the dental staff is concerned about tobacco use and can offer help. If youth admit using tobacco products, then TDI should be employed.

On community, state, and federal levels, dental professionals have many opportunities to become proactive in efforts to prevent tobacco use and to eliminate public exposure to second-hand smoke. In the 2000 report of the Surgeon General, *Reducing Tobacco Use*,[61] the CDC identified four primary strategies that have been proven to reduce youth tobacco initiation and discontinuance of tobacco products.

1. Provide effective educational tobacco-prevention strategies for youth. School educational programs should emphasize refusal and decision-making strategies. Public health messages should include hard-hitting counteradvertising venues such as those found in the *TRUTH* campaign at http://www.thetruth.com.

2. Provide tobacco-dependence assistance adapted to the needs of youth.

3. Enact regulatory and policy measures that restrict youth access to tobacco products and eliminate smoking in public spaces. These measures counter the generally held assumption that smoking is OK because it is legal and everybody is doing it.

4. Raise taxes on tobacco products. This action restricts access by youth because of the high cost.

According to the Surgeon General's report, effective tobacco-prevention programs take a comprehensive approach and should include tobacco control policy and regulations preventing smoking in public places, educational, and cessation components. Clearly, this scope of action requires collaboration among many private, governmental, public health, and business entities. The CDC offers extensive resources including fact sheets, educational DVDs, posters, printed material, research articles, and links to organizations actively involved in tobacco prevention at http://www.cdc.gov/tobacco. A dental-specific tobacco dependence curriculum, *Tobacco Free! Curriculum* contains many of the resources and information discussed in this chapter (http://tobaccofree.siu.edu).

SELF-STUDY QUESTIONS

1. The percentage of adult smokers in the United States steadily declined beginning in 1964 and then leveled off in recent years. What is the current percentage of adults who smoke?

   a. 20.6%

   b. 26.8%

   c. 38.2%

   d. 46.4%

   Rationale: In 2011, approximately 20.6% of adults in the United States smoked.

2. Smoking was once thought of as just a bad habit. Today smoking is understood as a nicotine-dependent action and is considered a:

   a. Temporary, relapsing disorder

   b. Chronic, relapsing disorder

   c. Disorder that is easily treated with medication

   d. Condition most people get over with minimal help

   Rationale: The APA *DSM-IV* and the PHS 2008 guideline identify nicotine dependence as a chronic relapsing disease.

3. For which of the following oral conditions is smoking *not* considered a significant risk factor?

   a. Increased bone loss

   b. Increased probing depths

   c. Exaggerated tori development

   d. Increased tooth loss

   Rationale: The exaggerated development of mandibular tori is *not* associated with the use of tobacco products. Smoking is a strong risk factor in tooth loss, increased bone loss, and increased probing depths.

4. Which one of the following represents the U.S Public Health Service 5A's tobacco dependence intervention?

   a. Arrange, assist, assess, ask, advise

   b. Ask, assist, assess, advise, arrange

   c. Ask, advise, assess, assist, arrange

   d. Ask, arrange assist, advise, assess

   Rationale: The correct sequence for the PHS guideline's 5A's recommend a tobacco intervention is ask, advise, assess, assist, and arrange, depending on the patient's readiness to make a quit attempt.

5. Cessation medications should be discussed with and recommended to patients as a part of a tobacco-dependency intervention because they are able to:

   a. Eliminate all withdrawal symptoms

   b. Aid in the reduction of withdrawal symptoms

   c. Continue the positive effects of nicotine

   d. Provide healing to the cells damaged by tobacco use

   Rationale: While cessation medications provide needed relief from the withdrawal from the drug nicotine, they are often not able to eliminate all cravings or withdrawal symptoms. The combination of medications with behavioral interventions provides the patient the best chance of successfully quitting long-term.

REFERENCES

1. Centers for Disease Control and Prevention. (2008). Annual smoking-attributable mortality, years of potential life lost, and economic costs—United States: 2000–2004. *MMWR Morb Mortal Wkly Rep,* 57:1226–28.

2. U.S. Department of Health and Human Services. (2010). *How tobacco smoke causes disease: The biology and behavioral basis for smoking-attributable disease.* Rockville, MD: Public Health Service, Office of Surgeon General.

3. Centers for Disease Control and Prevention. (2010). Vital signs: Current cigarette smoking among adults aged ≥ 18 years—United States, 2009. *MMWR Morb Mortal Wkly Rep,* 59:1–12.

4. Centers for Disease Control and Prevention. (2010). Adult Tobacco Survey—19 states, 2003–2007. *MMWR Morb Mortal Wkly Rep,* 59:1–25.

5. Thun, M. J., & Jemal, A. (2006). How much of the decrease in cancer death rates in the United States is attributable to reductions in tobacco smoking? *Tob Control,* 15:345–47.

6. U.S. Department of Health and Human Services. (2020). *Healthy People 2020.* Washington, DC: U.S. Government Printing Office. Retrieved February 12, 2011, from http://www.healthypeople.gov/2020/default.aspx.

7. Centers for Disease Control and Prevention. (2010). Youth risk behavior surveillance—United States, 2009. *MMWR Morb Mortal Wkly Rep,* 59:1–148.

8. Centers for Disease Control and Prevention. (2010). Cigarette use among high school students—United States, 1991–2009. *MMWR Morb Mortal Wkly Rep,* 59:797–801.

9. U.S. Department of Health and Human Services. (2006). *The health consequences of involuntary exposure to tobacco smoke—A report of the Surgeon General.* Atlanta, GA: U.S. Department of Health and Human Services, Centers for Disease Control and Prevention.

10. Mecklenburg, R. E., Greenspan, D., Kleinman, D. V., Manley, M. W., Niessen, L. C., Robertson, P. B., & Winn, D. E. (1996). *Tobacco effects in the mouth.* (NIH Publication No. 96-3330). Bethesda, MD: U.S. Department of Health and Human Services, Public Health Service, National Institutes of Health.

11. Gelskey, S. C. (1999). Cigarette smoking and periodontitis: Methodology to assess the strength of evidence in support of a causal association. *Community Dent Oral Epidemiol,* 27(1):16–24.

12. American Cancer Society. (2010). *Cancer facts and figures 2010.* Atlanta, GA: American Cancer Society.

13. Blott, W. J., Mclaughlin, J. K., Winn, D. M., Austin, D. F., Greenberg, R. S., Preston-Martin, S., Berstein, L., Schoenberg, J. B., Stemhagen, A., & Fraumeni, J. R., Jr. (1988). Smoking and drinking in relation to oral and pharyngeal cancer. *Cancer Res,* 48:3282–87.

14. Danaei, G., Vander Hoorn, S., Lopez, A. D., Murray, C. J., & Ezzati, M. (2005). Causes of cancer in the world: Comparative risk assessment on nine behavioural and environmental risk factors. *Lancet,* 366:1784–93.

15. Rodriguez, T., Altieri, A., Chatenoud, L., Gallus, S., Bosetti, C., Negri, E., Franceschi, S., Levi, F., Talamini, R., & La Vecchia, C. (2004). Risk factors for oral and pharyngeal cancer in young adults. *Oral Oncol,* 40:207–13.

16. Banoczy, J., Ginter, Z., & Dombi, C. (2001). Tobacco use and oral leukoplakia. *J Dent Educ,* 65:322–27.

17. Silverman, S., Gorsky, M., & Lozada, F. (1984). Oral leukoplakia and malignant transformation. *Cancer,* 53:563–68.

18. Department of Health and Human Services. (1986). *The health consequences of using smokeless tobacco.* (NIH Publication No. 86-2874). Bethesda, MD: Department of Health and Human Services.

19. Bates, C., Fagerstrom, K., Jarvis, M., Kinze, M., McNeil, A., & Ramstrom, L. (2003). European Union policy on smokeless tobacco: A statement in favor of evidence-based regulation for public health. *Tob Control,* 12:360–67.

20. Accortt, N., Waterbor, J. W., Beall, C., & Howard, G. (2002). Chronic disease mortality in a cohort of smokeless tobacco users. *Am J Epidemiol,* 156:730–37.

21. Cobb, C. M., Williams, K. B., Gerkovich, W., & Gerkovich, M. (2009). Is the prevalence of periodontitis in the USA in decline? *J Periodontol,* 50:13–24.

22. Tomar, S., & Asma, S. (2000). Smoking-attributable periodontitis in the United States: Findings from NHANES III. *J Periodontol,* 71:743–51.

23. Calsina, G., Ramon, J. M., & Echeverria, J. J. (2002). Effects of smoking on periodontal tissues. *J Clin Periodontol,* 29:771–76.

24. Bergstrom, J. (2003). Tobacco smoking and risk for periodontal disease. *J Clin Periodontol,* 30:107–13.

25. Jansson, L., & Lavstedt, S. (2002). Influence of smoking on marginal bone loss and tooth loss—A prospective study over 20 years. *J Clin Periodontol,* 29:750–56.

26. Kowolik, M. J., & Nisbet, T. (1983). Smoking and acute ulcerative gingivitis. *Br Dent J,* 154:241–42.

27. Krall, E. A., Abreau Sosa, C., Garcia, C., Nunn, M. E., Caplan, D. J., & Garcia, R. I. (2006). Cigarette smoking increases the risk of root canal treatment. *J Dent Res,* 85:313–37.

28. Strietzel, F. P., Reichart, P. A., Kale, A., Kulkarni M., Wegner, B., & Kuchler, I. (2007). Smoking interferes with the prognosis of dental implant treatment: A systemic review and meta-analysis. *J Cln Periodontol,* 34: 523–44.

29. Kinane, D. E., & Chestnutt, I. G. (2000). Smoking and periodontal disease. *Crit Rev Oral Biol Med,* 11:356–65.

30. Bergstrom, J., & Bostrom, L. (2001). Tobacco smoking and periodontal hemorrhagic responsiveness. *J Clin Periodontol,* 30:107–13.

31. Hanioka, T., Tanaka, M., Takaya, K., Matsumori, Y., & Shizukuishi, S. (2000). Pocket oxygen tension in smokers and non-smokers with periodontal disease. *J Periodontol,* 71:550–54.

32. Ryder, M. I., Saghizadeh, M., Ding, Y., Nguyen, N., & Soskoline, A. (2002). Effects of tobacco smoke on the secretion of interleukin-1β, tumor necrosis factor-α, and transforming growth factor β from peripheral blood mononuclear cells. *Oral Microbiol Immunol,* 17:331–36.

33. Giannopoulou, C., Cappuyns, I., & Mombelli, A. (2003). Effect of smoking on gingival crevicular fluid cytokine profile during experimental gingivitis. *J Clin Periodontol,* 30:996–1002.

34. Kamma, J. J., Giannopoulou, C., Vasdekis, V. G. S., & Mombelli, A. (2004). Cytokine profile in gingival crevicular fluid of aggressive periodontitis: Influence of smoking and stress. *J Clin Periodontol,* 31:894–902.

35. Mantyla, P., Stenman, M., Kinane, D., Salo, T., Suomalainen, K., Tikanoja, S., & Sorsa, T. (2006). Monitoring periodontal disease status in smokers and nonsmokers using a gingival crevicular fluid matrix metalloproteinase-8-specific chair-side test. *J Periodont Res,* 41:503–12.

36. Gamal, A. Y., & Bayomy, M. M. (2002). Effect of cigarette smoking on human PDL fibroblasts attachment to periodontally involved root surfaces in vitro. *J Clin Periodontol,* 29:763–70.

37. Johnson, G. K., & Hill, M. (2004). Cigarette smoking and the periodontal patient. *J Periodontol,* 75:196–209.

38. Palmer, R. M., Wilson, R. F., Hasan, A.S., & Scott, D. A. (2005). Mechanism of action of environmental factors—Tobacco smoking. *J Clin Periodontol,* 32(Suppl 6):180–95.

39. Labriola, A., & Needleman, I. (2005). Systematic review of the effect of smoking on nonsurgical periodontal therapy. *Periodontology 2000,* 37:124–37.

40. Morozumi, T., Kubota, T., Sato, T., Okuda, K., & Yoshie, H. (2004). Smoking cessation increases gingival blood flow and gingival crevicular fluid. *J Clin Periodontol,* 31:267–72.

41. Robertson, P. B., Walsh, M., Green, J., Ernster, V., Grady, D., & Hauch, W. (1990). Periodontal effects associated with the use of smokeless tobacco. *J Periodontol,* 61:438–43.

42. Sinusas, K., Coroso, J. G., Sopher, M. D., & Crabtree, B. F. (1992). Smokeless tobacco use and oral pathology in a professional baseball organization. *J Fam Pract,* 34:713–18.

43. Bergstrom, J., Keilani, H., Lundholm, C., & Radestad, U. (2006). Smokeless tobacco (snuff) use and periodontal bone loss. *J Clin Periodontol,* 33:549–54.

44. Fisher, M. A., Taylor, G. W., & Tilashalshi, K. R. (2005). Smokeless tobacco and severe active periodontal disease, NHANES III. *J Dent Res,* 84:705–10.

45. American Academy of Periodontology. (1999). Tobacco use and the periodontal patient. *J Periodontol,* 70:1419–27.

46. Substance Abuse and Mental Health Services Administration. (2010). *Results from the 2009 national survey on drug use and health: Volume I. Summary of National findings.* U.S. Department of Health and Human Services. Accessed March 4, 2011, at http://www.oas.samhsa.gov/NSDUH/2k9NSDUH/2k9 ResultsP.pdf.

47. Green, C. R., & Rodgman, A. (1996). The Tobacco Chemists' Research Conference: A half-century of advances in analytical methodology of tobacco and its products. *Recent Adv Tob Sci,* 22:131–304.

48. Hoffmann, D., & Hoffmann, I. (1997). The changing cigarette, 1950–1995. *J Toxicol Environ Health,* 50:307–64.

49. National Cancer Institute, Smoking and Tobacco Control. (1998). *Cigars, health effects and trends.* (Monograph 9, NIH Publication No. 98-4302). Bethesda, MD: U.S. Department of Health and Human Services, National Institutes of Health, National Cancer Institute, 73–97.

50. National Toxicology Program. (2000). *9th report on carcinogens* (11th ed.). Bethesda, MD: U.S. Department of Health and Human Sciences, National Institute of Environmental Health Sciences. Retrieved November 21, 2006, from http://www.cdc.gov/tobacco/ETS_Toolkit/PublicPlaces/secondhand-smoke.

51. Johnson G. K., & Guthmiller, J. M. (2007). The impact of cigarette smoking on periodontal disease and treatment. *Periodontol 2000,* 44:178–94.

52. National Cancer Institute, Smoking and Tobacco Control. (2002). *Risks associated with smoking cigarettes with low machine-measured yields of tar and nicotine.* (Monograph 13, NIH Publication No. 02-5047). Bethesda, MD: U.S. Department of Health and Human Services, National Institutes of Health, National Cancer Institute, 13–63.

53. Centers for Disease Control and Prevention. (2010). Tobacco use among middle and high school students—United States, 2000–2009. *Morb Mortal Wkly Rep,* 59(33):1063–68.

54. Watson, C. H., Polzin, G. M., Calafat, A. M., & Ashley, D. L. (2003). Determination of the tar, nicotine, and carbon monoxide yields in the smoke of bidi cigarettes. *Nicotine Tob Res,* 5:747–53.

55. Malson, J. L., Lee, E. M., Murty, R., Moolchan, E. T., & Pickworth, W. B. (2003). Clove cigarette smoking: Biochemical, physiological, and subjective effects. *Pharmacol Biochem Behav,* 74:739–45.

56. Asorta, K. (2005). Hooked on hookah? What you don't know can kill you. *Burning Issues: Hottest Topics: Tobacco-Related Disease Research Program Newsletter,* 7:1–11.

57. Shihadeh, A., & Saleh, R. (2005). Polycyclic aromatic hydrocarbons, carbon monoxide, "tar," and nicotine in the mainstream smoke aerosol of the narghile water pipe. *Food Chem Toxicol,* 43:655–61.

58. U.S. Department of Health and Human Services. (1986). *The health consequences of using smokeless tobacco: A report of the Advisory Committee to the Surgeon General.* (NIH Publication No. 86-2874). Bethesda, MD: U.S. Department of Health and Human Services, Public Health Service.

59. Hoffman, D., Djordjecic, M. V., Fran, J., Zang, E., Glynn, T., & Connolly, G. N. (1995). Five leading U.S. commercial brands of moist snuff in 1994: Assessment of carcinogenic N-nitrosamines. *J Natl Cancer Inst,* 87:1862–69.

60. Hoffman, D., & Djordjecic, M. V. (1997). Chemical composition and carcinogenicity of smokeless tobacco. *Adv Den Res,* 11:322–29.

61. U.S. Department of Health and Human Services. (2000). *Reducing tobacco use: A report of the Surgeon General.* Atlanta, GA: U.S. Department of Health and Human Services, Centers for Disease Control and Prevention.

62. Centers for Disease Control and Prevention. (1999). Nicotine, pH, and moisture of smokeless tobacco—Florida, January–February. *MMWR Morb Mortal Wkly Rep,* 48:398–401.

63. Going, R. E., Hsu, S. C., Pollack, R. L., & Haugh, L. D. (1980). Sugar and fluoride content of various forms of tobacco. *J Am Dent Assoc,* 100:27–33.

64. Tomar, S. L., & Winn, D. M. (1999). Chew-tobacco use and dental caries among U.S. men. *J Am Dent Assoc,* 130:1601–10.

65. Rubinstein, I., & Pedersen, G. W. (2002). Bacillus species are present in chewing tobacco sold in the United States and evoke plasma exudation from the oral mucosa. *Clin Diag Lab Immunol,* 9:1057–60.

66. Bowles, W. H., Wilkinson, M. R., Wagner, M. J., & Woody, R. D. (1995). Abrasive particles in tobacco products: A possible factor in dental attrition. *J Am Dent Assoc,* 126:327–31.

67. National Cancer Institute, Centers for Disease Control and Prevention. (2002, September). Smokeless tobacco fact sheets. Paper presented at the 3rd International Conference on Smokeless Tobacco, Stockholm Center of Public Health, Stockholm, Sweden.

68. International Agency for Research on Cancer (2004). Betel-quid and areca-nut chewing and some areca-nut-derived nitrosamines (vol. 84). Retrieved March 4, 2011 from http://monographs.iarc.fr/ENG/Monographs/vol85/volume85.pdf.

69. Critchley, J. A., & Unal, B. (2003). Health effects associated with smokeless tobacco: A systemic review. *Thorax,* 58:435–43.

70. Fiore, M. C., Jaen, C. R., Baker, T. B., Bailey, W. C., Benowitz, N. L., & Curry, S. J. (2008). *Treating tobacco use and dependence: 2008 Update.* (Clinical Practice Guideline). Rockville, MD: US Department of Health and Human Services.

71. U.S. Department of Health and Human Services. (1988). *Nicotine addiction: The health consequences of smoking: A report of the Surgeon General.* Rockville, MD: Centers for Disease Control and Prevention, National Center for Chronic Disease Prevention and Health Promotion, Office on Smoking and Health.

72. Benowitz, N. L. (1996). Pharmacology of nicotine: Addiction and therapeutics. *Annu Rev Pharmacol Toxicol, 36:*597–613.

73. Benowitz, N. L. (1997). Systemic absorption and effects of nicotine from smokeless tobacco. *Adv Dent Res,* 11:336–40.

74. Perkins, K. A. (1993). Weight gain following smoking cessation. *J Consult Clin Psychol,* 61:768–77.

75. Benwell, M. E. M., Balfour, D. K. J., & Birrell, C. E. (1995). Desensitization of the nicotine-induced mesolimbic dopamine responses during constant infusion with nicotine. *Br J Pharmacol,* 114:454–60.

76. Groman, E., & Fagerstrom, K. (2003). Nicotine dependence: Development, mechanisms, individual differences, and links to possible neurophysiological correlates. *Wein Klim Wochenschr,* 115:155–60.

77. Dodgen, C. E. (2005). *Nicotine dependence: Understanding and applying the most effective treatment interventions.* Washington, DC: American Psychological Association.

78. Hatsukami, D. K., Stead, L. F., & Gupta, P. C. (2008). Tobacco addiction. *Lancet,* 371:2027–38.

79. American Psychiatric Association. (2000). *Diagnostic criteria from diagnostic statistical manual of mental disorders* (4th ed.). Washington, DC: American Psychiatric Association.

80. National Survey on Drug Use and Health. (2008). *Nicotine dependence: 2006.* Retrieved March 4, 2011 from http://www.oas.samhsa.gov/2k8/nicotine/nicotine.htm.

81. Tong, E. K., Ong, M. K., Vittinghoff, E., & Perez-Stable, E. J. (2006). Non-daily smokers should be asked and advised to quit. *Am J Prev Med,* 30:23–30.

82. Munafo, M. R., Clark, T. G., Johnstone, E. C., Murphy, M. F. G., & Walton, R. T. (2004). The genetic basis for smoking behavior: A systemic review and meta-analysis. *Nicotine Tob Res,* 6:583–97.

83. Benowitz, N. L., Pomerleau, O. F., Pomerleau, C. S., & Jacob, P., III. (2003). Nicotine metabolite ratio as a predictor of cigarette consumption. *Nicotine Tob Res,* 5:621–24.

84. Henningfield, J. E., Pankow, J. F., & Garrett, B. E. (2004). Ammonia and other chemical base tobacco additives and cigarette nicotine delivery: Issues and research needs. *Nicotine Tob Res,* 6:199–205.

85. Kotlyar, M., & Hatsukami, D. K. (2002). Managing nicotine addiction. *J Dent Educ,* 66:1061–73.

86. Ellerbeck, E. F., Mahnken, J. D., Cupertino, A. P, Cox, L. S., Greiner, K. A., & Mussulman, L. M. (2009). Effect of varying levels of disease management of smoking cessation. *Ann Intern Med,* 150: 437–46.

87. Hughes, J. (2008). An algorithm for choosing among smoking cessation treatments. *J Subst Abuse Treat,* 34:426–32.

88. Cepeda-Benito, A., Reynoso, J. T., & Erath, S. (2004). Meta-analysis of the efficacy of nicotine-replacement therapy for smoking cessation: Differences between men and women. *J Consult Clin Pharm,* 72:712–22.

89. Schneider, N. G., Olmstead, R. E., Franzon, M. A., & Lunell, E. (2001). The nicotine inhaler: Clinical pharmacokinetics and comparison with other nicotine treatments. *Clin Pharmacokinet,* 40:661–84.

90. Le Houezec, J. (2003). Role of nicotine pharmacokinetics in nicotine addiction and nicotine-replacement therapy: A review. *Int J Tuberc Lung Dis,* 7:811–19.

91. Stead, L. F., Perera, R., Bullen, C., Mant, D., & Lancaster, T. (2008). Nicotine replacement therapy for smoking cessation (Review). *The Cochrane Library,* 3:1–163.

92. Heatherton, T. F., Kozlowski, L. T., Frecker, R. C., & Fagerstrom, K. (1991). The Fagerstrom test for nicotine dependence: A revision of the Fagerstrom tolerance questionnaire. *Br J Addict,* 86:1119–27.

93. Heatherton, T. F., Kozlowski, L. T., Frecker, R. C., Rickert, R. C., & Robinson, W. S. (1989). Measuring the heaviness of smoking using self-reported time to first cigarette of the day and the number of cigarettes smoked per day. *Br J Addict,* 84:791–800.

94. Ebbert, J. O., Patten, C. A., & Schroeder, D. R. (2006). The Fagerstrom test for nicotine dependence—Smokeless tobacco (FTND-ST). *Addict Behav,* 31:1716–21.

95. Warner, C., & Shoaib, M. (2005). How does bupropion work as a smoking-cessation aid? *Addict Biol,* 10:219–31.

96. Benowitz, N. L. (2008). Neurobiology of nicotine addiction: Implications for smoking cessation treatment. *Amer J Med,* 121:S3-S10.

97. Hays, J. T., Ebbert, J. O., & Sood, A. (2008). Efficacy and safety of varenicline for smoking cessation. *Amer J Med,* 121:S32-S42.

98. U.S. Food and Drug Administration. (2009). Varenicline and bupropion. *Drug Safety Newsletter,* 2:1–4.

99. Ebbert, J. O., Croghan, I. T., Sood, A., Schroeder, D. R., Hays, J. T., & Hurt, R. D. (2009). Varenicline and bupropion sustained-release combination therapy for smoking cessation. *Nic Tob Research,* 11:234–39.

100. Zevin, S., & Benowitz, N. L. (1999). Drug interactions with tobacco smoking: An update. *Clin Pharmacokinet,* 36:425–38.

101. Tremblay, M., Cournoyer, D., & O'Loghlin, J. (2009). Do correlates of smoking cessation counseling differ across health professional groups? *Nic Tob Research,* 11:1330–38.

102. Applegate, B. W., Sheffer, C. E., Crews, K. M., Payne, T. J., & Smith, P. O. (2008). A survey of tobacco-related knowledge, attitudes and behaviors of primary care providers in Mississippi. *J Eval Clin Pract,* 14:537–44.

103. Solenberg, L. I., Boyle, R. G., Davidson, G., Magnan, S. J., & Link Carlson, C. (2001). Patient satisfaction and discussion of smoking cessation during clinical visits. *Mayo Clin Proc,* 78:138–43.

104. Rollnick, S., Miller, W. R., & Butler, C. (2008). *Motivational interviewing in health care.* New York, NY: Guilford Publications.

105. Rosseel, J. P., Jacobs, J. E., Hilberink, S. R., Maassen, I. M., & Allard, R. H. B., Plasschaert, A. J. M., et al. (2009). What determines the provision of smoking cessation advice and counseling by dental care teams? *Brit Dent J,* 206, doi:10.1038/sj.bdj.2009.272

106. Gonseth, S., Abarca, M., Madrid, C., & Cornuz, J. (2010). A pilot study combining individual-based smoking cessation counseling, pharmacotherapy, and dental hygiene intervention. *MBC Pub Health,* 10:348. Retrieved March 24, 2011, from http://www.biomedcentral.com/1471-2458/10/348.

107. Little, S. J., Hollis, J. F., Fellows, J. L., Snyder, J. L., Snyder, J. J., & Dickerson, J. F. (2009). Implementing a tobacco assisted referral program in dental practices. *J Public Health Dent,* 69: 149–55.

108. Davis, J. M., Ramseier, C. A., Mattheos, N., Schoonheim-Klein, M., Compton, S., Al-Hazimi N., et al. (2010). Education of tobacco use prevention and cessation for dental professionals—A paradigm shift. *Int Dent J,* 60:60–72.

PEARSON
myhealthprofessionskit

Visit www.myhealthprofessionskit.com to access the interactive Companion Website for this textbook. Simply select "Dental Hygiene" from the choice of disciplines. Find this book and log in by using your user name and password to access additional learning tools.

Athletic Mouthguards

Christine N. Nathe

OBJECTIVES

After studying this chapter, the student should be able to:

1. Describe the preventive aspects of athletic mouthguards.
2. Describe the historical aspects of athletic mouthguards.
3. Describe the prevalence of sports-related orofacial and head trauma.
4. List the promotional activities advocating the use of mouthguards.
5. List the sports and activities that should involve the use of athletic mouthguards.
6. Describe the types of athletic mouthguards.
7. Describe the fabrication of custom-made vacuum-formed mouthguards.
8. Describe the dental provider's role in the use of athletic mouthguards.

KEY TERMS

Athletic mouthguard, 362
Concussions, 363
Custom-made mouthguard, 365
Dental trauma, 363
Mouth-formed mouthguard, 364
Prognathic, 366
Repeated mild brain injuries, 363
Stock mouthguard, 364
Study model, 366

INTRODUCTION

Although many orofacial injuries can be prevented during participation in athletic activities, some individuals do not use athletic mouthguards. It is necessary for dental providers to promote the use of athletic mouthguards, educate the public on the value of mouth protection during contact sports, and fabricate mouthguards for athletes. In addition, dental providers should promote the use of mouthguards by implementing mouthguard programs in school sports and private athletic organizations.

An **athletic mouthguard** is a removable oral appliance that protects the hard and soft tissues of the oral cavity during contact sports; the appliance is sometimes referred to as a *mouth protector* (Figure 21–1 ■). Mouthguards protect by absorbing energy during an impact, thus decreasing the likelihood of trauma to the oral cavity and brain.

Interestingly, 36% of all of mouth injuries are related to sports activities.[1] Emergency department visits are highest among the school-age to young adult population, and more than one-third of school-age children will sustain an injury severe enough to be treated by a doctor or nurse, which drives the costs to be estimated as high as 1.8 billion dollars per year.[2] This issue of prevention is significant considering that a 2008 survey found that more than 44 million children participated in some form of youth sports in the United States, which is an increase from 38 million children in 2000.[3]

Some postulate that coaches and trainers have not been favorably disposed to mouthguard use in organized sports programs.[4–6] These data underscore the need for the promotion of athletic mouthguards by dental providers.

HISTORICAL PERSPECTIVE

Historically, boxers became the first athletes on record to use mouthguards.[7,8] Mouthguards, or "gum shields," were originally developed in 1890 by Woolf Krause, a London dentist, as a means of protecting boxers from lip lacerations.[7] Marks constructed an early mouthguard by fabricating a rubber strip that fit securely under the lip and over the outer surfaces of the teeth and gingiva.[9] Boxers also placed other materials such as cotton and gutta-percha between lips and teeth for protection.[9]

In 1941, a study revealed that 25% of all football injuries reported among high school players involved teeth, and in 1950, a study stated that dental injuries were the most common football injury reported by school sports programs.[10] A 1952 photograph of the Notre Dame football team, which appeared in *Life* magazine, visibly educated the public about the extent of orofacial injuries; the caption read "The Football Smile" since it showcased a toothless smile of a football player in uniform. This smile revealed many college football players with missing teeth and portrayed a natural correlation between the contact sport and orofacial trauma. However, after a letter was received from the president of Notre Dame, which indicated that at least one of the photographs was actually adjusted to make it look like a player was missing teeth (when he, in fact, had a full dentition), *Life* magazine ran a new photograph of the team. Evidently, it was

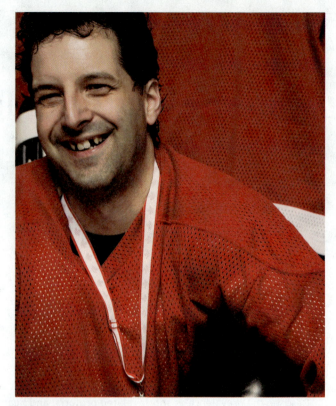

FIGURE ■ 21–1 The hockey smile
(*Source:* Radius Images/Alamy.)

a common perception that many individuals associated contact sports with dental injuries and perhaps even portrayed athletes with missing teeth as a side effect to extreme athleticism.

MOUTHGUARD USE

Recommendations have existed for the use of mouthguards dating back to the 1950s when the American Dental Association (ADA) became actively involved in promoting mouthguard use and in determining the extent of oral injuries in football.[11] Then, in 1962, the use of mouthguards was mandated in high school and junior college football by the National Alliance Football Rules Committee. By 1973, the National Collegiate Athletic Association (NCAA) followed suit. The Academy of Sports Dentistry was founded in 1983 to address the prevention of oral and facial injuries during athletic endeavors.[12] Then in the early 1990s, the NCAA expanded the mandated use of mouth protection to include additional sports.[13] The NCAA guidelines on mouthguards are listed in (Table 21–1 ■).

Although the majority of contact sports for youth, high school, and college athletes mandate the use of mouthguards, there is still controversy over their use. In 2007, Massachusetts coaches complained that the mouthguards inhibited communication on the court and said they were unsanitary because players would frequently drop them on the floor and have to put them back in their mouths. Subsequently, the Massachusetts Interscholastic Athletic Association voted to remove the mandatory use of the mouthguards.[14]

TABLE ■ 21–1 NCAA Guidelines for Mouthguards

1. Properly fitted mouthguards could reduce the potential chipping of tooth enamel surfaces and reduce fractures of teeth, roots, and bones.
2. Properly fitted mouthguards could protect the lip and cheek tissues from being impacted and lacerated against tooth edges.
3. Properly fitted mouthguards could reduce the incidence of fractured jaw caused by a blow delivered to the chin or head.
4. Properly fitted mouthguards could provide protection to toothless spaces; therefore, support is given to the missing dentition of the student athlete.

(*Source:* © National Collegiate Athletic Association 2011. All rights reserved.)

On the other side of the spectrum, the National Federation of High School Associations' Ice Hockey Rules Committee voted to eliminate a requirement for both boys and girls that a mouthguard be attached to a player's face mask. The committee noted that attached mouthguards make it easier for a player to let the guard dangle and believed their rule change would encourage more players to wear the mouthguards properly.[14]

DID YOU KNOW ?

Prior to implementation of the National Federation of State High School Association's mouthguard rule, an athlete participating in contact sports had a 10% chance of sustaining a significant oral-facial injury each season and better than a 50% chance during their secondary school careers.

On a professional level, the National Football League does not require the use of athletic mouthguards.[15] However, professional football players generally are seen on game day with team-colored mouthguards in place. This is an excellent example of an unintentional health promotional activity that naturally is geared toward young athletes and their parents on a consistent basis during football season.

One team from the National Hockey League recently collaborated with Delta Dental of Tennessee to kick off the "Protect Your Fangs" campaign. This intentional promotional activity involved professional athletes handing out mouthguards to local youth hockey players to encourage the use of mouthguards to prevent injury and maintain oral health.[16]

CONTACT SPORT INJURIES

Many types of orofacial injuries exist, including **dental trauma**, which is injury to the mouth, including teeth, periodontium, soft tissues, and the temporomandibular joint. The U.S. Surgeon General's report on oral health identified sporting activities as one of the major causes of craniofacial injuries.[17] Numerous studies have shown a link between athletic activities and dental

injuries; furthermore, almost one in six sports-related injuries is to the craniofacial area.[1,17] In fact, approximately 50% of children will sustain traumatic dental injury during childhood.[18] The National Youth Sports Foundation for the Prevention of Athletic Injuries reported that dental injuries are the most common type of injury sustained during participation in sports.[19]

DID YOU KNOW ?

Prior to the use of properly fitted mouthguards and face masks, more than 50% of football player's injuries were oral-facial, but now they represent less than 1% of injuries.

Chipped and avulsed incisor teeth are the most common sports-related orofacial injuries.[20] Mandibular fractures are the most common orofacial fracture, and 31% of all mandibular fractures are sports related; in contrast, 10% of all maxillofacial fractures are sports related.[20,21]

More than 300,000 people suffer traumatic brain injuries while playing sports, most of which are **concussions**.[22] What an athlete experiences during a concussion is actually a temporary trauma-induced alteration in mental status.[23] Many concussions occur without the individual ever losing consciousness, but researchers have determined that **repeated mild brain injuries** occurring over an extended period result in cumulative neurologic and cognitive deficits.[23] One article suggested that more than 90% of brain concussions resulting in unconsciousness to athletes are a result of a blow or trauma to the jaw.[24]

MOUTHGUARD PROTECTION AND INJURY PREVENTION

Studies have repeatedly revealed the protective value of mouthguards in reducing sports-related injuries to the teeth and soft tissues.[25–28] Mouthguards work by moving soft tissue in the oral cavity away from the teeth and into the upper jaw, preventing laceration and bruising of the lips and cheeks, especially for those individuals who wear orthodontic appliances. Additionally, mouthguards act as a simple protectant to the teeth by preventing chipping, fracturing, displacement, and avulsion.

Moreover, the dynamic properties of the mouthguard help absorb the energy associated with the blow the athlete receives. Mouthguards can prevent concussions, cerebral hemorrhages, unconsciousness, jaw fractures, and neck injuries by helping to avoid situations in which the mandible is jammed into the maxilla.[29,30] Mouthguards can work by providing cushioning between the maxilla and mandible and by lessening the severity of condylar-displacement injuries, which can subsequently reduce concussions as illustrated in (Figure 21–2 ■).

However, recent reports are suggesting that there is insufficient evidence that mouthguards reduce the occurrence of concussions and that more studies are recommended in this area.[7,8,31] The Centers for Disease Control and Prevention found insufficient evidence to issue a communitywide

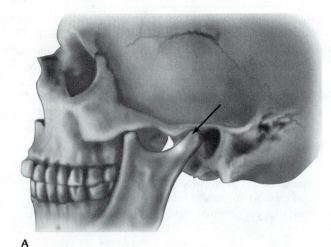

A

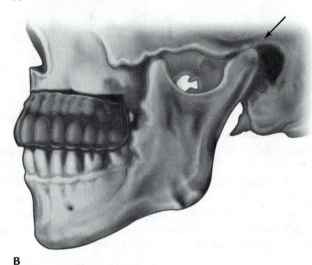

B

FIGURE ■ 21–2 **A. Note head of condyle and base of the skull without a properly fitted mouthguard. B. Note separation in space between the head of the condyle to the base of the skull with a properly fitted mouthguard in place.**

recommendation on the effectiveness of mouthguards as a preventive intervention and identified the need for more "high-quality research on their effectiveness."[31]

The ADA has promoted the use of properly fitted mouthguards as the primary means to protect against oral injuries during sports.[32] In particular, some sports are more likely to involve contact that could lead to sports injuries. For that reason, the American Academy of Pediatrics has classified sports according to the degree of contact. In addition, the American Academy of Pediatric Dentistry recommends the use of properly fitted mouthguards in organized sports.[33] Furthermore, the American Association of Orthodontics and the American Association of Oral and Maxillofacial Surgeons promote April as National Facial Protection Month. The American Dental Hygienists' Association supports mandating the use of mouth and head protection for participants during sports activities that involve risk of dental and/or craniofacial injuries.[34]

Interdisciplinary advocacy of mouthguard use was revealed in one study in which 93% of NCAA-certified athletic trainers reported that athletic mouthguards play a role in prevention.[35]

Studies suggest that athletic mouthguards improve the performance of the athletes by increasing concentration of their efforts on the execution of their sport.[36-38] These findings suggest that the use of mouthguards can have an unintended side effect of performance improvement.

Most athletes believe that mouthguards prevent injuries; however, some athletes do not want to wear a mouthguard because they believe that they would not be able to breathe as easily without one.[39] One study evaluated the oxygen consumption during exercise of athletes wearing mouthguards compared with those not wearing mouthguards; investigators found no difference in oxygen consumption between the two groups.[40]

One study has suggested the occurrence of more oral lesions on individuals routinely wearing athletic mouthguards.[41] The possibility exists that if an individual has sensitive skin, the skin around the mouth could react to the mouthguard material. This condition has not been described in the literature but has been reported in other venues.

TYPES OF MOUTHGUARDS

Three types of mouthguards are commonly available to the athlete: the stock, mouth-formed, and custom-made mouthguard (Table 21–2 ■). The role of any type of mouthguard is to provide protection and prevent orofacial injuries. Although there are inherent differences in types of mouthguards, the **mouth-formed mouthguards** are used most frequently (90%), but custom-made mouthguards (10%) are most effective at preventing injury.[9]

A **stock mouthguard** is available in different sizes. It is not custom made and is not preferred because of the poor fit and excess bulk. Many times athletes chew on this type to make it fit better; athletes also tend to be less compliant with this type of mouthguard because of the imperfect fit (Figure 21–3A ■ and B).

A mouth-formed guard, which is generally referred to as a *boil-n-bite* style, can be heated in water and then placed in the mouth. The athlete bites into the guard, producing an inexact

TABLE ■ 21–2   Types of Mouthguards

Type	Definition
Stock mouthguard	Available in different sizes. Not custom-made. Patients are generally not compliant about wearing this type because of its poor fit and excessive bulk.
Mouth-formed (Boil-n-bite)	Mouth-formed mouthguard that is heated in water and placed in the mouth, producing an inexact fit. Many young athletes use this type of mouthguard.
Custom-made mouthguard	A mouthguard that is made on a study model with the use of a vacuum-forming machine; is the most expensive. Can be made in the dental office or sent to a laboratory. Alginate impression is taken in the dental office. Compliance increases with this type of mouthguard.

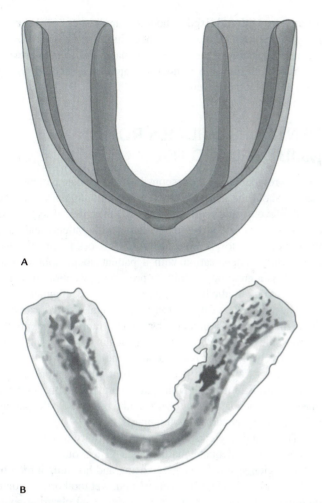

FIGURE ■ 21–3 A. Stock mouthguard. B. Stock mouthguard after several weeks of use.

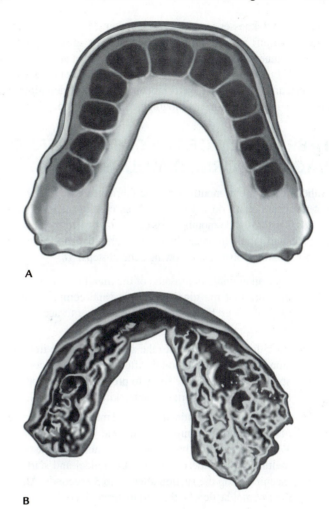

FIGURE ■ 21–4 A. Mouth-formed mouthguard. B. Mouth-formed mouthguard after it has been chewed by athlete.

fit. This type of mouthguard can become distorted and does not accommodate an individual athlete's unique oral features. Boil-n-bite mouthguards are the most widely used type (Figure 21–4A ■ and B).

Although there is limited research on the most-effective mouthguard, most dental organizations promote the use of the **custom-made mouthguard** (Figure 21–5 ■). One study reported no statistical difference between football players wearing boil-n-bite versus custom-made mouthguards in preventing concussions,[28] but another study suggested that custom-made mouthguards were significantly more protective in preventing head and oral injuries than boil-n-bite mouthguards.[42]

A study comparing the two different types of custom-made mouthguards reported that patients preferred the custom-made, double-layered, heat-and-pressure mouthguard to the custom-made, vacuum-formed type.[43] Furthermore, Winters suggested that custom-made laminated mouthguards do not break down with use, players do not tend to abuse or alter them, and this type of mouthguard increases separation of teeth, which is desirable to reduce concussions.[44]

Currently, there are two methods of fabricating custom-made mouthguards: vacuum formed and pressure laminated. These types of mouthguard are custom fabricated and fit precisely on the individual athlete's dentition. Because they are

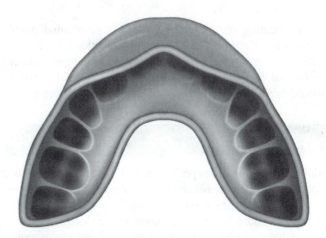

FIGURE ■ 21–5 Custom-made athletic mouthguard.

more comfortable and fit better, compliance increases; therefore, the custom-made mouthguard is more effective at reducing injuries. Both types can be fabricated in the dental office or sent to a laboratory. Many dental laboratories fabricate pressure-laminated mouthguards and use the sports team colors on the mouthguard to match the uniforms. Pressure-laminated mouthguards, compared with other mouthguards, seem to maintain minimal and consistent thicknesses in critical areas better. The thicker materials (3–4 mm) are more effective in absorbing impact energy, and the thinner materials show marked deformation at the site of impact.[12] In addition, this type of mouthguard does not need to be replaced unless the athlete has orthodontics or mixed dentition. If cost is an issue, a boil-n-bite mouthguard is recommended.

FABRICATION OF THE CUSTOM-MADE, VACUUM-FORMED MOUTHGUARD

Although boil-n-bite mouthguards are fabricated easily, they are not as accurate and do not fit as well as custom-made mouthguards. Custom-made mouthguards can be fabricated by a dental provider and should fit precisely over the dentition. Fabrication of a mouthguard involves the following general steps:

- Take an alginate impression of the maxillary arch, making sure that the gingival margins and complete anatomy of the arch are impressed. Take care to accurately reproduce the anatomy.

- Pour the dental stone into the accurate alginate impression to form a **study model**. After the model has cooled, spray it with a silicone spray to prevent the thermoplastic mouthguard material from sticking to the model.

- Place the thermoplastic mouthguard material in the frame of the vacuum-forming machine and heat the material. When the material has heated and slumped (plastic is melting), lower the frame onto the model and start the machine. Stop the suction after 20 to 30 seconds. Allow the thermoplastic mouthguard material to cool.

- Remove the mouthguard material from the model. Trim the mouthguard, making sure to trim above the gingival margin to help the mouthguard stay in place during the athletic event.

Fabricating athletic mouthguards for certain individuals requires a few special considerations. If an athlete has a **prognathic** (forward projecting) mandible, the mouthguard should be formed on the mandibular dentition.[45,46] Dental providers should fabricate maxillary and mandibular arch mouthguards for athletes with full fixed orthodontic appliances.[45,46] Silicone putty can be used on the study model during mouthguard fabrication and placed on the orthodontic band area to help prevent undercut.[46] Removable orthodontic appliances should not be worn during athletic events.

DENTAL PROVIDER'S ROLE IN MOUTHGUARD USE

Dental providers have the responsibility to educate patients and parents about the necessity of wearing a mouthguard in active sporting events and recreation. Many times, dental hygienists develop unique and close relationships with patients and have the opportunity to promote healthy behaviors frequently and consistently. Conversation with a patient about hobbies and interests is a great opportunity to promote prevention of dental trauma and traumatic brain injury by using a mouthguard.

During the dental appointment, the dental provider can take the alginate impression and subsequently fabricate the mouthguard in the office with the use of a vacuum-forming machine. Alternatively, dental providers could send the study model to a laboratory if fabrication is completed off-site. If a boil-n-bite mouthguard is requested by the patient, the dental provider can make recommendations of the size and type and help the patient locate a store that carries mouthguards.

The dental hygienist has the responsibility to instruct the patient on the adequate maintenance of a mouthguard. The dental hygienist should suggest rinsing and brushing a mouthguard after each use with a soft-bristled, wet toothbrush. Some mouthguards come with brushes. Professional cleaning solutions are also available, and specific directions are available when the product is purchased. One solution, in particular, contains chlorohexidine gluconate, which is to be used by rinsing the mouthguard and shaking off the excess cleaner before inserting into the mouth so it cannot be tasted when wearing the mouthguard. Mouthguards should be kept in a clean, dry area such as a well-ventilated protective case but should not be held in hot water or kept in unusually hot environments because the dimensions could change and lead to distortion.[47]

SUMMARY

Mouthguards are used to prevent oral trauma and possible brain injury during recreational and sporting events. Preventing these traumas could assist patients in having good oral health. Dental providers should be able to promote the use of mouthguards and instruct patients on their proper care and maintenance.

Dental hygienists can help create and implement programs for the education and promotion of athletic mouthguards and have the responsibility for promoting the use of mouthguards by patients who participate in school sports and private athletic events.

PRACTICE CONSIDERATIONS

Athletic mouthguards provide a mechanism to prevent oral-facial trauma and possibly concussions from occurring during sporting events. In clinical practice, the dental provider should question patients, especially school-age children, about sporting interests and activities.

Patients can be educated on the importance of athletic mouthguards, the types available, and mouthguard maintenance. The establishment of mouthguard programs for athletes of all age, is suggested.

SELF-STUDY QUESTIONS

1. Which teeth are most commonly affected by sports-related trauma?

   a. Incisors

   b. Canines

   c. Premolars

   d. Molars

   Rationale: Chipped and avulsed incisor teeth are the most common sports-related orofacial injuries.

2. Which of the following are two methods of fabricating custom-made mouthguards?

   a. Mouth formed and vacuum formed

   b. Vacuum formed and pressure laminated

   c. Pressure laminated and thermoplastic

   d. Thermoplastic and base formed

   Rationale: Currently, vacuum formation and pressure lamination are two methods of fabricating custom-made mouthguards.

3. On which arch(es) should a mouthguard for an athlete who has a prognathic mandible be formed?

   a. Maxillary

   b. Mandibular

   c. Both

Rationale: If an athlete has a prognathic (forward-projecting) mandible, the mouthguard should be formed on the mandibular dentition.

4. A mouthguard should provide protection during sporting events and prevent orofacial injuries to be effective.

   a. The first statement is true; the second statement is false.

   b. The first statement is false; the second statement is true.

   c. Both statements are true.

   d. Both statements are false.

   Rationale: The role of any type of mouthguard is to provide protection and prevent orofacial injuries.

5. Dental laboratories fabricate pressure-laminated mouthguards and pressure-laminated mouthguards that seem to be less effective at maintaining minimal and consistent thickness in critical areas.

   a. The first statement is true; the second statement is false.

   b. The first statement is false; the second statement is true.

   c. Both statements are true.

   d. Both statements are false.

   Rationale: Pressure-laminated mouthguards, compared with other mouthguards, seem to maintain minimal and consistent thicknesses in critical areas better.

REFERENCES

1. Bijur, P. E., Trumbel, A., Harel, Y., Overpeck, M. D., Jones, D., & Scheidt, P. C. (1995). Sports and recreation injuries in US children and adolescents. *Arch Pediatr Adolesc Med,* 149:1009–16.

2. Adirim T. A, & Cheng T. L. (2003). Overview of injuries in the young athlete. *Sports Med,* 33:75–81.

3. National Council of Youth Sports. (2008). *Reports of trends and participation in organized youth sports.* Stuart, FL: National Council of Youth Sports.

4. Berg, R., Berkey, D. B., Tang, J. M., Altman, D. S., & Londeree, K. A. (1998). Knowledge and attitudes of Arizona high school coaches regarding oro-facial injuries and mouthguard use among athletes. *J Am Dent Assoc,* 129:1425–35.

5. Kvittem, B., & Roettger, M. (1998). Prospective epidemiological study of oro-facial injuries in high school sports. *J Pub Health Dent,* 58:288–93.

6. Kumamoto D. P., & Maeda Y. (2004, May–June). A literature review of sports-related orofacial trauma. *Gen Den,* 52:270–80.

7. McCrory, P. (2001). Do mouthguards prevent concussion? *Br J Sports Med,* 35:81–82.

8. Knapik, J. J., Marshall, S. W., Lee, R. B., Darakjy, S. S., Jones, S. B., Mitchener, T. A., delaCruz, G. G., & Jones, B. H. (2007). Mouthguards in sport activities: History, physical properties and injury prevention effectiveness. *Sports Med,* 37:117–44.

9. Mouthguards: History. (2007). *Sports Dentistry on Web.* Retrieved September 13, 2907, from http://www.sportsdentistry.info/mouthguards.html.

10. Historical backgrounder: Mouthguard development. (2006). *Shock Doctor.* Retrieved July 21, 2006, from http://www.shockdoc.com/new/mgHistory.html.

11. Fogan, C. B. (1963). Mouth protection for football players. *J Am Dent Assoc,* 66:3354–55.

12. Academy of Sports Dentistry: About the organization. (2012). Retrieved September 18, 2012, from http://www.sportsdentistry.org.

13. Kleyman, M. & Vigil, A. (1996, Fall). Use of mouthguards: Review of the literature. *Discloser,* 4–8.

14. Bulletin Board: High school adjusts sports-medicine rules. (July/August 2007). Retrieved September 25, 2007, from http://www.training-conditioning.com.

15. *2011 Official Playing Rules of the National Football League.* (2011). Retrieved November 17, 2011, from http://www.nfl.com/rulebook.

16. National Hockey League. (2008). Predators and Delta Dental "Protect Your Fangs." Retrieved November 17, 2011, from http://www.usahockey.com/gnash/default.aspx.

17. U.S. Department of Health and Human Services. (2000). *Oral health in America: A report of the Surgeon General—Executive summary.* Rockville, MD: U.S. Department of Health and Human Services, National Institute of Dental and Craniofacial Research, National Institutes of Health.

18. Andreasen, J. O., & Andreasen, F. M. (1994). *Textbook and color atlas of traumatic injuries to the teeth* (3rd ed.). St. Louis, MO: Mosby.

19. National Youth Sports Foundation for the Prevention of Athletic Injuries, Inc. (2008). Retrieved on March 24, 2008, from http://www.sportsdentistry.com/sportsdentistry.html.

20. Emshoff, R., Shoning, H., Rothler, G., & Waldhart, E. (1997). Trends in incidence and cause of sports related mandibular fractures. A retrospective analysis. *J Oral Maxillofac Surg,* 55:585–92.

21. Tanaka, N., Hayashi, S., Amagasa, T., & Kohama, G. (1996). Maxillofacial fractures sustained during sports. *J Oral Maxillofac Surg,* 54:715–19.

22. Tyler, J. H., & Nelson, M. E., (2000, May 1). Second impact syndrome: Sports confront consequences of concussions. *USA Today.*

23. Common injuries. Maxxgard custom fit laminated mouthguards. (2007). Retrieved on September 13, 2007, from http://maxxgard.com/commoninjuries.htm.

24. Stewart, S., & Witzig, J. (1998). New findings of the importance of athletic mouthguards. *VIHJS Newsletter,* 7.

25. American Dental Association Division of Science (2012, March). For the dental patient. Keep sports safe–wear a mouthguard. *J Am Dent Assoc.* 143(3):312.

26. Newsome, P. R., Tran, D. C., & Cooke, M. S. (2001). The role of the mouthguard in the prevention of sports-related dental injuries: A review. *Int J Paediatr Dent,* 11:396–404.

27. Onyeaso, C. O. (2004). Secondary school athletes: A study of mouthguards. *J Natl Med Assoc,* 96:240–45.

28. Wisniewski, J. F., Guskiewicz, K., Trope, M., & Sigurdsson, A. (2004). Incidence of cerebral concussions associated with type of mouthguard used in college football. *Dent Traumatol,* 20:143–49.

29. Ranalli, D. (2002). Sports dentistry and dental traumatology. *Dent Traumatol,* 18:231–36.

30. Stenger, J., Lawson, E., Wright, J., et al. (1964). Mouthguards: Protection against shock to the head, neck and teeth. *J Am Dent Assoc,* 69:273–81.

31. Centers for Disease Control and Prevention. (2001). Promoting oral health: Interventions for preventing dental caries, oral and pharyngeal cancers, and sports-related craniofacial injuries—A report on recommendations of the task force on community preventive services. *MMWR Recomm Rep,* 50(RR-21):1–13.

32. American Dental Association Report. (2006). Using mouthguards to reduce the incidence and severity of sports-related oral injuries. *J Am Dent Assoc,* 37:1712–20.

33. American Academy of Pediatric Dentistry. (2010). Policy on prevention of sports-related orofacial injuries. Retrieved September 18, 2012, from http://www.aapd.org/pdf/sports.pdf.

34. American Dental Hygienists' Association. (2007). *American Dental Hygienists' Association policy manual, public health policy 7-04.* Chicago: American Dental Hygienists' Association.

35. Hawn, K. L., Visser, M. F., & Sexton, P. J. (2002). Enforcement of mouthguard use and athlete compliance in National Collegiate Athletic Association men's collegiate ice hockey competition. *J Athlet Train,* 37:204–8.

36. Stenger, J. M. (1977). Physiologic dentistry with Notre Dame athletes. *Basal Facts,* 2:8–18.

37. Smith, S. D. (1978). Muscular strength correlated to jaw posture and the temporomandibular joint. *NY State Dental J,* 44:279–82.

38. Garabee, W. F. (1981). Craniomandibular orthopedics and athletic performance in the long distance runner: A three year study. *Basal Facts,* 4:77–79.

39. The Academy of Sports Dentistry. (2006). Position statements for properly fitted mouthguard, on athletic mouthguard mandates, and on sports dentistry in the dental school curriculum. Retrieved March 23, 2008 from, http://www.sportsdentistry-asd.org/position_statement.asp#3.

40. Kececi, A. D., Çetin C., Eroglu, E., & Baydar, M. L. (2005). Do custom-made mouthguards have negative effects on aerobic performance capacity of athletes? *Dent Traumatol,* 21:276–80.

41. Glass, R. T, Conrad, R. S, Wood, C. R, Warren, A. J., Kohler, G. A., Bullard, J. W., Benson, G., & Gulden, J. M. (2009). Protective athletic mouthguards: Do they cause harm? *Sports Health: A Multidisciplinary Approach,* 1: 411.

42. Finch, C., Braham, R., McIntosh, A., McCrory, P., & Wolfe, R. (2005). Should football players wear custom fitted mouthguards? Results from a group randomized controlled trial. *Inj Prev,* 1:242–46.

43. Kenyon, B. J., & Loos, L. G. (2005). Comparing comfort and wearability between Type III single-layered and double-layered EVA mouthguards. *Gen Dent,* 53:261–64.

44. Winters, J. E. (2001, July/September). Role of properly fitted mouthguards in prevention of sport-related concussion. (Commentary). *J Athl Train,* 36:339–41.

45. Johnson, D. C., & Jackson, E. W. (1991). Prevention of intraoral trauma in sports. *Dent Clin North Am,* 35:657–66.

46. Chapman, P. J. (1989). Mouthguards and the role of sporting team dentists. *Aust Dent J,* 34:36–43.

47. Gladwin, M., & Bagby, M. (2011). *Clinical aspects of dental materials* (4th ed.). Philadelphia, PA: Lippincott Williams & Wilkins, 231.

Technological Advances in Primary Dental Care

Vicki Gianopoulos Pizanis

OBJECTIVES

After studying this chapter, the student should be able to:

1. Describe the current status and future of immunizations in oral health care.
2. Describe genetic evolution in oral health care.
3. Describe the current status and future of gene therapy in oral health care.
4. Describe the current status and future of stem cell use in oral health.
5. Describe the use of probiotics in oral health.

KEY TERMS

Active immunity, 370
Artificially acquired active
   immunity, 370
Artificially acquired passive
   immunity, 370
Chromosomes, 372
Gene polymorphisms, 374
Genome, 372
Immunity, 370
Naturally acquired active
   immunity, 370
Naturally acquired passive
   immunity, 370
Passive immunity, 370
Probiotics, 375
Proteome, 372
Specific immunity, 370
Stem cells, 374

INTRODUCTION

During the past century, society has benefited from tremendous advances in the primary dental sciences from community water fluoridation to the use of dental sealants in the pit-and-fissure surfaces of teeth, to the utilization of dental hygienists. The proliferation of information technology and the use of computers in dental care delivery will continue to impact the evolution of oral health science and practice (Table 22–1 ■). Dental providers must be equipped to study new innovations and treatment modalities; they also must strive to prevent diseases at their earliest stages. Current technological advances in the science of dental hygiene include the use of stem cells, immunizations, gene therapy, genetics, and oral probiotics (Table 22–2 ■).

IMMUNIZATIONS IN ORAL HEALTH

In 1777, a Gloucestershire milkmaid told her physician, Dr. Edward Jenner, that contracting cowpox had been a fortunate event because it conferred protection against smallpox. This bit of folk wisdom led Jenner to research the possibility of preventing smallpox, resulting in the advent of vaccinations. The incentives and rewards for questioning disease and health and, subsequently, for conducting clinical research were never clearer.[1] Since the first live vaccine was introduced by Edward Jenner, live vaccines have been used against a number of viral infections including polio, measles, mumps, rubella, chicken pox, hepatitis A, yellow fever, and influenza.[2]

Providing specific protection against the most common and damaging pathogens is accomplished by immunizations. Basically, immunizations work to prevent diseases from occurring by inducing **immunity**, which means that the body has biological defenses needed to avoid infection or disease.

Specific immunity can be acquired by either passive or active immunization; both modes can occur by natural or artificial means.[3] Immune cells from an immunized individual can be used to transfer immunity, which is termed

TABLE ■ 22–1 Primary Preventive Modalities

Toothbrushing
  Manual held toothbrush
  Mechanical toothbrush
Dentifrices/Toothpastes
Interdental Adjuncts
  Dental floss
  Interdental brushes
  Wooden interdental cleaners
Irrigation
Mouthrinses
Fluoride
Dental Sealants
Professional Dental Hygiene Treatment

TABLE ■ 22–2 Technological Advances in Primary Preventive Dental Care

Immunizations (refer to Table 22–3)
Genetics and their role in disease
Gene therapy (refer to Table 22–4)
Stem cell use
Oral probiotics

specific immunity. **Passive immunity** can be acquired without the immune system being challenged with an antigen. Passive immunity can be acquired naturally or artificially by transfer of serum or gamma-globulins from an immune donor to a nonimmune individual. **Naturally acquired passive immunity** occurs when immunity is transferred from mother to fetus through placental transfer of immunoglobulin G (IgG) or colostral transfer of IgA.[3] **Artificially acquired passive immunity** is often transferred artificially by injection with gamma-globulins from other individuals or gamma-globulin from an immune animal. Passive transfer of immunity with immune globulins or gamma-globulins is practiced in numerous acute situations of infections (diphtheria, tetanus, measles, rabies, etc.) and poisoning (insects, reptiles, botulism) and as a prophylactic measure (hypogammaglobulinemia). In these situations, gamma-globulins of human origin are preferable, although specific antibodies raised in other species are effective and used in some cases (poisoning, diphtheria, tetanus, gas gangrene, botulism).[3]

Active immunity refers to immunity produced by the body following exposure to antigens. **Naturally acquired active immunity** occurs through exposure to different pathogens, which leads to subclinical or clinical infections that result in a protective immune response against these pathogens. In contrast, **artificially acquired active immunity** can be achieved by administering live or dead pathogens or their components. Vaccines used for active immunization consist of live, attenuated, organisms; killed whole organisms; microbial components; or secreted toxins that have been detoxified[3] (Table 22–3 ■).

Dental Caries

Dental caries is a chronic, infectious disease that can cause severe pain without dental intervention and can result in tooth loss. In the United States, dental caries remains the most common childhood disease, five times more common than asthma.[4] How is this disease treated? Use of fluoride in its many forms, use of sugarless products (such as xylitol), sealants, and increased access to dental care are among the approaches that have had a significant impact on the amount of dental disease of the young and economically advantaged. Many of these approaches can be broadly effective. However, economic, behavioral, or cultural barriers to their use have continued the epidemic of dental disease in many populations. Could there be a solution to this disease? There are now studies on vaccinations for the prevention of carious lesions.

TABLE ■ 22–3   Types of Immunity

Immunity Type	Definition
Specific immunity	Immunity against a specific antigen or disease
Passive immunity	Immunity acquired by the transfer of antibodies from another individual as through injection or placental transfer to a fetus
Naturally acquired immunity	Immunity obtained either from the development of antibodies in response to exposure to an antigen as from vaccination or an attack of an infectious disease or from the transmission of antibodies as from mother to fetus through the placenta or the injection of antiserum
Artificially acquired immunity	Immunity obtained either from the development of antibodies in response to exposure to an antigen as from vaccination or an attack of an infectious disease or from the transmission of antibodies as from mother to fetus through the placenta or the injection of antiserum

DID YOU KNOW ?

Worldwide, 5 billion people suffer from tooth decay, and dental cavities affect 60% to 90% of U.S. schoolchildren and most adults.

Dental caries is a disease caused by a group of organisms called *Streptococcus mutans* (*S. mutans*) and occurs in 3 phases.[5] The first phase involves the initial attachment of the microorganism to the tooth or dental pellicle. This is mediated by an adhesion from *S. mutans* that is known as antigen I/II.[6] The second phase is the accumulation of the bacteria in a biofilm and the production of glucose and glucans by the bacterial enzyme glucosyltransferase (GTFs). The third phase occurs when the multiplication of these bacteria, known as *dental plaques,* are present with sugars, including sucrose and glucose. This combination produces large amounts of lactic acid, causing enamel dissolution and carious lesion formation.[5] Although other oral microorganisms can be cariogenic, mutans streptococci have unique biochemical features that make them efficient at accumulating and producing carious surfaces; therefore, they are good targets for therapies aimed at the prevention of dental caries. The characteristics that make mutans streptococci particularly efficient at causing dental caries include production of large amounts of lactic acid at a rapid rate and tolerance to extremes of sugar concentration, ionic strength, and pH.[7]

W. H. Bowen first introduced the principle of immunization against dental caries by showing that monkeys that were immunized intravenously with *S. mutans* developed little carious disease.[8] Later, studies were done on rats that were immunized subcutaneously in the vicinity of the salivary glands with mutans streptococci, which led to reductions in the number of mutans streptococci and the extent of dental caries.

In the past decade, several small clinical trials of active immunization with mutans streptococcal antigens have been carried out. Clinical trials have shown increased amounts of salivary secretory IgA specific for the mutans streptococcal antigen that was used for vaccination. In a clinical trial, the vaccine group members were immunized orally with GTF in capsules and showed substantially reduced re-accumulation of indigenous mutans streptococci for up to 42 days following tooth cleaning and vaccination. Similar delayed reaccumulation was observed after topical application of GTF to the buccal mucosa, which contains minor salivary glands and their ducts. In addition, when antigen, either in soluble form or incorporated in liposomes, was administered intranasally or by topical application to the tonsils, the production of antigen-specific salivary IgA was induced. The duration effects on mutans streptococci were short in the young adult populations that were studied. This indicates that immunizations of this population would not affect the accumulation of bacteria on a long-term basis (more than 42 days).[9] Therefore, adults are not the appropriate target population for this vaccine.

Passive-immunization techniques have been studied for dental caries as well. This uses transfer of milk antibody specific for whole mutans streptococci from mother to suckling infant. This has been investigated in animal models and has shown to be protective against dental caries.[5] However, it seems unlikely that this strategy would have significant impact, at least in Western societies, where breast-feeding, if given, usually terminates well before the "window of infectivity" for mutans streptococci opens.[10]

Although clinical trials have mostly been carried out in young adults (ages 18–23), this is not the target population of choice, primarily because young adults are already infected with mutans streptococci (mainly *S. mutans*). Infants represent the primary target population for caries vaccine. Immunization when infants are about one year old can establish effective immunity against colonization attempts by mutans streptococci.[6,11]

An ideal vaccine to alleviate dental caries should consist of an antigen that is involved in the molecular pathogenesis of dental caries, should be administered by a route that will reproducibly elicit mucosal antibodies, and should occur when infants are immunocompetent with respect to salivary IgA production and before infection with mutans streptococci occurs.[6] If these features are met, vaccines can be well suited for public health applications, especially in environments that do not lend themselves to regular health care.

Periodontal Diseases

Periodontitis is an oral chronic inflammatory condition that can result in tooth loss attributable to bone and tissue destruction. This disease is associated with pathogenic gram-negative bacteria; *Porphyromonas gingivalis* has been implicated as an important etiologic agent of adult periodontitis.[12,13]

To learn how immunization works, one must have a basic understanding of the method for progression of periodontal disease. It is recognized that the adherence of bacteria to host tissues is a prerequisite for colonization and an important factor in bacterial pathogenesis. An approach to protecting against periodontal diseases is to develop a passive immunization system that blocks two colonization factors of *P. gingivalis* cells involved in its attachment to human host tissues.

One of the colonization factors is the coaggregation factor, which plays a role in the colonization of *P. gingivalis* in the subgingival area through aggregation with other oral bacteria.[14] *Porphyromonas gingivalis* has the capability to adhere to the surfaces of several gram-positive bacteria such as *Actinomyces viscosus* and streptococci. Therefore, interbacterial adherence appears to be an essential step in colonization by *P. gingivalis*. It is well recognized that accumulation of bacteria on the tooth surface follows a sequence, beginning with gram-positive facultative species and shifting over time to gram-negative facultative and anaerobic species. In the earliest stages of dental plaque formation, *P. gingivalis* vesicles aggregate gram-positive bacteria such as *Actinomyces naeslundii*, which was formally named *A. viscosus;* these gram-positive bacteria are also regarded as potential pathogens in periodontal diseases.[15]

Another property of coaggregation factor is its relationship to pathogenicity as evidenced by more abscesses being formed by coaggregates of two strains than those caused by infection with a pure suspension of each microorganism. Furthermore, coaggregated cells were also more resistant to phagocytosis and killing by neutrophils in vitro and in vivo.[16]

Colonization of *P. gingivalis* at subgingival sites is critical in the pathogenic process of periodontal disease and tissue destruction. Bacterial coaggregation factors and hemagglutinins likely play major roles in colonization in the subgingival area. Emerging evidence suggests that inhibition of these virulent factors can protect the host against caries and periodontal disease. Recent advances in mucosal immunology and the introduction of novel strategies for inducing mucosal immune responses now raise the possibility that effective and safe vaccines can be constructed. In tests of these vaccines, some successful results were reported in animal experimental models.[16]

No vaccine is absolutely safe, and there is always risk when providing medical intervention in a healthy individual to alleviate future disease. Those who are opposed to immunizations for oral health conditions argue that a vaccination is not justifiable for a condition that is not life threatening. In the future, if dental caries and periodontal disease immunizations prove to have benefits that outweigh risks, this could be the needed solution of prevention to much disease.

GENETICS

Completed in 2003, the Human Genome Project (HGP) was a 13-year project coordinated by the U.S. Department of Energy and the National Institutes of Health (Table 22–4 ■). During the early years of the HGP, the Wellcome Trust (United Kingdom) became a major partner; additional contributions came from Japan, France, Germany, China, and others. Researchers also studied the genetic makeup of several nonhuman organisms, including the common human gut bacterium *Escherichia coli*, the fruit fly, and the laboratory mouse.[17]

An understanding of basic genetics language is needed to discuss the importance of genetics in dentistry. Cells are the fundamental working units of every living system. All the instructions needed to direct their activities are contained within the chemical DNA (deoxyribonucleic acid).[17]

DNA from all organisms is made up of the same chemical and physical components. The DNA sequence is the particular side-by-side arrangement of bases along the DNA strand (e.g., ATTCCGGA). This order spells out the exact instructions required to create a particular organism with its own unique traits. The **genome** is an organism's complete set of DNA (Figure 22–1 ■). Genomes vary widely in size: The smallest known genome for a free-living organism (a bacterium) contains about 600,000 DNA base pairs whereas human and mouse genomes have some 3 billion. Except for mature red blood cells, all human cells contain a complete genome.[17]

DNA in the human genome is arranged into 24 distinct **chromosomes**—physically separate molecules that range in length from about 50 million to 250 million base pairs. A few types of major chromosomal abnormalities, including missing or extra copies or gross breaks and rejoinings (translocations), can be detected by microscopic examination. Most changes in DNA, however, are subtler and require a closer analysis of the DNA molecule to find perhaps single-base differences.[17]

Each chromosome contains many genes, the basic physical and functional units of heredity. Genes are specific sequences of bases that encode instructions on how to make proteins. Genes compose only about 2% of the human genome; the remainder consists of noncoding regions, whose functions can include providing chromosomal structural integrity and regulating where, when, and in what quantity proteins are made. The human genome is estimated to contain 20,000 to 25,000 genes.[17]

Although genes receive a lot of attention, the proteins perform most life functions and even make up the majority of cellular structures. Proteins are large, complex molecules made up of smaller subunits called *amino acids*. Chemical properties that distinguish the 20 different amino acids cause the protein chains to fold up into specific three-dimensional structures that define their particular functions in the cell. The constellation of all proteins in a cell is called its **proteome**. Unlike the relatively unchanging genome, the dynamic proteome changes from minute to minute in response to tens of thousands of intra- and extracellular environmental signals. A protein's chemistry and behavior are specified by the gene sequence and by the number

TABLE ■ 22–4   Human Genome Project Goals and Completion Dates

Area	HGP Goal	Standard Achieved	Date Achieved
Genetic map	2- to 5-cM resolution map (600–1,500 markers)	1-cM resolution map (3,000 markers)	September 1994
Physical map	30,000 sequence-tagged sites (STSs)	52,000 STSs	October 1998
DNA sequence	95% of gene-containing part of human sequence finished to 99.99% accuracy	99% of gene-containing part of human sequence finished to 99.99% accuracy	April 2003
Capacity and cost of finished sequence	Sequence 500 Mb/year at < $0.25 per finished base	Sequence >1,400 Mb/year at <$0.09 per finished base	November 2002
Human sequence variation	100,000 mapped human SNPs	3.7 million mapped human SNPs	February 2003
Gene identification	Full-length human cDNAs	15,000 full-length human cDNAs	March 2003
Model organisms	Complete genome sequences of *E. coli, S. cerevisiae, C. elegans, D. melanogaster*	Finished genome sequences of *E. coli, S. cerevisiae, C. elegans, D. melanogaster,* plus whole-genome drafts of several others, including *C. briggsae, D. pseudoobscura,* mouse and rat	April 2003
Functional analysis	Develop genomic-scale technologies	High-throughput oligonucleotide synthesis	1994
		DNA microarrays	1996
		Eukaryotic, whole-genome knockouts (yeast)	1999
		Scale-up of two-hybrid system for protein-protein interaction	2002

(*Source:* The Human Genome Project. U.S. Department of Energy Office of Science, Office of Biological and Environmental Research, Human Genome Program. Found at, http://www.ornl.gov/hgmis/publicat/primer2001/)

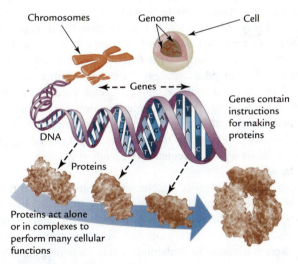

FIGURE ■ 22–1 Diagram of a gene.

(*Source:* The Human Genome Project. U.S. Department of Energy Office of Science, Office of Biological and Environmental Research, Human Genome Program. Found at, http://www.ornl.gov/hgmis/publicat/primer2001/)

and identities of other proteins made in the same cell at the same time and with which the protein associates and reacts.[17]

In 1995, the potential impact of gene therapy on dentistry was published; this finding was based on initial studies of gene transfer applications to salivary glands, keratinocytes, and cancer cells.[18] It is now evident that a genetic basis exists for most diseases including periodontal disease and dental caries.[18] In the past 6 years, remarkable progress has been made in the field of gene therapy, including seven areas relevant to dental practice: bone repair, salivary glands, autoimmune disease, pain, DNA vaccinations, keratinocytes, and cancer.[19] Decoding the genome completely depicts the molecular structure, and explains how genes build, maintain, and control all of the biological functions.[19]

Dental Caries

There has been convincing evidence for a number of years that host genetic factors contribute to an individual's susceptibility or resistance to dental caries. This study confirms this evidence and provides additional support for the concept that dental caries is a complex disorder with both environmental and genetic components.[20] This finding has important implications for the practice of dentistry because it demonstrates that there are additional risk factors for dental caries beyond those that have been traditionally understood. In practice, this finding means that the history of caries in siblings or parents should be evaluated as well as the individual's dietary and oral hygiene behaviors. It should also be recognized that a genetic susceptibility to caries does not imply that disease is unavoidable but that more intensive preventive interventions are required and that intervention should be started as early as possible.[20]

Periodontal Diseases

Genetic factors that influence an individual's risk for periodontal disease work similarly to environmental factors. The majority of genetic factors are also associated with an exaggerated inflammatory response to periodontal infection. A major genetic factor includes an individual's production of a proinflammatory cytokine interleukin-1B (IL-1B), which is associated with tissue destruction. Interleukin-1B is produced by many cell types but especially by monocytes in diseased patients.[21] Understanding the human genome and which genes are associated with exaggerated inflammatory response can help dental professionals with the prevention and control of periodontal disease.

In general, an individual's genetic background influences his or her susceptibility to many kinds of disease and conditions, including periodontitis. Familial aggregation of a trait or disease can suggest a genetic etiology. However, families also share many aspects of a common environment, including diet, nutrition, and behaviors such as smoking. In addition, certain infectious agents can cluster in families. Thus, familial aggregation can result from shared genes, environmental exposures, and similar socioeconomic influences.[22]

Many aspects of an individual's immune system are inherited and can contribute to a genetic susceptibility to periodontitis.[22] Genetic factors influence inflammatory and immune responses, and periodontitis is largely the result of an exaggerated inflammatory response.

Several studies have investigated genetic polymorphisms for cytokines as potential genetic markers for periodontitis. **Gene polymorphisms**, locations within the genome that vary in sequence for individuals, are very prevalent, affecting at least 1% of the population. The most common form of polymorphism is the single-nucleotide polymorphism, which is a change in a single base pair in the genomic DNA. The rationale for studying single-nucleotide polymorphisms is that they can be used to identify potential markers of susceptibility, severity, and clinical outcome. The results suggest that individuals carrying the positive genotype have significantly greater risk for developing periodontitis.[23]

The scientific literature during the decade has seen an increase in the number of reports claiming links for genetic polymorphisms with a variety of medical diseases, particularly chronic immune and inflammatory conditions. However, the literature reports of studies of periodontal diseases reveals that, despite major advances in the awareness of genetic risk factors for periodontal disease (with the exception of periodontitis associated with certain monogenetic conditions), research has not determined a genetic basis for aggressive or chronic periodontitis.[24] Periodontitis is a complex, multifactorial disease, and the susceptibility is genetically determined. There is no strong evidence for target genes and gene polymorphisms that play a key role in the susceptibility to and severity of periodontitis. Therefore, genetic testing for periodontitis is currently not indicated.[25]

GENE THERAPY

Gene therapy is the insertion of normal DNA directly into cells to correct a genetic defect;[26] the treatment of disease is addressed by replacing, altering, or supplementing a gene that is absent or abnormal and whose absence or abnormality is responsible for a disease.[26] Since the advent of gene therapy in dentistry, significant progress has been made to control periodontal disease and reconstruct the dentoalveolar apparatus. However, to date, gene therapy methods have not been developed to control periodontal disease because of its multifactorial origin, complex genetic predisposition, and associated risk.[27]

STEM CELLS IN ORAL HEALTH

Stem cells have the remarkable potential to develop into many different cell types in the body. Serving as a sort of repair system for the body, they can theoretically divide without limit to replenish other cells as long as the person or animal is still alive. When a stem cell divides, each new cell has the potential to either remain a stem cell or become another type of cell with a more specialized function, such as a muscle cell, a red blood cell, or a brain cell.[28] Stem cells have been the subject of heated ethical debates by those opposed to the use of human embryos for study. A new study has revealed a way to turn ordinary human skin cells into what appear to be embryonic stem cells without using a human embryo.[29]

Sharks of all species continually shed their teeth and regenerate new ones, in some cases with up to 50,000 in one lifetime.[30] Humans, on the other hand, are not as fortunate and frequently rely on the tertiary preventive services of dental providers to replace their teeth with implants or dental prosthetics. Many individuals with missing teeth faced making the decision of replacing them with implants, bridges, or dental prosthetics. Regeneration of a functional and living tooth is a promising therapeutic strategy for the replacement of a diseased or damaged tooth. Although dental implant therapies have achieved long-term success in the clinic for the recovery of tooth function, the implants require preexisting, high-quality bone structures to support the implants. Regeneration of teeth in individuals without adequate bone support would be a major dental advance.

In 2000, scientists of the National Institutes of Health discovered stem cells inside primary teeth. Dr. Shi took a lost primary tooth from his daughter, extracted the pulp, and cultured it. Amazingly, some of the tooth cells started to grow.[31]

Recent advances in dental stem cell biotechnology and cell-mediated murine (or rodent) tooth regeneration have encouraged researchers to explore the potential for regenerating living teeth with appropriate functional properties.[32] Murine teeth can be regenerated with the use of many different stem cells to collaboratively form dental structures in vivo. In addition, dentin and pulp tissue and cementum–periodontal complex have been regenerated by human dental pulp stem cells and periodontal ligament stem cells, respectively, when transplanted into immunocompromised mice.[32] However, because of the complexity of human tooth growth and development, the regeneration of a whole tooth structure including enamel, dentin–pulp complex, and periodontal tissues as a functional entity in humans is a promising challenge.[33]

The spatially and temporally organized microenvironment of the tooth bud and its surrounding tissues permits growth and development of the crown and roots, resulting in formation and eruption of the tooth. Root development involves dentin formation, cementum generation, instruction of epithelium, and tooth eruption. From a clinical perspective, the most important part of the tooth is the root, which supports a natural or artificial crown. The crown alone cannot fulfill normal tooth function without a viable root. In contrast, the wide use of synthetic crowns to replace damaged natural crowns has been widely applied in dental clinics with excellent therapeutic outcomes.

Stem cell–mediated root regeneration offers opportunities to regenerate a bio-root and its associated periodontal tissues, which are necessary for maintaining the physiological function of teeth.[34] This cell study reported that tooth regeneration is possible. A new population of stem cells was isolated from the root apical papilla of human teeth (extracted third molars from volunteers ages 18–20 years).[34] Human apical papilla and periodontal ligament stem cells were transplanted to generate a root–periodontal complex capable of supporting a porcelain crown, resulting in normal tooth function.[34] This work integrates a stem cell–mediated strategy for tissue regeneration, engineered materials for structure, and current dental crown technologies. This hybridized tissue-engineering approach led to recovery of tooth strength and appearance.

Probiotics in Oral Health

Ukrainian-born biologist and Nobel laureate Elie Metchnikoff discovered in1907 that Bulgarian yoghurt consumption (containing lactic acid bacteria) is good for health.[35] Today the term is referred to as probiotics, which has been found to aid in digestion in the gastrointestinal tract. **Probiotics**, by definition adopted by the International Scientific Association for Probiotics and Prebiotics, are "live organisms, which administered in adequate amounts, confer health benefit on the host."[36] Currently, this long ago discovered health benefit is sought to be an aid in achieving healthy flora in the oral cavity.

Probiotics can be another primary preventative treatment modality for the common chronic infectious disease dental caries. As previously mentioned, the evolution of a dental cavitation has three phases. There are also three specific elements that play a role in the progression of the disease: the host, bacteria, and nutrients. If one of these elements is not present, caries cannot exist. Probiotics in dentistry focuses on eliminating the harmful bacteria element by altering the flora in the oral cavity. The most well–publicized of these efforts is a substitution strategy developed by Hillman and colleagues.[37] They have genetically modified a *Streptococcus mutans* organism so that it no longer produces acid while competing aggressively for the ecological alcove where the wild type *S. mutans* is found. In theory and in laboratory animals, once this substitute organism is introduced, it entirely displaces the disease-causing wild type *S. mutans*. This not only stops the disease process but also

precludes the reemergence of the disease-causing organism and eliminates re-infection.[38]

Another form of probiotics that acts by removing harmful oral pathogens is called *targeted antimicrobials.* The technique is to develop an inexpensive targeting molecule that will reliably attach to only the organism of interest. This method of probiotics can be translated from caries prevention to periodontal disease prevention, yeasts prevention, and even halitosis prevention. Currently, the most common and traditional approach to caries-disease management in the oral cavity is the surgical model. This works by removing the demineralized portions of the tooth and replacing the missing tooth structure with inert restorative material. If effective and safe probiotic therapy is implemented, dental caries will be prevented, preserving natural tooth structure by inhibiting the accumulation of acid-causing bacteria in the mouth.

Along with the benefits of probiotics in dentistry, criticisms and concerns are also evident. One criticism of probiotic approaches is that they do not address the other pathogens that can be involved in a disease process such as dental caries. There are questions about the safety of probiotics and increasing probiotic supplementation to a host. Although currently this therapeutic approach appears safe, it is also evident that careful monitoring is still needed in future developments.

ADVANCES IN CARIES DETECTION

Traditional diagnostic tools used in dental caries detection are not sensitive enough to diagnose the disease process in its early stages; and frequently, once a diagnosis is made, restoration is the only effective means of treatment.[39] Currently, diagnostic methods are emerging for dental caries that are aimed at improving the detection and progress monitoring of caries in permanent and primary teeth. Examples of such methods include electrical conductance measurement, laser or light fluorescence, and digital imaging fiber optic transillumination.[39]

Electrical conductance measurement (ECM) utilizes the notion that different electrical conductivity exists in teeth of varied demineralization. Two devices have been developed for clinical use limited to occlusal surfaces that measure electrical conductance by placing the tip of the instrument on the fissure or groove and the connector on a high-conductivity area such as the skin. A review article by Huysmans concluded that there is variation among the results from using this method, but usually sensitivity is heightened compared with a visual examination, and specificity is lower.[40]

Laser fluorescence has been shown to detect occlusal caries in both in vivo and in vitro studies involving permanent teeth. Fluorescence can be used for caries detection with a device that detects differences in fluorescence observed between sound and demineralized enamel. When enamel is demineralized, the device illuminates the enamel with a colored light. This technology is limited, however, in its ability to determine the extent of the decay and to discriminate between active and inactive lesions.[41]

Fiber-optic transillumination (FOTI) allows for the detection of carious lesions by identifying the changes in the scattering and absorption of lightphoton. A carious lesion is detected when there is localized decrease of transillumination. To identify interproximal caries, a high-intensity light is placed on the buccal surface, and the interproximal surface is observed by transillumination through the occlusal surface. Enamel lesions appear as gray shadows, and dentinal lesions appear as orange-brown or bluish shadows.[41]

Primarily on the basis of in vitro and preclinical data, some of the reviewed methodologies showed promising results for the detection and monitoring of early caries lesions. However, very little clinical data are available to validate these emerging technologies. It was concluded that, although significant promise is apparent with these technologies, there is not enough evidence available at this time for any of the reviewed diagnostic techniques to be recommended as a substitute for traditional diagnostic techniques.[39]

SUMMARY

Many technologies are used to strive to prevent dental disease, and the development of further modalities continues to be an area of ongoing interest. Understanding more about the genetic makeup of an individual will lend information that can help dental providers to understand inherent risk factors and determine the best type of treatment for patients. The information encoded in a patient's genes can be invaluable in treating the patient through prevention of the initiation and the progression of disease. Although the genetic linkage to periodontal disease and the testing for it holds promise, it is more accurate to consider an individual's environmental and genetic factors in an assessment of risk for this disease.

Gene therapy can aid in altering the genetic makeup so that it will be more conducive to good health. Research into stem cells will aid in treating diseases and can enhance the practice of tertiary prevention. Immunizations can serve as primary prevention in individuals to prevent diseases from occurring. The development of probiotics in dentistry is a recent advancement sought to target specific pathogens in the oral cavity and create other, nonthreatening, microorganisms to aggressively take over the environment. Finally, further advances in noninvasive caries detection are becoming additions to traditional assessments. It is incumbent upon providers to keep up-to-date in the science of primary dental care so they can deliver the most optimum treatments available.

PRACTICAL CONSIDERATIONS

As a profession, we are slowly moving away from the purely surgical approach to treating oral disease. Science is providing us the tools to diagnose and treat infection before it causes damage. As oral healthcare providers, we need not to limit our focus to the oral cavity but to the overall systemic health of an individual. Interestingly, these newer technologies introduced in this chapter will serve other entire areas of health care as well. If a problem of specific infections such as dental caries and periodontal disease can be solved, then these solutions virtually can be implemented on all mucous membranes.

SELF-STUDY QUESTIONS

1. Immunizing an individual intravenously with *S. mutans* to prevent dental caries is an example of:

   a. Active immunization

   b. Passive immunization

   c. Specific immunization

   d. Both a and c

   Rationale: Active immunity is attained from an individual being exposed to an antigen.

   Because in this case the immunization is attempted against S. mutans specifically, this is also an example of specific immunization.

2. Current research on the genetic susceptibility of a host to periodontal disease focuses on the patient's:

   a. Diet

   b. Inflammatory response

   c. Oral hygiene

   d. Caries susceptibility

   Rationale: A patient can have a genetic predisposition to periodontal disease relating to how their bodies react with an exaggerated inflammatory response to the pathogen.

3. Probiotics in dentistry works by:

   a. Removing harmful bacteria from the mouth

   b. Encouraging nonpathogenic bacteria to culture in the oral cavity

   c. Assisting in the development of specific bacteria that will inhibit pathogenic bacteria from flourishing in the mouth

   d. Assisting the host in digesting the oral disease-causing bacteria

   Rationale: Probiotics works to develop genetically modified nonpathogenic strands of microorganisms to either compete for the ecological environment or attack the microorganism of interest.

4. The treatment of disease by replacing, altering, or supplementing a gene that is absent or abnormal and whose absence or abnormality is responsible for a disease is

   a. Immunizations

   b. Probiotics

   c. Stem cell implementation

   d. Gene therapy

Rationale: The treatment of disease by replacing, altering, or supplementing a gene that is absent or abnormal is gene therapy.

5. What would be the most effective age to administer a caries vaccine to a patient?

   a. Infant

   b. 2 years

   c. 4 years

   d. Adult

Rationale: A caries vaccine will be the most effective when administered prior to the patient being exposed to caries-causing bacteria in the oral cavity.

REFERENCES

1. Berg, A. O., Gordon, M. J., and Cherkin, D. C. (1986). *Practice-based research in family medicine.* Kansas City, MO: American Academy of Family Physicians.

2. Riedel, S. (2005, January). Edward Jenner and the history of smallpox and vaccination. *BUMC Proceedings,* 18:21–25

3. Ghaffar, A. (2002). Immunization. (MBIM 650/720 Medical Microbiology, Lecture 14. University of South Carolina), 2–4.

4. Dental vaccine could help billions. (2006, May). *United Press International.* Retrieved May 6, 2008, from http://www.upi.com.

5. (2003, January). Panel on caries vaccine. *National Institute for Dental and Craniofacial Research.*

6. Nash, D. A., & Taubman, M. A. (2006). The scientific and public health imperative for a vaccine against dental caries. *Science and Society,* 6:255–63.

7. Hamada, S., & Slade, H. D. (1980). Biology, immunology, and cariogenicity to *Streptococcus mutans. Microbiol Rev,* 44:331–84.

8. Bowen, W. H. A. (1969). Vaccine against dental caries.A pilot experiment in monkeys (*Macacairus*). *Br Dent J,* 126:159–66.

9. Smith, D. J., & Tuabman, M. A. (1987). Oral immunization of humans with *Streptococcus sobrinus* glucosyltransferase. *Infect Immu,* 55:2562–69.

10. Russell, M. W., Childers, N. K., Michalek, S. M., Smith, D. J., & Taubman, M. A. (2004). A caries vaccine? *Caries Research,* 38:230–35.

11. Hajishengallis, G., & Michalek, S. M. (1999). Caries vaccine. *Health Mantra,* 1–6.

12. Roberts, F. A., Houston, L. S., Lukehart, S. A., Mancl, L. A., Persson, R. G., & Page, R. C. (2004, February). Periodontitis vaccine decreases local prostaglandin E2 levels in primate model. *Infection and Immunity,* 72:1166–68.

13. Decarlo, A., Huang, Y., Collyer, A., Langley, D., & Katz, J. (2003, January). Feasibility of an HA2 domain-based periodontitis vaccine. *Infection and Immunity,* 71:562–66.

14. Booth, V., Ashley, P., & Lehner, T. (1996, February). Passive immunization with monoclonol antibodies against *Porphyromonas gingivalis* in patients with periodontitis. *Infect Immun.* 422–27.

15. Persson, R. G., (2005, October). Immune responses and vaccination against periodontal infections. *J Clin Periodontol,* 32:39–53.

16. Abiko, Y., (2000). Passive immunization against dental caries and periodontal disease: Development of recombinant and human monoclonal antibodies. *Crit Rev Oral Biol Med,* 11:140–58.

17. Collins, F. S., Morgan, M., & Patrinos, A. (2003). The Human Genome Project: Lessons from large-scale biology. *Science,* 300:286–90.

18. Baum, B. J., Kok, M., Tran, S. D., & Yamano, S. (2002). The impact of gene therapy on dentistry: A revisiting after six years. *J Am Dent Assoc,* 133:35–44.

19. Yeager, A. L. (2001). Where will the genome lead us? Dentistry in the 21st century. *J Am Dent Assoc,* 132:801–7.

20. Shuler, C. F. (2001). Inherited risks for susceptibility to dental caries. *J Dent Educ,* 65:1038–45.

21. Research, Science and Therapy Committee (2005). Implications of genetic technology for the management of periodontal diseases. *J Periodontol,* 76:850–57.

22. Hodge, P., & Michalowicz, B. (2000). Genetic predisposition to periodontitis in children and young adults. *Periodontology,* 26:113–34.

23. Takashiba, S., & Naruishi, K. (2006). Gene polymorphisms in periodontal health and disease. *Periodontology,* 40:94–106.

24. Kinane, D. F., & Hart, T. C. (2003). Genes and gene polymorphisms associated with periodontal disease. *Crit. Rev. in Oral Biol. Med,* 14:430–49.

25. Loos, B. G., van der Velden, U., & Laine, M. L. Genetics and periodontitis. (2008, February). *Ned Tijdschr Tandheelkd,* 115:87–92.

26. What is gene therapy? Genetic home reference. (2008). U.S. National Library of Medicine. Retrieved May 9, 2008 from http://ghr.nlm.nih.gov/handbook/therapy/genetherapy.

27. Karthikeyan, B. V., & Pradeep, A. R. (2006, July). Gene therapy in periodontics: A review and future implications. *J Contemp Dent Pract,* 7(3):83–91.

28. Murray, P. E., & Garcia-Godoy, F. (2004). Stem cell responses in tooth regeneration stem cells and development. Retrieved May 9, 2008 13:255–62. *Stem Cell Responses* doi:10.1089/154732804323099181.

29. University of Wisconsin-Madison. (2007, November). Scientists guide human skin cells to embryonic state. *Science Daily.* Retrieved May 9, 2008, from http://www.sciencedaily.com/releases/2007/11/071120092709.htm.

30. Sharks of the island. Nova online. (2002). Retrieved September 12, 2006, from http://www.pbs.org/wgbh/nova/sharks/world/click-ablesans.html.

31. National Institutes of Health, National Institute of Dental and Craniofacial Research. (2003, April 22). Scientists discover unique source of postnatal stem cells in "baby" teeth. *Science Daily*. Retrieved May 9, 2008, from http://www.sciencedaily.com/releases/2003/04/030422075224.htm.

32. Nakara, T., & Yoshiaki, I. D. E. (2007). Tooth regeneration: Implications for the use of bioengineered organs in the first-wave organ replacement. *Human Cell*, 20:63–70.

33. Chai Y., & Slavkin H. C. (2003, April). Prospects for tooth regeneration in the 21st century: A perspective. *Microsc Res Tech*, 60:469–79.

34. Sonoyama, W., Liu, Y., Fang, D., Yamaza, T., Seo, B., Zhang C., Liu H., Gronthos, S., Wang, C. Y., Shi, S., & Wang, S. (2006). Mesenchymalstem cell-mediated functional tooth regeneration in swine. *PloS ONE*, 1:e79.

35. Meurman, J. H. (2005). Probiotics: Do they have a role in oral medicine and dentistry? *Eur J Oral Sci*, 113:188–96.

36. Guarner F., Perdigon G., Coerthier G., Salminen S., Koletzko B., & Morelli L. (2005). Should yoghurt cultures be considered probiotic? *Br J Nutr*, 93:783–86.

37. Hillman J. D. (2002). Genetically modified *Streptococcus mutans* for the prevention of dental caries. *Antonie Van Leeuwenhoek*, 82:361–66.

38. Anderson M. H., & Shi, W., (2006). A probiotic approach to caries management. *Pediatr Dent*, 28:151–53.

39. Stookey, G. K., & González-Cabezas, C. (2001). Emerging methods of caries diagnosis. *J Dent Ed*, 65:1001-6.

40. Tam, L. E., & McComb, D. (2001). Diagnosis of occlusal caries: Part II. Recent diagnostic technologies. *J Can Dent Assoc*, 67:459–63.

41. Goel, A., Chawla, H. S., Gauba, K., & Goyal, A. (2009). Comparison of validity of DIAGNO dent with conventional methods for detection of occlusal caries in primary molars using the histological gold standard: An *in vivo* study. *J Ind Soc of Ped and Prev Dent*, 27: 22–34.

Pregnancy and Infancy

Sharon G. Peterson

OBJECTIVES

After reading this chapter, the student should be able to:

1. Describe and define pregnant women and infants as target populations.
2. Describe common oral conditions and diseases of pregnant and infant patients.
3. Describe specific preventive strategies to use with pregnant and infant patients.
4. Describe the role of the dental provider in treating pregnant and infant patients.

INTRODUCTION

Target population is a term used to represent a certain segment of the population that consists of groups of individuals with similarities of some sort, whether it be age, race, educational background, life situation, and/or health conditions. The term is broad and can represent 3-year-old children, a group of youths involved in a local church group, or even people who are elderly living in an assisted-living community. Basically, age can be a representative factor of a target group, but the group members usually have other commonalities as well. An example is, although children in a group are 3 years old, they may also share other characteristics because they attend the same Head Start program, live in the same geographic area, come from families in similar income sectors, have one parent, and live with extended families. In addition, many of the children have the same ethnic background. So, although dental providers know that these children are 3 years old, many factors are helpful when planning a dental hygiene in-service for this group. Infancy is a subcategory of childhood specifying a child who has not yet learned to walk on his own. Therefore, infancy can end as early as 9 months or up to 2 years of age. Toddlers delineate children who are walking. This chapter and the chapters that follow will discuss target populations, cultural diversity, and barriers to dental care that may be encountered.

INTRODUCTION TO PREGNANCY AND INFANCY

Pregnancy and infancy present significant risk for oral disease. Current trends show that the medical and dental disciplines are merging interests and expertise to improve access to oral health care services so as to deter the detrimental effects of dental decay, gingival inflammation, and periodontal destruction. These disease processes span the life of the individual and can be diminished or inhibited with well-constructed prevention programs.

The dental profession possesses the knowledge and technology to assist parents in raising children free of dental disease. In fact, the goal of dental care is to help infants and toddlers avoid the pain and devastation that accompanies **early childhood caries** (ECC); provide them with a pleasant, nonthreatening introduction to dental care; establish and reinforce the foundation of preventive oral habits. The inclusion of oral health in **anticipatory guidance**, which can be provided during well care visits, helps families understand what to expect during their infant's current and approaching stages of development and ensures that any oral health needs can be addressed in infancy. Recommendations indicate that the first dental risk assessment should occur as early as 6 months of age, and the establishment of a dental home should occur by approximately 1 year of age.[1]

As health professionals, dental care providers must identify the potential for the development of disease and institute effective measures for preventing disease; it is then a sound and logical practice to intervene before disease onset rather than treat the effects of the disease. The American Academy of Pediatrics recommends that an infant be evaluated by a pediatrician six times during the first year and four times during the second year of life. Although these visits are aimed at evaluating development, prevention, or early detection of disease, physicians should not be expected to provide a thorough oral evaluation or proper preventive oral health counseling. Dental professionals must be proactive and assume the responsibility.

POPULATION CHARACTERISTICS

Pregnant Women

In the short period after the diagnosis of pregnancy, an expectant mother is exposed to a barrage of information applicable to her health and that of her unborn child. Dental health information should be included in this routine. At the time of the oral health consultation, a dentist or dental hygienist should be the source of the essential information.

Women are particularly susceptible to periodontal disease because female hormones affect the periodontal structures. The increased risk of **pregnancy gingivitis** appears to be primarily the result of resistance changes that occur during pregnancy in the connective tissues composing the structure of the periodontium. If the pregnant woman does not have well-established oral self-care, she may not be aware of these changes. Figure 23–1 ■ shows predominant manifestations such as gingival enlargement, increased erythema, tissue sensitivity, and spontaneous bleeding. These manifestations of periodontal diseases can deter a pregnant woman from seeking effective oral care.

Shoba conducted an intervention trial of 60 pregnant women between 18 and 35 years of age with periodontal disease to determine the effects of periodontal intervention during pregnancy. All participants were provided periodontal scaling and root planing during the first trimester with 15 days of supplementary chemotherapeutics using Clorhexadine gluconate 0.12%. Participants also received periodontal maintenance and oral hygiene education during the second trimester. The pregnant women's periodontal status was assessed post-delivery. Results indicated a statistically significant impact on all periodontal indices. Shoba concluded that the study has shown that providing periodontal therapy and maintenance throughout the course of pregnancy results in a significant reduction in all

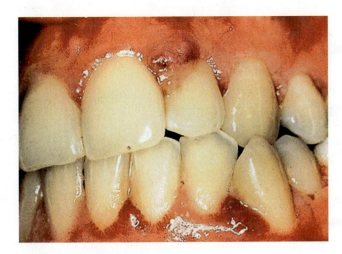

FIGURE ■ 23–1 **Pregnancy gingivitis.**
Predominant manifestations are gingival enlargement, increased erythema, tissue sensitivity, and spontaneous bleeding.
(*Source:* Courtesy of Sharon Peterson.)

clinical parameters, thus reducing the incidence of pregnancy-associated gingivitis. Gingival enlargements either localized or generalized can also be prevented.[2]

It is a common misunderstanding that bleeding is a sign of injury. With an increase in gingival inflammation, including bleeding, the pregnant woman often avoids flossing to reduce the incidence of bleeding. In addition, toothbrushing can be problematic if the woman is experiencing morning sickness. The placement or movement of the toothbrush in the posterior of the oral cavity can trigger an overactive gag reflex that is common in morning sickness. The increased acidity in the oral cavity as a result of frequent vomiting can irritate the mucosa and gingiva as well as increase the probability of demineralized tooth structures. Chronic avoidance of dental care during pregnancy is common; therefore, maintenance of oral health care should be a primary focus of oral health consultation from both the medical and dental professions.

DID YOU KNOW?

It is believed that periodontitis can contribute to adverse outcomes of pregnancy. Toxins or other products generated by periodontal bacteria in the pregnant mother can reach the blood circulation, cross the placenta, and harm the fetus. In addition, the response of the woman's immune system to the infection activates the release of inflammatory mediators, growth factors, and other potent cytokines, which can trigger preterm labor.

Research studies have consistently reported that oral disease has an effect on systemic diseases such as cardiovascular disease, stroke, endocarditis, and bacterial pneumonia. A relationship has been drawn between the incidence of periodontitis and of low-birth-weight and preterm babies. Researchers assert that the litany of inflammatory factors, as a result of the periodontitis process, is not limited to the oral environment.[3] Li, Kolltveit, Tronstad, and Olsen have identified three mechanisms in which oral infections can affect or manifest in a secondary site: "metastatic spread of infection from the oral cavity as a result of transient bacteremia, metastatic injury from the effects of circulating oral microbial toxins, and metastatic inflammation caused by immunological injury induced by oral microorganisms."[4] One or all of these processes probably exist in the expectant mother with periodontitis; however, the concept of injury, as a result of circulating endotoxins that cross the placental barrier, has been the most likely focus of the research.

Infection in the chorion and amniotic apparatus supports an association between **preterm birth** (PTB) or **low birth weight** (LBW) and infection during pregnancy.[5] In an abbreviated explanation, the presence of amniotic inflammatory factors promotes production of cytokines, which release prostaglandins. Once these prostaglandins have reached a threshold level, they appear to facilitate the onset of preterm labor through cervical dilation. In some cases in which periodontal disease is not the primary cause of premature delivery, it has been identified as a contributing factor to low-birth-weight babies. Figure 23–2 ■ shows the relationship between gestation and birth weight for a healthy pregnancy.

Preterm has been used to describe a birth that occurs on or before the end of the last day of the 37th week after determination of the woman's last menstrual period. Recent research has further defined the use of the term *preterm* and indicates the importance of identifying the fetus by gestational age. Furthermore, the use of more specific terminology can help to link medical complications, morbidity, and mortality by development weeks.

A variety of terms have been used to describe preterm infants born at a number of different intervals between 32 and 37 weeks' gestation ("late preterm," "near term," "marginally preterm," "moderately preterm," "minimally preterm," and "mildly preterm"). In contrast, preterm, term, and post term are mutually exclusive categories that have each been defined precisely according to week and day of gestation (counting the first day as day 1) by the American Academy of Pediatrics, the American College of Obstetricians and Gynecologists, and the World Health Organization.[6]

Infants

Significant progress has been made toward determining factors that contribute to poor birth outcomes. Rates for pregnant women receiving prenatal care have increased, tobacco use among pregnant women has decreased, and improvements have been made in neonatal intensive care units. But despite these improvements, PTB and LBW have not shown a corresponding decline. A pioneer in studying the association between

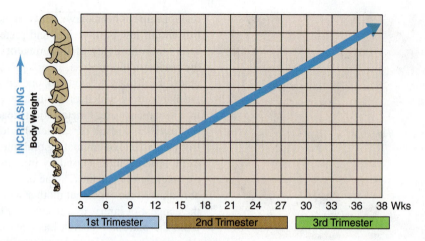

FIGURE ■ 23–2 Gestation and birth weight.
Pre-term delivery (births occurring prior to 37 weeks gestation) and low birth weight are among the adverse pregnancy outcomes that represent a significant public health concern (www.OralFetusConnection.com).

pregnancy and periodontal disease, Offenbacher and other researchers were the first to suggest the presence of maternal periodontal disease as a possible factor in delivery of a preterm/low-birth-weight infant. In a case-control study of 124 pregnant women, researchers observed that women who delivered an infant weighing less than 2500 grams or at less than 37 weeks' gestation had significantly worse periodontal disease than did control women.[7]

PTB and LBW have been shown to be the two most significant predictors of infant health and survival. In fact, LBW is a major worldwide public health problem; such infants confront a significant survival disadvantage that accounts for almost half of the nation's infant mortality. In addition, LBW babies can suffer from a number of medical disorders such as cerebral palsy, blindness, respiratory conditions, and cardiovascular malformations. Compared with term infants, PTB infants are nearly 7 times more likely to die before their first birthdays. Both PTB and LBW infants account for a large proportion of maternal and neonatal mortality and morbidity.[8]

Oral health counseling should come early because the first trimester of pregnancy is a critical time. All organ systems of the fetus are forming during this period. Tooth buds begin formation at the fourth to fifth weeks of gestation followed by the initial mineralization of bones and teeth from the ninth to twelfth weeks. Stress experienced by the fetus at this time can produce dento-oral deformities. For example, a cleft lip or palate results when the maxillae fail to unite between the fourth to sixth weeks. These changes can result from a variety of etiologic factors affecting the expectant mother, such as genetics, stress of an injury, severe virus infection, alcohol toxicity, or smoking. Excessive stress to the fetus at any critical time in development can result in a temporary, but often irreparable, arrest in cellular growth.

COMMON ORAL MANIFESTATIONS

Pregnant Women

A study of 903 pregnant women with periodontal disease conducted at the University of North Carolina showed a significant. increase in the numbers of women over the duration of their pregnancy who exhibited four or more sites with attachment loss measuring greater than or equal to 2 mm. A significant association between maternal periodontal disease, race, smoking, and insurance status was also found. Results showed that pregnant black women were more likely than white women to have periodontal disease.[9]

Research on saliva testing during pregnancy indicates that the change in hormones increases susceptibility to gingivitis because primary inflammatory regulating salivary proteinases (matrix metalloproteinases, or MMPs) are reduced. The presence of these proteinases were inversely proportionate to pregnancy ginigivitis; when increased, inflammatory factors decreased. It was also found that the highest levels of proteinases were found after lactation.[10]

The effect of periodontal interventions on pregnancy outcome was assessed in a prospective study designed to examine the relationship between periodontal disease and preterm LBW infants in a cohort of young, minority, pregnant, and postpartum women. Of 164 women for whom birth outcome data were available, 74 were subjected to oral prophylaxis during pregnancy, and 90 received no periodontal treatment. The preterm/LBW rate was lower among women who received periodontal treatment compared with those who did not (13.5% versus 18.9%).[11]

Research conducted to estimate whether maternal periodontal disease was predictive of preterm (less than 37 weeks) or very preterm (less than 32 weeks) births showed that the incidence of preterm birth was 11.2% among periodontally healthy women, compared with 28.6% in women with moderate-severe periodontal disease, and antepartum moderate-severe periodontal disease, was associated with an increased incidence of spontaneous preterm births. The unadjusted rate of very preterm delivery was 6.4% among women with periodontal disease progression, significantly higher than the 1.8% rate among women without disease progression.[12]

Jeffcoat et al. examined the relationship between periodontal disease and spontaneous PTB among 1,313 pregnant women; they found that moderate-severe maternal periodontal disease identified early in pregnancy was associated with an increased risk for spontaneous preterm birth, independent of other traditional risk factors.[13] Clearly periodontal health has an impact on the overall health of an infant and warrants the earliest intervention. All health care providers should establish routines of oral health counseling and referral for dental care in early pregnancy.

A pregnant woman is often at considerable risk of caries development. The expectant mother's teeth do not lose calcium as postulated in a number of myths; instead, the risk of dental caries probably increases because of changes in eating habits. For example, the sucking of hard candy to reduce nausea, dietary cravings, and frequent between-meal snacks of refined carbohydrates can raise the caries potential of the dental plaque. In addition, expectant women often experience nausea or morning sickness causing vomiting with a regurgitation of stomach acid, which can cause erosion and demineralization of the lingual surfaces of the teeth. Many times, only a toothbrush or a sudsy dentifrice is needed to trigger a gag reflex.

Avoidance of aberrant eating habits and snacking, exercise of sugar discipline, and use of xylitol products can greatly minimize the possibility of caries development. Primary teeth could benefit from prenatal exposure to dietary fluoride supplements taken by the mother-to-be; however, recent studies do not support maternal prenatal fluoride supplementation.[14] A study of prenatal and postnatal fluoride supplements compared to postnatal fluoride supplementation was conducted only to determine the existing amount of fluoride in enamel and dentin of deciduous teeth. The researchers concluded that "fluoride exposure during the prenatal period offered no additional measurable fluoride uptake by dental tissues beyond that attributable to postnatal fluoride alone."[15] The expectant woman should be provided appropriate treatment and recall appointments during the pregnancy. Professionally applied topical fluorides and systemic fluoride supplementation can benefit the pregnant woman's oral health in conjunction with additional daily self-care with fluoride dentifrices and mouthrinses. These measures will both prevent demineralization of the expectant mother's teeth and facilitate remineralization in the event of the development of an incipient lesion.

Infants

Dental caries can and does occur in infants and toddlers well before 3 years of age. Early infant caries has been observed in infants as young as 12 months of age.[16–22]

One of the first major hazards to an infant's primary dentition is ECC. This condition has also been referred to as *nursing caries, nursing bottle caries, nursing bottle mouth, baby-bottle syndrome, baby-bottle tooth decay,* and *bottle-mouth caries.* The caries pattern of this condition is highlighted by rampant dental caries initially involving the maxillary primary incisors and progressing to the first primary molars in later stages[19–27] (Figure 23–3 ■). The decay is caused by continual, prolonged exposure of the primary teeth to milk, infant formula, fruit juices, soft drinks, or other sugar/carbohydrate–containing fluids placed in the nursing bottle or sipping ("sippy") cup (Figure 23–4 ■).

Once teeth erupt, the practice of offering an infant a bottle filled with cariogenic fluid as a pacifier or at naptime or bedtime should be discouraged. Once teeth erupt and plaque accumulates, the ingestion of sugar-containing fluids during bedtime or naptime places the infant at considerable risk for dental caries because salivary flow decreases during sleep, and the fluid pools around the teeth, creating a highly acidic environment. The pooling of the oral fluids occurs around the maxillary anterior teeth.[20] Not all primary teeth are equally attacked. While an infant is sucking the nipple of either the bottle or the breast, the tongue overlies the lower incisors, which directs the sweetened liquid against the maxillary incisors and to the back of the palate. The mandibular incisors often are either completely intact or only slightly affected whereas the maxillary incisors bear the brunt of the repeated acid attacks. The other primary teeth are involved to various degrees, depending on the infant's suckling habits.

The caries attack begins with the appearance of white areas of demineralization around the gingival third of the teeth (Figure 23–5 ■). With time, these incipient lesions begin to turn brown as active caries progresses (Figure 23–6 ■). Eventually, the carious lesions that ring the cervical areas of the teeth can result in entire crowns being lost by either fracture of the undermined enamel or by the continuous action of the caries. In either event, only the exposed root is left in the alveolous.

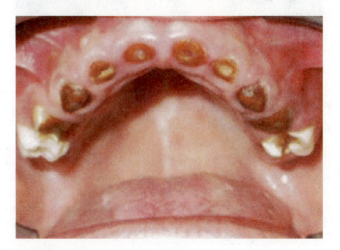

FIGURE ■ 23–3 Early childhood caries.
Early childhood caries is highlighted by rampant dental caries initially involving the maxillary primary incisors and progressing to the first primary molars in later stages.
(*Source:* Courtesy of Sharon Peterson.)

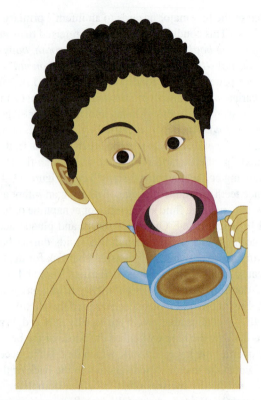

FIGURE ■ 23–4 Sippy cup.
Chronic use of a "sippy cup" to replace a bottle can have the same detrimental effect of early childhood caries.

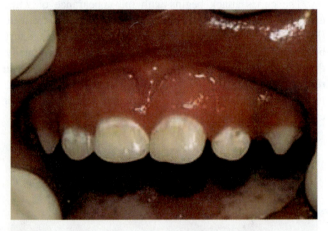

FIGURE ■ 23–5 Early childhood caries: "white spot" lesions.
(*Source:* Courtesy of Sharon Peterson.)

An infant should not be put to sleep with a bottle or no-spill sippy training cup. Frequent prolonged bottle feedings or use of a sippy cup containing beverages high in sugar (e.g., fruit drinks, soda, or fruit juice), milk, or formula during the day or at night should be avoided.[19] If a bottle is to be used as a pacifier, it should be filled only with water.[24]

Early childhood caries can also occur in some breast-fed infants who are nursed every time they indicate a desire for feeding (demand feeding, with 10 or more nursing events over a 24-hour period).[25] However, frequent bottle feeding at night, breast-feeding upon demand, and extended and repetitive use of

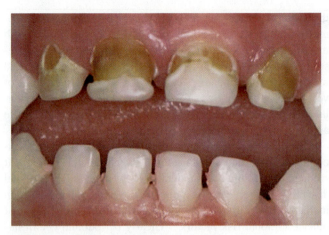

FIGURE ■ 23–6 Moderate early childhood caries: undermined enamel.
(*Source:* Courtesy of Sharon Peterson.)

a no-spill training cup are associated with, but not consistently implicated in, ECC.[26]

The loss of teeth resulting from ECC can have far-reaching effects on the infant's eventual face growth.[15] In addition, premature loss of primary molars predisposes infants to malocclusion (improper alignment of the jaws and teeth). The loss of tooth function, the ability to chew, or facial variance can result in low self-esteem for both the parent and infant.

On occasion, a toddler can have a pattern of multiple, severe caries without a substantiated history of early nursing patterns that placed him or her at an increased risk. The caries process is certainly multifactorial and, at times, a definite cause cannot be identifiable. Nevertheless, early, sound primary preventive strategies early on will provide the appropriate environment for the prevention of dental caries.

Evidence suggests that dental caries is an infectious disease process initiated via the transmission of *Streptococcus mutans* from parents to their infants.[29–33] The specific plaque hypothesis suggests microbial specificity in dental caries, and longitudinal evidence supports the role of *S. mutans* in caries initiation.[34,35] The following characteristics of *S. mutans* are important relative to dental caries in infants.

- Permanent *S. mutans* colonization of the oral cavity in infants can occur before the primary teeth erupt.[18,36]
- Sucrose facilitates the adherence of *S. mutans* to the tooth surface.[35–38]
- The source of infection of the infant with *S. mutans* is from within the family, most likely the mother.[15–19,39]
- Initial acquisition of infant caries takes place during the "window of infectivity."[39–41]

Transmission of *S. mutans* to the infant most likely occurs in the first year of life during a specific time period identified as the window of infectivity, between 6 and 30 months of age. Furthermore, there is higher risk between 18 and 30 months of age.[25,26] If the infant has a high-sucrose diet in the presence of *S. mutans,* the conditions are favorable for the initiation of caries. The early establishment of oral hygiene measures and the adoption of a low-cariogenic diet and low-risk feeding patterns should begin in infancy.

DID YOU KNOW

Mothers can transmit bacteria from their mouth to an infant by sharing utensils when feeding or when they insert the infant's pacifier into their own mouth in an attempt to "clean off" the pacifier when dropped on the floor and then replace it in the infant's mouth.

With the preceding bulleted points as a backdrop, it is possible to develop guidelines that minimize the possibility of transmittal of cariogenic flora from members of the family who will be most closely associated with the infant. The most important goal is to reduce the bacterial challenge to the point that the potential for transmission of *S. mutans* is minimal. For the expectant woman especially, this goal requires continual maintenance of a high level of oral hygiene. Preferably, such a program should commence no later than the sixth month of pregnancy and continue throughout until the time of the eruption of the infant's teeth and onward until a mature, stable, nonpathogenic plaque has been established (i.e., very low *S. mutans* count) on the infant's erupted primary teeth.[42] Such a program includes appropriately spaced professional visits for prophylaxis, bacterial counts, and monitoring of oral health. For the mother, the manual and chemical plaque control procedures can include, in addition to the toothbrushing, the use of irrigation devices and antiplaque rinses such as chlorhexidine, which can specifically target *S. mutans*. For the infant, the most important procedure from time of birth is a restriction of cariogenic foods and attention to oral hygiene as discussed later in this chapter. Recent studies have validated the use of xylitol products to suppress proliferation of *S. mutans* in both the mother and infant.[43,44] The long-term use of xylitol by the mother can prevent caries in the offspring by inhibiting bacterial transference from mother to infant and has been found to be very cost-effective.[45,46]

Another preventive treatment that is becoming more widespread is the application of fluoride varnish treatments on children under the age of 5. The U.S. Food and Drug Administration (FDA) has cleared the marketing of fluoride varnish for the treatment of dentin hypersensitivity associated with the exposure of root surfaces or as a cavity varnish but not for reducing caries. There is, however, an increasing body of evidence indicating that fluoride varnish is effective in caries prevention. Two or more applications of fluoride varnish per year are effective in preventing caries in high-risk populations.[47]

PREVENTIVE STRATEGIES

Preventive strategies for pregnant women and infants need to be initiated in a multifaceted approach that bridges oral health stakeholders. Cross-profession training in the oral disease process and prevention strategies ensures a diverse workforce who can better serve those at risk. The First Five Oral Health training program in the state of California, instituted by the First Five Commission, recognizes the need for cross-profession training. This is a statewide oral health project to provide various levels of training to oral health and other health providers about the prevention and treatment of dental disease for children ages zero to 5 years. The project's goals are to educate 30,000 dental professionals and 10,000 medical professionals and to deliver intensive training to 14,000 dental professionals and more than 3,500 medical professionals statewide. The program also provides education on the prevention of ECC to parents and caretakers of young children, including those with disabilities and other special needs.[48] Further research collaborations can draw together financial resources and create cohesive treatment protocols for early intervention programs.

DID YOU KNOW

The best time to start educating mothers about infant and child oral health care is during pregnancy. This is an appropriate time for an infant to begin a lifetime of dental prevention, decreasing the likelihood of complex dental issues and subsequent health problems.

Pregnant Women

It is important to provide oral health counseling throughout the pregnancy. The counseling should include dental hygiene and dental care as needed, which, it is hoped, would include at least one to two visits to the dental provider. Therefore, oral health counseling and assessment of existing oral conditions should be conducted in the medical office during obstetrical visits because the pregnant woman is seen more frequently (typically monthly) by her obstetrical doctor. This approach would provide her the most comprehensive prevention efforts during the scope of her pregnancy.

Proper nutrition during pregnancy is essential. Although nutritional deficiencies in the expectant mother usually must be severe to affect the fetus, a daily balanced diet provides the necessary proteins, fats, carbohydrates, vitamins, and minerals. The American Dietetic Association's position regarding pregnancy is that the key components of a health-promoting lifestyle during pregnancy include appropriate weight gain; consumption of a variety of foods in accordance with My Plate (http://www.choosemyplate.gov/); appropriate and timely vitamin and mineral supplementation; avoidance of alcohol, tobacco, and other harmful substances; and safe handling of food.[48]

All obstetric services should develop a positive referral system to ensure that expectant mothers receive an early dental examination, preventive oral health counseling for themselves and the fetus, and necessary treatment. The referral could be to a private practice, a hospital dental service, or a public health facility.

The mother-to-be should be encouraged to seek a flexible dental program, if available, in which prevention, monitoring, and therapy are commensurate with the severity of her dental condition. Many women who become pregnant are already

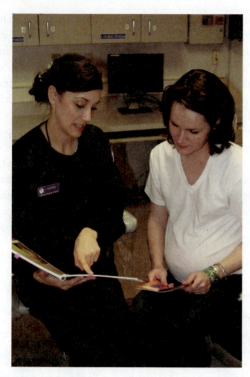

FIGURE ■ 23–7 Pregnancy counseling.
Counseling should include dental hygiene and dental care as needed, which, hopefully, would include at least one or two visits to the dental provider.

(*Source:* Courtesy of Sharon Peterson.)

long overdue for treatment; to postpone needed care for 9 more months could cause severe oral problems, leading to a potential premature birth or an LBW baby. During pregnancy, it would be ideal for the expectant woman to see a dental professional twice for preventive care and oral health counseling (Figure 23–7 ■). To accomplish this goal, she would need to be seen in the first and the last trimesters.

With pregnancy, modification in treatment necessitates alteration of the dental chair incline to accommodate comfort. It is recommended that the mother-to-be not be reclined completely in the last trimester because of the potential decrease in blood flow and increased pressure on the fetus. It is common for pregnant women to experience increased difficulty in breathing while reclining because of the pressure directed toward the diaphragm. With additional pressure directed toward the bladder, treatment might need to be presented in stages with frequent breaks. Dental radiographs for emergencies might be necessary but should be avoided whenever possible during the first trimester. If radiographs are necessary, careful gonadal and abdominal shielding is required as with all dental patients. According to the Food and Drug Administration (FDA), dental radiographs can be prescribed for pregnant patients as long as there is careful adherence to its selection criteria guidelines.[50–51] Dental disease left untreated during pregnancy can lead to problems for both the mother-to-be and the fetus, and dental radiographs could be required for proper diagnosis and management.[52]

All therapeutic or restorative dental treatment should be completed by the end of the second trimester because the position of the baby by the third trimester affects the pregnant woman's posture, making long dental appointments quite uncomfortable. When the treatment has been completed, the attending dentist should supply feedback to the obstetrician, indicating completion of the primary, secondary, and tertiary preventive dentistry treatment plans. The collaboration of medical and dental providers can ensure that both the pregnant woman and her fetus are being given the greatest opportunity for optimal oral health.

The New York State Health Department publishes *Oral Health Care During Pregnancy and Early Childhood Practice Guideline* to focus on the oral health needs of pregnant women. These recommendations have been developed to assist health care professionals in educating women about oral health and to improve their overall health and that of children. These guidelines can enable health care professionals to work as a team to improve the care delivered to mothers and children and to have significant health benefits.[53] An invaluable element of the guide is succinct recommendations for (1) prenatal care providers, (2) oral health professionals, and (3) child health professionals. The guidelines provide supplemental information to be made available to pregnant women on dietary habits, pediatric health and dental care, and resources for health professionals on referral for oral care, guidelines for prescribing dental radiographs, anticipatory guidance, and effective prevention programs. This proactive guide demonstrates the national trend to recognize overarching goals of medicine and dentistry.

The Prenatal Education and Treatment project, funded by the Osteopathic Heritage Foundation, is a current program that was initiated by the Columbus, Ohio Children's Hospital Dental Clinic to incorporate oral health into prenatal health. The program formed a partnership with three local prenatal clinics where low-income pregnant women receive their prenatal care. A hygienist conducts risk assessment, dental screening, and education during prenatal visits as part of overall prenatal care. Case management activities are incorporated to assist with transportation and establishment of a dental home for those needing treatment (including infants). Follow-up dental services, including comprehensive dental care, are provided at Columbus Children's Hospital Dental Clinic. In addition, the project educates nondental health professionals about the importance of oral health during pregnancy.[54]

This emphasis on excellent maternal oral health is required for three reasons: (1) to reduce the possibility of onset and/or progression of caries and periodontal disease throughout the pregnancy, (2) to provide an increased possibility of better care for the expected infant as a result of the woman's personal involvement with dental treatment, prevention, and counseling, and (3) to reduce the number of cariogenic organisms in the woman's mouth.

Infants

Early Dental Care

The newborn should become accustomed to oral care early. After feeding, the ridges where the teeth will later appear and the palate should be gently wiped with gauze or a soft washcloth. This removes leftover food and establishes a routine for the mother to clean inside the infant's mouth. Children, especially infants, need directly supervised oral hygiene care. It has traditionally been recommended that an infant should visit the dental office no later than 2 1/2 years of age. Ideally, the infant's first dental visit should occur at 6 months of age and no later than 1 year of age.[1] The purpose of this initial visit is to permit an evaluation of the mouth and jaws for proper formation and alignment of structures. A second objective is to allow the infant to become familiar with the dental office and its personnel under pleasant circumstances to forestall future apprehension.

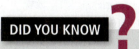

DID YOU KNOW

Ideally, the infant's first dental visit should occur at 6 months of age and no later than 1 year of age.

Because health professionals can identify the potential for the development of disease and have effective measures available for preventing the initiation of disease, it is a sound and logical practice to intervene before the onset of disease whenever possible rather than to wait and treat its effects. Examples of primary prevention exist in pediatric medicine with well-baby evaluations and immunization programs. Pediatricians recommend that the infant be evaluated five times during the first year and three times during the second year of life (Table 23–1 ■). Although these visits are aimed at evaluating development and prevention or early detection of disease, physicians are not adequately trained to provide a thorough dental evaluation or proper preventive dental health counseling. The dental profession must be proactive and assume this responsibility.

The education process can probably best start with the obstetrician and pediatrician explaining to the expectant or new parents the consequences of continued intake of sugary fluids. The physician can aid in reducing the problem by prescribing bottle formulas that contain the lowest amount of sugar. For instance, there is a considerable range in the amount of sugar found in the various commercially available baby foods. Finally, the dental profession should emphasize the need for high school and community dental education programs to alert would-be parents of their responsibilities in dental care for their infant.

Early Childhood Dental Information, Evaluation, and Programs

Because of problems such as ECC, parents of infants and toddlers increasingly desire an early dental evaluation for their children and want information on preventing dental diseases in them. According to parents, the major reasons they seek early dental evaluations are the desire

TABLE ■ 23–1 Infant and Toddler Oral Health Anticipatory Guidance Schedule

Age	Appropriate Guidance
Prenatal	Importance of good oral health for mother-to-be Signs of disease Disease prevention
1 month	Function of baby teeth Importance of baby teeth Process of decay
3 months	Appropriate bottle use Appropriate breast feeding Comforting tips
6 months	Characteristics of early childhood caries Causes of early childhood caries Effects of early childhood caries Prevention of early childhood caries
9 months	Importance of cleaning baby teeth Method of cleaning baby teeth Teaching of "lift the lip"
12 months	The change from breast or bottle to cup Importance of regular dental care Resources for dental care
18 months	Healthy eating
24 months	Implementation of healthy behaviors Screening for early childhood caries

(*Source:* Nevada State Health Division Office of Oral Health, Early Childhood Caries Anticipatory Guidance. February 2005. Used with permission.)

- For information on preventing tooth decay for their child.
- To prevent their children from having unpleasant experiences that the parents had suffered.
- To learn their role in their child's oral health.
- To obtain information and recommendations from their pediatrician or family physician.

The First Smiles Program in Vancouver, Washington, provides oral hygiene information, fluoride varnish applications, nutrition counseling, and dental referrals to interested clients of the Special Supplemental Nutrition Program for Women, Infants and Children (WIC) at the Clark County Health Department. The First Smiles Program began in 1995 to address the high incidence of decay in Head Start children. The program, which primarily operates from Medicaid reimbursement, is unique because it partners a dental hygienist and WIC staff to improve the oral health of the clients they serve. A nutritionist from WIC provides dietary risk assessment, and the dental hygienist provides dental screenings, fluoride varnish applications, and individualized oral health education. Frequency of return treatment for these children is based on the presence or absence of white spot lesions. Dental hygiene students from Clark Community College also provide oral health education and dental cleanings at the health department to pregnant women enrolled in WIC. The goal of the First Smiles Program is to prevent or reduce ECC in high-risk children. The program promotes xylitol in their dietary counseling and instructs clients on the benefits of xylitol. The program publishes a patient brochure on how xylitol prevents decay and how to use xylitol gum.[55]

According to the United Nations' Convention on "The Rights of the Child," articles 2 and 24, all children should have the same rights including the right to health and medical service. Early childhood caries is a lifestyle disease with biologic, behavioral, and social determinants. An early screening of all children at around 1 year of age is an excellent opportunity for early detection of risk factors and increases the possibilities for preventing them. The caries risk evaluation should form the base for appropriate recommendations of preventive measures.[56]

The American Academy of Pediatric Dentistry states, "Infant dental care begins with dental health counseling for the newborn, which should include a dental office visit for preventive oral health counseling no later than 12 months of age. However, for those children who are delayed in erupting teeth, the first visit may be postponed, but should occur within 6 months following the eruption of the first tooth."[14]

Early and Periodic Screening, Diagnosis, and Treatment (EPSDT), a federal program, mandates that medical and dental services be provided to children from low-income families and that children in the program receive a dental screening by 12 months of age. A survey of 54 dental school departments of pediatric dentistry showed that 86% teach students to see infants at 12 months of age or younger.[57]

One study evaluated a promotion program for oral health in which "health visitors" met with mothers of 8-month-old babies to address some of the risk factors associated with nursing caries. The program significantly improved the mothers' recall of advice given by health visitors that encouraged the use of a feeder cup, brushing of their babies' teeth with fluoride toothpaste, and restriction of sugary foods and drinks. Significant improvements were also found in recall of advice regarding the use of sugar-free medicine and registration of babies with a dentist. The program also encouraged more of the mothers to bring their children to clinics for a hearing check.[58]

The advantages of the infant oral health approach are:

- Identifying and modifying detrimental feeding habits, thus reducing potential risk of caries.
- Assisting parents in establishing for their children dietary and snack patterns that have a low risk of caries.
- Explaining and demonstrating tooth-cleaning procedures for infants and toddlers.
- Determining fluoride status and recommending an optimum fluoride program.
- Introducing dentistry to the child in a pleasant, nonthreatening manner.
- Preparing parents for upcoming dental events for their child (anticipatory guidance).

A Protocol for Early Preventive Intervention

The Interview

The interview process and counseling session should be thorough and specific yet concise. The infant's attention span is limited: Once they become bored and seek attention from the parent(s), parent's attentiveness to the dental provider's discussion will be limited at best. Experience shows that the interview and preventive counseling are best accomplished before the examination of the infant for the following reasons:

- The infant can be kept busy with toys or other distractions before the examination in a nonthreatening environment, and the parent(s) will be better able to direct their attention to the dentist.
- Should the infant fuss during the examination (normal behavior) and/or during the ensuing discussion, the infant, not the dental provider, usually receives the parent's attention.
- Specific parental concerns can be identified and addressed during the examination.

The interview should begin with a discussion of the parents' reason for seeking care. Historical information gathered at the initial interview assists the practitioner in developing the most appropriate and individualized preventive program for the family. Categories of helpful information follow.

1. **Growth and development:** An abnormal pattern of oral development could be discovered or suspected, prompting a referral to the dentist for further evaluation. Also, the date of the eruption of the first tooth provides a baseline

for determining patterns of dental development and assists in answering parents' questions in the future regarding their infant's dental development.

2. **Feeding history:** Knowledge of the feeding patterns during infancy is critical to (1) assist the dentist in assessing the infant's risk for developing ECC by discovering potentially harmful feeding habits and (2) help form a basis for recommendations regarding proper feeding practices that minimize the potential for dental disease.

3. **Medical history:** A complete medical history is important. Knowledge of any systemic conditions that could adversely affect dental health will assist the dental provider in developing appropriate preventive strategies. For example, long-term, frequent intake of sucrose-based medications could require additional recommendations for tooth cleaning to offset the increased caries risk from the sucrose intake.

4. **Preventive assessment:** Information regarding dental development and dental health attitudes in addition to current oral hygiene practices serves as a starting point for counseling parents about an appropriate preventive program for their infant. A history of tooth decay in the family ("soft teeth") will provide insight into the environmental influences as well as parental attitudes about dental health and guide the dental provider's discussion regarding preventive strategies.

5. **Fluoride supplementation:** It is important for the dentist to know whether the infant has access to fluoride in drinking water. It is not sufficient to establish that a family lives in a fluoridated community. On occasion, the family might drink bottled water, which contains an unknown amount of fluoride. On the other hand, a family drinking well water might or might not be receiving systemic fluoride depending on the concentration of fluoride in the water. Before any fluoride supplements should be prescribed, the water should be tested for fluoride concentration, and supplements should be prescribed accordingly. Some families live in rural settings with well water, but the infant spends the majority of the day in a location such as a day care facility or school with fluoridated water. Therefore, an accurate assessment of all potential sources of fluoride intake should be explored before making any recommendations regarding fluoride supplementation.

If the daily intake of fluoride is insufficient, parents should be informed that small daily dosages are beneficial to an infant's teeth. Initially, supplementation is best accomplished by the use of fluoride drops. Around the age of 3 years when the child gains skill in chewing tablets, the drops can be replaced by fluoride tablets. Later, as the infant gains skill in chewing the tablet, the fluoride-laden saliva can be swished around the mouth and then swallowed to provide a topical application as well as systemic benefits. The practice of using a tablet a day should continue from infancy through childhood to at least 12 years of age, although many believe that fluoride supplementation should be considered as long as the individual—child or adult—has a fluoride-deficient intake.

6. **Oral hygiene:** An assessment of current tooth-cleaning activities is important to establish the parents' role in oral hygiene for their infant. Many parents think incorrectly that allowing an infant or toddler to brush their own teeth is adequate. If the infant's teeth are being brushed, it is important for the dental practitioner to establish how, when, and by whom and to inquire whether the parents experience any difficulties during the process.

The education process can probably best start with the obstetrician and pediatrician explaining to the expectant or new parents the consequences of continued intake of sugary fluids. The physician can further aid in reducing the problem by prescribing bottle formulas that contain the lowest amount of sugar. For instance, there is a considerable range in the amount of sugar found in the various commercially available baby foods. Finally, the dental profession should emphasize the need for high school and community dental education programs to alert would-be parents of their responsibilities in dental care for their infant.

In one study, almost half of the parents interviewed had started toothbrushing programs for their infants at 12 months, and 75% had done so by 18 months.[59] With such infant and toddler toothbrushing programs, only a small amount of a fluoridated dentifrice, approximately the size of a pea, should be used to avoid the possibility of the infant's ingesting an excess of fluoride. Around the age of 6 years, the infant can begin daily fluoride mouthrinses as part of the total lifelong program for oral health.

The following is a recommended set of interview questions to ask pregnant women and new mothers within the first 30 months of the infants's life[60]:

- Do you have any problems with your teeth?
- Does your family have any inherited problems/diseases affecting the teeth?
- Do you know the fluoride status of your drinking water?
- Are you brushing and flossing regularly?
- As your infant grows up, do you think you can help her or him prevent tooth decay? What kinds of things do you want to do to protect your infant's teeth?

Counseling

On the basis of the information gathered to this point, the practitioner is ready to provide recommendations on how parents can play an active role in preventing dental disease in their infant by assuming responsibility for the his or her oral hygiene and diet.

Parents should be educated regarding the following tooth-cleaning recommendations:

- A parent, other adult, or older sibling must assume total responsibility for tooth cleaning in infants and young children. Many children are unable to perform adequate plaque removal until they are 6 to 8 years of age.

- Tooth cleaning should be done in a comfortable location and pleasant environment. Positioning will be demonstrated during the dental examination.

- A dentifrice is not necessary for infants. In many cases, its taste and foaming action may be unpleasant.

- If a dentifrice is used, only a pea-sized amount should be placed on the brush to avoid ingestion of excess fluoride.

- Tooth cleaning should be accomplished with a small, soft-bristled toothbrush.

- Tooth cleaning should be accomplished at least once daily.

- The evening tooth cleaning may be easier to accomplish after the infant's last feeding instead of waiting until just before bedtime because a tired infant can frequently be fussy during the procedure.

Parents have control, for the most part, over their infant's diet during the early years. The exceptions include time spent with babysitters and in day care settings. Parents can have some influence in those situations, however, if they make their wishes known. Medical and dental professionals should share the following information with parents.

- Infants should be weaned from the bottle around 12 months of age.

- The bottle should not be used as a pacifier or given during bedtime or naptime.

- Only water, formula, or milk should be offered in the bottle.

- Frequent, prolonged episodes of breast-feeding could be a caries risk.

- Sleeping with the infant and allowing nursing through the night should be avoided.

- Infants and young children generally eat more frequently than three times daily.

- Between-meal snacks should consist of foods that have a low cariogenic potential.

- Total amount of cariogenic foods is not the issue; rather, the frequency of ingestion and retentiveness of the food are the factors that contribute to the caries risk.

Conducting the Examination

Once the interview and counseling aspects of the visit have been completed, the practitioner is ready to proceed with the examination of the infant or toddler. The dental chair and overhead light are neither required nor very useful for examining infants this young. Because one of the prime objectives is to provide a dental examination in a pleasant, nonthreatening manner, the procedure is best accomplished in the knee-to-knee position for children under 3 years of age (Figure 23–8 ■). This position

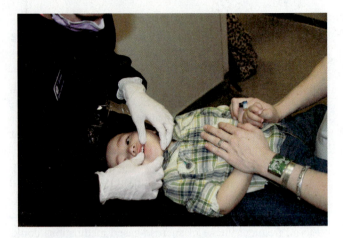

FIGURE ■ 23–8 Knee-to-knee positioning.
Practitioner and parent hold the child in their lap with the parent stabilizing the child's legs and hands.
(*Source:* Courtesy of Sharon Peterson.)

provides a stable, yet comfortable, environment that incorporates the security of parental involvement, which could produce a calming effect on infants and toddlers who lack the cognitive ability to cooperate. Should the infant offer resistance, his or her mouth and head can be gently stabilized while cradled in the practitioner's lap. The parent can hold the infant's hands and, if needed, stabilize his or her legs by cradling them with the elbows. Many of the infants and toddlers accept the examination procedures in this position without resistance. It is important in those instances in which the infants resist or cry that the parents be assured that the behavior is normal (and expected) for his or her age and should not be considered "bad" or "uncooperative."

The examination should begin with a soft touch, evaluating the extraoral head and neck conditions first, allowing the infant to become accustomed to the practitioner's actions. The examination of the oral cavity should begin by using the fingers to palpate the oral structures before introducing the dental instruments. Illumination can be provided with a penlight or flashlight held by the dental assistant. Access and stabilization of the mouth can be obtained by placing a finger on the gum pad distal to the most posterior tooth in a maxillary quadrant. After inspection of the oral soft and hard tissues, the practitioner can perform a dental cleaning (plaque removal) with a soft-bristled, moist, infant-size toothbrush. Rarely will a rubber cup and polishing paste be required for stain removal. The tooth-cleaning process is discussed and demonstrated while removing the plaque. At this point, it is very important that the infant be repositioned with the head cradled in the parent's lap and the parent given the opportunity to practice the tooth-cleaning process with the practitioner's supervision and guidance. This approach will help some parents overcome their reluctance to clean their infant's teeth, especially when the infant resists. Occasionally, some infants and toddlers exhibit tight contacts between the anterior as well as the posterior teeth, which accumulate considerable plaque. The parent can be shown how to clean these areas using dental floss in a holder with relative ease. The parents are advised that they need to perform tooth cleaning for their infant at least once per day, but preferably after each meal. The most critical time to clean the teeth is after the last meal or snack of the day. It is emphasized that toothpaste is not required and is usually objectionable to the infant. If it is used, only a minimal quantity should be placed on the brush.

It should also be emphasized early that, when the infant is becoming accustomed to the routine of having a parent brush the teeth, the process should not become an unpleasant struggle for those infants and toddlers who initially resist the procedure. When the infant struggles considerably, the procedure should not be abandoned. Rather, less attention can be placed on performing thorough plaque removal while maintaining a consistent effort to establish a routine with the infant. A more thorough tooth cleaning can be performed another day when the infant is more cooperative. Parents can be reminded of other routines that are accomplished despite the infant's objections, such as hair washing. If the tooth-cleaning routine is established during the first 12 months of age, strong objections and resistance to the procedure during the "terrible twos" can usually be avoided.

Concluding the Appointment

The practitioner concludes the appointmentwith the following:

- Provides a summary of clinical findings to the parents.
- Makes appropriate recommendations based on clinical findings.

- Solicits and answers any remaining questions that the parents may have.
- Reinforces the parents' role and responsibilities in their infant's oral health care.
- Establishes an optimal fluoride program (pending any water analysis).
- Provides educational pamphlets/brochures as desired.
- Provides anticipatory guidance information.
- Establishes an appropriate recall schedule.

Providing Anticipatory Guidance

Anticipatory guidance is a process for preparing parents for upcoming developmental changes and concerns that may arise before the next scheduled dental visit to minimize the any problems that arise. Wherever possible, information on preventive oral health should be provided to expectant parents during prenatal education programs.

Establishing a Recall Schedule

The recall appointment may be scheduled for 3, 6, or 12 months depending on the infant's potential risk for developing dental disease, which is based on clinical findings, stage of dental development, and feeding or diet patterns. See Table 23–2 ■ for examples for determining appropriate recall schedules.

TABLE ■ 23–2   Clinical Findings According to Infant Age and Expected Feeding or Diet Patterns and Dental Development Characteristics

	Clinical Findings	Feeding or Diet Patterns	Dental Development
3 months	Enamel decalcification Considerable plaque buildup Amelogenesis imperfecta Dentinogenesis imperfecta	Bottle used at bedtime or naptime Bottle used as a pacifier Bottle used beyond 12 months of age Frequent cariogenic diet or snacks	Stage of dental development has minimal influence on decision for a 3-month recall
6 months	Posterior proximal contacts No previous tooth cleaning Primary dentition crowding Moderate plaque build-up	Relatively cariogenic diet or frequent snacking on cariogenic foods	Second primary molar eruption anticipated within 6 months
12 months	Generalized spacing Good oral hygiene exhibited Shallow occlusal anatomy	Good dietary habits exhibiting a low cariogenic potential	Second primary molar eruption anticipated within 12 months

SUMMARY

The potential exists today for dental health professionals to assist parents in raising caries-free infants. The knowledge and technology are available, and the request for this service is growing. The dental professional has the opportunity to accept this role with enthusiasm and continue to be a leader among the health professions in disease prevention. Dental providers must not ignore the oral health needs of infants and toddlers less than 3 years of age. They must instead take advantage of their knowledge and technology to begin disease prevention efforts with infants and to educate parents-to-be and new parents about their important role in the oral health of their infants. By doing so, dental providers can provide a pleasant and logical introduction to dentistry and promote the profession in a most positive way.

PRACTICAL CONSIDERATIONS

Practitioners and staff should develop an office policy for management of pregnant patients. Policies should include recommended prophylaxis or periodontal maintenance visits, essential radiographic exposures, and treatment modifications.

Team members can practice the essential elements of counseling a pregnant woman about her own oral health and methods of infant tooth management to accustom her infant to daily plaque removal. It is best to practice the knee-to-knee examination method so that health professionals will feel comfortable with managing the infant and providing examination procedures without the aid of lighting and instruments. "Lift-the-lip" examinations should be taught to the parents with instructions on recognizing the manifestations of early childhood caries. Several national organizations offer informative brochures that can be obtained relating to nutrition, oral manifestations of pregnancy, and the oral care and maintenance of the infant to supplement counseling sessions.

SELF-STUDY QUESTIONS

1. What is the recommended time frame for an infant's first dental risk assessment?

   a. 6 months

   b. 1 year

   c. 4 years

   d. 6 years

   Rationale: It is recommended that the first dental risk assessment should occur as early as 6 months of age, and the establishment of a dental home should occur by approximately 1 year of age.

2. In following anticipatory guidance, at which stage should "lift the lip" be demonstrated and taught to the caregivers?

   a. 5 to 7 months regardless of breast or bottle feeding

   b. 9 months when discussing the importance of cleaning baby teeth

   c. 1 year when counseling the parent to switch from bottle to cup

   d. 18 months during explanation of nutrition and oral health

   Rationale: Although some infants have deciduous teeth prior to 6 months of age, most of them usually acquire at least one tooth by 9 months. When deciduous teeth first erupt, they are not completely mineralized and are more susceptible to decay. Older infants are more apt to be tolerant with daily oral care at this age and therefore parents need to be diligent and consistent.

3. Which of the following is *not* associated with pregnancy gingivitis?

   a. Increase in erythema

   b. Tissue sensitivity

   c. Spontaneous bleeding

   d. Tissue sloughing

   Rationale: Predominant manifestations of pregnancy gingivitis include gingival enlargement, increased erythema, tissue sensitivity, and spontaneous bleeding. Tissue sloughing is not a typical manifestation.

4. All of the following are characteristics of *S. mutans* relative to dental caries in infants *except* one. Which statement is the exception?

   a. Permanent *S. mutans* colonization of the oral cavity in infants does not occur before the primary teeth erupt.

   b. Initial acquisition of infant caries takes place during the "window of infectivity."

   c. Sucrose facilitates the adherence of *S. mutans* to the tooth surface.

   d. The source of an infant's infection from *S. mutans* is from within the family, most likely the mother.

   Rational: Permanent *S. mutans* colonization of the oral cavity in infants can occur before the primary teeth erupt.

5. Initially, which of the following fluoride supplementation methods is the *best* for an area that does not have community water fluoridation?

   a. 5% dissolvable fluoride tablets

   b. Topical fluoride applications

   c. Fluoride drops

   d. 25% dissolvable fluoride tablets

   Rationale: Initially, supplementation is best accomplished by the use of fluoride drops. Around the age of 3 years, the drops can be replaced by fluoride tablets, which are swallowed. Later, as as the infant progresses into childhood, they gain skill in chewing the tablet. The fluoride-laden saliva can be swished around the mouth and then swallowed to provide a topical application as well as systemic benefits. The practice of using a tablet a day should continue until the child is at least 12 years old,

REFERENCES

1. New York State Department of Health. (2006, August). *Oral health care during pregnancy and early childhood practice guidelines.* Albany, NY: New York State Department of Health, 6–9, 15. Retrieved from http://www.health.state.ny.us/publications/0824.pdf.

2. Shoba, C. (2006). The effect of supportive periodontal therapy in reducing the risk of pre-term low birth weight in women with periodontal disease. *Dissertation.* Rajiv Ghandi University of Health Sciences, Bangalore, India.

3. Thoden van Velzen, S. K., Abraham-Inpijn, L., & Moorer, W. R. (1984). Plaque and systemic disease: A reappraisal of the focal infection concept. *J ClinPeriodontol,* 11:209–20.

4. Li, X., Kolltveit, K. M., Tronstad, L., & Olsen, I. (2000, October). Systemic diseases caused by oral infection. *Clin Micrbiol Rev,* 13:547–58.

5. Offenbacher, S., Beck, J. D., Lieff, S., & Slade, G. (1998). Role of periodontitis in systemic health: Spontaneous preterm birth. *J Dent Educ,* 62:852–58.

6. Engle, W. A., Tornashek, K. M., Wallman, C., and the Committee on Fetus and Newborn. (2007). Late-preterm infants: A population at Risk. *Pediatrics,* 120:1390–1401.

7. Offenbacher, S., Katz, V., Fertik, G., Collins, J., Boyd, D., Maynor, G., McKaig, R., & Beck, J. (1996). Periodontal infection as a possible risk factor for preterm low birth weight. *J Periodontol,* 67:1103–13.

8. ACOG Practice Bulletin. (2001, October). Assessment of risk factors for preterm birth. Clinical management guidelines for obstetrician-gynecologists. *Obstet Gynecol,* 98:709–16.

9. Jared, H. L., Lieff, S., Wilder, R. S., & Offenbacher, S. (1999, March). Periondontal disease and low birth weight: A critical link. *Access,* 13:32–37.

10. Gursoy, M., Kononen, E., Tervahartiala, T., Gursoy, U., Pajukanta, R., & Sorsa, T. (2010). Longitudinal study of salivary proteinases during pregnancy and postpartum. *J Periodont Res,* 45:496–503.

11. Lieff, S., Boggess, K. A., Murtha, A. P., Jared, H., Madianos, P. N., Moss, K., Beck, J., & Offenbacher, S. (2004). The oral conditions and pregnancy study: Periodontal status of a cohort of pregnant women. *J Periodontol,* 75:116–26.

12. Offenbacher, S., Boggess, K. A., Murtha, A. P., Jared, H. L., Lieff, S., McKaig, R. G., Mauriello, S. M., Moss, K. L., & Beck, J. D. (2006, January). Progressive periodontal disease and risk of very preterm delivery. *Obstet Gynecol,* 107:29–36.

13. Jeffcoat, M. K., Geurs, N. C., Reddy, M. S., Cliver, S. P., Goldenerg, R. L., & Hauth, J. C. (2001). Periodontal infection and preterm birth: Results of a prospective study. *J Am Dent Assoc,* 132:875–80.

14. Moss, S. J. (1988).The year 2000 health objectives for the nation. *Pediatr Dent,* 10:228–33.

15. Sā Roriz Fonteles, C., Zero, D. T., Moss, M. E., & Fu, J. (2005, November-December). Fluoride concentrations in enamel and dentin of primary teeth after pre- and postnatal fluoride exposure. *Caries Res,* 39 (6):505–8.

16. Dimitrova, M. M., Kukleva, M. P., & Kondeva, V. K. (2000). A study of caries polarization in 1-, 2- and 3-year-old children. *Folia Med* (Plovdiv), 42:55–59.

17. Dimitrova, M. M., Kukleva, M. P., & Kondeva, V. K. (2000). Specificity of caries attack in early childhood. *Folia Med* (Plovdiv), 42:50–54.

18. Dimitrova, M. M., Kukleva, M. P., & Kondeva, V. K. (2000). Early childhood caries—Incidence and need for treatment. *Folia Med* (Plovdiv), 42:46–49.

19. Behrendt, A., Sziegoleit, F., Muler-Lessmann, V., Ipek-Ozdemir, G., & Wetzel, W. E. (2001). Nursing-bottle syndrome caused by prolonged drinking from vessels with bill-shaped extensions. *ASDC J Dent Child,* 68:47–50.

20. Petti, S., Cairella, G., & Tarsitani, G. (2000). Rampant early childhood dental decay: An example from Italy. *J Public Health Dent,* 60:159–66.

21. Faye, M., Ba, A. A., Yam, A. A., Ba, I. (2006). Caries patterns and diet in early childhood caries. *Dakar Med.* 51(2):72–77.

22. Psoter, W. J., Pendrys, D. G., Morse, D. E., Zhang, H., Mayne, S. T. (2006 Winter). Associations of ethnicity/race and socioeconomic status with early childhood caries patterns. *J Public Health Dent,* 66:23–29.

23. Dini, E. L., Holt, R. D., & Bedi, R. (2000). Caries and its association with infant feeding and oral health-related behaviours in 3–4-year-old Brazilian children. *Community Dent Oral Epidemiol,* 28:241–48.

24. National Maternal and Child Oral Health Resource Center. (2006). Open wide: Oral health training for health professionals. Retrieved March 7, 2010, from http://www.mchoralhealth.org/OpenWide/index.htm.

25. Valaitis, R., Hesch, R., Passarelli, C., Sheehan, D., & Sinton, J. (2000). A systematic review of the relationship between breastfeeding and early childhood caries. *Can J Public Health,* 91:411–17.

26. Mouradian, W. E., Huebner, C. E., Ramos-Gomez, F., & Slavkin, H. C. (2007, May). Beyond access: The role of family and community in children's oral health. *J Dent Educ,* 71:619–31.

27. Herbert, F. L., Lenchner, V., & Pinkham, J. R. (1994). In Starkey, P. A., Ed. *The answer book.* Chicago: American Society of Dentistry for Children.

28. Thorild, I., Lindau-Jonson, B., & Twetman, S. (2002). Prevalence of salivary *Streptococcus mutans* in mothers and in their preschool children. *Int J Paediatr Dent,* 12:2–7.

29. Li, Y., Wang, W., & Caufield, P. W. (2000). The fidelity of mutans streptococci transmission and caries status correlate with breast-feeding experience among Chinese families. *Caries Res,* 34:123–32.

30. Ercan, E., Dülgergil, C. T., Yildirim, I., & Dalli, M. (2007, August). Prevention of maternal bacterial transmission on children's dental-caries-development: 4-year results of a pilot study in a rural-child population. *Arch Oral Biol,* 52(8):748–52.

31. Berkowitz, R. (2006). *Mutans streptococci:* Acquisition and transmission. *Pediatr Dent,* 28:106–9.

32. Lindquist, B., & Emilson, C. (2004) Colonization of *Streptococcus mutans* and *Streptococcus sobrinus* genotypes and caries development in children to mothers harboring both species. *Caries Res,* 38(2):95–103.

33. Li, S., Liu, T. J., Xiao, X. R., Ye, W. W. (2004, November). Acquisition of Mutans streptococci by children of 3-4 years with possible source of the pathogen from their mothers. *Sichuan Da Xue Xue Bao Yi Xue Ban,* 35:818–20.

34. Tanzer, J. M., Livingston, J., & Thompson, A. M. (2001).The microbiology of primary dental caries in humans. *J Dent Educ,* 65:1028–37.

35. Ooshima, T., Matsumura, M., Hoshino, T., Kawabata, S., Sobue, S., & Fujiwara, T. (2001). Contributions of three glycosyltransferases to sucrose-dependent adherence of *Streptococcus mutans. J Dent Res*, 80:1672–77.

36. Bowen W. H., & Koo H. (2011). (Epub 2011, February 23). Biology of *Streptococcus mutans*-derived glucosyltransferases: Role in extracellular matrix formation of cariogenic biofilms. *Caries Res*, 45(1), 69–86

37. Sheiham, A. (2001). Dietary effects on dental diseases. *Public Health Nutr*, 4:569–91.

38. Shemesh, M., Tam, A., & Steinberg, D. (2007, November). Expression of biofilm-associated genes of *Streptococcus mutans* in response to glucose and sucrose. *J Med Microbiol*, 56(Pt 11): 1528–35.

39. Caufield, P. W., Dasanayake, A. P., Li, Y., Pan, Y., Hsu, J., & Hardin, J. M. (2000). Natural history of *Streptococcus sanguinis* in the oral cavity of infants: Evidence for a discrete window of infectivity. *Infect Immun*, 68:4018–23.

40. Carletto, K. F., Cornejo, L., & Gimenez, M., (2005). Early acquisition of *Streptococcus mutans* for children. *Acta Odontol Latinoam*, 18:69–74.

41. Brambilla, E., Felloni, A., Gagliani, M., Malerba, A., García-Godoy, F., & Strohmenger, L. (1998). Caries prevention during pregnancy. Results of a 30-month study. *J Am Dent Assoc*, 129:871–77.

42. Russell, S. L., & Mayberry, L. J. (2008, January–February). Pregnancy and oral health: A review and recommendations to reduce gaps in practice and research. *MCN Am J Matern Child Nurs*, 33:32–37.

43. Caglar, E., Kavaloglu, S. C., Kuscu, O. O., Sandalli, N., Holgerson, P. L., & Twetman, S. (2007, December). (Epub 2007 June 16). Effect of chewing gums containing xylitol or probiotic bacteria on salivary mutans streptococci and lactobacilli. *Clin Oral Investig*, 11:425–29.

44. Haresaku, S., Hanioka, T., Tsutsui, A., Yamamoto, M., Chou, T., & Gunjishima, Y. (2007). Long-term effect of xylitol gum use on mutans streptococci in adults. *Caries Res*, 41:198–203.

45. Soderling, E., Isokangas, P., Pienihakkinen, K., Tenovuo, J., & Alanen, P. (2001). Influence of maternal xylitol consumption on mother-child transmission of mutans streptococci: 6-year follow-up. *Caries Res*, 35(3):173–77.

46. Thorild, I., Lindau, B., & Twetman, S. (2003). Effect of maternal use of chewing gums containing xylitol, chlorhexidine or fluoride on mutans streptococci colonization in the mothers' infant children. *Oral Health Prev Dent*, 1:53–57.

47. American Dental Association Council on Scientific Affairs. (2006). Professionally applied topical fluoride: Evidence-based clinical recommendations. *J Am Dent Assoc*, 137:1151–59.

48. First Five Training Program. Healthy teeth begin at birth. (Position paper). Retrieved March 28, 2008, from http://www.first5oralhealth.org/downloads/brochure_May_25_2005.pdf.

49. Kaiser, L. L., & Allen, L. American Dietetics Association. (2002). (Position paper on Nutrition and Pregnancy). Nutrition and lifestyle for a healthy pregnancy outcome. *J Am Diet Assoc*, 102:1470–90.

50. National Council for Radiation Protection & Measurements. (2003). *Radiation protection in dentistry.* Bethesda, MD: National Council for Radiation Protection & Measurements.

51. U.S. Department of Health and Human Services, Public Health Service, Food and Drug Administration; & American Dental Association, Council on Dental Benefit Programs, Council on Scientific Affairs. (2004). The selection of patients for dental radiographic examinations. (rev. ed.). Retrieved November 17, 2010 from http://www.ada.org/prof/resources/topics/radiography.

52. Little, J. W., Falace, D. A., Miller, C. S., & Rhodus, N. L. (2002). *Dental management of the medically compromised patient* (6th ed.). St. Louis, MO: Mosby, 306.

53. New York State Department of Health. (2006, August). *Oral health care during pregnancy and early childhood practice guidelines.* Albany, NY: New York State Department of Health, 31–38. Also available at http://www.health.state.ny.us/publications/0824.pdf.

54. Homa, A., & Casamassimo, P. S. (2007, November). Access to dental care during pregnancy: An innovative approach. *APHA 135th Annual Meeting and Expo.Poster Abstract.* Program information at http://apha.confex.com/apha/135am/techprogram/paper_147787.htm.

55. First Smiles Program. (1995). *Xylitol gum.* Vancouver, WA: Clark County Public Health. Retrieved March 26, 2008, from http://www.co.clark.wa.us/health/oralhealth/documents/xylitol-eng-1.pdf.

56. Twetman, S., Garcia-Godoy, F., & Goepferd, S. J. (2000). Infant oral health. *Dent Clin North Am*, 44:487–505.

57. McWhorter, A. G., Seale, N. S., & King, S. A. (2001). Infant oral health education in U.S. dental school curricula. *Pediatr Dent*, 23:407–9.

58. Hamilton, F. A., Davis, K. E., & Blinkhorn, A. S. (1999). An oral health promotion programme for nursing caries. *Int J Paediatr Dent*, 9:195–200.

59. Davies, G. M., Duxbury, J. T., Boothman, N. J., Davies, R. M., & Blinkhorn, A. S. (2005, June). A staged intervention dental health promotion programme to reduce early childhood caries. *Community Dent Health* 22:118–22.

60. Holt, K., & Barzel, R. (2006). *Health professional's guide to pediatric oral health management.* National Maternal and Child Oral Health Resource Center (OHRC). Retrieved March 3, 2007, from.

Pediatrics

Christine N. Nathe

OBJECTIVES

After reading this chapter, the student should be able to:

1. Describe and define this pediatric population.
2. Describe common oral conditions and diseases of pediatric patients.
3. Describe specific preventive strategies to use with pediatric patients.
4. Describe the role of the dental provider in treating pediatric patients.

INTRODUCTION

Oral health is essential in children's overall health, functional capacity, and social welfare.[1] Dental care is an indispensable health service for children because dental caries and untreated dental disease can have significant consequences for children's health and well-being. Children can experience pain, infection, dysfunction, poor appearance, and low self-esteem as well as drastic alterations to their ability to eat, communicate, sleep, and play.[1–3] Furthermore, dental caries and untreated dental disease provide a reservoir of infection for systemic spread and have been associated with low social functioning and failure to thrive.[4,5]

For a child, dental experiences are unique psychological and behavioral experiences, which can cause distinct challenges to the delivery of treatment. These challenges place unique demands on dental providers.[6] The highest level of technical skill and knowledge is used when treating child patients. To ensure effective treatment, dental professionals need familiarity with the developmental norms of different ages and an understanding of the underlying dynamics of childhood. As this requirement indicates, treating children is different. One reason more progress is not being made in eradicating common oral diseases in childhood could be a narrow interpretation of their needs, which fails to consider the broader social, developmental, and environmental context of children's lives.[5]

POPULATION CHARACTERISTICS

Dental care has been identified as the most prevalent unmet health need in U.S. children.[4] Millions of children continue to suffer needlessly from preventable oral diseases as a result of extensive disparities existing in oral health and access to care.[1,2,4,7] Furthermore, dental caries remains the preeminent oral disease of childhood.[1,2,7,8]

The vast majority of children are affected by dental caries to some degree by the time they reach adulthood.[8] Children from lower-income households and ethnic minority families are disproportionately affected by dental caries because prevalence and severity of childhood dental caries are linked to socioeconomic status across all age groups.[1,2,5,7] Consequently, this group of children experiences 80% of all dental caries.[1,4]

U.S. children experience an estimated 52 million hours lost from school in addition to problems with schoolwork completion and deterioration of school performance because of dental problems.[2,3,5] Children also experience costly emergency room visits and hospital-based medical and surgical treatments because of pain or dental problems.[1,5] Moreover, children with poor oral health could be subjected to acute or chronic pain; the impact of pain on each child varies depending on his or her developmental level.[9]

Many changes have evolved since dental care for children was predominately secondary and tertiary care.[7,8,10] Today, however, pediatric dental care is prevention oriented. Limiting children's experience of dental pain and infection enhances their capacity to function well, grow normally, and engage in normal activities.[1] Accordingly, dental professionals possess the potential to reduce oral disease in children and establish a healthy functioning dentition through the provision of preventive dental services.

In childhood, changes occur rapidly, particularly in children's abilities to think, reason, understand, and consequently make thoughtful decisions about their behavior. The rapidity and power of such changes make knowledge imperative for anyone wishing to understand the health care needs of any child at any given age.[11]

Each period of development is characterized by specific, sequentially developing skills and traits. Dental providers must consider child patients' ability or readiness to perform a given task and assess their capacity for understanding information and cooperating with care.[5,12]

DID YOU KNOW

Flossing should be taught only when children are physically able to accomplish this skill.

It is critical that dental providers be competent in approaching children during different stages of development to build a trusting relationship.[13] Although adult patients require a one-to-one relationship involving the dental provider and patient, children necessitate a one-to-two relationship consisting of the dental provider, child, and parents.[12] Consequently, every time a child patient presents for treatment, parental concerns must be considered as well.[14]

This section focuses on the pediatric patient involving the **early childhood** (2–5 years), **school age** (6–11 years), and **adolescence** (12–19 years) stages of development. Although each stage illustrates the behavior trends for each age group, the information is given as a guide to anticipated abilities and behaviors in children because each child has an individual pattern of growth.

Child Development

Children are not little adults; they are dynamic beings who are in a state of constant development.[15,16] During each developmental stage, children encounter diverse challenges and specific needs that require fulfillment so they can progress to the next stage. Therefore, to better understand children's behavior and respond to their age-related needs, dental providers must have a philosophical appreciation of child development and must recognize that the major changes taking place in the various stages of growth and development are important considerations that impact preventive care and treatment.[6]

Child development theories can provide a framework for understanding many issues related to children, such as behaviors, their own understanding of their illness process and treatments, their interaction with peers and family members, and their ability to cope in other settings.[17] This understanding can help guide the dental professionals in planning, implementing, and evaluating patient care while fostering the healthy development of children.

Piaget's Cognitive Developmental Theory

Jean Piaget theorized that children actively construct their understanding of the world and go through four stages of **cognitive development** (Table 24–1 ■): sensorimotor (birth to 2 years of age), preoperational (2 to 7 years of age), concrete operational (7 to 11 years of age), and formal operational (11 years of age through adulthood).[13,18,19] The stages occur in a fixed sequence in which the accomplishments of one stage provide the foundation for the next stage, and the transition from one stage to another is gradual, not abrupt; children often show aspects of two stages while going through these transitions.[20]

Piaget's stages of cognitive development provide additional aspects of development to consider when treating child patients: their intellectual capabilities and level of understanding.[13] This cognitive development is crucial to a child's ability to understand the relationships between behavior and health and to make decisions about their own health behavior. Children's understanding can affect how they interpret and comply with treatment. Children's increasing cognitive sophistication leads them toward an increased ability to engage in self-protective behavior and to assume responsibility for preventing problems and promoting health. Age can influence the psychological and behavioral responses to illness and treatment.[11]

Social Learning Theory

Albert Bandura studied how learning through observation (modeling and imitation) affects behavior and thought. He contended that many behaviors or responses are acquired through observational learning.[20] Bandura's **social learning theory** emphasizes reciprocal interactions among the person, behavior, and environment.[19] It maintains that children can learn through observations of others or from vicarious experience through others.[21] An example is a child watching another child patient cry or scream during dental treatment. The very act of observing a negative reaction to dental treatment could cause the observing child to become fearful of dental treatment. Essentially, by observing that patient's experience, that particular experience also becomes the observing child's.[21]

Pavlov's Classical Conditioning

Ivan Pavlov's theory was based on the principle of **classical conditioning** in which a neutral stimulus acquires the ability to produce a response originally produced by another stimulus, that is, learning by association. It occurs when a person makes a mental association between two events or stimuli, and a simple encounter with the first stimulus produces a response once associated only with the second stimulus.[19] For instance, many children have developed a dental phobia after having painful dental procedures. These children fear a dental drill and a wide range of stimuli associated with it—the waiting room, the dental chair, the dental operatory. In the conditioning of fear, a conditioned stimulus, such as the dental drill, is associated with an aversive stimulus, such as the pain that can happen in the course of a dental procedure, in a new or unfamiliar environment. After one such pairing (dental drill and pain), children can develop a long-lasting fear of the conditioned stimulus and of the context.

Skinner's Operant Conditioning

B. F. Skinner's theory says the consequences of a behavior produce changes in the probability of the behavior's occurrence, a process of trial and error known as **operant conditioning**.[18,22] Skinner claimed that the inner mental events such as thoughts,

---

TABLE ■ 24–1 **Piaget's Four Stages of Cognitive Development**

Age Range	Stage of Development	Primary Points of Development
Birth–2 years	Sensorimotor stage	The infant constructs an understanding of the world by coordinating sensory experiences with physical actions. An infant progresses from reflexive, instinctual action at birth to the beginning of symbolic thought toward the end of the stage.
2–7 years	Preoperational stage	The child begins to represent the world with words and images that reflect increased symbolic thinking and go beyond the connection of sensory information and physical action.
7–11 years	Concrete operational stage	The child can now reason logically about concrete events and classify objects into different sets.
11 years–adulthood	Formal operational stage	The adolescent reasons in more abstract, idealistic, and logical ways.

(*Source:* Based on Santrock, J. W. (2004). *Life-span development* (9th ed.). Boston, MA: McGraw-Hill Higher Education, 1–435; Beauman, 2001;[13] Child Development Institute, 1998–2005;[15] and Microsoft Corporation, 2005.[19])

feelings, or perceptions are themselves behaviors and, like any other behaviors, are shaped and determined by environmental forces.[20] Reinforcement is a key concept in operant conditioning; this concept may be defined as any event that follows a response and strengthens or increases the probability of the response being repeated.[20] Positive reinforcement (toys, stickers, handshakes, verbal praise) increases the probability that behavior will be repeated, and a negative reinforcement (punishment, omission, avoidance) decreases the probability that it will be repeated.[19,22]

Just as individuals engage in behaviors to get positive reinforcement, they also engage in behaviors to avoid or escape unpleasant conditions. Therefore, it is important to reinforce only desired behavior, and it is equally important to avoid reinforcing behavior that is not desired.[22] For instance, halting treatment because of a child's behavioral resistance (negative reinforcement) is likely to reinforce undesirable behavior for subsequent visits because the child has now established that the previous response (behavioral resistance) successfully ended the perceived unpleasant condition (treatment).

Erikson's Psychosocial Theory

Erikson's theory describes **psychosocial development** as a series of eight stages (Table 24–2 ■). Each stage consists of a unique developmental task that confronts individuals with a crisis that must be resolved.[18] Erikson's first five stages are related to child patients. These stages and their associated psychosocial crises are trust versus mistrust (birth to 1 year of age); autonomy versus shame and doubt (1 to 3 years); initiative versus guilt (3 to 6 years); industry versus inferiority (7 to 12 years); and identity versus identity confusion (adolescence to early adulthood).[13,18,23]

Erikson's stages of psychosocial development provide a framework for approaching children at different ages and stages with consideration for their emotional needs. *Psychosocial development* refers to the changes in children's relationships with other people, especially their ability to function as autonomous individuals. Enhancements in psychosocial development influence each child's behavior with regard to health promotion and prevention, his or her psychological response to illness, and the ability to assume personal responsibility for his or her health.[13,23]

TABLE ■ 24–2   Erickson's Psychosocial Developmental Stages

Stage of Development and Basic Conflict	Age Range	Important Events and Primary Points of Development
Trust versus mistrust (hope)	Birth–1 year	A sense of trust requires infants' basic physical needs to be met and a loving, nurturing, relationship to be formed with parents or caregiver. If requirements are not met, infants will develop insecurity and mistrust. Trust in infancy allows a lifelong expectation that the world will be a good and pleasant place to live.
Autonomy versus shame and doubt (will)	1–3 years	Infants begin to discover that their behavior is their own. Their energies are centered on developing physical skills, controlling body functions, and making decisions. They develop an ability to do things for themselves and assert their sense of autonomy. They realize their *will*. "Well-parented" children emerge from this stage sure of themselves, elated, and proud of their newly found control. If children are restrained too much or punished too harshly, they can develop shame and doubt.
Initiative versus guilt (purpose)	3–6 years	Children develop a vigorous curiosity, foster a strong imagination, and use fantasy and play to broaden their skills. They use active, purposeful behavior to cope with the challenges of the widening social world. They are asked to assume responsibility for their bodies, their behavior, and their possessions, which develops their sense of initiative. Uncomfortable guilt feelings can arise if a child's curiosity or sense of initiative is restricted.
Industry versus inferiority (competence)	7–12 years	Children are mastering knowledge and intellectual skill. They learn to compete and cooperate with others. They are enthusiastic about learning and want real achievement to be industrious. They can be reasoned with and can understand explanations. These "school-age" children must deal with demands to learn new skills or experience feelings of defeat, failure, incompetence, or inferiority.
Identity versus identity confusion (fidelity)	Adolescence	Adolescents experiment with various roles, trying to find out who they are, what they are all about, and where they are going in life. They are confronted with many new adult responsibilities and statuses. They seek someone to inspire or lead them. They establish sexual identity and gradually develop socially agreeable and desirable ideals. Adolescents will face identity confusion if self-certainty is not achieved.

(*Source:* Based on Santrock, 2004;[18] Beauman, 2001;[13] and Child Development Institute, 1998–2005.[15])

Early Childhood Development: 2 to 5 Years of Age

Physical

Physical growth during early childhood is characterized by a steady rate of change. Children typically grow about 3 inches in height and approximately 4.5 pounds annually with a broad range of variation for normal height and weight. During this time, children become taller, slimmer, heavier, and less top-heavy. Also, their gross motor skills (Table 24–3 ■) continue to increase dramatically as children master the standing posture, walking becomes instinctive, and reaching and throwing are refined. Furthermore, their fine motor skills (Table 24–4 ■) improve substantially from sophistication of reaching, grasping, and manipulating small objects. Moreover, there is an increase in brain maturation, which contributes to improved cognitive abilities.[18]

TABLE ■ 24–3   Gross Motor Skills in Early Childhood

Age	Examples of Gross Motor Skills
2 years	Running Kicking a ball Picking up an object without falling down
3 years	Walking up stairs by alternating feet Pedaling a tricycle Throwing a ball forward Jumping in place
4 years	Preforming a standing broad jump Catching a large ball Hopping on one foot
5 years	Skipping smoothly Balancing on one foot

(*Source:* Dworkin, P. H. (1988). The preschool child: Developmental themes and clinical issues. *CurrProblPediatr*, 18:73–134.)[32]

TABLE ■ 24–4   Fine Motor Skills of Early Childhood

Age	Examples of Fine Motor Skills
2 years	Turning pages of a book Eating well with a spoon Holding a glass securely Building a tower of six blocks
3 years	Scribbling with a crayon Building a tower of nine to ten blocks Using a fork Pouring from a pitcher
4 years	Buttoning clothing Lacing shoes Cutting with scissors
5 years	Brushing teeth Combing hair Washing face

(*Source:* Dworkin, P. H. (1988). The preschool child: Developmental themes and clinical issues. *CurrProblPediatr*, 18:73–134.)[32]

Cognitive

Early in this period of intellectual growth, children constantly ask questions because of their curiosity and exploration of surroundings and perceived objects. They can recall specific past experiences; however, if they are not given appropriate cues and prompts, the information can be unreliable and incomplete because they can remember only the features of an experience that capture their attention instead of the relevant dimensions. Furthermore, there is an increase in children's attention span and vocabulary, as well as dramatic enhancements in language development during this time.

Socioemotional

Children become more proficient at talking about their own emotions as well as the emotions of others during early childhood. The amount of terms used to describe emotion increases as they learn more about the causes and consequences of feelings—along with the understanding that a single event can generate different emotions in different people.[18] Children's rich imagination leads to magical thinking and pretend play, causing them to interpret what they are told quite literally. It is this vivid fantasy that aids children in emotional development by allowing them to experiment with strong feelings, work through areas of tension, and assume aspects of identification of those around them.[24] During this period, children struggle to ascertain autonomy and independence as well as to establish self-identity, self-awareness, and a capacity for self-monitoring.[25] Their emotional attachments to parents and other caregivers, however, still remain a vital source of emotional well-being because the strongest fears at this time are those of separation from parents and self-injury.[25] Children also begin to experience self-referential emotions such as pride, guilt, shame, and embarrassment in addition to developing an awareness of gender and a sense of gender-specific behavior.[19] Moreover, early childhood is a time when cooperative play and group play are possible because of the increased development of impulse control. Children will actively seek social contact with their peers, although there are wide ranges of how aggressively they will pursue such contacts, depending on each child's temperament, or behavioral style.[25]

School-Age Development: 6 to 11 Years of Age

Physical

Children grow more slowly and gradually during the school-age period. They gain 2 to 3 inches in height and about 5 pounds in weight each year. Body proportions change: They become slimmer as "baby fat" begins to decrease, and muscle mass and strength steadily increase.[18] Motor development becomes much smoother and more coordinated because of improved myelination of the central nervous system, enabling children to use their hands more dexterously for fine motor skills such as handwriting, producing arts and crafts, and playing instruments. In addition, they can perform gross motor skills such as running, climbing, skipping rope, swimming, bicycle riding, batting a ball, and skating. These skills allow them to participate in organized sports. School-age children gain increased control over their bodies and experience energetic physical health during this period; however, they are far from having physical maturity and possess a need to be active.[18]

Cognitive

During this period of development, children's cognitive skills are well suited to begin a formal education by attending school; therefore, the stage is called *school-age.* These children can concentrate better and longer than before, and their capacity for thought and reasoning significantly increases with more systematic and selective learning that is applied with increasing ease to a variety of contexts.[19] Also, school-age children gain improved verbal reasoning and use of symbolic and graphic representations through a refined use of language and advances in reading, vocabulary, grammatical skills, science, and mathematics.[25] They begin to master and appreciate their intellect by becoming more consciously aware of their mental processes and are capable of attaining cognitive skills to accomplish goals. By the end of this stage, children have the intellectual skills to function competently in the adult world; however, abstract and hypothetical issues remain difficult to understand because this stage is characterized by concrete operational thinking.[18,19]

Socioemotional

The emotional development of school-age children is a period when the child learns about the outside world and becomes increasingly independent of his parents.[25] Children develop a conscience or a sense of responsibility about matters of importance to them. These are the years when closely knit groups are formed, such as clubs and gangs, to fulfill children's need for peer acceptance. During this period, children are introduced to the culture of society through the public or private school. These years are important for learning how to get along with other people and to abide by the rules of society. During this time, children link achievement with self-concept and are constantly measuring themselves and their achievements against others.[24] They have an increased understanding of complex emotions such as pride and shame as well as the ability to detect that more than one emotion can be experienced in particular situations and the capability to consider the circumstances that led up to the emotional reaction. In addition, school-age children improve their ability to suppress and conceal emotions and use self-initiated strategies to redirect emotions.

This period is marked by children's quest for social involvement and social acceptance.[24] Doing the "in thing" becomes extremely important, and most school-age children pursue gender-stereotyped activities with same-gender friendship groupings. Their success in maintaining a positive sense of self during the many changing friendships depends on the resilience of their coping and social skills, which encompass a good sense of humor, an ability to make others feel wanted, a willingness to share, a positive mood, creativity, leadership, and negotiation abilities. Finally, children with positive peer relations tend to give and receive positive attention, conform to classroom rules, and perform well academically; they also initiate social contact in a positive manner and develop pleasant social interchanges with others.

Adolescent Development: 12 to 19 Years of Age

Physical

The most important marker of the beginning of adolescence is puberty. During this time, accelerated growth in height and weight as well as a process of "filling out" occurs that is largely under the influence of the sex hormones and gives the appearance of sexual characteristics and ability to reproduce.[25] Throughout this sexual maturation, major changes occur in the distribution of body fat and musculature, genitals enlarge, breasts develop, and skin becomes oily.

Cognitive

Adolescents move toward the stage of cognitive development known as *formal operational thinking.* In this stage, they develop critical thinking, conceptual thinking, and introspection through their increased speed, automaticity, and capacity of information processing; they also have more breadth of content knowledge in a variety of domains, increased ability to construct new combinations of knowledge, and an increased range and spontaneous use of strategies or procedures for applying or obtaining knowledge.[18] They also have the cognitive ability to develop hypotheses followed by deduction or conclusion for solving problems. Furthermore, adolescents are capable of making competent decisions as well as moral judgments.

At this time, adolescents can apply a set of solutions to a specific problem as well as contemplate the effect of all possible variables. Furthermore, having reached this stage, adolescents can now think in abstract terms and deal with hypothetical situations. They give consideration to the *possible* and *what might be.*[25] They begin to ask and answer the question, "What if?" Adolescents begin to think about things that cannot be seen, heard, or touched, such as faith, trust, beliefs, and spirituality as they journey toward self-reflection and self-identity.[26,27]

Socioemotional

Adolescence is the period of transition from childhood to adulthood; the transition is accompanied by a series of baffling and sometimes highly disturbing emotional and social problems attributable to the structural and physiologic changes occurring as a process of physical alterations and sexual maturation.[25] Personal appearance becomes a source of great conflict because of adolescents' heightened interest in body image and agonizing self-consciousness. Furthermore, adolescents develop a need to separate from parents and establish their own identities as individuals, which requires the support of a peer group for the safe psychological shelter in which to grow outside the family.[25] Separation from the family need not be physical, although it often is, but refers to confidence in adolescents' decision making and ability to perform socially on an equal basis with peers.[25] Moreover, there is a dramatic increase in the emotional importance and intimacy of close friends because peers are looked to as role models for dress, music, entertainment, and lifestyle; nonetheless, adolescents need reassurance, support, and physical affection from their parents.

Children's Development and Behavior

Temperament

Temperament is an individual's behavioral style and characteristic way of emotionally responding.[18] It is the foundation for the child's distinct personality because personality is determined by the interaction of temperament traits with the environment.[24,28] Temperamental characteristics influence all aspects of development and behavior. The three basic types, or clusters, of temperament are (1) easy child, (2) difficult child, and (3) slow-to-warm-up child.[18,24,25,28] The **easy child** is characterized by regularity, easy adaptability, and a positive mood in the approach to new situations. The **difficult child** demonstrates considerable irregularity, many negative mood expressions, slow adaptability, and frequently reacts negatively to new situations. Lastly, the **slow-to-warm-up child** has a low activity level and mild reactions, is somewhat negative, and shows low adaptability.

Parents

Parents influence how children think, socialize, and become self-aware.[19] Consequently, parents play an important role in the dental experience of their children because they decide the importance they will place on the dental health of their child and the role they will take in supervising oral hygiene, scheduling regular dental appointments, and monitoring the child's diet.[29] Furthermore, a child looks to the parents for information on appropriate and inappropriate behavior in a strange situation.[30] The level of anxiety a child experiences children is often a reflection of parental fears; parental anxiety (mostly maternal) correlates with a child's mood, cooperativity, anxiety, and anxious behavior during treatment.[12,14,29,31] Thus, a child's behavior during the dental appointment is affected significantly by the parents.

Economics

Children from low-income families can experience excessive domestic turmoil, nutritional deficiencies, child abuse, neglect, or the lack of role models and an intellectually stimulating environment.[32] Furthermore, children who identify with their poor families are vulnerable to feelings of shame, anxiety, anger, or psychological impotence that can portray as a chronic mental stress.[33] Consequently, these children have an inability to coordinate behavior with identified authority, which causes a more compromised ability to work well with adults, particularly adults who are authoritative and seek compliance. Moreover, these children could harbor rejection and resentment of the dental professional during an appointment.[29]

The abilities of children from low-income families to learn and communicate are adversely affected. For example, when children grow up in impoverished circumstances and when their parents do not use a large number of vocabulary words in communicating with them, their vocabulary development suffers; they also acquire language more slowly, retain immature pronunciations longer, and speak in shorter sentences.[18,25,29] Thus, it is suggested that a clinician speak slowly, repeat information more often than usual, and use visual aids when communicating with children from low-income families.[29]

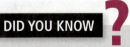

DID YOU KNOW

The provision of community-based oral health programs may be an effective way to increase access to prevention dental care for children.

Culture

Child development is powerfully influenced by the cultural context in which it occurs. Culture is the complex internal psychological structures that determine values, sense of self and others, and expected patterns of behavior. It establishes ideas about health and illness, personal responsibility in health and disease, and nature of healing, which influence the experience of a health care encounter as well as dental hygiene treatment.[24]

Setting

Protective equipment such as goggles and a facemask can elicit anxiety if worn during the initial contact with child patients. Also, wearing plain white clothing or a white coat can elicit fear from a small number of them.[34] Furthermore, if the dental professional shows insecurity around children, these patients could demonstrate increased behavioral problems compared with their reaction to experienced clinicians.[29] It is reported that providers who express increased confidence perform more effectively and experience less uncooperative behavior from children.[35]

COMMON ORAL MANIFESTATIONS

The more common oral conditions of early childhood are dental caries, oral mucosal infections, accidental and intentional dental and oral trauma, developmental disturbances associated with teething or tooth formation, and developmental clefts of the lip and/or palate. In addition, parents frequently request information on additional concerns including sucking habits, tooth alignment, timing and order of tooth eruption, and tooth coloration. Of these conditions, dental caries is the preeminent concern because of its tremendous prevalence and consequences.[1]

Early Childhood Caries

Dental caries among very young children is referred to as **early childhood caries (ECC)** (Figure 24–1 ■). This condition is defined as the presence of one or more decayed, missing, or filled tooth surfaces in any primary tooth in a young child. This unique pattern of dental caries affects the smooth surfaces of primary maxillary incisors and occlusal fissures of the first molar teeth.

PREVENTIVE STRATEGIES

Children exhibit a broad range of physical, cognitive, and socioemotional development as well as diverse behavioral characteristics; therefore, maintaining children's compliance in the dental environment could require behavior-management techniques. **Behavior management** can be described as

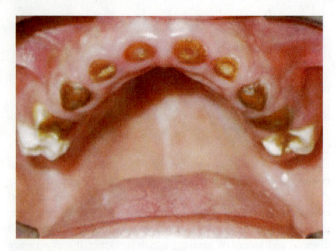

FIGURE ■ 24–1 Early Childhood Caries

(*Source:* Courtesy of Sharon Peterson.)

a continuum of interaction with a child/parent directed toward communication and education. Its goal is to ease fear and anxiety while promoting an understanding of the need for good dental health and the process by which it is achieved.[36]

Cooperative behavioral management with children and families can assist in promoting optimal dental care because a number of specific dental and dental hygiene procedures can cause anxiety or discomfort.[37]

Tables 24–5 ■ through 24–7 ■ outline implications of dental treatments for the three developmental stages. The following behavior-management techniques are communication based; therefore, no specific consent or documentation is necessary before use.

Communication

Communication is the most fundamental form of behavior management. It is the foundation for cooperation and trust as well as the basis for establishing a relationship with the child that can allow for successful completion of dental procedures, and at the same time, help the child develop a positive attitude toward dental health.[36]

Communication is the process by which a person sends a message to another person with the intention of evoking a response; the objective of communication is understanding.[37,38] Communication can be applied with both cooperative and uncooperative pediatric patients; many different approaches are required to communicate with the variety of children who enter the dental operatory because they need communication, teaching, and guidance in the new environment.[39]

TABLE ■ 24–5   Implications for Dental Treatment during Early Childhood

- Develop rapport with child and parent as a foundation for cooperation and trust.
- Regard the parent as a partner in the child's oral health care.
- Talk to a child in short sentences using simple words without double meanings; do not use metaphors because children interpret language literally.
- Maintain a calm, slow, reassuring voice that does not intimidate the child.
- Explain all procedures in simple, concrete terms.
- Clarify what the child's role is during treatment, and set acceptable rules for behavior.
- Demonstrate the use of equipment, and involve the child in the dental care as much as possible.
- Use substitution words (e.g., refer to the suction as a "straw"; describe the handpiece as a "tooth tickler"; portray x-rays as using a "camera" to take "pictures" of the teeth).
- Give simple instructions and directions one at a time.
- Use gestures and facial expressions.
- Use a confident manner and positive voice when inviting a child to sit in the dental chair independently.
- Consider allowing the child to sit on his or her parents' lap, depending on parental attachment.
- Allow the child to explore the environment through smell, taste, touch, sight, and sound (e.g., smelling the fluoride, hearing the compressed air, handling a mirror, tasting prophylactic paste).
- Do not lie to a child about pain; describe exactly what the procedure will feel like.
- Avoid logic because the child lacks reasoning skills during this stage.
- Allow a child to make choices whenever possible, and give her or him a means to interrupt treatment, such as raising a hand to signal discomfort.
- Answer questions and encourage curiosity.
- Avoid overdirecting the very cooperative child.
- Be aware that negativism (saying "no") might be the child's only way of control and that temper tantrums are a possibility.
- Teach parent and child appropriate oral hygiene care according to the child's needs.
- Offer suggestions and/or recommendations to parents concerning risk factors and their assistance of the child with oral hygiene activities.
- Ignore inappropriate behaviors while praising appropriate behaviors and cooperation.
- Reward good behavior with a tangible gift (e.g., toothbrush, sticker, toy).

TABLE ■ 24–6   Implications for Dental Treatment for School-Age Children

- Develop rapport with children as a foundation for cooperation and trust.
- Talk with children about their friends, school, and outside interests.
- Direct questions toward the children first, indicating that they are your patient.
- Develop rapport with the parents, and consider them partners in children's oral health care.
- Dispel myths that children could have learned from other children and/or adults about dental visits.[6]
- Clarify what the children's role is during treatment, and set acceptable rules for behavior.
- Encourage questions and give straight answers.
- Explain procedures using simple vocabulary.
- Regularly ask children to repeat (in their own words) what has just been said or explained to them to ensure understanding.
- Describe the operation of equipment and reasons for its use.
- Give clear explanations of what the patients will experience in terms of pain or discomfort; do not mislead children.
- Help child patients retain control by including them in decision making, soliciting their help, giving them the opportunity to make choices involving their care when possible, and providing them a means to interrupt treatment, such as raising a hand to signal discomfort.
- Introduce children to routine care of their teeth and gums, including regular brushing, flossing, and reductions in sugar consumption (e.g., candy, sodas).
- Teach parents to monitor their children's oral hygiene activities, and offer suggestions to parents who struggle with their children regarding these issues.
- Be positive and supportive to children, thus avoiding judgment and embarrassment.
- Be aware that children in this stage can have temper tantrums that are difficult to control, and their behavior can be unpredictable—from cooperative to obstructive to withdrawn to enthusiastic.
- Distinguish between emotional crying (pain, fear) and crying used to control the environment (tantrums); handle emotional crying with patience and empathy; tantrums require behavior-management techniques.
- Understand that praise becomes a stronger reinforcer and that "rewards" used for appropriate behaviors can become less tangible.

TABLE ■ 24–7   Implications for Dental Treatment of the Adolescent

- Develop rapport with the adolescent as a foundation for cooperation and trust.
- Talk with the adolescent about friends, school, interests, and hobbies.
- Allow sufficient time for the adolescent patient to adjust before asking demanding questions because she or he can at first be mistrustful of authority.[6]
- Reassure the adolescent about confidentiality and privacy issues.
- Set reasonable limits and standards for cooperation and behavior.
- Help these patients retain control by including the adolescent in decision making, soliciting his or her help, giving him or her the opportunity to make choices involving care when possible, and providing him or her a way to interrupt treatment, such as raising a hand to signal discomfort.
- Allow self-expression and avoid being judgmental.
- Listen, be attentive, and attempt to understand the adolescent while making sure to respond in consistent standard English.[43]
- Be supportive and be a good role model and resource.
- Set goals for oral hygiene activities and future recall appointments.
- Appeal to the adolescents regarding the impact of oral health on social interactions (e.g., plaque and oral bacteria can cause bad breath).
- Dispel myths of idealized media images of dental health (e.g., extremely white teeth).
- Understand that the adolescent can exhibit arrogant and disrespectful attitudes.
- Treat all questions seriously and provide full explanations.
- Discuss oral health in terms of disease and infections; give explanations and consequences, especially physical consequences.
- Give clear explanations of what the patient will experience in terms of pain or discomfort; do not lie to or mislead the patient.
- Include dietary habits, tobacco, alcohol, and drug use in health education messages.
- Strive for a positive dental hygiene experience, allowing the adolescent to gain more self-esteem.

Communicating with children takes skill, thoughtfulness, and practice.[40] In addition, working with and educating children successfully require the dental professional to analyze each child's developmental level and comprehension skills to communicate according to age, behavior, and the context of the interaction.[22,36–38,40] The intellectual development of children sets absolute limits on what can be communicated with young patients; a good understanding of their developmental stage—their cognitive and personality development, their fears and desires, their individual backgrounds—will enable the dental professional to communicate more successfully in terms the children will understand.[38] Consequently, if a dental professional uses language the patient cannot understand, the children lose attention and desire to cooperate, decreasing the chances that goals will be achieved.[37]

A child's essential link to parents emphasizes the need for effective communication with parents. Moreover, parents' behavior and attitudes can have a key effect on their children's behavior during treatment. Anything that can be done to improve communication with parents will likely lead to better dental experiences for the parent and child because well-informed parents will likely be more relaxed and, therefore, can influence their child in a positive way.[36]

Tell-Show-Do

The **tell-show-do technique** is a basic and straightforward strategy used to help introduce a new experience in conjunction with helping to minimize fear of the unknown.[34] This method of behavior shaping involves the following concepts:

- *Tell:* Give verbal explanations of procedures in phrases appropriate to the patient's developmental level.
- *Show:* Demonstrate for the patient the visual, auditory, olfactory, and tactile aspects of the procedures in a carefully defined, nonthreatening setting.

- *Do:* Completion of the procedure without deviating from the explanation and demonstration.

The tell-show-do method is indicated for all patients to teach them important aspects of the dental visit, to gain positive behavior at the subsequent appointments, and to shape their response to procedures through desensitization; this method grants patients the ability to learn new and more pleasant associations with anxiety-provoking stimuli.[22,36]

Voice Control

Voice control refers to a measured alteration of voice volume, tone, or pace to influence and direct the patients' behavior to gain their attention and compliance, avert negative or avoidance behavior, and establish appropriate adult–child roles.[36] It has been reported that the contingent and specific use of firm commands when children were beginning to lose control and drift away from communication led to much more control, compliance, and good behavior during dental treatment; this tactic also led to patients' increased sense of self-worth after treatment.[41]

Positive Reinforcement

Positive reinforcement refers to the presentation of a stimulus immediately after desirable patient behavior that results in an increase in the frequency of the behavior.[41] Social reinforcers can be the most influential consequences for increasing the occurrence of adaptive behaviors. They include verbal reinforcers (e.g., "good job keeping your mouth open"), appropriate physical demonstrations (e.g., patting the child's shoulder, shaking the child's hand), or through nonverbal gestures (e.g., smile, thumbs-up). Tangible reinforcers (e.g., toys, stickers) can also be used to reinforce desired behaviors; however, access to these "rewards" should occur only after the appropriate behavior in order for the behavior to remain effective.[36,42]

Distraction

Distraction is the technique of diverting the patient's attention (e.g., listening to music with earphones) from what may be perceived as an unpleasant procedure by decreasing children's perceptions and expectations of unpleasantness, thus preventing negative behavior.[36]

A positive dental setting with child-themed waiting areas and patient education areas can be an excellent distraction for fearful pediatric patients and serve as a positive reminder of a dental visit.

SUMMARY

For all children, oral health is an essential component of overall health, and dental care is an essential health service. Dental professionals need to understand several dimensions of a child's psychological development to relate effectively to and guide the child patient. The dental professional needs to know what emotional and social behaviors to expect from children in different age groups. The dental professional also must be able to communicate on a level consistent with the child's view of the world. In addition, knowledge about how children learn is needed so that the dental professional can teach the child desirable behavior. The definitive achievement of oral health care for a child is the prevention of oral disease.

PRACTICAL CONSIDERATIONS

It is imperative for dental providers to understand the culture and changes that occur in children during development. These changes include developmental mastery of skills that are important to understand when providing individualized instruction.

The provision of preventive oral health services is the best defense the dental provider has when planning treatment regimens for a lifetime of dental health.

SELF-STUDY QUESTIONS

1. Although adult patients require a one-to-one relationship involving the dental provider and patient, children necessitate a one-to-two relationship consisting of the dental provider, child patient, and parent.

   a. The first statement is true; the second statement is false.

   b. The first statement is false; the second statement is true.

   c. Both statements are true.

   d. Both statements are false.

   Rationale: Although adult patients require a one-to-one relationship involving themselves and the dental provider, a child necessitates a one-to-two relationship consisting of the dental provider, child patient, and the parent.

2. Pediatric dental care should focus on the provision of which type of dental care?

   a. Restorative

   b. Preventive

   c. Urgent

   d. Emergency

   Rationale: Limiting children's experience of dental pain and infection enhances their capacity to function well, grow normally, and engage in normal activities and the need to focus on preventive dental care.

3. Which of the following refers to the presentation of a stimulus immediately after desirable patient behavior that results in an increase in the frequency of behavior?

   a. Positive assessment

   b. Positive reinforcement

   c. Negative confirmation

   d. Negative reinforcement

   Rationale: *Positive reinforcement* refers to the presentation of a stimulus immediately after desirable patient behavior that results in an increase in the frequency of the behavior.

4. The specific use of firm commands when children were beginning to lose control and drift away from communication leads to which of the following?

   a. Patient control

   b. Better outcomes with treatment

   c. Patient apprehension

   d. Both a and b

   Rationale: Contingent and specific use of firm commands when children were beginning to lose control and drift away from communication led to much more control, compliance, and good behavior during dental treatment; this tactic also led to the patients' better sense of self-worth after treatment.

5. Whose behavior and attitudes can have a key effect on children's behavior during treatment?

   a. Teachers

   b. Principals

   c. Providers

   d. Parents

   Rationale: Parents' behavior and attitudes can have a key effect on their children's behavior during treatment.

REFERENCES

1. Edelstein, B. L. (2002). Dental care considerations for young children. *Spec Care Dent,* 22 (Suppl 3):11S–25S.
2. U.S. Department of Health and Human Services. (2000). *Oral health in America: A report of the Surgeon General—Executive summary.* Rockville, MD: U.S. Department of Health and Human Services, National Institute of Dental and Craniofacial Research, National Institutes of Health.
3. Kanellis, M. J. (2000). The impact of poor oral health on children's ability to function. *J Southeastern Soc Pediatr Dent,* 6:12–13.
4. Mouradian, W. E., Wehr, E., & Crall, J. J. (2000). Disparities in children's oral health and access to dental care. *JAMA,* 284:2625–31.
5. Mouradian, W. E. (2001). The face of a child: Children's oral health and dental education. *J Dent Educ,* 65:821–31.
6. Windmer, R. (2002). Implications of child development on the practice of oral care. *Compend Contin Educ Dent,* 23(Suppl 2):4–9.
7. Crall, J. J. (2002). Children's oral health services: Organization and financing considerations. *AmbulPediatr,* 2 (Suppl 2):148–53.

8. Edelstein, B. L. (2002). Disparities in oral health and access to care: Findings of national surveys. *AmbulPediatr,* 2 (Suppl 2):141–47.

9. Schechter, N. (2000). The impact of acute and chronic dental pain on child development. *J Southeastern SocPediatr Dent,* 6:16–17.

10. American Dental Education Association. (2003). Improving the oral health status of all Americans: Roles and responsibilities of academic dental institutions. *The report of the ADEA president's commission.* Washington, DC: American Dental Education Association, ADEA Center for Educational Policy and Research.

11. Maddux, J. E., Roberts, M. C., Sledden, E. A., & Wright, L. (1986). Developmental Issues in child health psychology. *Am Psychol,* 41:25–34.

12. McDonald, R. E., Avery, D. R., & Dean, J. A. (2004). Nonpharmacologic management of children's behaviors. *Dentistry for the child and adolescent* (8th ed.). St. Louis, MO: Mosby, 35–49.

13. Beauman, S. S. (2001). Didactic components of a comprehensive pediatric competency program. *J Infus Nurs,* 24:367–74.

14. Mallin, K., & Lazarus, M. C. (2005). Treating children is different. *Dermatol Clin,* 23:171–80.

15. Child Development Institute. *Stages of intellectual development in children and teenagers.*Retrieved January 7, 2006 from http://childdevelopmentinfo.com/child-development/piaget.shtml. Copyright © 1998–2005 by Child Development Institute.

16. Price, S. (1994). The special needs of children. *J AdvNurs,* 20:227–32.

17. Revell, G. M., & Liptalk, G. S. (1991). Understanding the child with special health care needs: A developmental perspective. *J Pediatr Nurs,* 6:258–67.

18. Santrock, J. W. (2004). *Life-span development* (9th ed.). Boston, MA: McGraw-Hill Higher Education, 1–435.

19. Thompson, R. A. (2005). Child development. Microsoft® Encarta® Encyclopedia 1993–2004. Redmond, WA: Microsoft Corporation.

20. Wood, S. E., Wood, E. G., & Boyd, D. (2006). *Mastering the world of psychology* (2nd ed.). Boston, MA: Pearson Education, 136–67.

21. Do, C. (2004). Applying the social learning theory to children with dental anxiety. *J Contemp Dent Pract,* 5:126–35.

22. Baghdadi, Z. D. (2001). Principles and application of learning theory in child patient management.*Quintessence Int,* 32:134–41.

23. George, J. M., & McIver, F. T. (1983). Three theories of psychological development: Implications for children's dentistry. *J Dent Educ,* 47:112–13.

24. Dixon, S. D., & Stein, M. T. (2000). *Encounters with children: Pediatric behavior and development* (3rd ed.). St. Louis, MO: Mosby, 14–22.

25. Lowrey, G. H. (1986). *Growth and development of children* (8th ed.). Chicago-London: Year Book Medical Publishers, Chs 6, 9.

26. Huebner, A. (2000, March). *Adolescent growth and development.* (Family and Child Development, Publication 350-850). Virginia Cooperative Extension, Virginia Polytechnic Institute and State University; Virginia State University; U.S. Department of Agriculture.Retrieved April 25, 2006, from http://www.ext.vt.edu/pubs/family/350-850/350-850.html.

27. Barnett, R. V. (2005). *Helping teens answer the question "Who am I": Cognitive development in adolescents.* (Document FCS2241). Family Youth and Community Sciences Department, Florida Cooperative Extension Service, Institute of Food and Agricultural Sciences, University of Florida. Retrieved April 25, 2006, from http://www.edis.ifas.ufl.edu/FY769.

28. Child Development Institute. *Temperament and your child's personality.* Retrieved January 7, 2006, from http://childdevelopmentinfo.com/child-development/piaget.shtml. Copyright © 1998–2005 by Child Development Institute.

29. Pinkham, J. R. (1995). Personality development: Managing behavior of the cooperative prweschool child. *Dent Clin North Am,* 39:771–87.

30. Newton, J. T., & Harrison, V. (2005). The cognitive and social development of the child. *Dent Update,* 32:33–34.

31. Kagan, J. (1999). The role of parents in children's psychological development. *Pediatrics* 104:164–67.

32. Dworkin, P. H. (1988). The preschool child: Developmental themes and clinical issues. *CurrProblPediatr,* 18:73–134.

33. Fayle, S. A., & Tabmassebi, J. F. (2003). Pediatric dentistry in the new millennium: 2. Behaviour management—Helping children to accept dentistry. *Dent Update,* 30:294–98.

34. Musselman, R. J. (1991). Considerations in behavior management of the pediatric dental patient: Helping children cope with dental treatment. *PediatrClin North Am,* 38:1309–23.

35. Wurster, C. A., Wenstein, P., & Cohen, A. J. (1979). Communication patterns in pedodontics. *Percept Mot Skills,* 48:159–66.

36. American Academy of Pediatric Dentistry. (2004). Reference manual, 2004–2005: Clinical guideline on behavior management. *Pediatr Dent,* 26:89–94.

37. Darby, M. L., & Walsh, M. M. *Dental hygiene theory and practice.* Philadelphia, PA: W.B. Saunders, 75–101.

38. Chambers, D. W. (1976). Communicating with the young dental patient. *J Am Dent Assoc,* 93:793–99.

39. Feigal, R. J. (2001). Guiding and managing the child dental patient: A fresh look at old pedagogy. *J Dent Educ,* 65:1369–77.

40. Deering, C. G., & Cody, D. J. (2002). Communicating with children and adolescents. *Am J Nurs,* 102:34–41.

41. Greenbaum, P. E., Turner, C., Cook, E. W., & Melamed, B. G. (1990). Dentists's voice control: Effects on children's disruptive and affective behavior. *Health Psychol,* 9:546–58.

42. MacDonald, E. K. (2003). Principles of behavioral assessment and management. *Pediatr Clin North Am,* 50:801–16.

Adult Dental Care

Maria Perno Goldie

OBJECTIVES

After reading this chapter, the student should be able to:

1. Describe and define this adult population.
2. Describe common oral conditions and diseases of adult patients.
3. Describe specific preventive strategies to use with adult patients.
4. Describe the role of the dental provider in treating adult patients.

INTRODUCTION

Oral diseases continue to be among the most prevalent problems in our society despite the importance of oral health to personal overall health and well-being. **Oral health** is defined as being without oral cancer, dental caries, periodontal diseases, or other forms of oral problems.[1] The general level of oral health has improved steadily in recent decades. The baby boomer generation will be the first in which the majority will maintain their natural teeth over their entire lifetime, having benefited from water fluoridation and fluoride toothpastes. Over the past 10 years, the number of adults missing all their natural teeth has declined from 31% to 25% for those ages 60 years and older and from 9% to 5% for those adults between 40 and 59 years. However, 5% means a surprising one of twenty middle-age adults are missing all their teeth. More than 40% of poor adults (20 years and older) have at least one untreated decayed tooth compared with 16% of nonpoor adults.[2] Dental caries and periodontal diseases are preventable and controllable. Dental caries can be prevented by a combination of fluoride, dental sealants, and other new technologies. Periodontal diseases can be prevented mainly by personal and professional control of plaque biofilm.

POPULATION CHARACTERISTICS

Humans go through a variety of life stages from birth to old age. Changes usually begin at puberty when the adult life cycle begins. The following sections illustrate the characteristics of specific age groups of adults.

Adolescence to Young Adulthood: 13–20 Years of Age

There is no standard definition of *adolescent,* according to the American Psychological Association.[3] Adolescents are defined very broadly as youths between the ages of 10 to 18. Using this definition, there were approximately 41.5 million adolescents in the United States in 2008, according to the U.S. Census Bureau.[4] **Adolescence** is a period of transition from the dependence of childhood to the independence of adulthood. It can be identified in terms of sexual maturity, identity development, and a period of social transition into adulthood. Puberty and associated physical changes can occur between the ages of 9 and 17 years. The pituitary gland is responsible for the control of the production of estrogen from the ovaries in females and androgen from the testes in males. These hormones, responsible for the development of sex organs, continue to cause profound physical and emotional influences during this life stage. Physically, both males and females experience accelerated growth, height, weight, and muscle mass. Because of the pattern of growth spurts, adolescents can appear clumsy and awkward. Lack of physical coordination can become an issue and can affect self-esteem. Dermatological changes are often evident in this life stage and can cause immense concern in teens.

Early Adulthood: 21–39 Years of Age

The transition from adolescence to adulthood is marked by the ability to make independent choices, a sense of identity, and psychological and social adjustments that ready one for marriage, parenthood, and career choice. Although this is a period in which individuals are generally in good health (i.e., peak bone mass, stabilized hormones), lifestyle choices made during this time can cause chronic disease later in life. During this life stage, many females can take oral contraceptives. Individuals also can marry and start families, so oral care of expectant mothers and unborn children becomes a relevant issue.

Mature Adulthood: 40–60 Years of Age

As the middle years of adulthood approach, many people are established, have definite lifestyles, and have found their role within the societal structure. This is also a time of reflection and slowing of the pace of their life. An important trend seen in this age group is the increasing role as a caregiver. Individuals could now have to care for aging parents, adult children who have returned home, or grandchildren.[5] Hair begins to gray and thin, weight gain is more apparent, and physical inabilities due to arthritis or other conditions can surface. Lifestyle choices, such as lack of exercise, poor nutrition, increased stress, tobacco use, obesity, and alcohol abuse, can have consequences not seen before. The risk for disease increases, orally and systemically. Numerous physiologic changes that have an effect on oral health occur during this life stage. Conversely, many oral conditions can affect other aspects of physiologic health. A patient's understanding of the impact of oral health on overall health is extremely important. Initially, the link of periodontal diseases to systemic diseases was thought to be unidirectional, but growing evidence shows that the relationship can be bidirectional.

As women approach midlife, **hormonal imbalances** become evident in the cessation of menstruation and presentation of various symptoms indicative of the changing hormone levels during perimenopause and menopause. Some females choose hormone replacement therapy or estrogen replacement therapy to control symptoms such as vaginal dryness, hot flashes, and increased urinary frequency. However, because of the release of the results of the Women's Health Initiative

DID YOU KNOW? **?**

The WHI was launched in 1991 and consisted of a set of clinical trials and an observational study, which together involved 161,808 generally healthy postmenopausal women. The clinical trials were designed to test the effects of postmenopausal hormone therapy, diet modification, and calcium and vitamin D supplements on heart disease, fractures, and breast and colorectal cancer. Those studies have now ended. The women in these studies are now participating in a follow-up phase, which will last until 2010.

(WHI) Study, fewer women are taking oral hormones because of their potential deleterious effects.[6] These effects include, but are not limited to, increased risk of breast cancer, heart disease, and stroke.[6] Having lower levels of circulating sex hormones causes systemic and oral symptoms.

More information on the WHI is available at http://www .nhlbi.nih.gov/whi/.

COMMON ORAL MANIFESTATIONS

Systemic conditions that affect oral health include **hormonal changes** and **imbalances.** Oral disease can affect a patient's life in many ways. Certain oral conditions can undermine self-image and self-esteem, discourage social interaction, and be noteworthy chronic stressors.[5] Some conditions can also lead to or contribute to other health issues, such as heart disease, diabetes, and low-birth-weight babies, and interference with vital functions, such as food selection, chewing, and swallowing. Just as physical–physiologic factors demonstrate some crossover, psychosocial–behavioral factors can, in turn, affect diagnosis and therapy. For example, a psychiatric disorder can influence oral health (e.g., bulimia, which causes tooth destruction through regurgitation, or depression, which can impair oral hygiene), or fear of dental procedures can impair communication or otherwise interferes with the provision of care.

DID YOU KNOW

The strong connection between oral health and a person's overall well-being emphasizes the importance of the dental provider's interaction with patients on many psychosocial–behavioral levels: attitude, health beliefs, motivating factors, living situation, and previous dental experiences.

Dental Caries

Dental caries is still as prevalent as ever.[7] Dental caries affects not only children but also teens and adults (Table 25–1 ■; Figures 25–1 ■ and 25–2 ■). Adolescence is a period of significant caries activity formany individuals. Current research suggests that the overall caries rate is declining yet remains highest during adolescence.[8] Immature permanent tooth enamel, a total increase in susceptible tooth surfaces, and environmental factors such as diet, independence to seek care or avoid it, a low priority for oral hygiene, and additional social factors also can contribute to the upward slope of caries in adolescence.[9] Recurrent caries and root caries are prevalent among adults and the elderly. Again, the segment of the general population most prone to caries is also the most vulnerable. In the adult population it is the poor, ethnic minorities, and those with certain medical conditions or disabilities. Ongoing investigation is needed to identify the most effective health education messages for the prevention of caries, particularly for the vulnerable populations. New methods to diagnose, control, and prevent caries throughout the life span could be on the horizon as more is understood about the molecular consequences of the interaction between host and microbes, and about the genomic makeup of bacteria implicated in dental caries.

Periodontal Diseases

Periodontal diseases result from infections caused by bacteria in the biofilm that forms on the teeth and in the periodontal pocket.[10] The mildest form, gingivitis, is the only reversible stage. Gingivitis can lead to periodontitis, a more severe form of the disease that can destroy the periodontal ligament and surrounding bone and, in some cases, lead to the loss of teeth. Almost half of U.S. adults ages 35 to 44 years have gingivitis, and about one-fourth have periodontitis.[11] Severe periodontal diseases affect 14% of adults age 45 to 54 years and 23% of those age 65 to 74 years.[11] Tobacco use is a major risk factor for the development and progression of periodontal diseases.[12] There also is significant substantiation that diabetes, particularly if poorly controlled, increases the risk for periodontal disease (Table 25–2 ■).

Treatment of periodontal diseases includes surgical as well as nonsurgical methods, and advances in regeneration of tissues have increased through the years. Specific treatment for periodontal disease will be determined by a number of factors including age, overall health, and medical history; extent of the disease; tolerance for specific medications, procedures, or therapies; expectations for the course of the disease and treatment outcomes; and patient opinion or preference. Treatment can include any or a combination of the following: scaling and root planing; pharmaceuticals; or surgery, including pocket reduction, regeneration procedures, soft tissue grafts, crown lengthening, or dental implants. As with all diseases, prevention is the best way to manage this problem.

Oral and Pharyngeal Cancer

Oral and pharyngeal cancer is the sixth most common cancer in the developed world.[13] Each year, an estimated 37,000 Americans are diagnosed with this disease, and more than 8,000 die each year from it.[14] The most disturbing aspect about oral and pharyngeal cancer is the survival rate. In the United States, the 5-year survival rate is approximately 50%, a statistic that has not improved over the past 20 years.[15] African American men suffer the highest incidence of these cancers and have a much poorer 5-year survival rate than do white men, regardless of diagnostic stage.[16] Despite the devastating consequences of oral cancer, which include impaired ability to chew, swallow, speak, and often disfigurement from extensive surgery to remove parts of the face and oral structures, only 14% of U.S. adults report receiving oral cancer examinations that can detect early disease. Reconstruction and management of the oral cancer survivor come at a high price, both economically and socially. More efforts are needed to increase public and professional knowledge about oral cancer and its prevention. A critical need involves developing biomarkers and diagnostic tests that can be used to improve cancer diagnosis and more accurately

TABLE ■ 25–1 Prevalence of Coronal Caries in Permanent Teeth among Dentate Adults[a] Aged 20 Years or Older, by Selected Characteristics—United States, National Health and Nutrition Examination Survey, 1988–1994 and 1999–2002

Characteristic	1988–1994		1999–2002		Difference in %[d]	% Change[d]
	%[b]	SE[c]	%	SE		
Age group (years)						
20–39	93.11	0.52	86.76	0.85	−6.35	−6.82
40–59	96.25	0.43	95.07	0.44	−1.18	−1.23
≥ 60	94.58	0.53	93.10	0.56	−1.48	−1.56
Sex						
Male	93.83	0.45	90.34	0.64	−3.49	−3.72
Female	95.41	0.27	92.27	0.51	−3.14	−3.29
Race/Ethnicity[e]						
White, non-Hispanic	96.37	0.28	93.32	0.38	−3.05	−3.17
Black, non-Hispanic	88.35	0.68	84.61	0.85	−3.74	−4.24
Mexican-American	87.29	0.70	83.50	1.62	−3.79	−4.34
Poverty status?[f]						
<100% FPL	86.89	1.17	86.65	1.28	−0.24	−0.28
100%–199% FPL	92.75	0.73	89.06	0.93	−3.69	−3.98
≥ 200% FPL	96.27	0.28	93.17	0.47	−3.10	−3.22
Education						
<High school	89.65	0.59	84.53	1.11	−5.12	−5.71
High school	96.01	0.33	92.63	0.85	−3.38	−3.52
>High school	96.11	0.37	93.16	0.39	−2.95	−3.07
Smoking history						
Current smoker	93.45	0.64	90.19	0.85	−3.26	−3.49
Former smoker	95.15	0.71	92.47	0.93	−2.68	−2.82
Never smoked	94.66	0.42	90.96	0.46	−3.70	−3.91
Total	94.62	0.27	91.30	0.36	− 3.32	− 3.51

[a] Defined as having one or more decayed or filled surfaces (DFS > 0) in the tooth crowns of adults with at least one permanent tooth (dentate). All estimates are adjusted by age (10-year groups) and sex to the U.S. 2000 standard population, except sex, which is adjusted only by age.
[b] Weighted prevalence estimates.
[c] Standard error.
[d] Between the two surveys and using 1988–1994 as reference. A positive value indicates an increase, a negative value a decrease.
[e] Calculated using "other race/ethnicity" and "other Hispanic" in the denominator.
[f] Percentage of the federal poverty level (FPL), which varies by income and number of persons living in the household.
(*Source:* Beltrán-Aguilar, E. D., Barker, L. K., Canto, M. T., Dye, B. A., Gooch, B. F., Griffin, S. O., Hyman, J., Jaramillo, F., Kingman, A., Nowjack-Raymer, R., Selwitz, R. H., & Wu, T. (2005, August). Surveillance for dental caries, dental sealants, tooth retention, edentulism, and enamel fluorosis—United States, 1988–1994 and 1999–2002. *MMWR Surveillance Summaries*, 54: 1–44.

predict the course of the disease. There also is a pressing need to develop more effective, individualized treatments that spare healthy tissues and improve quality of life.

Studies have been examining the association between the **human papillomavirus (HPV)** and head and neck squamous cell carcinomas (HNSCC), especially in young people who do not smoke or drink.[17] HPV is responsible, or plays a part, in the etiology of some oropharyngeal carcinomas.[18] HPV16 DNA has been found in cancer of the oral cavity and oropharynx, primarily in the tonsillar region and base of the tongue.[19]

DID YOU KNOW ?

Engaging in sexual intercourse, including oral sex, at a young age and having multiple partners are risk factors for oral cancer and should be assessed. These factors are due to increased risk for HPV infection of genital and oropharynx regions. Patients should be encouraged to have regular physical examinations with a family practitioner and/or gynecologist, have the HPV vaccine (both for boys and girls), and have oral cancer examinations performed at all dental and dental hygiene appointments.

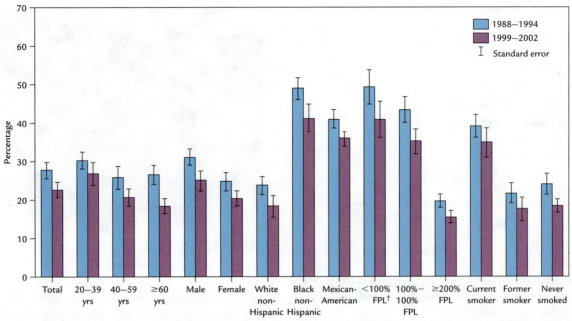

*Defined as having one or more decayed surfaces (DS>0) in the tooth crowns of adults with at least one permanent tooth (dentate). All estimates are adjusted by age (10-year groups) and sex to the U.S. 2000 standard population, except sex, which is adjusted only by age.
†Percentage of the Federal Poverty Level (FPL), which varies by income and number of persons living in the household.

FIGURE ■ 25–1 Prevalence of untreated dental decay among dentate adults age 20 years and older, by selected characteristics—United States, National Health and Nutrition Examination Survey, 1988–1994 and 1999–2002.

(*Source:* Based on Beltrán-Aguilar, E. D., Barker, L. K., Canto, M. T., Dye, B. A., Gooch, B. F., Griffin, S. O., Hyman, J., Jaramillo, F., Kingman, A., Nowjack-Raymer, R., Selwitz, R. H., & Wu, T. (2005, August). Surveillance for dental caries, dental sealants, tooth retention, edentulism, and enamel fluorosis—United States, 1988–1994 and 1999–2002. *MMWR Surveillance Summaries,* 54: 1–44.)

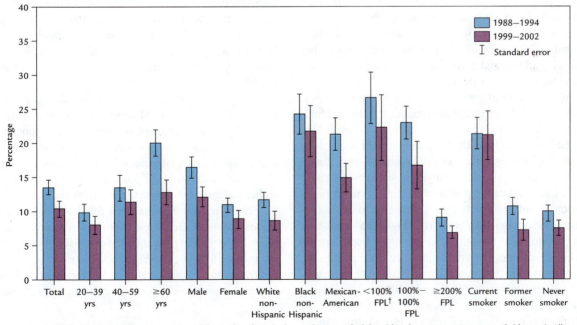

*Defined as having one or more untreated decayed surfaces in the tooth roots of adults with at least one permanent tooth (dentate). All estimates are adjusted by age (10-year groups) and sex to the U.S. 2000 standard population, except sex, which is adjusted only by age.
†Percentage of the Federal Poverty Level (FPL), which varies by income and number of persons living in the household.

FIGURE ■ 25–2 Prevalence of untreated root caries in dentate adults age 20 years and older, by selected characteristics—United States, National Health and Nutrition Examination Survey, 1988–1994 and 1999–2002.

(*Source:* Based on Beltrán-Aguilar, E. D., Barker, L. K., Canto, M. T., Dye, B. A., Gooch, B. F., Griffin, S. O., Hyman, J., Jaramillo, F., Kingman, A., Nowjack-Raymer, R., Selwitz, R. H., & Wu, T. (2005, August). Surveillance for dental caries, dental sealants, tooth retention, edentulism, and enamel fluorosis—United States, 1988–1994 and 1999–2002. *MMWR Surveillance Summaries,* 54: 1–44.)

TABLE ■ 25–2   Risk Factors for Periodontal Diseases

- Genetics
- Lifestyle choices
- Diet low in nutrients
- Smoking and use of smokeless tobacco
- Autoimmune and systemic diseases
- Diabetes
- Hormonal changes in the body
- Bruxism
- Certain medications

Women's Oral Health

Puberty marks the intitial time when hormonal changes can take place in the mouth. Women taking oral contraceptives and pregnant women experience significant hormonal changes. The woman who uses **oral contraceptives (OCs)** will experience hormonal imbalances similar to those in pregnancy. The hormones contained in OCs inhibit the release of the ovum from the ovary, thereby preventing fertilization. These hormonal changes can result in oral manifestations such as hormonal gingivitis, an important topic for oral care education. The relative proportion of the *Bacteroides* species, implicated in periodontitis, is increased 55-fold in pregnant women and 16-fold in women taking oral contraceptives over the control group.[20] We see a shift in bacteria from those that cause gingivitis to those that cause periodontitis when circulating sex hormones are high. Both the hormones estrogen and progesterone have been shown to be a substitute for naphthoquinone, which is an essential growth factor for the *Bacteroides* species and *Prevotella intermedia*.[20] Also, the bacteria and the lipopolysaccharide elicit a host response, including production of cytokines and proinflammatory mediators, which contribute to the negative tissue response.[21] Synthesis of prostaglandins (mediators of inflammation) is high during pregnancy, and it is suggested that progesterone functions as an immunosuppressant in the gingival tissues of pregnant women.[22] This effect can be observed clinically as an exaggerated appearance of inflammation. Progesterone-induced inhibition of collagenase, superimposed on vascular changes, is stated as the cause of **pregnancy granulomas**. These combined effects result in the accumulation of collagen within the connective tissue, sometimes causing these tumor-like growths[23] (Figure 25–3 ■).

Young adults who needed orthodontic treatment during adolescence but did not receive it can have that orthodontic treatment performed at this time. Patients of this age are beginning to realize the importance of their teeth from an aesthetic standpoint and as an important element of their general health. The aesthetic appearance of their teeth is indeed important to their overall oral health.

The oral health of patients in this group increases in complexity as they age. They also begin to experience the onset of various chronic conditions. These conditions or often the therapies used to treat them can have significant effect on the oral tissues. For example, the onset of diabetes in someone with previously excellent plaque control can result in significant

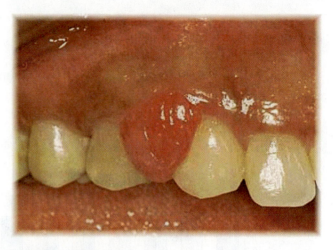

FIGURE ■ 25–3 **Pregnancy granuloma.**
(*Source:* Courtesy of Maria Perno Goldie.)

bleeding, which can frighten the patient, and the clinician should consider this in treatment planning and observation.

During this time frame, most women experience perimenopause and menopause. With the accompanying decline of estrogen, women are more susceptible to reduced bone density, called **osteoporosis**, which also can affect the dental alveolar structure.[24,25] The patient usually does not expect loss of dental alveolar bone that often can accompany osteoporosis. The effect of reduced estrogen levels on bone density must be considered a potential contributing factor in the onset of periodontal disease[26] (Figure 25–4 ■).

Cosmetic options to restore a more youthful smile range from cosmetic whitening with a peroxide-based product to more significant procedures, including veneers, replacement of amalgam restorations with composite materials, and porcelain crowns. The patient is more likely to feel comfortable discussing these topics with the dental hygienist, at least initially, before consultation with the dentist.

The female patient approaching middle age faces hormonal changes inevitably brought about with the onset of **menopause**. These changes often present as alterations in emotions because the hormonal changes can cause mood swings, depression, anxiety, and a general feeling of malaise.[27] Clinicians must be alert to these changes in addition to the potential physiologic ones mentioned earlier and approach the patient in a calm and courteous manner.

These transitional years are filled with psychologic milestones that the clinician must consider in determining treatment plans and providing treatment. Awareness of and sensitivity to the major life changes people face can make a tremendous difference in the relationship that develops between patient and clinician, which can be rewarding and enriching to both parties.

PREVENTIVE STRATEGIES

Adolescence to Young Adulthood: 13–20 Years of Age

Dental hygiene and dental providers can experience some difficulty when trying to relay oral health messages to individuals in this age group. The importance of good oral hygiene and

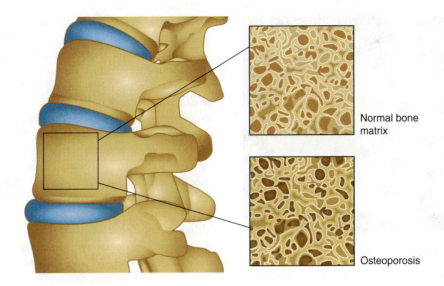

FIGURE ■ 25–4 Osteoporosis.

plaque biofilm control must be stressed to minimize caries and periodontal disease. Contributing to periodontal diseases in this age group are the abundant sex hormones circulating in the bloodstream.[28] Females are particularly sensitive because they have high levels of circulating estrogen and progesterone. Oral tissue has many receptors for these hormones and will most likely be affected as they accumulate in the tissue. Effects include increased vascularity, decreased cell-mediated immunity, increased subgingival bacteria, increased gingival swelling, increased redness, bleeding on probing, increased vascular effects/edema, and increased number of *Prevotella intermedia*.[29] Increased efficacy and frequency of self-care are vital during this life phase.

An oral condition that becomes evident and has increased importance during adolescence is malocclusion,[30] a condition or variation from proper alignment of the teeth and jaw; minor alignment problems have very little impact on patient health.[31] Conversely, some malocclusions can be aesthetically displeasing, can affect chewing and speaking, and can necessitate treatment to maintain health and function. This is also a life stage when orthodontic treatment is considered; risk factors, potential benefits, and costs should be taken into account. A noteworthy psychologic advantage often realized with orthodontic treatment is an enhanced self-image, which can have a positive effect on an adolescent's life.

Eating disorders are more prevalent in this stage of life.[32] Purging behavior of those with eating disorders could result in **perimolysis** in which the acid produced by repeated vomiting dissolves the enamel of teeth.[33] The teeth can have a dull, chalky enamel surface. Often the lingual/palatal surfaces appear eroded, and restorations appeared raised from the tooth (**floating amalgams**). An oral examination indicating disordered eating should result in a frank discussion with the patient and a referral to the appropriate health care professional. This

particular psychologic problem should be approached from a medical–dental team perspective. The psychiatrist or other mental health professional should be aware of and involved in the progress or deterioration of the patient's oral health as it relates to recovery from this eating disorder.[34]

Early Adulthood: 21–39 Years of Age

The dental provider can expect to educate pregnant women about their oral health before and after conception as well as the impact that certain lifestyle choices can have on the oral health of the fetus. Dispelling myths such as "you lose one tooth for every child you have" is another aspect in the education of the patient in this life stage. An expectant woman should not fear damage to her teeth during pregnancy if she maintains adequate care and takes the necessary vitamins and minerals for both herself and her unborn child. Explaining the relationship between gingivitis during pregnancy and its effects on fetal development (e.g., preterm low birth weight) can significantly elevate the importance of oral self-care during this phase of adult life.[35] What was once called **pregnancy gingivitis** is now called *hormonal gingivitis* (Figure 25–5 ■) and is present in more than 30% of pregnant women.[36] Clinically, the gingival tissues appear bright red and edematous at the marginal gingiva and interdental papilla with an increased tendency to bleed. This is a period of great receptivity to medical–dental knowledge because expectant parents generally seek and appreciate information regarding health changes during this very important period of their life.

The current focus on wellness can be a powerful motivational strategy for patients and can provide dental providers opportunities for patient education about oral health. Health promotion theory indicates that people are often more willing to comply with health instruction if a visually pleasing advantage

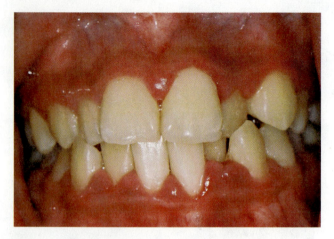

FIGURE ■ 25–5 Hormonal gingivitis.
(*Source:* Courtesy of Maria Perno Goldie.)

is realized versus only a health improvement.[37] An example can be tobacco cessation. Although a significant health benefit exists when one ceases use of tobacco products, it can be the lack of stain on the teeth or fewer facial wrinkles that are the true motivators behind the change in behavior. Knowledge of health promotion theory allows the dental hygienist to present information about oral self-care or treatment options to patients in terms that are relevant to their needs and desires—and beyond expected health benefits.

Mature Adulthood: 40–60 Years of Age

As the U.S. population ages, life expectancy is increasing and has increased from 47.3 years of age in 1900 to 77.8 years of age in 2004.[38] It was estimated in 2011 to be 78.37 in the United States.[39] This increase is accompanied by an expectation of a good quality of life. Oral problems have a negative effect on quality of life because difficulty with the oral cavity can affect the ability to eat, digest food, and communicate. Diet, nutrition, sleep, psychologic status, and social interaction are all affected by impaired oral health. Oral health and disease also have a significant impact on general health and disease.

To understand an individual patient's attitudes, one must evaluate the cultural, psychologic, educational, social, economic, dietary, and chronologically specific cohort experiences that could have influenced that patient's life.[40] Oral health status is affected by these same factors and is the sum of an individual's life experiences with oral health care as well as caries, periodontal disease, and **iatrogenic disease** (caused inadvertently by a medical provider, a medical treatment, or a diagnostic procedure).

A comprehensive approach to the provision of preventive services, counseling, education, and disease screening for average-risk, asymptomatic adults includes regular assessments of health risks. Individuals who have chronic disorders or are members of high-risk populations could need additional interventions. Screening and counseling include risk stratification and health assessment; screening for tobacco use, hypertension via blood pressure measurement, problem drinking,

osteoporosis via bone mineral density testing; and, of course, oral health for periodontal disease, dental caries, xerostomia, oral cancer, and other diseases and conditions.[41]

About 25% of adults 60 years old and older no longer have any natural teeth.[42] Periodontal disease or dental caries is the most frequent cause of tooth loss. Older Americans continue to experience dental decay, and older adults can have new tooth decay at higher rates than children.[43]

Severity of periodontal disease increases with age. At all ages, men are more likely than women to have more severe disease. In addition, at all life stages, people at the lowest socioeconomic level have the most severe periodontal disease.

Root decay is a common problem among the elderly. It afflicts a large percentage of geriatric patients and is difficult to manage. The dental hygienist or dental provider should conduct a detailed history and clinical examination, including a check of salivary flow, medication history for hyposalivatory medications, and the possibility of a high sugar intake (sucking candies; consuming sweetened tea or coffee, soft drinks, candy, gum, ice cream).[44] The etiology of root decay includes dietary habits, microbial plaque biofilm, and decreased salivary flow.[45] To rule out xerostomia as an etiologic factor, a salivary volume study as well as a buffering capacity test can be performed[46].

> **DID YOU KNOW ?**
>
> The bacterial infection that causes tooth decay is called the *caries process.* The resulting lesion in the tooth is called *decay* or *carious lesion.* Caries and decay are not synonymous.

Root lesions are often very difficult to restore because of their location, problems with moisture control, and proximity to the pulp; therefore, they are prone to high recurrence rates. Prevention is the best treatment. As a primary, secondary, or tertiary intervention, chewing gum can be used as an adjunct to preventive therapy because it has been shown to increase pH of the plaque and saliva, thereby assisting in neutralization of plaque acid formation.[46] Xylitol-containing gum stimulates saliva, inhibits bacterial plaque biofilm, and is a five carbon sugar alcohol that cariogenic bacteria cannot metabolize for energy production.[48] Antimicrobial agents are effective against the infective process of caries: Chlorhexidine is extensively used as a mouthrinse to reduce the bacterial load intraorally.[49]

Fluoride is the primary preventive measure because it has an antimicrobial effect on the bacteria that cause dental caries, and it supports remineralization of tooth structure.[50] Fluoride can be delivered to a patient in different forms including rinses, pastes, gels, varnishes, lozenges, tablets, and drinking water. Low-dose fluoride (1000 to 11,100 ppm) in a dentifrice has been reported to reduce caries by maintaining a low concentration of salivary fluoride available for remineralization with daily uses.[51] Mouthrinses (0.05% sodium fluoride) available for purchase over the counter are also retained in the saliva and dental plaque and, when used daily or weekly, help to prevent dental caries. Prescription-strength fluoride is available at a higher potency (5000 ppm dentifrice or 2.0% sodium fluoride rinse) for added caries protection. The effectiveness of all at-home products depends on patient compliance.

Professionally applied topical fluoride in the form of acidulated phosphate fluoride (1.23%) provides a long-term, low-fluoride-release source of calcium fluoride. This agent can slowly release fluoride and maintain the salivary fluoride level. Varnishes offer a high concentration of fluoride (5% sodium fluoride at 22,600 ppm) that adheres to the tooth structure, is applied professionally, and creates a film of calcium fluoride, which is then released in a timed manner.

DID YOU KNOW ?

The use of specific fluoride therapies are dependent upon the caries risk of the individual.

Products containing calcium phosphates are now available. These products support remineralization by increasing calcium and phosphate in saliva, thus changing the pH balance toward remineralization. Ming S. Tung at the American Dental Research Association's Paffenbarger Research Center developed amorphous calcium phosphate (ACP) technology using a two-phase delivery system that prevents the calcium and phosphate from reacting. NovaMin is a synthetic mineral composed of calcium, sodium, phosphorous, and silica, which binds to the tooth surface and releases rapid, continuous deposition of a natural crystalline hydroxyl carbonate.[52] Recaldent (ACP-CPP) contains casein phosphopeptide, a milk-derived peptide, that is bound to amorphous calcium phosphate. Casein phosphopeptide binds the compound to the tooth structure, and amorphous calcium phosphate is released during acidic challenges.[53] Studies have shown this compound to be effective in remineralizing carious lesions and interfering with the adhesion of some bacteria to the tooth surface.[54]

Enabling individuals to maintain good oral hygiene is an important preventive strategy for reducing gingival inflammation, particularly for dependent older people and others who might have difficulty maintaining adequate self-care. Aids such as power toothbrushes provide a useful approach for individuals with decreased dexterity and visual acuity. Dietary modification suitable to the oral condition is another health promotion strategy among the elderly.

In summary, the use of fluoridated water and of fluoride toothpaste provides protection against dental decay at all ages. Practicing effective oral hygiene will reduce dental plaque biofilm and can help prevent periodontal disease and dental caries. Regular professional visits to the dental provider are vital even if a person has no natural teeth and wears dentures. Professional care helps to maintain the overall health of the teeth and mouth and provides for early detection of precancerous or cancerous lesions. Tobacco-cessation counseling is vital to reduce general health risks that tobacco use poses. Smokers have 7 times the risk of developing periodontal disease compared with non smokers. The Smoking Cessation Leadership Center is an excellent resource for tobacco counseling education.[54] Tobacco use in any form increases the risk for periodontal disease, oral and throat cancers, and oral fungal infection, namely oral candidiasis.[56] Spit tobacco containing sugar also increases the risk of dental caries.[57] Limiting alcoholic beverages reduces the risk for oral and throat cancers because alcohol and tobacco used together are the primary risk factors for these cancers. Decreasing exposure to HPV by practicing safe sex can also decrease risk of oral and pharyngeal cancers. Oral care before cancer chemotherapy or radiation to the head or neck is important because these therapies can damage or destroy oral tissues and result in severe irritation of the oral tissues, mouth ulcers, loss of salivary function, rampant tooth decay, and destruction of bone. Caregivers should reinforce the daily oral hygiene routines of elders who are unable to perform these activities independently.

DID YOU KNOW ?

It is important to know which medications adults are taking and to ask them at each appointment about medication changes, since medications can impact oral health.

Individuals taking bisphosphonates for cancer or osteoporosis must be evaluated thoroughly. The development of bisphosphonate-related osteonecrotic lesions of the jaw is a clinical problem in which spontaneous exposure of alveolar bone occurs or, much worse, the patient presenting for routine dental extractions or periodontal curettage develops an area of necrotic bone that does not respond to conservative treatment or surgical management. The burden now falls on dental providers to consider the ramifications of bisphosphonate therapy on the patient population carefully before undertaking what might seem to be routine dental care.[58] If osteonecrosis is suspected, panoramic and tomographic imaging can be performed; however, radiographic changes are not evident until there is significant bone involvement. A thorough history and intraoral clinical examination is the most effective way to establish the diagnosis.

SUMMARY

The challenge to enhance public knowledge of oral health care remains for health care professionals in the private and public sectors, for developers of school programs, and for the news media. These groups can join forces to develop and implement a variety of relevant, culturally sensitive, and effective approaches for the appropriate use of fluorides and dental sealants, control of gingival conditions, and increasing awareness of the value of community water fluoridation, specifically for adults in their roles as eligible voters or parents.

Barriers to oral health care include availability, accessibility, affordability, and acceptability in addition to the individual's functional and medical status, previous patterns of use of dental treatment, lack of knowledge, and fear.

Dental providers must be aware that the demand for oral health care, especially geriatric care, will soon far exceed the number of dentists currently willing and able to provide such care. Alternative providers, such as dental hygienists, offer a viable option to increase access to preventive and therapeutic care.

PRACTICAL CONSIDERATIONS

Risk assessment is vital when implementing the suggestions in the chapter. Assessment is a part of the dental hygiene process of care. The six components to the dental hygiene process of care are assessment, dental hygiene diagnosis, planning, implementation, evaluation, and documentation. Risk assessment is a qualitative and quantitative evaluation gathered from the assessment process to identify any risks to general and oral health. The data provide the clinician the information for developing and designing strategies for preventing or limiting disease and promoting health.

SELF-STUDY QUESTIONS

1. *Risk assessment* is
   a. A qualitative evaluation
   b. A quantitative evaluation
   c. Gathered from the assessment process to identify any risks to general and oral health
   d. All of the above

   Rationale: Risk assessment is a qualitative and quantitative evaluation gathered from the assessment process to identify any risks to general and oral health. The data provide the clinician the information to develop and design strategies for preventing or limiting disease and promoting health.

2. Risk factors for HPV related oral and pharyngeal cancer are
   a. Tobacco
   b. Alcohol
   c. Chewing betel nuts
   d. Multiple sexual partners

   Rationale: Engaging in sexual intercourse, including oral sex at a young age, and having multiple partners are risk factors for oral cancer and should be assessed. These factors are due to increased risk for HPV infection of genital and oropharynx regions. Patients should be encouraged to have regular physical examinations with a family practitioner

   and/or gynecologist, have the HPV vaccine (both for boys and girls), and have oral cancer examinations performed at all dental and dental hygiene appointments.

3. There is a connection between oral health and overall health and oral disease may lead to systemic infection.
   a. The first statement is true, the second statement is false
   b. The first statement is false, the second statement is true
   c. Both statements are true
   d. Both statements are false

   Rationale: The strong connection between oral health and a person's overall well-being emphasizes the importance of the dental hygienist's interaction with patients on many psychosocial–behavioral levels: attitude, health beliefs, motivating factors, living situation, and previous dental experiences. Oral disease, left untreated may lead to systemic infection

4. Are the dental caries process and subsequent dental decay preventable?
   a. No, they are genetic.
   b. No, they are controllable but not preventable.
   c. Yes, they are preventable and controllable.
   d. No, because this is a bacterial disease originating in the biofilm.

Rationale: Dental caries and subsequent dental decay are preventable and controllable. Dental caries can be prevented by a combination of fluoride, dental sealants, and other new technologies.

5. Hormonal changes from pregnancy or oral contraceptive use, that result in gingivitis are a result of:

   a. A shift in bacteria from those that cause periodontitis to those that cause gingivitis

   b. Estrogen and progesterone becoming a substitute for naphthoquinone

   c. A decrease in the proportion of the *Bacteroides* species

   d. The *Bacteroides* species, implicated in gingivitis

Rationale: These hormonal changes can result in oral manifestations such as hormonal gingivitis. The relative proportion of the *Bacteroides* species, implicated in periodontitis, is increased 55-fold in pregnant women and 16-fold in women taking oral contraceptives over the control group.[13] We see a shift in bacteria from those that cause gingivitis to those that cause periodontitis when circulating sex hormones are high. Both estrogen and progesterone hormones have been shown to be a substitute for naphthoquinone, which is an essential growth factor for the *Bacteroides* species and *Prevotella intermedia*.[13]

REFERENCES

1. Barker, B. D., & Gift, H. C. (1990). Oral health problems in the second fifty. In Berg, R. L., & Cassells, J. S., Eds. *The second fifty years: Promoting health and preventing disability,* Washington, DC: National Academy Press, 119–135.

2. United States Department of Health and Human Services, Centers for Disease Control and Prevention. (2006). Oral health for adults. Retrieved October 5, 2012, from http://www.cdc.gov/OralHealth/publications/factsheets/adult.htm. Accessed June 30, 2011.

3. American Psychological Association. (2002). *Developing adolescents: A reference for professionals.* Washington, DC: American Psychological Association.

4. MacKay, A. P., & Duran C. Adolescent health in the United States, 2007. National Center for Health Statistics, 2007. Retrieved from http://www.cdc.gov/nchs/data/misc/adolescent2007.pdf on June 30, 2012.

5. U.S. Department of Health and Human Services. (2002). *Oral health in America: A report of the surgeon general.* Rockville, MD: U.S. Department of Health and Human Services, National Institute of Dental and Craniofacial Research, National Institutes of Health. Retrieved June 30, 2011, from.

6. The Writing Group for the WHI Investigators. (2002). Risks and benefits of estrogen plus progestin in healthy post-menopausal women: Principal results of the Women's Health Initiative randomized controlled trial. *JAMA,* 288:321–33.

7. Hopcraft, M. S., & Morgan, M. V. (2006). Pattern of dental caries experience on tooth surfaces in an adult population. *Community Dent Oral Epidemiol,* 34:174–83.

8. Kaste L. M., Selwitz R. H., Oldakowski J. A., Brunelle J. A., Winn D. M., & Brown L. J. (1996). Coronal caries in the primary and permanent dentition of children and adolescents 1–17 years of age: United States, 1988–1991. *J Dent Res,* 75 (special issue):631-41.

9. Kirkham J., Robinson C., Strong M., & Shore R. C. (1994). Effects of frequency of acid exposure on demineralization/remineralization behavior of human enamel in vitro. *Caries Res,* 28(1):9–13.

10. NIDCR/CDC Dental, Oral and Craniofacial Data Resource Center. (2002). Oral health, U.S. 2002 annual report. Retrieved June 30, 2011, from http://drc.hhs.gov/report/3_0.HTM.

11. Brown, L. J., & Löe, H. (2000). Prevalence, extent, severity and progression of periodontal disease. *Periodontology,* 2:57–71.

12. Johnson, G. K., & Slach, N. A. (2001). Impact of tobacco use on periodontal status. *J Dent Educ,* 65:313–21.

13. Horowitz, A., Drury, T. F., Goodman, H. S., & Yellowitz, J. A. (2000, April). Oral pharyngeal cancer prevention and early detection—Dentists' opinions and practices. *J Am Dent Assoc,* 131:453–62.

14. Oral Cancer Foundation. (2011). Oral cancer facts. Retrieved June 30, 2011, from http://oralcancerfoundation.org/facts/index.htm.

15. Swango, P. A. (1996). Cancer of the oral cavity and pharynx in the United States: An epidemiologic review. *J Public Health Dent,* 56:309–18.

16. National Cancer Institute. (1999). *SEER cancer statistics review, 1973–1996.* Bethesda, MD: National Cancer Institute.

17. Marur S., D'Souza G., Westra W. H., & Forastierre A. A. (2010). HPV-associated head and neck cancer: a virus related cancer epidemic. *Lancet Oncol,* 11:781–789.

18. The HPV Connection—the human papillomavirus related to oral cancer. Oral Cancer Foundation. Retrieve from http://oralcancerfoundation.orgon June 30, 2011.

19. D'Souza G., Freimer A. R., Viscidi R., Pawlita M., et al. (2007). Case-control study of human papillomavirus and oropharyngeal cancer. *N Engl J Med,* 356:1944–1956.

20. Sooriyamoorthy, M., & Gower, D. B. (1989, April). Hormonal influences on gingival tissue: Relationship to periodontal disease. *J Clin Periodontol,* 16:201.

21. Roberts, F. A., & Darveau, R. P. (2000). Beneficial bacteria of the periodontium. *Periodontology,* 30:40–50.

22. Majerus, P. W. (1998, January). Prostaglandins: Critical roles in pregnancy and colon cancer. *Curr Biol,* 8:R87–R89.

23. Amar, S., & Chung, K. M. (1994). Influence of hormonal variation on the periodontium in women. *Periodontol 2000,* 6:79–87.

24. Willing, M., Sowers, M., Aron, D., Clark, M. K., Burns, T., Bunten, C., Crutchfield, M., D'Agostino, D., & Jannausch, M. (1998, April). Bone mineral density and its change in white women: Estrogen and vitamin D receptor genotypes and their interaction. *J BoneMiner Res,* 13:695–705.

25. Anbinder, A. L., Prado, M., Spalding, M., Balducci, I., Carvalho, Y. R., & da Rocha, R. F. (2006). Estrogen deficiency and periodontal condition in rats: A radiographic and macroscopic study. *Braz Dent J,* 17:201–7.

26. Yoshihara, A., Seida, Y., Hanada, N., & Miyazaki, H. (2004). A longitudinal study of the relationship between periodontal disease and bone mineral density in community-dwelling older adults. *J Clin Periodontol*, 31:680–84.

27. Halbreich, U., & Kahn, L. S. (2001). Role of estrogen in the aetiology and treatment of mood disorders. *CNS Drugs* (Review article), 15:797–817.

28. Mariotti, A. (1994). Sex steroid hormones and cell dynamics in the periodontium. *Critical Rev Oral Biol Med*, 5:27–53.

29. Machtei, E. E. (2004). The effect of menstrual cycle on periodontal health. *J Periodontol*, 75:408–12.

30. Feldmann, I., Lundström, F., & Peck, S. (1999). Occlusal changes from adolescence to adulthood in untreated patients with Class II Division 1 deepbite malocclusion. *Angle Orthodont*, 69:33–38.

31. Siegel, M. A. (2002). A matter of class: Interpreting subdivision in a malocclusion. *Am J Orthod Dentofacial Orthop*, 122:582–86.

32. Sheiham, A., Steele, J. G., Marcenes, W., Tsakos, G., Finch, S., & Walls, A. W. (2001). Prevalence of impacts of dental and oral disorders and their effects on eating among older people: A national survey in Great Britain. *Community Dent Oral Epidemiol*, 29:195–203.

33. Little, J. W. (2002). Eating disorders: Dental implications. *Oral Surg Oral Med Oral Pathol Oral Radiol Endod*, 93:138–43.

34. Fairburn, C., & Harrison, P. (2003, February) Eating disorders. *Lancet*, 361:407–16.

35. Pirie, M., Cooke, I., Linden, G., & Irwin, C. (2007). Dental manifestations of pregnancy. *Obstetrician Gynaecologist*, 9:21–26.

36. California Dental Association Foundation. (2010). Oral health during pregnancy & early childhood: Evidence-based guidelines for health professionals. Retrieved June 30, 2011, from http://www.cdafoundation.org/library/docs/poh_guidelines.pdf.

37. Earp, J. A., & Ennett, S. T. (1991). Conceptual models for health education research and practice. *Health Educ Res*, 6:163–71.

38. National Center for Health Statistics. (2006). *Health, United States, 2006 with chartbook on trends in the health of Americans*. Hyattsville, MD: National Center for Health Statistics.

39. Central Intelligence Agency. World fact Book. Retrieved from https://www.cia.gov/library/publications/the-world-factbook/rankorder/2102rank.html on June 30, 2011.

40. John, J., Mani, S. A., & Azizah, Y. (2004). Oral health care in the elderly population in Malaysia—A review. *Med J Malaysia*, 59:433–39.

41. Institute for Clinical Systems Improvement (ICSI). (2006, October). *Preventive services for adults*. Bloomington, MN: Institute for Clinical Systems Improvement, 1–48.

42. Centers for Disease Control and Prevention. (2006, modified November 21, 2006). *CDC fact sheet. Oral health for older Americans*. Retrieved March 24, 2008, from http://www.cdc.gov/OralHealth/factsheets/adult-older.htm.

43. Faine, M. P., Allender, M. S., Baab, D., Persson, R., & Lamont, R. J. (1992). Dietary and salivary factors associated with root caries. *Spec Care Dent*, 12:177–82.

44. Cohen, G., Negron, R. J., Bocker, M. A. clinical approach to the treatment and management of rampant root caries. Retrieved from http://www.cumc.columbia.edu/news/dental/cdr96/cohen.html. on March 24, 2008.

45. Berg, R. L., & Cassells, J. S. (1990). *Oral health problems in the The second 50 years: Promoting health and preventing disability*. Washington DC: National Academy Press.

46. Guzmán-Armstrong, S., & Warren, J. J. (2007). Management of high caries risk and high caries activity patients: Rampant Caries Control Program (RCCP). *J Dent Educ*, 71:767–75.

47. Park, K. K., Schemehorn, B. R., Bolton, J. W., & Stookey, J. K. (1990). Effect of sorbitol gum chewing on plaque pH response after ingesting snacks containing predominantly sucrose or starch. *Am J Dent*, 3:185–91.

48. Anderson, M. H., Bratthall, D., Einwag, J., Eldertom, R. J., Ernst, C.-P., Levin, R. P., Tynelius-Bratthall, G., & Willershausen-Zonnchen, B. (1994). *Professional prevention in dentistry*. Baltimore, MD: Williams & Wilkins.

49. Santos, S., Herrera, D., López, E., O'Connor, A., González, I., & Sanz, M. (2004). A randomized clinical trial on the short-term clinical and microbiological effects of the adjunctive use of a 0.05% chlorhexidine mouth rinse for patients in supportive periodontal care. *J Clin Periodontol*, 31:45–51.

50. Rozier, R. G. (2001). Effectiveness of methods used by dental professionals for the primary prevention of dental caries. *J Dent Educ*, 65:1063–72.

51. Wolfgang, H. A. (2006). Effect of fluoride tooth pastes on enamel demineralization. *BMC Oral Health*, 6:8.

52. Burwell, A., Jennings, D., Muscle, D., & Greenspan, D. C. (2010). NovaMin and dentin hypersensitivity—in vitro evidence of efficacy. *J Clin Dent*, 21(3):66–71.

53. Aimutis, W. R. (2004, April). Bioactive properties of milk proteins with particular focus on anticariogenesis. Supplement: The emerging role of dairy proteins and bioactive peptides in nutrition and health. *J. Nutr*, 134:989S–95S.

54. Reynolds, E. C. (1997). Remineralization of enamel subsurface lesions by casein phosphopeptide-stabilized calcium phosphate solutions. *J Dent Res*, 76:1587–95.

55. The Smoking Cessation Leadership Center. Retrieved June 30, 2011.

56. Barbour, S. E., Nakashima, K., Zhang, J. B., Tangada, S., Hahn, C. L., Schenkein, H. A. & Tew, J. G. (1997). Tobacco and smoking: Environmental factors that modify the host response (immune system) and have an impact on periodontal health. *Crit Rev Oral Biol Med*, 8:437–60.

57. Tomar, S. L., & Winn, D. (1999). Chewing tobabcco use and dental caries among U.S. men. *J Am Dent Assoc*, 130:1601–10.

58. Salmassy, D. (2007, July). Fosamax: Bad to the bone? *Mod Hyg*, 3:7.

Geriatrics

Charles D. Tatlock

OBJECTIVES

After reading this chapter, the student should be able to:

1. Describe and define the geriatric population.
2. Describe common oral conditions and diseases of geriatric patients.
3. Describe specific preventive strategies to use with geriatric patients.
4. Describe the role of the dental provider in treating geriatric patients.

KEY TERMS

Dementia, 425
Elderly, 421
Frail elderly, 422
Functional dentition, 426
Functionally independent, 422
Functional status, 424
Kyphosis, 424
Long-term care, 427

INTRODUCTION

"One of the undeniable facts about living is that every day we are getting older."[1] The good news is that people in the United States are living longer and healthier lives than ever before. The current "baby boomer" generation—the cohort representing those born between the years 1946 and 1964—demonstrates a strong and consuming desire to stem the tide of the aging process. Yet as hard as this generation has tried to counteract the aging process, the first baby boomers inevitably joined the ranks of those 65 years and older in 2011.[1]

The numbers in this cohort are not insignificant. What trends are expected to be seen among our older population? The U.S. population of people age 65 and older is expected to double in size within the next 25 years. By 2030, almost one of every five Americans—some 72 million people—will be 65 years or older compared to 12% of the population in 2003.[2]

As seniors, baby boomers will continue to need dental care more than previous generations of seniors.[3] What trends will likely be seen in the dental care given by dental providers to this age group? As will be discussed in this chapter, with the associations between oral and systemic health becoming clearer, dental practitioners will become increasingly involved in promoting their patients' *overall* health.[3]

A number of significant changes occur during aging. Fortunately, most of these normal changes do not cause oral diseases.[4,5] Instead, the cumulative effects of both oral and systemic diseases result in the prevalence of oral disease among those who are elderly.[4] It is interesting to note that increasing numbers of "well people who are elderly" are able to retain their natural teeth and enjoy normal oral function throughout old age. The current baby boomer generation is becoming increasingly aware of the fact that oral health is important, both in terms of one's general health status and the effects oral health has on physical appearance and the development of positive self-concepts.[6]

Looking ahead, older adults by the year 2040 are expected to account for approximately 23% of the population in the United States, a significant increase from 4% in 1900 and 12% in 1990.[7] The 85-and-older age group will be the most rapidly growing segment in the U.S. population. Projections by the U.S. Census Bureau suggest that this population could grow from about 4 million in 2000 to 19 million by 2050.[7]

POPULATION CHARACTERISTICS

The U.S. older population grew rapidly for most of the 20th century, from 3.1 million in 1900 to 35 million in 2000. In addition, the number of centenarians, people at least 100 years old, has increased from about 37,000 in 1990 to more than 50,000 in 2000. By 2010, more than 79,000 Americans reached this age plateau. It is projected that this number will surpass 175,000 by the year 2025 and will exceed 600,000 in 2050.[8] About 80% of centenarians are women (Figure 26–1 ■). Except during the 1990s, the growth of the older population has outpaced that of the total population, prompting social observers to describe the older population as being on the threshold of a boom.[9]

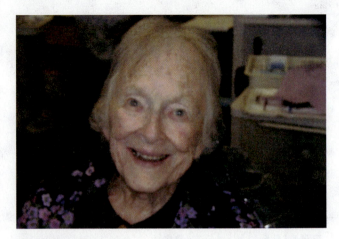

FIGURE ■ 26–1 Heloise A. Arnold, RDH and centenarian, graduate of the first school of dental hygiene, Fones School of Dental Hygiene in Bridgeport, Connecticut.

(*Source:* Courtesy of Charles D. Tatlock, D.D.S., M.P.H.)

The baby boomer cohorts' impact on the country's age structure will continue into the first half of the 21st century. By 2020, the baby boomer cohorts will be 56 to 74 years old (Figure 26–2 ■). The size of the older population (those over 74 years of age) is projected to double over the next 30 years, growing to 70 million by 2030. After 2030 the baby boomers will become the oldest old, and the country's age structure is expected to change (Figures 26–3 ■ through 26–6 ■).[9]

DID YOU KNOW **?**

The current age structure is unprecedented in U.S. history. Baby boomers now include more than 76 million people, 25% of whom have a college education. In addition, they are the first generation to have benefited from widespread community water fluoridation and fluoride in toothpaste. As a result, many will reach older adulthood with their dentition virtually intact.[10]

In response to this changing U.S. and world demographic, the World Health Organization (WHO) issued in 2002 *Active Ageing: A Policy Framework,*[11] which outlines essential approaches toward healthy aging. As a way for people to enjoy longevity and sustain health-related quality of life with age, this document emphasizes the importance of minimizing risk factors that contribute to chronic disease and functional decline while maximizing protective factors against such problems.

It is important to recognize that *oral health* is an identified component of "active aging" and is included in the WHO policy proposals. In many ways, this is a visionary statement. Although it generally has been agreed that good oral health care should begin at birth, relatively few have argued and advocated for oral health among people who are elderly. Slowly, and thanks in part to advocacy by former U.S. Surgeons General, a national realization that oral health is important to overall health for people of all ages is emerging.

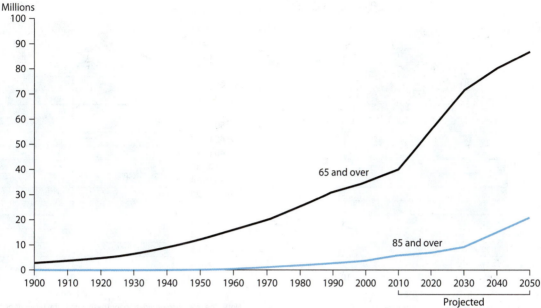

FIGURE ■ **26–2** Number of people in the United States age 65 and over, by age group, selected years 1900–2000 and projected 2010–2050.

(*Source:* U.S. Census Bureau, Decennial Census and Projections.)

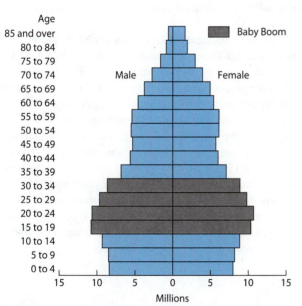

Note: The reference population for these data is the resident population.

FIGURE ■ **26–3** U. S. population by age and sex: 1980.

(*Source:* U.S. Bureau of the Census, 1983, Table 44. For full citation, see references at end of chapter.)

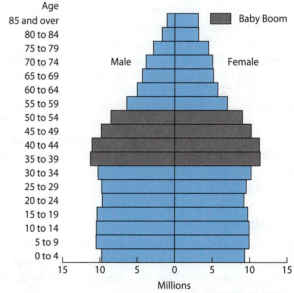

Note: The reference population for these data is the resident population.

FIGURE ■ **26–4** U.S. population by age and sex: 2000.

(*Source:* U.S. Census Bureau, 2001, Table PCT12. For full citation, see references at end of chapter.)

The WHO defines the population between 65 and 75 years as **elderly**. The word *"old"* is used for individuals between 76 and 90 years, and *"very old"* is the term for those older than age 90. Individuals who are elderly and those who are old are often very different with respect to their physiologic function, burden of illness, and any associated disability.[12] In essence, when we describe the geriatric population, we are dealing with a very heterogeneous group.

Changing demographics, including an increase in life expectancy and the growing numbers of individuals who are elderly has recently focused attention on the need for geriatric dental care. Aging affects oral tissues in addition to other parts

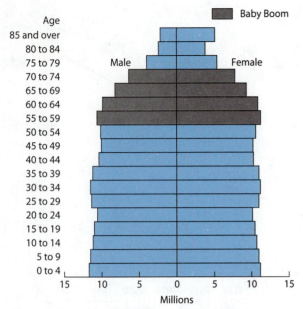

Note: The reference population for these data is the resident population.

FIGURE ■ 26–5 U.S. population by age and sex: 2020.
(*Source:* U.S. Census Bureau, 2004. For full citation, see references at end of chapter.)

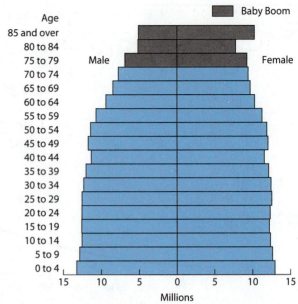

Note: The reference population for these data is the resident population.

FIGURE ■ 26–6 Population by age and sex: 2040.
(*Source:* U.S. Census Bureau, 2004. For full citation, see references at end of chapter.)

of the human body, and oral health (including oral mucosa, lips, teeth, and associated structures and their functional activity) is an integral component of general health; indeed, oral disease can cause pain, difficulty in speaking, mastication, swallowing, and maintaining a balanced diet, not to mention aesthetical considerations and facial alterations leading to anxiety and depression.[4,13]

Although oral health problems are not usually associated with death, oral cancers represent approximately 2% of all cancers with approximately 30,000 new cases in the United States each year. These result in nearly 8,000 deaths each year, and more than half of these occur at an age of 65 years plus.[4,5,13]

Frail Elderly

Ettinger and Beck[14] developed a functional definition of the elderly based upon an older person's ability to seek dental services. The categorization that they developed can be divided into three groups:

- The functionally independent older adult.
- The frail older adult.
- The functionally dependent older adult.[15]

According to this description, the vast majority of older adults can get to the dentist and are categorized as **functionally independent**. About 14% of community-dwelling people who are elderly are in the **frail elderly** category. These are persons with chronic conditions contributing to major limitations in mobility. About 5% of community dwelling elderly adults are homebound or functionally dependent. Another group of

functionally dependent older adults are those who live in nursing homes.[2,15,16]

Living arrangements of U.S. older adults are closely linked to income, health status, and the availability of caregivers. Those who live alone are more likely to be in poverty and experience health problems, compared with those who live with a spouse or a relative. Currently, 1.57 million older adults live in long-term care facilities and more than 1.00 million older adults reside in assisted living facilities.[16] The percentage of the population who live in nursing homes also increases dramatically with age, ranging from 1% for persons 65 to 74 years, to 5% for persons 75 to 84 years, to 19% for persons 85 years and older.[1] The use of assisted-living facilities, board and care homes, continuing-care retirement communities, and other types of facilities in addition to long-term care in a nursing home has increased over the last 15 years[1,2,9,16–21] (Figure 26–7 ■).

Health

About 80% of seniors have at least one chronic health condition, and 50% have at least two chronic health conditions, which often lead to disability. Arthritis, hypertension, heart disease, diabetes, and respiratory disorders are some of the leading causes of activity limitations among older people.[2,19] Most chronic systemic conditions (heart disease, cardiovascular disease, pulmonary disease, and chronic kidney disease) share common risk factors with oral disease. Oral health is an integral part of total health and affects salivary flow, altered sense of taste, smell, orofacial pain, gingival enlargement, alveolar bone resorption, tooth mobility, speech, social mobility, employment, self-esteem, and quality of life.[16]

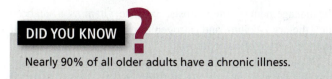

DID YOU KNOW

Nearly 90% of all older adults have a chronic illness.

The most common chronic illnesses found in older American adults are hypertension, arthritis, heart disease, cancer, and diabetes (Table 26–1 ■). At present, 30% of the individuals over age 65 have three or more chronic illnesses,[14,22] yet, almost 71% of noninstitutionalized older adults describe their general health to be excellent, very good, or good compared with others their age.[6,23]

As one ages, diagnoses of chronic disorders frequently multiply. These co-existing conditions are termed *comorbidities*.

To the older person with chronic illness in the 21st century, a longer life expectancy may mean periods of disability, vulnerability to other health problems, financial expense, and increasing care concerns.[24] Presently, the medical costs of people who have chronic diseases account for more than 75% of the nation's $1.4 trillion medical care costs.[23]

The leading causes of death in adults over the age of 65, which account for approximately 75% of all the deaths, are heart disease, cancer, stroke, and Alzheimer's disease or dementing illnesses.[6,14] Cardiovascular disease remains the leading cause of death in older adults but has experienced a significant reduction since 1940 (since a marked reduction in cardiovascular deaths for all age groups has occurred). The 85-years-and-older group has had the least reduction, with more than 20%.[14,20,25]

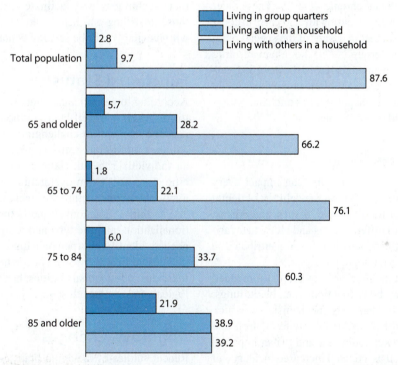

FIGURE ■ 26–7 **Living arrangements in the U.S.: 2000 (percent distribution data based on sample).**
(*Source:* U.S. Census Bureau, Census 2000 special tabulation. For information on confidentiality protection, sampling error, nonsampling error, and definitions, see www.census.gov/prod/cen2000/sf4.pdf)

TABLE ■ 26–1 **Top Five Chronic Health Conditions Among the Population age 65 and over, by sex**

Men	*Women*
1. Hypertension	**1.** Hypertension
2. Arthritis	**2.** Arthritis
3. Heart disease	**3.** Heart disease
4. Cancer	**4.** Cancer
5. Diabetes	**5.** Diabetes

Note: Data are based on a 2-year average from 2007–2008.

(*Source:* From U.S. Census Bureau, Statistical Abstract of the United States, 1996 (118th Edition), Washington DC, 1998.)

Cancer (lung, breast, prostate, and colon) is the second most common cause of death in older adults. Since 1940, a 20% increase has occurred in cancer deaths for persons 55 years of age and older. Statistics show that 37% of men and 22% of women ages 60 to 79 years will develop invasive cancer. The risk for invasive cancer from birth to death is 50% in men and 30% in women. The most marked increase has been in cancer of the lung in both men and women.[14,19,20] The third leading cause of death in older adults is cerebrovascular disease (stroke). The incidence has been decreasing since 1960.[19,20] Approximately 10 stroke patients exist per 1,000 people in the United States. Prevalence rises in men from 14.6 per 1,000 adults at 45 to 64 years to 77.5 per 1,000 for men ages 75 and older and from 15.9 to 79.6, respectively, in the age groups in women.[14,19,20]

The preceding information leads to the expectation of a dramatic increase in the number of older adults in this country and in the proportion with significant chronic illnesses. These older adults will need dental care at an increasing level in years to come and oral health professionals must be aware of the special management needed to treat this group.[4,5,14,16] For example, drug dosages and duration of treatment might have to be modified, certain drugs might have to be avoided, antibiotic prophylaxis might have to be administered, and special precautions might have to be made before surgery to avoid excessive bleeding.[4,5,14,16]

Physiologic Changes

Physiologic changes associated with aging can impact every system in the body and have an effect on the delivery of dental care. Overall, changes occur for all people, tissues, and organs, but these changes occur with different rates and individual variability. However, many of the deficits traditionally attributed to aging are actually signs of pathologic processes.[4,6]

The major results of the aging process are (1) a reduced physiologic reserve of many body functions (i.e., heart, lungs, kidney); (2) an impaired homeostasis mechanism by which bodily activities (i.e., fluid balance, temperature control, and blood pressure control) are kept adjusted; and (3) an impaired immunologic system, as well as a related increased incidence of neoplastic and age-related autoimmune conditions.[4,6]

Bone remains metabolically active throughout life. Age-related bone loss is extremely common, reflecting an imbalance between bone resorption by osteoclasts and bone formation by osteoblasts. *Osteoporosis,* a common problem in people who are elderly, is an age-related disorder characterized by a decrease in bone mass and an increase in susceptibility to bone fractures.[26,27] Clinically, advanced osteoporosis can present with chronic back pain from mechanical strain caused by kyphosis or vertebral compression fractures.[6,28] **Kyphosis** is the condition that generally results in the affected elder's stooping posture and rounded-shoulder appearance.

Recent studies indicate that changes in alveolar bone as a result of osteoporosis could contribute to the progression of periodontal disease.[4,6,29] Also, a significant decrease in bone mass of the mandible could lead to fragility and increased resorption, risk of fracture, and failure of osseointegration of dental implants. Prevention rather than treatment is the key to the management of osteoporosis. Exercise, vitamins, a balanced diet, dietary calcium, and estrogen play a role in the treatment and prevention of osteoporosis.[4,6]

Osteoporosis is extremely common in the United States; one in two women and one in three or four men experience fragility fracture after age 50. The U.S. Surgeon General estimates that approximately 44 million Americans have low bone mass including 10 million with osteoporosis. As a result, at age 50 years, the likelihood of osteoporotic fracture in remaining life is approximately 50% in women and 25% to 30% in men.[28] Osteoporosis increases the risk of mandibular fracture. Some studies suggest that systemic osteoporosis can contribute to periodontal attachment loss in the form of gingival recession.[4] It is incumbent upon the dental team to be aware of and adaptable to the commonly seen age-related changes in their patients. Modifications of office design and patient management techniques will facilitate and enhance the practices of those providing oral health care to a growing older population who inevitably will be seeking dental care.

Functional Status

According to geriatricians, functional status is a critical indicator of health and well-being in the older person. Furthermore, it is one of the most challenging issues in health care of older adults. **Functional status** is often used as a way to describe an individual's health status rather than the presence of specific diseases.[6] As an overarching concept, the term describes a more complete picture that includes impairments in physical and cognitive functioning and helps predict mortality, institutionalization, and the type and amount of health care services needed. Identifying a person's functional status requires a comprehensive health assessment, including an assessment of the individual's functional abilities, health status, physical, psychological, and oral health status.[6]

Cognitive Changes

Recent studies of the aging brain demonstrate that major cognitive declines do not occur in the absence of disease, trauma, or stress. These studies suggest that developmental transitions, life events, and environmental changes can interfere with older adults' ability to concentrate and to think clearly.[6] Research has indicated that a person's intellect does not decline as an outcome of aging, but as a result of many conditions including poor nutrition, vitamin deficiencies, disease, and hormonal changes.[26,27,30] An older person usually takes longer than a younger adult to learn the same information, but when given sufficient time, the end result is similar for both individuals. In general, an older person needs more time to encode—that is, to retrieve or to recall information. In later life, mental health is measured by the capacity to cope effectively with relationships and environment and by the satisfaction experienced in doing so.[6]

Because of the multiplicity of factors that relate to the treatment of individuals who are elderly, evaluating the patient's ability to communicate and to understand, consent to, and participate in the treatment is important. The practitioner must determine, either through an interview or professional services, an individual's capacity to respond to treatment.[6]

Dementia is the loss of established intellectual activity that interferes with occupational and social function. It includes impairment of memory, language, perception, calculation, abstract thinking, judgment, and executive function.[14,30,31] The most common type of dementia in people who are elderly is senile dementia of the Alzheimer's type (SDAT), accounting for more than 50% of all dementias seen in them.[6,30,31] The second most common cause of dementia in this group is multi-infarct dementia, or vascular dementia, accounting for 15% to 25% of cases.[30,31] Both of these types of dementia are irreversible. Between 10% and 20% of the cases of dementia are classified as reversible.[14,30,31] The reversible dementias can be associated with the following medical diseases: hepatic encephalopathy, acid–base disturbances, hypoglycemia, thyroid disease, uremia, AIDS, trauma, syphilis, multiple sclerosis, and stroke.[14]

Alzheimer's disease is discussed here briefly because it is the most common type of dementia seen in elders. SDAT is a progressive, degenerative, dementing illness that attacks the brain and leads to the loss of memory, intellectual capacity, ability to think, and changes in behavior. Approximately 10% of adults 65 years of age and older and 45% more than 85 years old have SDAT. In its early stages, the individual generally maintains good social skills and is often able to "disguise" the presence of the disease. At this stage, the disease is often very difficult to assess, and family members generally deny its existence.[6]

Fourteen million Americans will have SDAT by 2050 unless a cure or preventive treatment is found.[24] The cause of SDAT is not known; however, several possibilities are under investigation, including genetics, nutrition, environment, and infectious agents.[14,30–33] Currently, there is no cure for SDAT. A relatively new drug, tacrine (Cognex), has shown short-term benefit but has a high rate of toxicity.[30,31] Another new drug, donepezil (Aricept), has shown about the same level of benefit as tacrine but without the high rate of toxicity.[30,31] Velnacrine, a metabolite of tacrine, also has been used to treat SDAT with limited results.[34]

Among the group of ACE (or angiotensin-converting-enzyme) inhibitors in addition to donepezil are three other drugs showing promise. Memantine (sold as Namenda) is the first drug in this group to aid in preserving memory in patients with moderate-to-severe forms of SDAT. The other two drugs showng promise as being relatively safe and effective are galantamine and rivastigmine.[30,31]

Despite treatment, the disease progresses over a period of from 2 to 20 years and presents as a complex picture of overlapping symptoms that reflect a continuous decline in memory, ability to think, and behavior control. Cognitive skills and competency in life skills decline. There is loss of memory, language, intellectual prowess, concentration, and emotionality, as well as altered spatial motor performance. Both verbal and nonverbal communication is affected.[6]

Alzheimer's patients are managed best by an understanding and empathetic approach. The oral health professional should keep the patient's attention and explain what is going to happen before doing it. The provider should communicate using short words and sentences and should repeat instructions and explanations. Nonverbal

communication can be very helpful. Facial motion and body posture of the dental professional should show support, willingness to care, and cues that the patient is understood. Positive nonverbal communication includes direct eye contact, smiling, touching the arm, patting the hand, and so on.[14] Patients with SDAT should be placed on an aggressive preventive dentistry program including 3-month recall, oral examination, prophylaxis, fluoride gel application, oral hygiene instruction, and adjustment of prosthesis.[35]

COMMON ORAL MANIFESTATIONS

Healthy older people can expect to keep their teeth throughout their lifetime. However, in the presence of one or more medical conditions and/or their treatments, oral functions can be altered, which can then impact the patients' general and oral health status.[2,5,6]

During the past 50 years, one of the major changes in patterns of oral disease in the United States has been a steady decrease in the rate of edentulism. (Figures 26–8 ■ and 26–9 ■). It is likely that, for the first time in recorded history, there are now more older adults with natural teeth than those without

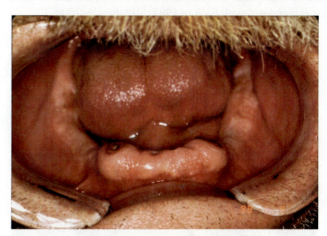

FIGURE ■ 26–8 Edentulous mandibular ridge. Geriatric dentists advocate keeping endodontically treated roots when possible for preservation of the alveolar ridged. Note the ridge resorption of the posterior ridges compared to the anterior areas.
(*Source:* Courtesy of Charles D. Tatlock, D.D.S., M.P.H.)

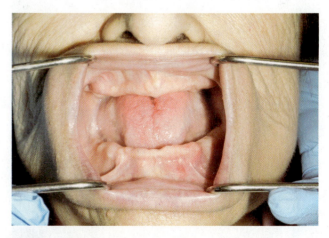

FIGURE ■ 26–9 Edentulous maxillary and mandibular ridges.
(*Source:* Courtesy of Dr. Stephen Wagner, D.D.S., M.S.)

teeth.[2,6] In 1986, almost 30% of those 65 to 74 years were edentulous, whereas it was predicted in 2024 that only 10% of this group will be edentulous.[2,8,17,18,20,21] This decline in edentulism appears to be the result of water fluoridation, increased public awareness of preventive approaches, improved access to services, and a decrease in early tooth loss.[4-6,9,18]

Consequently, older adults today retain more teeth than did earlier generations. They also often maintain so-called **functional dentitions**, defined as the presence of at least 20 natural teeth, many of which may be heavily restored with fillings, crowns, and bridges[12] (Figures 26–10 ■ and 26–11 ■).

Although the prevalence of edentulism increases in older age groups who are not institutionalized, these rates have steadily decreased over time.[4,5,16,20] At the same time that more teeth are being retained, this decline in tooth loss results in more natural teeth at risk for caries (coronal, recurrent, and root) and periodontal diseases. As these trends continue, future dental practices will need to perform more restorative and preventive services.[4,5,6,16] This need is already evident in the fact that 60% of adults 65 years and older visited a dental office in 2009 compared with 54% in 1997[23] (Figure 26–12 ■).

According to recent reports, the prevalence of coronal caries is decreasing for children and young adults in middle to high socioeconomic status. Although dental caries has not traditionally been perceived as a problem for individuals who are elderly, decay rates have been found to be higher in some adult groups than in children. As long as teeth are present, individuals remain at risk of dental caries.[2,4,5,9,14,16,36] Unfortunately, many older adults do not place a priority on oral health care; they think the only reason to see a dentist is to relieve pain and discomfort. This effect, coupled with a reduced sensory ability, means that many older adults tend to seek care only when their decay is in a late stage.[6] Root caries is common and frequently occurs in this age group (Figure 26–13 ■). A 2010 survey in the state of Massachusetts reported that statewide, root caries was found in 35% of seniors screened at meal sites with 17% having major to urgent dental needs while 59% of seniors in long-term care facilities had untreated decay with 24% having major to urgent dental needs.[37] With the use of new preventive approaches and restorative materials, the dilemma associated with restoring root-carious lesions is expected to diminish in the future.[6,10]

Contrary to many long-held views, periodontal disease is not age related. Although the prevalence of periodontal

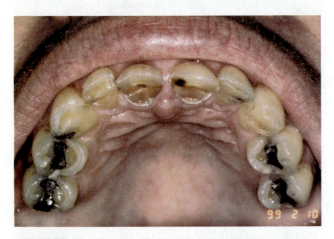

FIGURE ■ 26–10 Functional dentition in people who are elderly.

(*Source:* Courtesy of Charles D. Tatlock, D.D.S., M.P.H.)

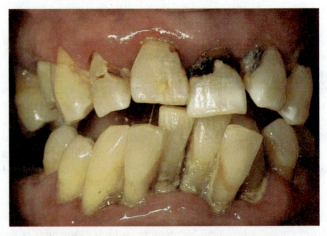

FIGURE ■ 26–12 Periodontal disease and root caries.

(*Source:* Courtesy of Dr. Stephen Wagner, D.D.S., M.S.)

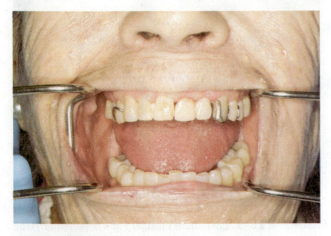

FIGURE ■ 26–11 Functional dentition in the elderly.

(*Source:* Courtesy of Dr. Stephen Wagner, D.D.S., M.S.)

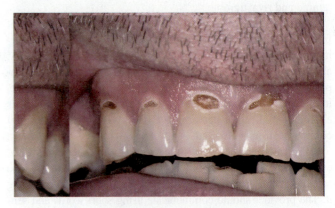

FIGURE ■ 26–13 Root caries.

(*Source:* Courtesy of Charles D. Tatlock, D.D.S., M.P.H.)

disease appears to increase with age, this is likely due to the long-standing cumulative nature of the disease with its onset earlier in adulthood. It is estimated that 90% of adults aged more than 65 years need periodontal treatment and 15% of them need complex treatment.[4,7,13,29] With new diagnostic methods complementing traditional clinical techniques, earlier identification of periodontal disease and risk factors will be possible as well as early treatment to help reduce disease progression and subsequent loss of teeth.[6,38] Fortunately, most evidence indicates that geriatric patients with periodontal disease respond to periodontal therapy as well as younger adults do.[36]

Like most cancers, oral cancer occurs primarily in the older age segments of the population; the majority of cases are diagnosed after age 65, and more than 95% occur after age 40.[2,18,20,25] The key issue related to oral cancer problems is the need for early and effective diagnosis. Although the primary risk factors for the development of oral squamous cell carcinoma, the most-common form of oral cancer, have traditionally included alcohol abuse and use of tobacco products, these risk factors do not have to be present for a lesion to develop.[16,39] Thus, it is vitally important for the oral health care professional to provide oral cancer examinations to all patients on a regular (at least annual) basis. Early diagnosis of oral cancer greatly improves the prognosis of recovery from the disease. Many factors, such as lack of access to care and patient delay in seeing treatment, influence the timing at which oral cancers are diagnosed.[4,16] Therefore, oral health professionals must provide, when appropriate, routine comprehensive intra- and extraoral examinations of their patient population[6] (Figure 26–14 ■).

Through frequent recall visits and regular professional examinations, adults will be able to better maintain their dentition throughout their life. Prevention of oral disease is the critical component for oral health maintenance. In addition to promoting and monitoring basic oral hygiene practices, the practitioner needs to be aware of the changing physical, psychological, socioeconomic, and medication status of their older adult patients[6,16] to be ready and willing to intervene, to make necessary modifications to treatment, and to make referrals to community resources. Older adults and their caregivers need to be educated and have their education reinforced to enhance their knowledge of oral care protocols.[10,16]

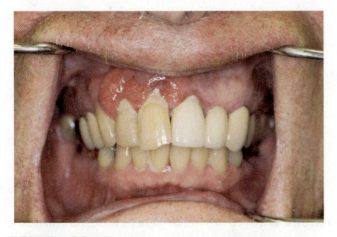

FIGURE ■ 26–14 **Oral cancer: squamous cell carcinoma.**

(*Source:* Courtesy of Dr. Stephen Wagner, D.D.S., M.S.)

Long-Term Care

Long-term care refers to health, social, and residential services provided to chronically disabled persons over an extended time.[6,40] Population studies in the United States suggest that persons 65 years and older have a 40% chance of spending some time in a long-term care facility before they die. Of those who enter nursing homes, 55% will spend at least 1 year there, and more than 20% will spend more than 5 years there. Two of the most-common symptoms that lead to nursing home placement are incontinence and behavioral problems such as wandering or disruptive actions often associated with dementia and Alzheimer's disease.[6,40]

The long-term care population has been characterized as having high levels of edentulism, coronal and root caries, poor oral hygiene, periodontal diseases, and soft tissue lesions.[1,6,7,13,14,36] Residents of long-term care facilities could have their oral health needs met on-site with the use of new technological advances in portable and mobile dental equipment. An increasing number of oral health professionals are willing to provide mobile services, so comprehensive oral health programs could become feasible and logical activities in this setting.

Surgeon General's Report

The U.S. Surgeon General's report, *Oral Health in America,* emphasizes the fact that oral health is integral to general health and describes the disparities in the availability of dental care, especially for very young and very old populations.[41] The report uses the phrase "silent epidemic" to characterize the disparity between the epidemic of oral disease and the silence from those who need care. Although this seminal report was issued in 2000, it is still recognized as the most significant monograph that addresses the inclusion of oral health as an integral component of overall health. In this respect, the U.S. Surgeon General's report highlights many reasons that dental care is of particular importance for frail older adults:

- Oral diseases are cumulative and become more complex over time. The older adult population has high rates of oral diseases. This is complicated additionally by the fact that many senior adults lose their dental insurance when they retire. Medicare does not reimburse for routine dental services, and many states do not have Medicaid dental coverage for the adult population.[1]

- Oral problems have a negative effect on quality of life. Oral–facial pain and tooth loss can greatly reduce the quality of life and restrict major functions. Problems with the teeth and mouth can affect the ability to eat and communicate. Individuals with facial disfigurements due to oral diseases often experience loss of self-esteem, anxiety, depression, and social stigma. Impaired oral health affects diet, nutrition, sleep, psychological status, and social interaction.[1]

- Dental disease has a significant impact on general health. The oral cavity can be a portal of entry for microbial infections that affect the whole body. Oral diseases give rise to pathogens, which can be blood-borne or aspirated into the lungs,[2] bringing about severe, even life-threatening, consequences. Recent research findings have linked possible associations between chronic oral infections and diabetes, heart and lung disease, and stroke.[1]

Older adults suffer from the cumulative effects of oral diseases over their lifetime resulting in extensive oral disease.[2] In a review of oral health studies of elderly people who are institutionalized published between 2005 and 2010, researchers described the compromised oral health status of nursing home residents. Up to 70% had unmet oral needs, exhibiting high rates of edentulism (complete tooth loss), dental caries (decay), poor oral hygiene, periodontal disease (diseases of the supporting structures of the teeth), and soft tissue lesions.[42–44] More than 30% of community-dwelling elderly individuals in 1997 were edentulous; the rate rose to 43% of those older than 85 years.[1] This is a significant finding because a common perception is that with the loss of teeth, a decreased need for oral health care necessarily follows. In fact, more than 25% of the U.S. population more than 65 years old has not seen a dental professional in the past 5 years. In addition, elderly persons who wear complete dentures are four times less likely to visit a dentist than are those with remaining teeth.[23,39] A study published in the August 2010 issue of the *International Journal of Dental Hygiene* found that among 71 denture wearers, hygiene was good in only about 21%, fair in about 43%, and poor in about 35% This same study also revealed that denture-induced stomatitis (DIS) was higher in elderly patients, and a "significant association was found between the presence of DIS and denture hygiene habits and sleeping with dentures"[36] (Figure 26–15 ■).

Among those who are not edentulous, approximately one-third of community-dwelling elderly individuals have untreated coronal or root caries and other oral health problems including periodontal disease, attrition, unreplaced missing teeth, abrasion and erosion, broken or failing older dental restorations, dry mouth, mucosal diseases, oral cancer, and alveolar ridge atrophy.[1] Among people who are elderly receiving community-based health services noted in one study, the majority (more than 55%) reported their oral health was "fair" or "poor," and nearly 80% were treatment planned for dental needs which

had not yet been initiated. In addition, more than half (52.5%) reported not having been to the dentist within the year.[45]

A major impact of systemic diseases on the oral health of older adults is caused by the side effects of medications. With increasing age and associated chronic disease, people who are elderly are prescribed an ever-expanding variety of medications. By year 2030, 40% of all retail drugs will be consumed by persons age 65 or older.[4] More than 400 prescribed and over-the-counter drugs can lead to a decrease in salivary flow, which alone can result in rampant oral disease without early intervention.[36]

Besides the desired therapeutic outcome of these medications, adverse side effects could alter the integrity of the oral mucosa. Problems such as xerostomia (persistent dry mouth), bleeding disorders of the tissues, lichenoid reactions (oral tissue changes), tissue overgrowth, and hypersensitivity reactions could occur as a result of drug therapy.[46]

The dental treatment needs of people who are elderly differ from those of younger adults, and newer cohorts of elderly people have significantly different needs than do older cohorts. Shay reports that in 1957, 70% of adults aged 75 years were fully edentulous, where as today the number has dropped to less than 40%. This finding means that, more than 50 years ago, most dental treatment for older adults involved making and repairing full dentures. Today the picture has changed dramatically; far more natural teeth are present, and newer cohorts of people who are elderly have significantly different attitudes toward oral health and dental care Those who are elderly now receive a full range of dental services from examinations and preventive services to complex restorative and periodontal services.[10,16,36,47]

Aging has an impact on oral tissues just as it has on other tissues throughout the body. As teeth age, the enamel, dentin, and pulp undergo progressive changes. The enamel becomes less hydrated (drier). In addition, the thickness of the enamel decreases from abrasion and attrition. Dentin changes more profoundly over a lifetime. The dentin volume expands into the pulp chamber as secondary dentin forms in response to decay and mastication. Many dentinal tubules narrow, and others close altogether, forming sclerotic dentin. These changes make the older tooth more brittle, less resilient, less soluble, less permeable, and darker in color.[1] (See Figure 26–16 ■.)

FIGURE ■ 26–15 Denture induced stomatitis.
(*Source:* Courtesy of Dr. Stephen Wagner, D.D.S., M.S.)

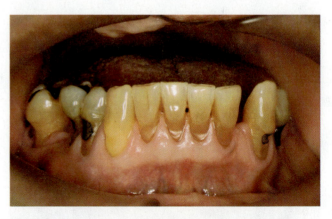

FIGURE ■ 26–16 Age-related changes to natural dentition.
(*Source:* Courtesy of Dr. Andrew Brunner, D.M.D., M.S.)

The pulp chamber, where the blood vessels and nerves of the teeth are located, also undergoes significant changes. The volume of the chamber declines as secondary dentin is deposited. The blood vessels and nerves in the pulp decline, losing myelinated nerve fibers and gaining dystrophic calcium.[48,49]

PREVENTIVE STRATEGIES

It has been said that the greatest failure in modern dentistry is the failure to treat. At the same time that dentistry is able to provide implants, aesthetic veneers, and other "high-tech" treatments that would have been unimaginable only a few years ago, large segments of the population, including frail elderly individuals, lack access to necessary basic care.[1]

A major question is whether older adults today, as well as baby boomers who will be entering their seventies within the next decade, will demand dental care as part of their overall well-being. The current cohort of elders varies widely in its use of dental services from regular preventive users to nonusers who report that they have not been to a dentist in more than 20 years. In 1999, 53.5% of older adults reported that they had visited a dentist, the lowest rate of any age group beyond 18 years of age.[46]

Perhaps one should not expect current cohorts of older adults—born before 1940—to value oral health and dental aesthetics in the same way younger generations do. Several researchers have reported significant differences between younger and older adults in oral health status and utilization patterns.[50] In studies in which age groups are compared, significant differences generally emerge. Older adults are more likely to report not seeking dental care within the most recent 5 or more years. Utilization appears to peak in middle age, and then declines dramatically by age 65. The 2009 National Health Interview Survey (NHIS) data revealed that only 53.5% of adults aged 65 and older had seen a dentist in the past year compared with 67% of those aged 35 to 54 years. More than a quarter (28%) of the older group had not been to a dentist in more than 10 years.[50–52]

Senior-Friendly Dental Practice

Many frail older adults can be seen at a regular dental office if they are mobile and the office is accessible and senior friendly. In some instances, modifications are needed to accommodate frail older adults. Erickson developed a list of essentials for the senior-friendly office to make a dental office more accessible to older adults.[53] The list includes the following features that a dental office might want to consider incorporating:

1. To ensure ease of access to the office, there should be no stairs (a ramp, or perhaps an elevator, instead) and adequate, safe parking.
2. For ease of being seated and standing again, reception room furniture should not be low to the floor, but should be firm and with arm rests.
3. To reduce the risk of falls, flooring should have consistency throughout the office with no deep pile carpeting, no throw rugs or clutter on the floors, and no slippery areas or surfaces.
4. Provide adequate lighting without glare and consistent lighting throughout the office.
5. Avoid small print in written materials.
6. Stand closer to the patient for verbal communication. To enhance visual and oral instructions, remove the dental mask; establish face-to-face eye level contact. Drop the pitch of the voice and speak distinctly, possibly increasing the volume of voice but avoid yelling. Minimize background noise. Whenever possible, turn off dental equipment.
7. To enhance communication, use titles and surnames unless asked specifically to use first name. Provide written instructions to reinforce verbal ones that are easily readable with bold, large font and suitably contrasting paper and ink. Communicate with caregivers as appropriate. Do not communicate with caregivers at the expense of speaking to the patient.[53]

Health Promotion

Health promotion has become an important means of improving older adults' behaviors in a variety of areas, including exercise, weight loss, and management of diabetes and hypertension.[54] Unfortunately, it has received less attention in dentistry except for some early efforts 20 or more years ago. With the rapid advances in materials and methods for home-based oral hygiene as well as in the materials and techniques in dental practice, it is important to educate the general population on an ongoing basis. Even those who make semiannual dental visits generally do not receive oral health education. Many patients would welcome such efforts, as noted by the findings of Abrams and colleagues that 73% of adults younger than 55 years and 62% of those 55 and older indicated a desire for educational programs in their dentist's office.[54] For those who do not seek regular dental care, this information is even more critical and should be provided in alternative settings such as senior centers, assisted-living facilities, and adult day health centers as well as nontraditional settings such as malls and faith community centers. Advocates of oral health care for current and future cohorts of elders can adopt many of the techniques used by the medical community to assist patients with chronic systemic diseases. The dental care community must find creative ways to reach out to underserved segments of older adults.[53]

Although one expects to observe an increase in dentures among people who are elderly, a question remains as to whether the non-edentulous individuals receive an array of dental care similar to other adults.[54] Having examinations and preventive care on a continuing and regular basis over the life span is essential for good oral health and for reducing the incidence of periodontal disease and requirements for dentures.

In other words, this population represents those for whom the broader range of dental services is appropriate. The diminished use of preventive services (cleaning and examinations) currently experienced by the older adult population, however, suggests that a special effort could be needed to encourage older adults to use preventive dentistry and to develop assurances that improved access to dental care will be extended to all ages in the life span.[54]

Public Policy

Although preventive dentistry has increased in the United States in recent years, the gains have been most dramatic among the younger cohorts. Programs to encourage and support access to dental care for individuals who are elderly are needed to reduce the age-based utilization gap and to improve the oral health of elders.

What can health care policy makers do to ensure that there are enough trained health professionals for the future of the United States? As the dental needs of adults who are frail and elderly discussed in this chapter become more apparent, some recommendations have been proposed. See Table 26–2 ■ for action steps proposed by Helgeson and colleagues, which are among the most concise and far-reaching recommendations that the author has encountered regarding the issue of increased access to oral health care for the geriatric population.[1]

Dental Providers

The role of the oral health professional will focus more on the diagnosis and treatment of oral diseases and disorders and the use of new modalities. As diseases of the hard tissues are resolved, more emphasis will be placed on the diagnosis and treatment of soft tissue lesions. With new and improved diagnostic skills, older adults, the group identified as having the highest risk of oral cancer, might no longer require the extensive and often disfiguring surgical remedies currently being administered. These projected oral health outcomes justify that preventive oral health approaches need to be maintained throughout the life span.[6]

To provide optimal care to the aging population, oral health professionals must remain current on oral medicine, pharmacotherapeutics, and changing technologies and must address how this aging population will manage in a variety of dental settings and, at a minimum, have accessible, senior-friendly offices, medical history forms printed in large type, and easy-to-read signs, health literature, and appointment cards.[6]

Oral health is important to overall health for people of all ages. Definitive research shows the connections between poor oral health and systemic diseases, such as diabetes, cardiovascular disease, and respiratory disease, particularly among older adults. Oral cancers are known to be more prevalent in people over the age of 50.[14] New research is pointing to potential connections between oral health and other systemic conditions.[55] Researchers are still learning about the links between oral health and general health, but in itself, oral disease can cause pain, tooth loss, and bad breath. Seniors living in long-term care facilities, as well as some seniors being cared for in their home, are at particular risk of complications from poor oral health because of frailty, poor health, and increased dependence on others for personal care. In many cases, oral health problems of residents of long-term care facilities go undetected until there are acute symptoms, such as pain or infection.

The changing marital and family composition occurring in the United States is likely to change the types of familial support that are available to people at older ages. The future older population is likely to be better educated than the current older population, especially when baby boomers start reaching age 65. Their increased levels of education can result in better health, higher incomes, more wealth, and, consequently, higher standards of living in retirement. Research on genetic, biologic, and physiologic aspects of aging is likely to change the future for the older population. In the medical and public health arenas, research to understand chronic diseases, such as diabetes and Alzheimer disease, could produce significant improvements for treatment and prevention.[55]

TABLE ■ 26–2   Policy Strategies to Change Perceptions toward Oral Health Care for People Who Are Elderly

Work to change perceptions regarding oral health and disease so that oral health becomes an accepted component of general health

Include oral health services in all health promotion, disease prevention, and care delivery programs. Develop training programs for nondental health professionals to emphasize how they can and should work to enhance oral health.

Accelerate the building of the science and evidence base and apply science effectively to improve oral health

Survey dental needs among older adults living in a variety of settings, including senior housing, board and care homes, assisted living facilities, nursing homes, and other long-term care facilities.

Build an effective oral health infrastructure that meets the needs of all Americans

Develop community-based dental care delivery systems at regional and state levels to reduce gaps in prevention and care for low-income older adults, nursing home residents, and older people with disabilities.

Remove known barriers between people and oral health services

Increase the number of dental professionals who are trained to provide mobile, on-site dental care for frail elderly adults and other groups with special dental access needs.

Provide oral health benefits in all public health programs, especially those for adults who are elderly.

Use public–private partnerships to improve the oral health of those who still suffer disproportionately from oral diseases

Increase the number of dental, medical, and nursing programs with active partnerships or cooperative working agreements with public and private community-based organizations that serve people with special access needs, such as frail elderly adults.

(*Source:* From Helgeson, M. et.al., (2001). Frail Elderly Adults. Dental Care Considerations of Disadvantaged and Special Care Populations. Proceedings of the Conference Held April 18–19, 2001, in Baltimore, Maryland. U.S. Department of Health and Human Services, Health Resources and Services Administration. Rockville, Md.)

SUMMARY

Today's oral health professional and the one of the future will be called on to treat an ever-increasing number of older adults. The future for people who are elderly will differ from the cohort seen today. The oral health status group will have more teeth, visit the dental professional more often, and have a higher level of education, better finances, and a dramatically different perspective on needs. They are, and will continue to be, a heterogeneous mix of individuals with various levels of functional, socioeconomic, and oral health status. Advances in materials and technology combined with the changing patterns of oral diseases will continue to have dramatic effects on the practice of dentistry.[6]

The social and economic implications of the aging of the baby boomer generation will be a significant concern for policy makers, the public health and private sectors, and individuals. The size and longevity of this group will trigger debate about possible modifications to Social Security, Medicaid, Medicare, and disability and retirement benefits among other issues.[9] And to think this was the generation that once vowed never to trust anyone over 30.[57]

This chapter has underscored the notion that oral health is important to overall health for people of all ages. Ideally, this important component of health care should continue past retirement into the twilight years. Proper dental care must now be understood as a lifetime commitment. As we learn more about the link between oral and systemic health and as more people keep their natural teeth into old age, it is critical to help adults who are older learn and practice preventive oral health care.

PRACTICAL CONSIDERATIONS

Dental providers will be treating more patients with more teeth (which means more teeth at risk) in an upward trend for decades. Oral health professionals can play a key role in helping seniors to achieve optimum quality of life. Most changes in the oral health of seniors are the consequences of chronic disease and medications, in addition to physical disability and/or cognitive impairment. Of even greater concern than the link between chronic disease and poor oral health is the reverse connection—the one that suggests poor oral health can create a higher risk for other diseases.[36] Current research suggests that oral microorganisms are associated with diabetes, respiratory disease, stroke, and myocardial infarction. Poor oral health also appears to be connected to chronic diseases including osteoporosis, arthritis, and Alzheimer's disease. In light of the dramatic demographic shift in the aging U.S. population as evidenced in this chapter, it is highly likely that dental practitioners in the next several decades will interact more frequently with older dental patients who present with one or more chronic conditions. Addressing the oral health needs of this rapidly emerging subgroup will call for an increasing dental workforce willing and competent to participate in the promotion of their overall health and quality of life.

SELF-STUDY QUESTIONS

1. Which of the following statements is correct?

   a. Elderly people today are declining in proportion to the general population.

   b. There are fewer centenarians now than a decade ago.

   c. The majority of individuals over 85 live in nursing homes.

   d. The older population is on the verge of a population boom.

   Rationale: Social scientists in the U.S. are describing a population boom among cohorts of the older population.

2. Which of the following statements is correct?

   a. All of the following are major signs of the aging process: (1) reduced physiologic reserve of many body functions; (2) impaired homeostasis; (3) impaired immunologic system; (4) increased number of neoplastic conditions; (5) heart conditions, and (6) stroke.

   b. In counseling an older individual, it is advisable speak with a caregiver about the treatment regimen.

   c. The advent of dementia is inevitable in people who are elderly.

   d. SDAT and vascular dementias are reversible conditions.

   Rationale: All of the following are major signs of the aging process: (1) reduced physiologic reserve of many body functions; (2) impaired homeostasis; (3) impaired immunologic system; (4) increased number of neoplastic conditions; (5) heart conditions, and (6) stroke.

3. Which of the following statements is correct?

   a. Dental providers will be treating less elderly in the future, due to medical complications.

   b. Periodontal disease is associated with the older individual; but is not caused by aging; it is caused by oral neglect while aging.

c. *Kyphosis* refers to an infectious disease process afflicting the elderly.

d. Oral cancer is more prevalent in younger cohorts than in those in cohorts who are over age 65.

Rationale: Periodontal disease is associated with the older individual; but is not caused by aging; it is caused primarily by oral neglect while aging.

4. Which of the following statements is NOT correct?

a. Dental care is of particular importance to people who are elderly and frail because oral diseases are cumulative and become more complex over time.

b. Dental disease has a negligible impact on general health.

c. The proportion of edentulism in adults over age 65 is declining in the United States.

d. Teeth become less hydrated and more brittle with advancing age.

Rationale: Research has clearly established an association between oral health and overall health.

5. Which of the following statements is correct?

a. Periodontal therapy in senior adults is futile, and thus, contraindicated, since there is no apparent connection between periodontal disease and systemic disease.

b. It is incumbent upon the dental workforce to anticipate an increasingly larger component of an aging patient population.

c. Denture care for institutionalized elders is not an issue that dental practitioners should be concerned about.

d. In reviewing medical histories of older adults, an assessment of over-the-counter medications need not be addressed because they have no effect on oral health.

Rationale: Statistically, dental practitioners will likely encounter a larger representation of older patients.

REFERENCES

1. Helgeson, M., Smith, B. J., Johnsen, M., & Ebert, C. (2001). Frail elderly adults. In Health Resources and Services Administration. *Proceedings of a conference on dental care considerations of disadvantaged and special care populations.* Rockville, MD: U.S. Department of Health and Human Services, Health Resources and Services Administration, U. S. Government Printing Office.

2. National Institute on Aging. (2006) Dramatic changes in U.S. aging highlighted in new census (NIH Report). Retrieved January 22, 2010, from www.nia,nih.gov/NewsAndEvents/PressReleases.

3. Ferguson, D. A., Steinberg, B. J., & Schwien, T. (2010). Dental economics and the aging population, *Comp Contin Educ Dent,* 31:418–20.

4. Ship, J. A. (2006). *Clinician's guide Oral health in geriatric patients* (2nd ed.). In Atkinson, J. C., Jacobson, P. L., Mohammad, A. R., Navazesh, M., & Patton, L. L., Eds. Hamilton, Ontario, Canada: BC Becker.

5. Allen, P. F. (2002). Changing times: the dentate elderly In Wilson, N. H. F., *Teeth for life for older adults.* London: Quintessence, 1–17.

6. Yellowitz, J. A., & Strayer, M. S. (2004). Geriatric dental care. In Harris, N. O., & Garcia-Godoy, F., Eds. *Primary preventive dentistry* (6th ed.). Upper Saddle River, NJ: Prentice Hall, 589–604.

7. De Rossi, S. S., & Slaughter, Y. A. (2007). Oral changes in older patients: Aclinician's guide. *Quintessence Int,* 38:773–80.

8. U.S. Census Bureau. (2008). *Projections of the population by selected age groups and sex for the United States: 2010 to 2050.* Washington, DC: Population Division, U.S. Census Bureau.

9. U.S. Census Bureau. (2005). *65+ in the United State: 2005* Washington, DC: U.S. Census Bureau; Retrieved January 22, 2010 from www.census.gov/prod/2005 pubs.

10. Niessen, L. C., & Gibson, G. (2000). Aging and oral health for the 21st century. *Gen Dent,* 48: 544–49.

11. World Health Organization. (2002). Active ageing: A policy frame work. *Aging Male,* 5:1–37.

12. Alian, A. Y., McNally, M. E., Fure, S., & Birkhed, D. (2006). Assessment of caries risk in elderly patients using the Cariogram model. *J Can Dent Assoc,* 72:459–63.

13. Guiglia, R., Musciotto, A., Compilato, D., Procaccini, M., Lo Russo, L., Ciavarella, D., & Lo Muzio L. (2010). Aging and oral health: Effects in hard and soft tissues. *Curr Pharm Des,* 16:619–30.

14. Ettinger, R. L., & Beck, J. D. (1984). Geriatric dental curriculum and the needs of the elderly. *Spec Care Dent,* 4:207–13.

15. Little, J. W., Falace, D. A., Miller, C. S., & Rhodus, N. L. (2002). Dental management of older adults. *Dental management of the medically compromised patient.* St. Louis, MO: Mosby, 526–40.

16. Dounis, G., Ditmyer, M. M., McClain, M. A., Cappelli, D.P., & Mobley, C.C. (2010). Preparing the dental workforce for oral disease prevention in an aging population. *J Dent Educ,* 74:1086–1094.

17. U.S. Census Bureau. (2004). We the people: Aging in the United States. Retrieved December 1, 2006, from http://www.census.gov/prod/2001pubs/c2kbr01-10.pdf.

18. U.S. Department of Health and Human Services. (2006). *Advance data from vital and health statistics.* (Number 370). Rockville, MD: U.S. Department of Health and Human Services.

19. American Hospital Association, First Consulting Group. (2007) *When I'm 64: How boomers will change health care.* Chicago, IL: American Hospital Association.

20. Federal Interagency Forum on Aging-Related Statistics. (2010). *Older Americans 2010: Key indicators of well-being.* (Key Indicator 16 of the Federal Interagency Forum on Aging Related Statistics). Washington, DC: U.S. Government Printing Office. Retrieved January19, 2011, from http://www.agingstats.gov/.

21. U.S. Department of Health and Human Services. (2011). *Healthy people 2020.* Washington, DC: U.S. Government Printing Office. Retrieved January 19, 2011, from http://www.healthypeople.gov/.

22. Hardin, S. R. (2006). Financial impcat. In Lubkin, I. M, & Larsen, P. D., Eds. *Chronic illness. Impact and interventions* (6th ed.). Sudbury, MA: Jones & Bartlett, 639–56.

23. U.S. Department of Health and Human Services, National Center for Health Statistics. (2009) *National health interview survey, sample adult questionnaires.* Retrieved January 19, 2011 from http://www.cdc.gov/pub/Health_Statistics/nchs/survey_Questionnaires/nhis/English/qadult.pdfCenters for Disease Control and Prevention. United States.

24. Larsen, P. D. (2006). Chronicity. In Lubkin, I. M., & Larsen, P. D., Eds. *Chronic illness. Impact and interventions* (6th ed.). Sudbury, MA, Jones & Bartlett, 3–22.

25. U.S. Department of Health and Human Services. (2004). *The burden of chronic diseases and their risk factors.* Atlanta, GA: National and State Perspectives, Center for Disease Control and Prevention

26. Halter, J. B., Ouslander, J. G., Tinetti, M. E., Studenski, S., High, K. P., & Asthana, Eds. (2009). In *Hazzard's geriatric medicine and gerontology* (6th ed.). New York: McGraw-Hill

27. Duthie, E. H., Katz, P. R., & Malone, M. L., Eds. (2007). *Practice of geriatrics* (4th ed.). St. Louis, MO: W. B. Saunders.

28. Hansen, K., & Binkley, N. (2007). Osteoporosis. In Duthie, E. H., Katz, P. R., & Malone, M. L., (Eds). *Practice of geriatrics* (4th ed) St. Louis, MO: W. B. Saunders

29. Rose, L. F., Steinberg, B. J., & Minsk, L. (2000). The relationship between periodontal disease and systemic conditions. *Compend Continu Educ Dent,* 21: 870–77.

30. Mobius, H. J. (2004). Alzheimer's disease In Richter, W. R., & Richter, B. Z., Eds. *A physician's guide to practical management.* Totowa, NJ: Humana Press

31. Klein, W. L. (2008). Synaptic plasticity and the mechanism of A!zheimer's disease. In Selkoe, D. J., Triller, A., & Christen, Y., Eds. *Research and perspectives in Alzheimer's disease.* Berlin & Heidelberg, Germany: SpringerVerlag.

32. Katz, M. S., & Gerety, M. B. (1998). Gerontology and geriatric medicine. In Stein, J. H., Ed. *Internal medicine.* St. Louis, MO: Mosby, 2282-93.

33. Thornburg, J. E. (1994). Gerontological pharmacology. In Brody, T. M., Larner, J., & Minneman, K. P., Eds. *Human pharmacology: Molecularto clinical.* St. Louis, MO: Mosby, 855–60.

34. Antunono, P. G. (1995). Effectiveness and safety of velnacrine for the treatment of Alzheimer's disease: A double-blind placebo-controlled study. *Arch Intern Med,* 155:1766–73.

35. Friedlander, A. H., & Jarvik, L. F. (1987). The dental management of the patient with dementia. *Oral Surg,* 64:549–53.

36. Asa, R. (2010). The age of dentistry: Oral-systemic health with emphasis on the geriatric population. *AGD Impact,* 38:30–34.

37. Massachusetts Department of Public Health. (2010). *The Commonwealth's high-risk senior population. Results and recommendations from a 2009 statewide oral health assessment.* Boston, MA: Office of Oral Health.

38. Katz, J., Wallet, S., & Cha, S. (2010). Periodontal disease and the oral-systemic connection: "Is it all the RAGE?" *Quintessence Int,* 41: 229–37.

39. Ship, J. A. (2009) Oral cavity. In Halter, J. B., Ouslander, J. G., Tinetti, M. E., Studenski, S., High, K. P., & Asthana, S., Eds. *Hazzard's geriatric medicine and gerontology* (6th ed.). New York: McGraw-Hill.

40. Ship, J. A. (2009). *Clinician's guide: Oral health in geriatric patients.* In Ship, J. A., Ed. Hamilton, Ontario, Canada: BC Decker.

41. Satcher, D. (2000). *Oral health in America: A report of the Surgeon General.* Rockville, MD: U.S. Department of Health and Human Services, National Institutes of Health, National Institute of Dental and Craniofacial Research.

42. Barnes, S. J. (2006). Long-term care. In Lubkin, I. M., & Larsen, P. D, Eds., *Chronic illness. Impact and interventions* (6th ed.). Sudbury, MA: Jones & Bartlett, 555–78.

43. Pyle, M. A., Jasinevicius, T. R., Sawyer, D. R., & Madsen, J. (2005). Nursing home executive directors' perception of oral care in long-term care facilities. *Spec Care Dent,* 25: 111–17.

44. Thole, K., Chalmers, J., Ettinger, R. L., & Warren, J.(2010). Iowa intermediate care facilities: An evaluation of care providers' attitudes toward oral hygiene care. *Spec Care Dent,* 30: 99–105.

45. Smith, B. J., Ghezzi, E. M., Manz, M. C., & Markova, C. P. (2010). Oral healthcare access and adequacy in alternative long-term care facilities. *Spec Care Dent,* 30: 85–94.

46. Ettinger, R. L., Watkins, C., & Cowen, H. (2000). Reflections on changes in geriatric dentistry. *J Dent Educ,* 64: 715–22.

47. Marshall, S., Northridge, M. E., De La Cruz, L. D., Vaughan, R. D., O'Neil-Dunne, J., & Lamster, I. B., (2009). ElderSmile: A comprehensive approach to improving oral health for seniors. *Am J Public Health,* 99: 595–99.

48. Shay, K. (2000). Restorative considerations in the dental treatment of the older patient. *Gen Dent,* 48: 550–53.

49. Burke, F. M., & Samarawickrama, D. Y. D. (1995). Progressive changes in the pulpo-dentinal complex and their clinical consequences. *Gerodontology,* 12:57.

50. Wall, T. P., & Brown, L. J. (2003). Recent trends in dental visits and private dental insurance, 1989 and 1999. *J Am Dent Assoc,* 134: 621–27.

51. Ettinger, R. L. (1992). Attitudes and values concerning oral health utilization of services among the elderly. *Int Dent J,* 42: 373–84.

52. Manski, R. J., Goodman, H. S., Reid, B. C., & Macek, M. D. (2004). Dental insurance visits and expenditures among older adults, 1995–1997. *MMWR CDC SurveillSumm,* 48:51–88.

53. Erickson, L. (2000). The senior friendly office. *Gen Dent,* 48:562.

54. Kiyak, H. A., & Reichmuth, M. (2005). Barriers and enablers of older adults' use of dental services. *J Dent Educ,* 69:975–86.

55. Abrams, R. A., Ayers, C. S., & Lloyd, P. M. (1992). Attitudes of older versus younger adults toward dentistry and dentists. *Med Care,* 12:67–70.

56. Crozier, S. (2006). Elder care. Resolution addresses oral health news of "vulnerable" older adults. *ADA News,* 37:24.

57. Vorenberg, S. (2007, January). Going out with a boom: A generation faces its mortality. *Albuquerque Tribune,* 1. Retrieved January 27, 2007, from http://www.abqtrib.com.

Medically Compromised Populations

Diana Burnham Aboytes

OBJECTIVES

After reading this chapter, the student should be able to:

1. Describe and define characteristics of each condition.

2. Describe common oral conditions and diseases of medically compromised patients.

3. Describe preventive treatment strategies to use with medically compromised patients.

4. Describe the role of the dental provider in treating medically compromised patients.

INTRODUCTION

The dental practitioner encounters patients with various types of medical conditions. It is important for professionals to understand what oral changes can occur as a result of an altered medical state. Furthermore, in an attempt to provide the patient the proper methods of preventive care, the dental professional should be aware of approaches unique to each patient and his or her condition. This chapter briefly addresses the characteristics of several conditions, their oral manifestations, and preventive strategies for each.

ARTHRITIS

Characteristics and Common Oral Manifestations

Arthritis literally means joint inflammation.[1-3] The word is used to describe more than 100 rheumatic diseases and conditions such as rheumatoid arthritis, gout, fibromyalgia and systemic lupus erythematosus; however, osteoarthritis is the most common form.[4,5] These diseases and conditions affect joints, the surrounding tissues of the joints, and other related connective tissues. Generally, arthritic states are characterized by pain, stiffness, aching, and swelling of the affected areas.[2,6] Arthritis can have a gradual or sudden onset.[2] According to the Centers for Disease Control and Prevention, data from the National Health Interview Survey (NHIS) in 2007–2009 reported that 50 million American adults had self-reported doctor diagnosed arthritis, and an estimated 67 million adults will be diagnosed with arthritis by 2030.[4]

Preventive Treatment Strategies

Rheumatoid arthritis is generally seen as a systemic inflammatory disease that affects the connective tissue of multiple joints in the body, whereas osteoarthritis is considered a degenerative joint disease typically affecting the cartilage in a few select joints. In both conditions, the dental practitioner should be aware of the possible effects on the temporomandibular joint (TMJ). If the TMJ is involved, the dental professional should consider several factors including decreased jaw function, possible need for a soft-food diet, and any medication the patient is taking to manage discomfort.[7] Dental practitioners need to consider the use of either heat or cold therapy to relax and soothe the joint during and after treatment. The dental provider also needs to assess the possible benefits of an oral appliance to decrease pressure exerted on the TMJ.

DID YOU KNOW ?

Patients with arthritis can benefit from a toothbrush with a modified handle to help brush more effectively and with less discomfort.

Patients with an arthritic condition need individualized treatment plans. These plans need to consider the need for shorter visits. Another consideration when assessing appointment length are visits with enough time to allow the patient to walk around as needed, adjust any physical supports, or change position frequently while in the dental chair. Plans for personalized oral hygiene instruction should also be addressed. The patient with an arthritic condition might not have the strength, movement, or dexterity to perform typical self-care regimens.

EATING DISORDERS

Characteristics of Anorexia and Bulimia and Common Oral Manifestations

The two most common eating disorders are anorexia nervosa (AN) and bulimia nervosa (BN). Anorexia nervosa is a psychiatric eating disorder characterized by unrealistic fear of weight gain and the refusal to maintain a normal health body weight. Anorexia patients can present with two subtypes of the disorder, the restricting type or the binge/purge type. The restricting type maintains their low body weight by purely restricting intake and increasing activity. A person with the binge/purge type usually restricts food intake but also engages in binge eating and purging behaviors.

Bulimia nervosa is a psychiatric eating disorder characterized by recurrent episodes of overeating, otherwise known as *binge eating*. These episodes are generally associated with a feeling of loss of control. Individuals with this disorder then use some means to "get rid" of the food by vomiting or engaging in excessive exercise or by using diuretics, laxatives, and enemas to prevent weight gain.[8]

Bulimia has been associated with both depression and overachieving behaviors.[5,9] These conditions can be effectively treated by antidepressant medication, cognitive-behavior therapy, and interpersonal therapy.

The repeated insult of acid from purging as well as from high carbohydrate foods taken during a binging episode can damage teeth. Both factors increase the likelihood of multiple caries. Injuries to the soft palate or pharynx may also be visible, due to the repeated force of a finger or object used to stimulate the gag reflex and initiate the purging cycle.

Characteristics of Pica and Common Oral Manifestations

Pica is an eating disorder characterized as persistent ingestion of non-nutritive substances. This variety of nonfood substances includes, but is not limited to clay, dirt, sand, stones, pebbles, hair, feces, lead, laundry starch, vinyl gloves, plastic, pencil erasers, ice, fingernails, paper, paint chips, coal, chalk, wood, plaster, light bulbs, needles, string, cigarette butts, wire, and burned matches.[10] Pica is common in those with developmental disabilities but can be frequently observed in children and pregnant women. Pica should be considered when ingestion occurs for a period of one month or longer at an age when pica is developmentally inappropriate and is not part of cultural, ethnic, or religious practice. Dental abnormalities, including severe tooth abrasion, abfraction, and tooth surface loss, could be evident on physical examination.[11,12] In addition, trauma such as chemical burns or lacerations to the lining of the oral mucosa and pharynx can be apparent depending on items ingested.

Preventive Treatment Strategies

When a patient with anorexia or bulimia is in the dental chair, the practitioner must pay special attention to the condition of the teeth. A person with even the slightest evidence of this acid erosion damage should be placed on a home-care fluoride regimen in addition to professionally applied fluoride. Also, the dental provider should highly stress the oral hygiene instruction after each purging episode. Patients should be instructed to use a teaspoon of sodium bicarbonate (baking soda) mixed with a cup of water to rinse and expectorate immediately after each purging episode. This will help neutralize the acidic environment. Brushing should be placed on hold for at least 1 hour to avoid creating additional damage to the tooth enamel. Lastly, the dental provider should refer these individuals for further medical consultations.

CANCER

Characteristics and Common Oral Manifestations

There are multiple types of cancer, each type having its own unique characteristics. This section discusses cancer in very general terms in an attempt to address concerns the dental provider can encounter. Cancer is characterized by an out-of-control growth of abnormal cells that have the ability to outlive normal cells. The development of these abnormal cells is due to damage to DNA. The proliferation of the abnormal cells allows them to spread relatively easily from the organ of origin to other sites throughout the body.[13] In addressing cancer issues, the dental professional should complete a thorough health history of each patient at every visit followed by an oral cancer screening.

When cancer is diagnosed, it is categorized according to a stage (see Chapter 7). The stage I, II, III, or IV is based on the size of the tumor and how far it has spread. In stage I, the cancer remains in the original organ. In stage II, the cancer is in a regional area, having spread to nearby structures. In stage III, the cells have moved even farther away from the site of origin. If the cancer has been diagnosed as stage IV, it can be found throughout the body. Depending on the type and stage of the cancer, various treatments can be recommended. The most common treatments are surgical removal of the affected tissues, radiation therapy, chemotherapy, and biologic therapies.[14]

As a result of both the cancer itself and the treatments, the patient may experience several dental manifestations. These manifestations include mucositis, xerostomia, ulcers, increased susceptibility to infection, and poor healing, to name a few.[5]

Preventive Treatment Strategies

The dental professional should consider placing a patient who has encountered any of the cancer manifestations on an antimicrobial mouthrinse to decrease the numbers of oral pathogens present. This measure will help the patient's body fight off any possible infection, hopefully averting any need for additional healing. Saliva substitutes should also be recommended to keep the oral cavity moist. These products will increase general comfort as well as reduce the propensity toward caries and periodontal disease.

A patient who is suffering with ulcers of the oral cavity can be prescribed a rinse with diphenhydramine to decrease oral pain. Patients might also experience oral burning sensations, which can be reduced by a rinse with sodium bicarbonate and water. An antifungal agent can be prescribed to eliminate candidiasis, which is also prevalent in individuals undergoing cancer treatments. Use of mouth exercises and tongue depressors can assist in opening the mouth and can be recommended for the patient who is suffering from **trismus** (involuntary contraction of the muscles used in chewing). With all of these potential culprits damaging the oral cavity, the one component of the individual treatment plan that would be most beneficial for patients with cancer is to place them on self-care fluoride treatments. Having soft, custom-fit trays for daily application of a fluoride gel can help protect the teeth.

Patient education is another important area in which a dental professional can help to prevent cancer. Information about risk factors can be easily included during patient education. Some of the most common risk factors are tobacco use, unprotected sun exposure, poor diet, infectious diseases, chemicals, and radiation exposure.[15]

CARDIAC ARRHYTHMIAS

Characteristics and Common Oral Manifestations

Cardiac arrhythmias occur when electrical impulses in the heart do not function properly.[16] This condition can be any change from a normal sequence of electrical impulses.[17] A proper heartbeat needs a rhythmic coordination of impulses. A lack of this rhythmic coordination can result in many types of ailments. The most common are an inadequate circulation of the blood supply, damage to or death of the heart tissues, coronary artery disease, cardiomyopathy, and valvular heart disease.[18] The two types of cardiac arrhythmias are tachycardia and bradycardia. **Tachycardia** is an abnormally rapid heartbeat for an individual whereas **bradycardia** is an atypically slow heartbeat.[19]

Cardiac arrhythmia might not have any signs or symptoms. Some things to look for are a fluttering feeling, racing or slow pulse rate, chest pain, shortness of breath, and light-headedness with dizziness and possible fainting. Although there are no specific oral manifestations of a cardiac arrhythmia, the *medications* used to treat an arrhythmia can induce some manifestations. Drug-induced xerostomia and ulcerations can be seen.

Preventive Treatment Strategies

Patients with cardiac arrhythmias should use saliva substitutes and stimulants, and self-care fluoride treatments are recommended. If oral signs of the condition are causing pain, a diphenhydramine rinse may be helpful. In addition to maintaining a low-stress environment, use of a local anesthetic with epinephrine should be considered. Excessive amounts of epinephrine, however, could cause a life-threatening arrhythmia.

CONGESTIVE HEART FAILURE

Characteristics and Common Oral Manifestations

Congestive heart failure (CHF) is a life-threatening condition in which the heart can no longer pump enough blood to the rest of the body. Organs that do not receive enough blood are not getting adequate oxygen or nutrients. This deficiency results in damage to the organs, which in turn reduces their function. The most common causes of CHF are hypertension and coronary heart disease.[20] Congestive heart failure can also result after a heart attack from the scar tissue that it produced, coronary artery disease, heart valve disease, and other heart defects.[21]

The symptoms associated with CHF are weight gain; swelling of the feet, ankles, and abdomen; and pronounced neck veins. In addition, a person experiencing CHF may have shortness of breath, general weakness, and decreased urine production.[20]

Preventive Treatment Strategies

Patients with well-controlled CHF can have routine dental treatment. However, the dental professional should remember that these patients are more susceptible to infections. Stressing the importance of good oral hygiene is imperative. These patients also most likely take medications related to the causative factors of CHF and can cause xerostomia. Saliva substitutes and stimulants can help relieve the dry mouth. If the patient is taking digitalis, the amount of epinephrine used should be carefully determined. Digitalis also exacerbates the gag reflex. In addition, dental appointments should be short and stress free.

DEPRESSION

Characteristics and Common Oral Manifestations

Depressive disorders are illnesses involving the body, mood, and thoughts. The three most common types of depressive disorders are major depression, dysthymia, and bipolar disorder.[22] *Major depression* is characterized by a feeling of sadness or hopelessness most of the day, decreased energy, change in weight, difficulty concentrating, and either insomnia or hypersomnia. These symptoms must last longer than 2 weeks to be classified as depression. **Dysthymia** has similar symptoms, but they are less severe and last longer than 2 years. *Bipolar disorder* manifests as episodes of mania, a euphoric high, mixed with episodes of major depression. The causes of depression are not totally clear. Depression is

thought to be tied to low self-esteem, an inherited trait, or some major physical change that leads to a brain–mental change.[22]

Preventive Treatment Strategies

All of these types of depression can have effects on dental patients. They can experience drug induced xerostomia, which could be helped with saliva substitutes and stimulants. In addition, patients experiencing depressive states could have little or no interest in maintaining proper oral hygiene. Providing proper oral hygiene education and referring patients to other medical professionals could help reduce the frequency or severity of these depressive episodes. Patients experiencing a manic phase could do damage to their oral tissues by aggressively cleaning their mouths. Reinforcing the proper techniques and proper dental adjuncts could prevent these injuries.

DIABETES MELLITUS

Characteristics and Common Oral Manifestations

Diabetes mellitus is a group of metabolic diseases in which the body does not produce or properly use insulin.[23,24] *Insulin* is a hormone produced by the pancreas that helps convert sugars, starches, and other food into energy.[23,25] Approximately 25.5 million, or 8.3%, of the U.S. population has diabetes. The most current data rank diabetes as the seventh leading cause of death in the United States.[26]

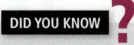

DID YOU KNOW

Overall, the risk for death among people with diabetes is about twice that of people of similar age but without diabetes.[26]

The three basic types of diabetes are type 1, type 2, and gestational diabetes. Type 1 diabetes occurs when the body fails to produce insulin.[23] This type most commonly presents in childhood or adolescence but can occur at any age and requires daily insulin injections. Individuals with type 1 diabetes tend to be slender in stature, have thick saliva, and are prone to other autoimmune diseases.

Individuals with type 2 diabetes produce insulin, but their bodies are unable to use it properly. This diabetic type has a gradual onset. Eighty-five percent of these patients are obese or have increased abdominal fat. Most frequently, type 2 diabetes occurs in adults, but recently been seen more often in overweight, underactive children.[23]

Gestational diabetes is a temporary condition that occurs in 2% to 10% of pregnancies.[26] Although this condition can resolve after pregnancy, women who had gestational diabetes have a 35% to 60% chance of developing type 2 diabetes in the next 10 to 20 years.[26]

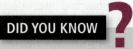

DID YOU KNOW

Uncontrolled diabetics have a compromised ability to respond to infections; therefore, they are at greater risk for periodontal disease.

Preventive Treatment Strategies

With any type of uncontrolled diabetes, oral complications increase; both candidiasis and angular cheilitis are seen. The increased glucose levels provide a favorable environment for fungal organisms. Treatment with a topical antifungal medication can help alleviate these conditions. An altered immune response is the primary culprit behind an increase in caries and periodontal disease. The goal of the dental professional is to educate patients on the oral effects of diabetes and ensure that patients manage their diabetic condition appropriately. Patients who experience ulcerations, numbness, burning, or pain of the oral tissues can try to reduce these symptoms with a sodium bicarbonate and water rinse or a diphenhydramine rinse.

EPILEPSY

Characteristics and Common Oral Manifestations

Epilepsy is a disorder of the brain in which cells create abnormal electricity that causes a seizure.[27] Seizures can manifest in several different ways. In addition to the well-known jerky movements, a seizure can be a loss of consciousness, a period of confusion, a staring spell, or muscle spasms.[27–29] Seizures can occur as the result of stress, sleep deprivation, fever, alcohol or drug withdrawal, and syncope (fainting).[5,29] The two basic types of seizures are partial and generalized. A *partial seizure* involves only one part of the brain, whereas a *generalized seizure* engages most or all of the brain.[30] Not all seizures are considered epilepsy. See Table 27–1 ■ for a brief description of each type. A true diagnosis of epilepsy indicates that the individual has recurrent seizures.[28,29]

Preventive Treatment Strategies

Phenytoin-induced gingival hyperplasia is the major oral complication associated with epilepsy. This gingival overgrow, which contributes to an increase in periodontal pocket depth and plaque retention, can be reduced and controlled with thorough daily oral hygiene routines. In addition, any overhanging restorations and calculus must be removed in an attempt to control the overgrowth. If these relatively mild treatments do not work, surgical reduction of the gingival tissues could be necessary.

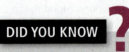

DID YOU KNOW

Recommending the use of a mouth guard for children with uncontrolled epilepsy might help to prevent oral-facial trauma.

A dental provider must stress the importance of regular examinations for the patient with epilepsy. Early identification of any oral injury could prevent severe discomfort later. Grand mal seizures are severe and are initially tonic (prolonged contraction of muscles occurs) but become clonic (alternating contractions and partial relaxations of muscles occur) and usually result in loss of consciousness. With this type of seizure, fractured teeth and injuries to the lips and tongue may occur.[31]

BLOOD DISORDERS

Blood is a connective tissue of the body made up of both liquid and solid components. The liquid component is known as plasma, while the solid components are the red blood cells, white blood cells, and platelets. Red blood cells are vital

TABLE ■ 27–1 Types of Epileptic Seizures

Category	Types	Description
Partial	• Simple partial seizures	Typically no loss of consciousness; last 30–60 seconds; motor and sensory function affected
	• Complex partial seizures	Loss of consciousness; last 1–2 minutes; accompanied by automatisms or purposeless involuntary movements
Generalized	• Petit mal (also known as *absence seizures*)	No aura or subjective sensation that precedes an epileptic episode; brief impairment of consciousness lasting only a few seconds; vacant stare; affects young children primarily; rare past 20 years of age
	• Gran mal (also known as clonic-tonic seizure)	Best known type; known for stiffening and then jerking of limbs; loss of consciousness can occur; recovery in minutes to hours with lethargy
	• Atonic (also known as akinetic or drop attacks)	No aura; abrupt loss of muscle/postural tone; brief loss of consciousness
	• Myoclonic	Brief, involuntary muscle contractions, often occurring bilaterally

for transporting oxygen, white blood cells are crucial to the immune system and are responsible for fighting infection, and platelets play an important role in blood clotting. All are needed for the body to function properly.

Characteristics and Common Oral Manifestations of Red Blood Cell Disorders

Polycythemia results when excessive red blood cells are present in the blood. *Anemia* is a condition in which the body does not have enough healthy red blood cells, resulting in an insufficient amount of hemoglobin, which is required for transporting oxygen through the body. Of the approximately 400 types of anemia, each has its own etiology; thus, anemia is often thought of as a symptom rather than its own disease. Iron-deficiency anemia results when the body is lacking in iron, which is necessary for hemoglobin production. *Pernicious anemia* occurs when the body is lacking vitamin B_{12}, which is vital for the proper development of red blood cells. *Instrinsic factor* is a protein produced in the stomach, and if enough is not being produced, Vitamin B_{12} is unable to be absorbed from the gastrointestinal tract. *Sickle cell anemia* is an inherited condition in which the body synthesizes abnormal hemoglobin. This inability to properly carry oxygen causes the red blood cells to take on a sickled or cresent shape, resulting in a decrease of circulating oxygen.

Presentation of oral manifestations of anemia depend slightly on the etiology, and in many cases, patients are asymptomatic. In general, depending on the severity, patients can exhibit pallor of the oral tissues, angular cheilitis, and changes to the papillae of the tongue, causing a smooth appearance often accompanied with soreness or burning. In polycythemia, the oral mucosa appears deep red in color and is often accompanied with multiple submucosal petechiae, ecchymosis, or hematomas.

Characteristics and Common Oral Manifestations of White Blood Cell Disorders

The total number of white blood cells in a given volume typically ranges from $4,000/mm^3$ to $11,000/mm^3$. When there is an increase above normal in the number of circulating white blood cells this is referred to as leukocytosis, while a decrease is referred to as leukopenia.

Leukemia is cancer of the body's blood-forming tissues. The type of leukemia is dependent on which cells, the myeloid or lymphoid cells, are being affected and whether the disease is in the chronic or acute form. These cells are produced in the bone marrow, but with leukemia, the cells are abnormal or immature, and too many are produced. Oral manifestations of both the chronic and acute forms of leukemia include increased risk for infection, necrotizing periodontal conditions, ulcerations, petechiae, and ecchymosis. Chronic forms may present with lymphandenopathy, which means swollen or enlarged lymph nodes. Gingival enlargement is a common oral manifestation but is seen more commonly in acute forms of leukemia.

Preventive Treatment Strategies

Consultation with a patient's physician may be necessary to confirm that the patient is stable enough for dental treatment. These patients should be recommended to follow routine preventive dental hygiene care with consideration for shorter appointment times.

Characteristics and Common Oral Manifestations of Bleeding Disorders

A majority of bleeding disorders results from a platelet disorder or a deficiency in blood clotting factors. The term *thrombocytopenia* describes a disorder in which the number of platelets is abnormally low. *Hemophilia* is a disorder of the body's blood-clotting system. The body has difficulty changing blood from a liquid to a solid state to stop bleeding.[32,33] Hemophilia may be considered if a patient answers positively to having unexplained bleeding or bruising; blood in the urine or stool, large, deep bruises, or prolonged bleeding from a cut. A medical evaluation should be obtained for an individual who has spontaneous nosebleeds or tightness in the joints.[34]

Preventive Treatment Strategies

When a patient with a bleeding disorder presents for dental care, the most important thing to stress is the need for impeccable oral hygiene. The patient cannot risk unnecessary infection.[35] Patients with mild-to-moderate hemophilia can typically be treated in a traditional dental setting. Those with severe cases should have their dental treatment in a hospital setting.[33,36] If a person with hemophilia is scheduled for multiple extractions, it is important that a splint be made to cover and protect the extraction sites. In mild and moderate hemophiliac patients, pressure packs can be used alongside a product containing thrombin to control bleeding.

HIV AND AIDS

Characteristics and Common Oral Manifestations

Human immunodeficiency virus (HIV) infects and attacks human cells, primarily the CD4 cells. HIV causes decreased and disordered immunity that progresses over time. As the CD4 cell count drops over time, the patient becomes more susceptible to opportunistic infections. When HIV advances, it develops into acquired immune deficiency syndrome or acquired immunodeficiency syndrome (AIDS). Treatments are available for HIV and AIDS, but they only control the disease; there is no cure.

HIV is transmitted several ways. The virus can be acquired through sexual contact, including anal, vaginal, and oral sexual encounters with an HIV-positive person. In addition, a mother can infect her child with HIV in utero (in the uterus), during birth, and through breast-feeding. This type of transmission is preventable with medications; therefore, all pregnant women should be tested. HIV is also transferred in blood-to-blood contacts. This type of transference is very pertinent to the dental professional because contaminated instruments and needle sticks are a method of transmitting blood. Although small amounts of the virus are detectable in saliva, there is very little concern about it being a primary infective factor.[37]

Many oral manifestations are associated with HIV and AIDS. See Table 27–2 ■ for various categories of associated oral conditions. The development of oral candidiasis suggests an immune dysfunction of some type. In the HIV-positive patient, it usually indicated a low CD4 count. Candidiasis can have a range of presentations in the mouth (Figures 27–1 ■ through 27–3 ■). The three most commonly seen types of oral candidiasis are angular cheilitis, erythematous candidiasis, and psuedomembranous candidiasis.[38–40] They can be treated with several antifungal drugs.

Additional common findings include oral hairy leukoplakia (OHL) (Figure 27–4 ■), which is caused by the Epstein-Barr virus; herpes simplex virus; and major aphthous-like ulcers.[39,40] Although OHL is rarely treated, the herpes virus

TABLE ■ 27–2 HIV Oral Manifestations

Mucosal	*Hyperplastic*	*Ulcers*	*Gingival Disease*	*Other*
Candidiasis	Papillomavirus warts	Aphthous ulcers	Linear erythema	Caries
Oral hairy leukoplakia	Kaposi sarcoma	Herpes simplex	Gingivitis	Xerostomia
Hyperpigmentation	Bacillary angiomatosis	Varicella-zoster	Necrotizing periodontal disease	Lymphadenopathy
	Other malignancies and fungi	Cytomegalovirus		Parotid disease

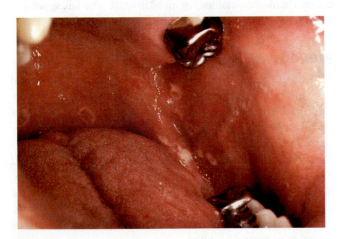

FIGURE ■ 27–1 Candidiasis.
(*Source:* Centers for Disease Control and Prevention [CDC].)

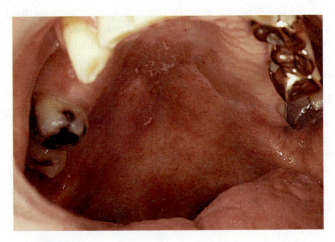

FIGURE ■ 27–3 Acute oral pseudomembranous candidiasis of an HIV-positive patient.
(*Source:* Centers for Disease Control and Prevention [CDC].)

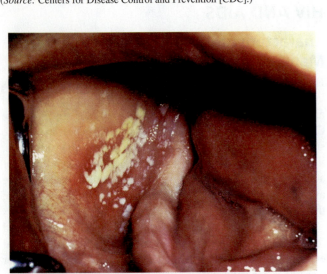

FIGURE ■ 27–2 Erythematous candidiasis.
(*Source:* Centers for Disease Control and Prevention [CDC].)

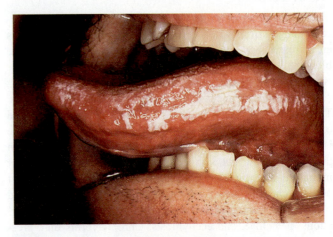

FIGURE ■ 27–4 Oral hairy leukoplakia of an HIV-positive patient.
(*Source:* Centers for Disease Control and Prevention [CDC].)

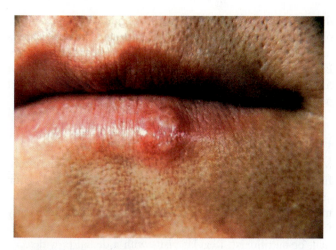

FIGURE ■ 27–5 Herpes simplex lesion.
(*Source:* Centers for Disease Control and Prevention [CDC].)

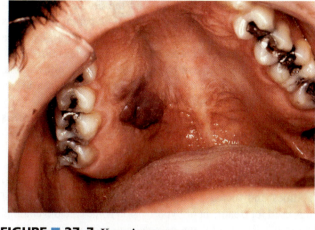

FIGURE ■ 27–7 Kaposi sarcoma.
(*Source:* Centers for Disease Control and Prevention [CDC].)

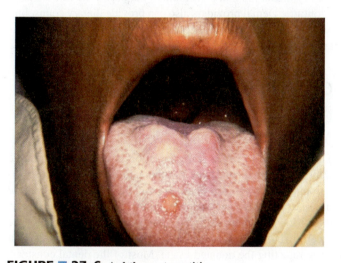

FIGURE ■ 27–6 Aphthous stomatitis.
(*Source:* Centers for Disease Control and Prevention [CDC].)

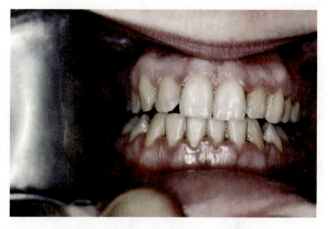

FIGURE ■ 27–8 Necrotizing ulcerative gingivitis.
(*Source:* Centers for Disease Control and Prevention [CDC].)

(Figure 27–5 ■) can be treated with an antiviral drug such as acyclovir (Zovirax), famciclovir (Famvir), or valacyclovir (Valtrex).[41] Major aphthous like ulcers (Figure 27–6 ■) tend to respond well to both systemic or topical corticosteroid therapy. Kaposi sarcoma is also widely seen[39] (Figure 27–7 ■). It typically presents on the skin first, and then intraorally. As a lesion becomes more severe and internally located, the body corresponds with a decreasing CD4 count. Kaposi sarcoma can be treated with an antiretroviral therapy and chemotherapy or radiation for refractory cases.

Periodontal involvement in the HIV-positive patient can advance rapidly compared with that in the general population. This advancement is thought to be associated with the immunocompromised state. Two specific states more frequently seen in the HIV patient are linear gingival erythema and necrotizing ulcerative periodontitis (NUP) (Figure 27–8 ■). Both states can be prevented and treated with debridement of the plaque and calculus followed by a regimen of chlorhexidine 0.12% rinses for several weeks. In addition, the patient experiencing NUP will most likely need systemic antibiotic therapy.[38]

Strategies to Prevent Oral Manifestations

HIV and AIDS patients benefit the most from prevention and control of the microbial buildup in the oral cavity. Adequate professional care and self-knowledge of how to maintain a plaque- and calculus-free environment can help these patients avoid getting secondary oral infections. HIV/AIDS patients must seek regular dental examinations and treatments because most common lesions are easily detected.

HYPERTENSION

Characteristics and Common Oral Manifestations

Hypertension is commonly known as high blood pressure. Blood pressure is determined by the amount of blood the heart pumps and the amount of resistance to blood flow in the arteries. Normal blood pressure measures 120/80 mm Hg or below.

As the heart pumps more blood and the arteries narrow, the blood pressure increases. Diagnosis of hypertension begins when blood pressure reaches 140/90 mm Hg.[42] Typically, there are no signs or symptoms associated with hypertension.[43]

Although hypertension has no direct oral manifestations, several of the medications to treat this condition can affect the oral cavity.[44] Some antihypertensive drugs, especially diuretics, can cause a dry mouth. Several different medications to treat high blood pressure can give the patient a **lichenoid reaction** characterized by the eruption of shiny, violet-colored, flat-topped elevations of mucosal tissue. Angiotensin-converting enzyme inhibitors have been known to delay healing times and increase gingival bleeding. Another class of drugs used for treatment of hypertension is the calcium channel blocker (CCB), also known as *calcium antagonist,* which has been associated with gingival enlargement. Research reviews identified nifidepine as having the highest prevalence whereas verapamil, diltiazem, and amlodipine had significantly lower prevalence.[5]

Preventive Treatment Strategies

Patients taking these medications need to follow a meticulous oral hygiene routine to minimize plaque accumulation and help to eliminate any irritating local factors found on the teeth or gingiva. The use of salivary stimulators and substitutes can treat irritation caused by xerostomia. If gingival enlargement is experienced, patients should be encouraged to follow a 3-month continuing care with their dental office.

OBESITY

Characteristics and Common Oral Manifestations

Obesity describes a range of weight that is greater than what is considered healthy and is associated with an increase in health problems and conditions. According to the Centers for Disease Control and Prevention, about one-third of U.S adults are obese, and approximately 17% of children and adolescents aged 2–19 are obese.[45] In fact, in 2010, no state had a prevalence of obesity less than 20%.[45] Recent guidelines use a person's body mass index (BMI) to determine obesity, which is calculated using a patient's height and weight. Although BMI is not a diagnostic tool and does not measure body fat directly, it has been shown to be a fairly good indicator of a person's body fat.

Various systemic complications are associated with excessive weight gain such as type 2 diabetes mellitus, hypertension, hyperlipidemia, coronary artery disease, cerebrovascular disease, sleep apnea, and certain cancers. Each of these conditions presents with its own set of oral manifestations as previously mentioned in the chapter. Specifically with obesity, a patient's oral health is affected by drugs used to control weight as well as the medications that treat the comorbidities of obesity. Different varieties of these drugs have shown to cause xerostomia, mouth ulcers, carious lesions, and gingivitis.[46] It has also been shown that obesity is a risk factor for periodontitis; a high prevalence of periodontitis is seen among obese patients.[47] Increased levels of TNF-α in gingival crevice fluid have been shown to correlate with increased body mass index.[47] Analysis of data from a national health survey (NHANES III) indicated that BMI and periodontal attachment loss are positively correlated.[48]

Preventive Treatment Strategies

Maintaining a healthy weight and lifestyle takes time and effort. Individuals must make conscious decisions in meal selection and engage in regular physical activity. Eating well-balanced meals in correct proportion can be achieved by keeping a daily food journal and with the help of the patient's physician, dietitian, or nutritionist. Regular visits with a dental provider can help to maintain an obese person's oral health by removing harmful pathogens that contribute to the release of the inflammatory mediators that contribute to the destruction of the periodontium. Dental providers also can provide dietary counseling regarding food choices that potentially increase the risk of dental caries.

ORGAN TRANSPLANTS

Characteristics and Common Oral Manifestations

The first type of organ transplantation is a solid organ/tissue transplant; the second type is a hematopoietic cell transplantation, also known as a *bone marrow transplant.* Solid organ/tissue transplants include the heart, lungs, kidneys, liver, intestines, pancreas, skin, eye components, and limbs.[49] The greatest risk of failure with a transplant is the recipient's own body rejecting the donated tissue. Most of the dental considerations begin with this rejection. The immunosuppressive drugs administered to a patient are typically the cause of many oral manifestations.

In general, excessive immunosuppression can lead to mucositis, herpes infections, ulcerations, candidiasis, and alveolar bone loss. Gingival overgrowth has also been indicated with immunosuppression and poor oral hygiene.[50] Cyclosporine (Gengraf®, Neoral®, Sandimmune®) continues to be the primary agent associated with gingival overgrowth in some patients. Tacrolimus is another immunosuppressant agent used increasingly in place of cyclosporine, and although it causes less gingival overgrowth, it is associated with oral ulcerations and numbness or tingling, especially around the mouth.[50]

Preventive Treatment Strategies

Patients with an organ transplant need to ensure that their periodontal health is stable by undergoing a professional dental hygiene evaluation. Increasing the frequency of dental hygiene visits can help to maintain plaque and calculus control in deeper gingival pockets thus helping to prevent the progression of periodontal disease. Thorough oral hygiene instruction can help the patient keep the oral cavity as plaque free as possible while at home.

PULMONARY DISEASE

Characteristics and Common Oral Manifestations

Chronic obstructive pulmonary disease (COPD) is a generic term used to describe damage to the lungs that makes it difficult to breathe.[52] The two most common diseases named under the classification of COPD are bronchitis and emphysema. Although these diseases have considerations during dental treatment, no specific oral manifestations are found as a direct result of the disease. However, the typical causative factor leading to the development of COPD is cigarette smoking.[53] The oral manifestations and preventive strategies related to smoking are discussed later in this section.

DID YOU KNOW ?

Although pulmonary diseases do not present a specific oral manifestation, the presence of periodontal disease can increase the risk of respiratory infections such as pneumonia.

Asthma is a disease of the respiratory system in which the airway constricts, becomes inflamed, or is lined with excessive amounts of mucus. Several different stimuli including allergens, respiratory infections, exercise, and certain drugs can trigger an asthma attack.

Asthma itself does not cause oral disease; however, some of the asthma treatments can. Beta$_2$-agonist inhalers decrease salivary flow and plaque pH levels. These conditions are related to an increase in the number of caries and the prevalence of gingivitis. Asthmatics tend to have a higher than-than-average amount of acid reflux, which can cause increased enamel erosion.

Inhaled steroids are common treatments for asthma and COPD.[54] These steroids decrease the normal immune function in the oral cavity, which is associated with increased cases of candidiasis.

Preventive Treatment Strategies

Individuals with caries and erosion can benefit from self-care fluoride regimens. All of the oral conditions mentioned benefit from thorough oral hygiene, which should be planned and taught by the dental professional.

Candidiasis can be treated with an antifungal medication; however, patients can take preventive measures to reduce the outbreak of the *Candida* species. Patients who rinse with water after using their inhalers can reduce the incidence of candidiasis. Also, using inhalers with a "space" chamber will reduce the likelihood of developing candidiasis.[55]

RENAL DISEASE/FAILURE

Characteristics and Common Oral Manifestations

The function of the kidneys is to excrete wastes, concentrate urine, and regulate electrolytes.[56] Kidney or renal disease and failure causes the kidneys to stop effectively removing metabolic end products from the blood and be unable to regulate the fluid level, electrolyte balance, and pH balance of the extracellular fluid. Systemic symptoms of kidney failure are weight loss, fatigue, decreased urine production, easy bruising, yellowing of the skin, and a decreased sensation in the extremities. The only treatments for renal failure or end-stage kidney disease are dialysis or kidney transplantation.[57,58]

A very common oral manifestation of someone in chronic renal failure is pallor (paleness) of the oral mucosa, which is due to the decrease in the number of red blood cells present.[59] Patients also could complain of a metallic taste in their mouths caused by a high concentration of urea in the saliva.[59] A high concentration of urea, however, inhibits the growth of lactobacilli, which in turn decreases the caries rate.[60] Xerostomia and candidal infections are also prevalent. A lack of vitamin C gives the gingiva an abnormal red appearance; the gingiva is also spongy and bleeds easily.[61,63] In addition to these oral manifestations, evidence of chronic renal failure is seen in radiographs. A loss of the lamina dura, demineralized bone, and radiolucent jaw lesions could be present.[64,65]

Preventive Treatment Strategies

The first step for the dental professional in preventing oral manifestations is to prescribe individualized oral hygiene for patients with renal disease/failure. Because of increased susceptibility for infection, the number of oral pathogens must be controlled. Moreover, the patient's general comfort must be considered. Conditions such as xerostomia and ulcerations can cause discomfort that can be controlled by saliva substitutes, fluoride treatments, or diphenhydramine rinses. If the patient has candidiasis, an antifungal agent can be prescribed.

SUBSTANCE ABUSE DISORDERS

Substance abuse refers to the overindulgence in and dependence on a **psychoactive** (substance that affects the mind and/or behavior), leading to effects that are detrimental to the individual's physical health and/or mental health, or the welfare of others.[66] Although several types of substances can be abused, this section focuses on a few frequently encountered substances with associated oral manifestations. The most important strategy for a dental provider regarding these substance abuse disorders is to encourage patients to obtain the proper help required to control and eventually stop the habitual cycle of the abuse.

Characteristics of Alcohol Abuse and Common Oral Manifestations

Alcoholism is defined as a primary, chronic disease characterized by impaired control of drinking alcohol, preoccupation with the drug alcohol, use of alcohol despite adverse consequences, and distortions in thinking.[67] In the United States, approximately 75,000 deaths per year are caused by excessive alcohol use.[68] Over time, abusive alcohol consumption can lead to many physical problems including, but not limited to, strokes, cardiovascular issues, depression, liver diseases, and gastrointestinal problems in addition to social problems.[69,78]

Direct oral manifestations of alcohol abuse are xerostomia, petechiae (localized hemorrhaging of skin or mucosal surfaces characterized by small reddish/purplish spots), **ecchymoses** (escape of blood into tissues from ruptured blood vessels), and increased gingival bleeding. Tooth erosion is also evident, predominately from vomiting that may follow episodes of binge drinking.[79] An overall neglect of the body leads to poor oral hygiene, increasing the risk of dental caries and periodontal disease.[80] Increases in stress levels add to bruxism and allow for opportunistic infections such as candidiasis to develop.[81] A chronic alcoholic is 10 to 15 times more likely to develop oral squamous cell carcinomas than nonalcoholics.[81]

DID YOU KNOW ?

People who combine the use of alcohol and tobacco are at an especially high risk of oral cancer because these substances are believed to act synergistically, increasing each other's harmful effects.

Characteristics of Tobacco Use and Common Oral Manifestations

Cigarette smoking is the most popular means of tobacco use; however, smokeless tobacco products such as snuff and chewing tobacco are also very popular. Cigars and pipes are other ways to smoke tobacco. Nicotine, a highly addictive chemical in tobacco, is absorbed through mucous membranes. As the nicotine enters the bloodstream, the body releases adrenaline, which stimulates a release of blood glucose, an increase of blood pressure, respiration, and heart rates.[83] The National Center for Health Statistics reports that, in 2009, approximately 21% of the U.S. adults aged $\geq$ 18 were current cigarette smokers.[84]

DID YOU KNOW ?

Each year, approximately 3,000 nonsmokers die of lung cancer from second-hand smoke.

Oral effects such as oral cancer, leukoplakia, nicotine stomatitis, and hairy tongue may result from tobacco use. Tobacco users have a 4 times higher chance of developing oral cancer than people who do not use it.[85] Leukoplakia, which can

become cancerous, develops from tobacco contacting the oral mucosa for long periods of time.[86] Nicotine stomatitis is a precancerous mucosal change of the hard palate. It is caused by the heat of smoking tobacco, not to the chemicals in the tobacco.[87] Hairy tongue is a result of the elongation of the filiform papillae of the tongue. It is thought that the tobacco causes the epithelial cells of the tongue to stop shedding.[85] Patients who use tobacco also have a higher incidence of periodontitis and a higher caries rate.[88,89] Contributing to these conditions is xerostomia, which is a decrease of salivary production.[89]

Characteristics of Marijuana Use and Common Oral Manifestations

Marijuana is a mix of flowers, stems, seeds, and leaves of the hemp plant *Cannabis sativa*. It is usually smoked either as a cigarette or through a pipe. Delta-9-tetrahydrocannabinol (THC) is the addictive chemical in marijuana. Users experience a high from the binding of certain nerve cells to THC.[90] In 2004, approximately 14.6 million Americans used marijuana at least once a month.[91] Many terms used for marijuana include *pot, herb, weed, grass, ganja,* and *hash.*

In general, the oral health of marijuana abusers is poorer than that of nonusers; abusers have an increased risk of caries and periodontal diseases.[92] Xerostomia, a major effect of marijuana, can also increase the risk of caries and periodontitis.[93] Marijuana smoke acts as a carcinogen and is associated with dysplastic changes and premalignant lesions in oral mucosas.[94] Marijuana users are prone to oral infections, such as benign epithelial tumors that project from the surrounding oral mucosa, called *oral papillomas,* which are most likely due to the immunosuppressive effects of marijuana.[93,95] These effects may also be the link to the increased prevalence of candidiasis.[96]

Characteristics of Cocaine Abuse and Common Oral Manifestations

Cocaine, and alkaloid ester extracted from the leaves of the plants,[97] is a highly addictive stimulant of the central nervous system. The two basic forms of cocaine are hydrochloride salt and freebase, which is also called "crack cocaine." Hydrochloride salt, the powdered form of cocaine, is dissolved in water and can be taken intravenously or intranasally. *Freebase* refers to a compound that has not been neutralized by an acid to make the salt. This drug is smoked.[98] Cocaine has several street names including *blow, nose candy, snowball, tornado, wicky stick,* and *Perico.*[99]

Cocaine interferes with the reabsorption process of dopamine whose buildup causes continuous stimulation of the receiving neurons resulting in feelings of euphoria.[100,101]

Topically applied cocaine can be locally destructive to the oral mucosa and dentition. Ulceration, necrosis, and rapid recession occur, as does erosion of both enamel and dentin.[102] These oral manifestations can be attributed to addicts checking the purity of the cocaine on these areas of the mouth.[103] When crack cocaine is smoked, the crack pipe directs extremely hot smoke to the midline of the hard palate. This heat can lead to ulcerations or, in extreme cases, perforation of the hard palate.[104,105] Necrotic ulcers of the tongue and epiglottis are also related to smoking freebase cocaine.[106] Candidiasis can be seen as a result of the weakened immune system. Craving sweets during cocaine use leads to an increased caries rate. Prolonged periods of stimulation of the central nervous system leads to long periods of bruxism, giving way to severe tooth wear.[103] Aggressive toothbrushing while on a cocaine high has been implicated as the cause of both cervical and tooth abrasion and gingival lacerations.[102]

Characteristics of Methamphetamine Abuse and Common Oral Manifestations

Methamphetamine is a potent stimulant that releases high levels of dopamine, norepinephrine, and serotonin. This drug also blocks the reuptake of these same substances. Similar to cocaine, the dopamine stimulates brain cells, which in turn enhance mood and body movements.[106] Cocaine has been found to increase dopamine units by 350, and methamphetamine increases it by 1,250 units compared with base levels of dopamine.[107] Excessive norepinephrine may be responsible for the alertness and lack of fatigue felt by methamphetamine users. The extra serotonin is thought to cause cognitive impairment and eventual depression.[108]

Methamphetamine is an odorless, white, bitter-tasting crystalline powder that dissolves in water or alcohol. The drug can be taken orally or intranasally, smoked, or injected. Methamphetamine is known on the streets by names such as *speed* and *chalk*. Methamphetamine hydrochloride is the form that can be smoked. Because it presents in crystals that resemble ice, methamphetamine hydrochloride is also referred to as *ice, crystal, glass,* and *tina*.[109] Crank is the less pure form of methamphetamine.

DID YOU KNOW ?

"Meth mouth" is an actual term used to describe the mouth of a methamphetamine user who exhibits serious damage resulting in rampant decay and tooth loss.

The most common and related oral manifestation of methamphetamine use is rampant caries. This rapid decay process begins between the teeth and moves around the teeth at the cervical junction[110] (Figure 27–9 ■). One cause of this destructive process is said to be the caustic substances used in the production of methamphetamine. Methamphetamines have also been implicated in slowing salivary production, an extreme desire for sugary soda consumption, and a lack of desire for good oral hygiene. It is thought that smokers have worse dental effects, because the chemicals are brought in direct contact with the oral cavity, causing sores and infections. Injectors of methamphetamine do not experience the same severe tooth decay; however, they do experience more severe clenching and grinding. The increased bruxism is attributed to the more powerful effects of the injected drug.[111]

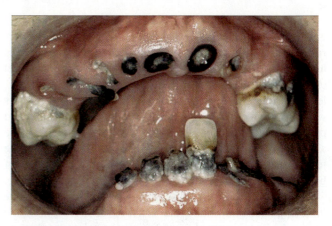

FIGURE ■ 27–9 Methamphetamine mouth.
(*Source:* Courtesy of Charles D. Tatlock, D.D.S., M.P.H.)

Preventive Treatment Strategies

As previously stated, one the most important roles of the dental provider is to educate patients as to why they should not engage in these types of damaging activities. However, if a patient is a substance abuser, the dental professional should direct them to a safe environment to receive the necessary care to get clean and sober.

Encouraging these patients to seek consistent dental visits is of top priority. These visits will allow the patients to be taught appropriate, individualized self-care regimens. Proper self-care allows patients to keep the oral environment less conducive to the bacteria that cause caries and periodontal diseases. In addition, the patients need regular screenings for oral cancer. Early detection increases the likelihood of successful treatment of an oral cancer lesion. Patients who have xerostomia should be directed to consider the integration of saliva substitutes and stimulants into the daily dental routines. Topical fluoride treatment could help with this problem as well as prevent caries. An antifungal medication may be prescribed to lessen the insult of the *Candida* species if present in the patient's mouth. Patients who feel discomfort from ulcerative lesions could find a diphenhydramine rinse beneficial. If attrition from clenching and grinding is present, a mouthguard can be recommended to stop the progression of the tooth wear.

THYROID DYSFUNCTION

Characteristics and Common Oral Manifestations

The thyroid gland is an endocrine gland that secretes three hormones: thyroxine, triiodothyronine, and calcitonin. Thyroxine, also known as *T4,* contains four iodine molecules and is produced only by the thyroid. Triiodothyronine, referred to as *T3,* is a variation of T4 and contains three iodine molecules.[112] These hormones are transported through the blood by binding to plasma proteins and are regulated by the hypothalamic–pituitary–thyroid axis.[112]

The two basic types of thyroid dysfunction are hypothyroidism and hyperthyroidism. *Hyperthyroidism,* also known as **thyrotoxicosis**, is an overactivity of the thyroid gland, which causes high levels of T4 or T3 in the blood.[112,113] This excessive level of hormone results in an acceleration of vital body functions, leading to higher physical and mental activity.[113–115] Patients with hyperthyroidism have an increased rate of dental caries and periodontal disease. Contributing to this, is osteoporosis of the alveolar ridges,[117,118] which is characterized by decreased bone mass resulting from decreased bone density and enlargement of bone spaces. The bone is more porous and susceptible to fracture.

Hypothyroidism, by contrast, is the underactivity of the thyroid gland. This subnormal secretion of the T4 hormone causes the body's normal functioning rate to slow, resulting in a decrease in overall mental and physical activity.[112,113,115,116]

Hypothyroidism has very different oral manifestations including macroglossia (enlarged tongue), glossitis, and delayed tooth eruption. Delayed wound healing contributes to the poor periodontal health seen in these individuals.[117]

Preventive Treatment Strategies

Demonstrating proper plaque control and then evaluating the patients' plaque-control technique will help increase the patients' ability to prevent the progression of oral diseases related to thyroid dysfunction. Excessive tissue on the lateral posterior tongue, called a *lingual thyroid,* can also be seen. Patients also commonly complain of a burning sensation in their mouths.[117] These patients could benefit from rinsing with sodium bicarbonate and water.

SUMMARY

Medically compromised patients are present every day in the dental practice. Dental providers need to help their patients find a means to prevent and care for oral conditions that may be associated with medical states. Each medical circumstance has unique oral manifestations. Being knowledgeable about these characteristics and associated preventive strategies will be beneficial to both the practitioner and the patients.

PRACTICAL CONSIDERATIONS

It is the responsibility of the dental provider to ensure that a complete, current health history is obtained and that updates are made at each continuing care appointment. The health history should allow patients the opportunity to disclose previous as well as current medical conditions. Patients should be asked about all prescription, over-the-counter, and herbal medications they take. Dental providers must be educated and remain knowledgeable about the various medical conditions and the medications used to treat them. They should be prepared to offer recommendations in preventing and treating oral manifestations related to one's systemic condition. Resources such as the current *Physician's Desk Reference* (*PDR*) or access to the Internet should be readily available to the provider in the event that they are unfamiliar with a condition or medication. Refer to Table 27–3 ■ as a reference for a synopsis of several medical conditions, their characteristics, associated oral manifestations and some preventive strategies.

SELF-STUDY QUESTIONS

1. Which of the following assessments would be the best at determining a patient's health status?

   a. Extraoral examination

   b. Radiographs

   c. Completed health history

   d. Intraoral examination

   Rationale: Although the other options give some clues as to a patient's health status, a completed health history is the most appropriate for obtaining information regarding past and present health conditions.

2. Which of the following medical conditions can directly involve oral manifestations?

   a. Hypertension

   b. Bulimia

   c. Epilepsy

   d. Congestive heart failure

   Rationale: The repeated insult of acid from purging will lead directly to damage of the tooth structure. The other medical conditions do not directly result in oral manifestations, but the medications associated with them cause the presentation of any oral manifestations.

3. Which of the following preventive treatment strategies should be used with substance abuse disorders?

   a. Educate patients on why not to engage in these types of damaging activities.

   b. Direct patients to a safe environment to receive necessary care to get clean and sober.

   c. Encourage patients to seek consistent dental visits.

   d. All of the above.

   Rationale: Each of these options is a critical preventive treatment strategy. Patients must be educated on the damage that can result from the use of such substances and where they can turn for help. Consistent dental visits will allow dental providers to identify problems and provide the needed dental treatment.

4. Which of the following preventive treatment strategies should be used when caring for a patient with arthritis?

   a. Assessment of temporomandibular joint at each continuing care visit

   b. Daily home fluoride therapy

   c. Periodic antifungal therapy to avoid candidiasis

   d. All of the above

   Rationale: Both types of arthritis have the potential to affect the temporomandibular joint. The TMJ should be assessed during each visit for decreased function and/or pain. Fluoride and antifungal therapy will not prevent any oral manifestations associated with this medical condition.

5. Which of the following is a common oral manifestation associated with HIV and AIDS?

   a. Candidiasis

   b. Xerostomia

   c. Linear gingival erythema

   d. All of the above

   Rationale: A diminished immune system causes these patients to be susceptible to opportunistic infections. Candidiasis is common due to the immune dysfunction. Periodontal bacteria are also able to thrive resulting in linear gingival erythema. Often the medications used to treat these infections result in xerostomia.

TABLE ■ 27–3   **Synopsis of Medical Conditions, Their Oral Manifestations, and Preventive Treatment Strategies**

Condition	Description	Oral Manifestations	Preventive Treatment Strategies
Alcohol abuse	Excessive consumption of ethanol	Oral cancer Poor oral hygiene Xerostomia Petechiae Ecchymoses Increased bleeding Candidiasis Tooth erosion	Individualized oral hygiene instruction Saliva stimulants and substitutes Self-care fluoride treatments Antifungal agent Diphenhydramine rinse
Arthritis	Damaged joints	Poor oral hygiene TMJ issues	Individualized oral hygiene instruction Short appointment times Oral appliance Alternative positioning during appointments
Asthma	Abnormal lung function	Candidiasis Increased caries Increased gingivitis	Antifungal agent Diphenhydramine rinse Individualized oral hygiene instruction
Bulimia	Binge eating followed by purging	Tooth erosion Increased caries and periodontitis Tooth sensitivity Trauma to soft palate and pharynx	Self-care fluoride treatments
Cancer	Out-of-control growth of abnormal cells	Mucositis Candidiasis Xerostomia Loss of taste Trismus Cervical caries Sensitive teeth Excessive/spontaneous bleeding Poor healing Increased susceptibility to infection	Antifungal agent Individualized oral hygiene instruction Saliva stimulants and substitutes Self-care fluoride treatments Antimicrobial rinse Mouth exercises Tongue depressors to open mouth

(Continued)

TABLE ■ 27–3 (Continued)

Condition	Description	Oral Manifestations	Preventive Treatment Strategies
Cardiac arrhythmias	Abnormal heartbeat or rate	Xerostomia Ulceration Petechiae	Diphenhydramine rinse Saliva stimulants and substitutes Self-care fluoride treatments
Cocaine use	Addictive stimulant of the central nervous system	Ulceration of mucosa Palatal perforation Necrosis of gingiva Bruxism Cervical tooth abrasion Tooth erosion	Individualized oral hygiene instruction Mouthguard use Diphenhydramine rinse
Congestive heart failure	Inability of heart to pump enough blood to the body's other organs	Infection Bleeding Petechiae Ecchymoses Xerostomia	Saliva stimulants and substitutes Self-care fluoride treatments
Depression	Illness of mind, body, and thoughts	Poor oral hygiene Xerostomia Damage to tissues due to "over"cleaning	Saliva stimulants and substitutes Self-care fluoride treatments
Diabetes	Metabolic disorder resulting in abnormal blood glucose levels	Impaired healing Increased susceptibility to infections Candidiasis Accelerated periodontal disease Xerostomia Ulcerations Numbness/burning/pain of oral tissues	Antifungal agent Diphenhydramine rinse Sodium bicarbonate and water rinse Saliva stimulants and substitutes Self-care fluoride treatments
Epilepsy	Neurologic disorder causing seizures	Gingival hyperplasia Fractured teeth Injury to lips and tongue	Individualized oral hygiene instruction Surgical reduction of gingival
Hemophilia	Bleeding disorder	Spontaneous bleeding Prolonged bleeding Hematomas	Individualized oral hygiene instruction
HIV/AIDS	Immune system failure	Candidiasis Kaposi sarcoma Hairy leukoplakia Linear gingival erythema NUG/NUP	Antifungal agent Individualized oral hygiene instruction Antibiotics Corticosteroid therapy
Hypertension	Elevation of blood pressure	Xerostomia Ulceration Lichenoid reactions Decreased healing Increased bleeding Gingival hyperplasia	Diphenhydramine rinse Saliva stimulants and substitutes Self-care fluoride treatments
Hyperthyroidism	Excessive release of thyroid hormone	Progressive periodontal disease Extensive caries Tumors on tongue Osteoporosis of alveolar ridge Premature loss of teeth Early eruption patterns Burning sensation	Sodium bicarbonate and water rinse Individualized oral hygiene instruction
Hypothyroidism	Thyroid failure	Increased tongue size Delayed eruption of teeth Delayed wound healing	Individualized oral hygiene instruction
Liver disease	Inflammation of the liver	Bleeding, lichenoid eruptions	Individualized oral hygiene instruction

TABLE ■ 27–3   (Continued)

Condition	Description	Oral Manifestations	Preventive Treatment Strategies
Marijuana use	Smoking of plant *Cannabis sativa*	Xerostomia Oral cancer Poor oral hygiene Candidiasis Increased gingivitis and periodontitis	Individualized oral hygiene instruction Antifungal agent Saliva stimulants and substitutes
Methamphetamine use	Use of addictive stimulant drug	Poor oral hygiene Xerostomia Rampant decay	Individualized oral hygiene instruction Saliva stimulants and substitutes Self-care fluoride treatments
Organ transplants	Solid organ/tissue or hematopoietic cell transplantation	Candidiasis Herpes (simplex and zoster) Hairy leukoplakia Kaposi sarcoma Aphthous stomatitis Spontaneous bleeding Increased infection Ulceration Petechiae Ecchymoses Gingival hyperplasia Salivary gland dysfunction Xerostomia	Individualized oral hygiene instruction Antifungal agent Saliva stimulants and substitutes
Pica	Ingestion of nonnutritive substances	Chipped/Broken teeth Trauma to oral mucosa and pharynx	Medical consultation Behavioral intervention
Renal disease	Complete or near failure of the kidneys	Mucosal pallor Xerostomia Metallic taste Ammonia breath Stomatitis Loss of lamina dura Bone radiolucencies Increased bleeding Ulcerations Candidiasis	Antifungal agent Diphenhydramine rinse Saliva stimulants and substitutes Self-care fluoride treatments Individualized oral hygiene instruction
Tobacco use	Use of plants in the genus *Nicotiana*	Oral cancer Leukoplakia Xerostomia Alveolar bone damage Gingival damage Hairy tongue Nicotine stomatitis Increased caries	Saliva stimulants and substitutes Self-care fluoride treatments

REFERENCES

1. What is arthritis? *The Arthritis Foundation guide to good living with rheumatoid arthritis.* Retrieved January 8, 2007, from www.arthritis.org

2. Centers for Disease Control and Prevention, National Center for Chronic Disease Prevention and Health Promotion. (2007, May 24). Arthritis overview. Retrieved November 22, 2006, from http://www.cdc.gov/arthritis/arthritis/index.htm.

3. Abramson, S. B., & Yazici, Y. (2006). Biologics in development for rheumatoid arthritis: Relevance to osteoarthritis. *Adv Drug Deliv Rev,* 58:212–25.

4. U.S. Department of Health and Human Services, Centers for Disease Control and Prevention. (2011, February 18). *Chronic disease—Arthritis—At a glance.* Retrieved March 23, 2011 from http://www.cdc.gov/chronicdisease/resources/publications/aag/arthritis.htm.

5. Dongari-Bagtzoglou, A. (2004) Drug associated gingival enlargement: Informational paper. *J Periodontol,* 75:1424–31.

6. Mahalik, J., Shigaki, C. L., Baldwin, D., & Johnstone, B. (2006). A review of employability and worksite interventions for persons with rheumatoid arthritis and osteoarthritis. *Work,* 26:303–11.

7. Ardic, F., Gokharman, D., Atsu, S., Guner, S., Yilmaz, M., & Yorgancioglu, R. (2006). The comprehensive evaluation of temporomandibular disorders seen in rheumatoid arthritis. *Aust Dent J,* 51:23–28.

8. Reba, L., Thornton, L., Tozzi, F., Klump, K.L., Brandt, H., Crawford, S., Crow, S., Fichter, M. M., Halmi, K. A., Johnson, C., Kaplan, A. S., Keel, P., LaVia, M., Mitchell, J., Strober, M., Woodside, D. B., Rotono, A., Berrettini, W. H., Kaye, W., & Bulik, C. M. (2005). Relationships between features associated with vomiting in purging-type eating disorders. *Int J Eat Disord,* 38:287–94.

9. Johnson, C. D., Koh, S. H., Shynett, B., Koh, J., & Johnson, C. (2006). An uncommon dental presentation during pregnancy resulting from multiple eating disorders: Pica and bulimia: Case report. *Gen Dent,* 54:198–200.

10. Ellis, C., & Schnoes, C. (2009, June 4) Eating disorders, pica. eMedicine. Retrieved March 23, 2011, from http://emedicine.medscape.com/article/914765-overview.

11. Barker, D. (2005). Tooth wear as a result of pica. *Br Dent J,* 199:271–73. Retrieved March 24, 2011 from http://www.nature.com/bdj/journal/v199/n5/full/4812651a.html.

12. Johnson, C.D., Shynett, B., Dosch, R., & Paulson, R. (2007). An unusual case of tooth loss, abrasion, and erosion associated with a culturally accepted habit. *Gen Dent,* 55:445–48.

13. American Cancer Society. (2006, February 6). *Cancer reference information: What is cancer?* Retrieved November 22, 2006 from http://www.cancer.org/docroot/CRI/content/CRI_2_4_1x_What_Is_Cancer.asp?sitearea.

14. American Cancer Society (n.d.) *Cancer reference information: How is cancer treated?* Retrieved November 22, 2006 from http://www.cancer.org/docroot/CRI/content/CRI_2_4_4x_How_Is_Cancer_Treated.asp?

15. American Cancer Society. *Cancer reference information: What are the risk factors for cancer?* Retrieved March 27, 2008 from http://www.cancer.org/docroot/CRI/content/CRI_2_4_2x_What_are_the_risk_factors_for_cancer_72.asp?sitearea=.

16. Mayo Clinic Staff. (2005, February). *Heart arrhythmias introduction.* Retrieved 2/16/08 from http://mayoclinic.com/health/heart-arrhythmias/DS00290.

17. American Heart Association. What are arrhythmias? Retrieved March 27, 2008, from http://www.americanheart.org/presenter.jhtml?identifier=4469.

18. Mayo Clinic Staff. (2005, February). *Heart arrhythmias causes.* Retrieved 2/16/08 from http://mayoclinic.com/health/heart-arrhythmias/DS00290.

19. Brasel, K. J., Guse, C., Gentilello, L. M., & Nirula, R. (2007). Heart rate: Is it truly a vital sign? *J Trauma,* 62:812–17.

20. Gandelman, G. (2006, July). Heart failure. In *MedlinePlus Medical Encyclopedia.* Retrieved November 22, 2006, from http://www.nlm.nih.gov/medlineplus/ency/article/000158.htm.

21. American Heart Association. (n.d.). *Congestive heart failure.* Retrieved November 22, 2006, from http://www.americanheart.org/presenter.jhtml?identifier=4585.

22. National Institutes of Health Depression. Retrieved March 20, 2008, from http://www.nimh.nih.gov/health/topics/depression/index.shtml.

23. American Diabetes Association. (n.d.). *All about diabetes.* Retrieved November 22, 2006, from http://www.diabetes.org/utils/printthispage.jsp?PageID=ALLABOUTDIABETES_233165.

24. American Diabetes Association. (2004). *American Diabetes Association: Clinical practice recommendations 2004. Report of the expert committee on the diagnosis and classification of diabetes mellitus.* Alexandria, VA: American Diabetes Association.

25. Centers for Disease Control and Prevention, National Center for Chronic Disease Prevention and Health Promotion. (2006, June 27). *CDC's diabetes program. What is diabetes?* Retrieved November 22, 2006, from http://www.cdc.gov/diabetes/faq/basics.htm.

26. Centers for Disease Control and Prevention. National Center for Chronic Disease Prevention and Health Promotion. (2011) *National diabetes fact sheet.* Retrieved March 23, 2011, from http://www.cdc.gov/diabetes/pubs/pdf/ndfs_2011.pdf.

27. American Academy of Family Physicians. (1994, September). *Epilepsy.* Retrieved November 22, 2006, from http://familydoctor.org/214.xml?printxml.

28. Mayo Clinic Staff. (2005, April). *Epilepsy.* Retrieved November 22, 2006, from http://www.mayoclinic.com/health/epilepsy/DS00342.

29. Kohrman, M. H. (2007). What is epilepsy? Clinical perspectives in the diagnosis and treatment. *J Clin Neurophysiol,* 24:87–95.

30. Mayo Clinic Staff. (2005, April). *Epilepsy signs and symptoms.* Retrieved November 22, 2006, from http://www.mayoclinic.com/health/epilepsy/DS00342/DSECTION=2.

31. Aragon, C. E., & Burneo, J. G. (2007). Understanding the patient with epilepsy and seizures in the dental practice. *J Can Dent Assoc,* 73:71–76.

32. Mayo Clinic Staff. (2005, May). *Hemophilia.* Retrieved November 22, 2006, from http://www.mayoclinic.com/health/hemophilia/DS00218.

33. Israels, S., Schwetz, N., Boyar, R., & McNicol, A. (2006). Bleeding disorders: Characterization, dental considerations and management. *J Can Dent Assoc,* 72:827.

34. Mayo Clinic Staff. (2005, May). *Hemophilia signs and symptoms.* Retrieved November 22, 2006 from http://www.mayoclinic.com/health/hemophilia/DS00218/DSECTION=2.

35. Hoots, W. K., & Nugent, D. J. (2006). Evidence for the benefits of prophylaxis in the management of hemophilia A. *Thromb Haemost,* 96:433–40.

36. Correa, M. E., Annicchino-Bizzacchi, J. M., Jorge, J., Paes de Almeida, O., Ozelo, M. C., Aranha, F. J., & Lourdes Barjas-Castro, M. (2006). Clinical impact of oral health indexes in dental extraction of hemophilic patients. *J Oral Maxillofac Surg,* 64:785–88.

37. Centers for Disease Control and Prevention. (1999, July). *HIV and its transmission.* Bethesda, MD: U.S. Department of Health and Human Services, Centers for Disease Control and Prevention.

38. Reznik, D. (2005, December–2006, January). Oral manifestations of HIV disease. *Perspective,* 13:143–48.

39. Baccaglini, L., Atkinson, J. C., Patton, L. L., Glick, M., Ficarra, G., & Peterson, D. E. (2007). Management of oral lesions in HIV-positive patients. *Oral Surg Oral Med Oral Pathol Oral Radiol Endod,* 103 (Suppl):S50.e1–23.

40. Sroussi, H. Y., Villines, D., Epstein, J., Alves, M. C., & Alves, M. E. (2007). Oral lesions in HIV-positive dental patients—One more argument for tobacco smoking cessation. *Oral Dis,* 13:324–28.

41. Emmert, D. (2000, March). Treatment of common cutaneous herpes simplex virus infections. *Am Fam Physicia,* 61:1697–704.

42. Mayo Clinic Staff. (2006, September). *High blood pressure (hypertension).* Retrieved March 27, 2008, from http://mayoclinic.com/health/high-blood-pressure/DS00100.

43. Mayo Clinic Staff. (2006, September). *High blood pressure (hypertension)—Signs and symptoms.* Retrieved March 27, 2008, from http://mayoclinic.com/health/high-blood-pressure/DS00100.

44. Gibson, R. M., & Meechan, J. G. (2007). The effects of antihypertensive medication on dental treatment. *Dent Update,* 34:70–72.

45. Centers for Disease Control and Prevention. (2011, July 21). *U.S. obesity trends.* Retrieved December 27, 2011, from http://www.cdc.gov/obesity/data/trends.html

46. Duley, S., & Fitzpatrick, P. (2006, November). The bariatric treatment team. *Dimensions of Dental Hygiene,* 4:14–16.

47. Lundin, M., Yucel-Lindberg, T., Dahllöf, G., Marcus, C., & Modéer, T. (2004). Correlation between TNF alpha in gingival crevicular fluid and body mass index in obese subjects. *Acta Odontol Scand,* 62:273–77.

48. Wood, N., Johnson, R. B., & Streckfus, C.F. (2003). Comparison of body composition and periodontal disease using nutritional assessment techniques: Third National Health and Nutrition Examination Survey (NHANES III). *J Clin Periodontol,* 30:321–27.

49. Sollecito, T. (2003). Transplantation medicine. *Burket's Oral Medicine Diagnosis and Treatment* (10th ed., Chapter 19) Lewiston, NY: BC Decker, 503–24.

50. Oliveira Costa, F., Ferreira, S. D., Lages, E. J., Costa, J. E., Oliveira, A. M., & Cota, L. O. (2007). Demographic, pharmacologic, and periodontal variables for gingival overgrowth in subjects medicated with cyclosporine in the absence of calcium channel blockers. *J Periodontol,* 78:254–61.

51. National Institute of Dental and Craniofacial Research. *Dental management of the organ transplant patient.* Retrieved November 23, 2011, from http://www.nidcr.nih.gov/OralHealth/Topics/OrganTransplantationOralHealth/OrganTransplantProf.htm.

52. Fehrenbach, C. Chronic obstructive pulmonary disease. (2002). *Nurs Stand,* 17:45–51.

53. Mannino, D. M., Gagnon, R. C., Petty, T. L., & Lydick, E. (2000). Obstructive lung disease and low lung function in adults in the United States: Data from the National Health and Nutrition Examination Survey 1988–1994. *Arch Intern Med,* 160:1683–89.

54. Antoniu, S. A., Mihaescu, T., & Donner, C. F. (2007). Inhaled therapy for stable chronic obstructive pulmonary disease. *Expert Opin Tharmacother,* 8:777–85.

55. Casiglia, J., & Mirowski, G. (2006, October 5). Oral manifestations of systemic diseases. Retrieved November 22, 2006, from http://www.emedicine.com/derm/topic887.htm#section~author_information.

56. U.S. National Library of Medicine, National Institutes of Health. End-stage kidney disease. In *MedlinePlus Medical Encyclopedia.* Retrieved November 22, 2006, from http://www.nlm.nih.gov/medlineplus/ency/article/000500.htm.

57. National Institute of Diabetes and Digestive and Kidney Diseases, National Institutes of Health. (2006, December). *Treatment methods for kidney failure: Hemodialysis.* Retrieved November 22, 2006, from http://kidney.niddk.nih.gov/kudiseases/pubs/hemodialysis/.

58. Sharma, D. C., & Pradeep, A. R. (2007, January). End stage renal disease and its dental management. *NY State Dent J,* 73:43–47.

59. DeRossi, S. S., & Glick, M. (1996). Dental considerations for the patient with chronic renal disease receiving hemodialysis. *J Am Dent Assoc,* 127:211–19.

60. Brescia, M. J., Cimino, J. E., & Appel, K. (1966). Chronic hemodialysis using venipuncture in a surgically created arteriovenous fistula. *N Engl J Med,* 275:1089–92.

61. Kerr, A. R. (2001). Update on renal disease for the dental practitioner. *Oral Surg Oral Med Oral Path,* 92:9–16.

62. Spielman, A. L., Bivona, P., & Rifkin, B. R. (1996). Halitosis. A common oral problem. *NY State Dent J,* 62:36–42.

63. Eigner, T. L., Jastak, J. T., & Bennet, W. M. (1986). Achieving oral health in patients with renal failure and renal transplants. *J Am Dent Assoc,* 113:612–16.

64. Gavalda, C., Bagan, J., Scully, C., Silvestre, F., Milian, M., & Jimenez, Y. (1999). Renal hemodialysis patients: Oral, salivary, dental and periodontal findings in 105 adult cases. *Oral Dis,* 5:299–302.

65. Syrjanen, S., & Lampainen, E. (1983). Mandibular changes in panoramic radiographs in patients with end-stage renal disease. *Dentomaxillofac Radiol,* 12:51–56.

66. Anderson, K. N., Anderson, L. E., & Glanze, W. D. (1998). *Mosby's medical, nursing, and allied health dictionary* (5th ed.). St. Louis, MO: C.V. Mosby.

67. The Joint Committee of the National Council on Alcoholism and Drug Dependence and the American Society of Addictive Medicine to Study the Definition and Criteria for the Diagnosis of Alcoholism. (1992). The definition of alcoholism. *JAMA,* 268(8):1012–14.

68. Stahre, M. A., Brewer, R. D., Naimi, T. S., & Miller, J. W. (2004). Alcohol-attributable deaths and years of potential life lost—United States, 2001. *MMWR Morb Mortal Wkly Rep,* 53:866–70.

69. Corrao, G., Rubbiati, L., Zambon, A., & Arico, S. (2002). Alcohol-attributable and alcohol-preventable mortality in Italy. *Eur J Public Health,* 12:214–23.

70. Corrao, G., Bagnardi, V., Zambon, A., & La Vecchia, C. (2004). A meta-analysis of alcohol consumption and the risk of 15 diseases. *Prev Med,* 38:613–19.

71. Rehm, J., Gmel, G., Sepos, C. T., & Trevisan, M. (2003). Alcohol-related morbidity and mortality. *Alcohol Res Health,* 27:39–51.

72. Castandeda, R., Sussman, N., Westreich, L., Levy, R., & O'Malley, M. (1996). A review of the effects of moderate alcohol intake on the treatment of anxiety and mood disorders. *J Clin Psychiatr,* 57:207–12.

73. Kochanek, K. E., Murphy, S. C., Anderson, R. N., & Scott, C. (2004). *Deaths: Final data for 2002* (National Vital Statistics Reports 53(5)). Hyattsville, MD: National Center for Health Statistics.

74. Schiff, E. R. (1997). Hepatitis C and alcohol. *Hepatology,* 26 (Suppl 1):39S–42S.

75. Lesher, S. D. H., & Lee, Y. T. M. (1989). Acute pancreatitis in a military hospital. *Military Med,* 154:559–64.

76. Kelly, J. P., Kaufman, D. W., Koff, R. S., Laslow, A., Wiholm, B. E., & Shapiro, S. (1995). Alcohol consumption and the risk of major upper gastrointestinal bleeding. *Am J Gastroenterol,* 90:1058–64.

77. Booth, B. M., & Feng, W. (2002). The impact of drinking and drinking consequences on short-term employment outcomes in at-risk drinkers in six southern states. *J Behav Health Serv Res,* 29:157–66.

78. Leonard, K. E., & Rothbard, J. C. (1999). Alcohol and the marriage effect. *J Stud Alcohol Suppl,* 13:139–46.

79. Olshan, A. F., Weissler, M. C., Watson, M. A., & Bell, D. A. (2001). Risk of head and neck cancer and the alcohol dehydrogenase 3 genotype. *Carcinogenesis,* 22:57–61.

80. Genco, R. J. (1999). Current view of risk factors for periodontal disease. *J Periodontol,* 67 (Suppl):1041–49.

81. Wynder, E. L., & Bross, I. J. (1998). Etiological factors in mouth cancer: An approach to its prevention. *BMJ,* 1:389–95.

82. Holbrook, T. L., & Barrett-Conner, E. (1998). A prospective study of alcohol consumption and bone density. *BMJ,* 306:1506–509.

83. National Institute on Drug Abuse. (2006—Revised). *Tobacco addiction* (Research Report Series). Bethesda, MD: U.S. Department of Health and Human Services, National Institutes of Health, National Institute on Drug Abuse.

84. Centers for Disease Control and Prevention (2011, September 11). Vital signs: Current cigarette smoking among adults aged ≥ 18 years-2005–2010. *MMWR.* 60(35):1207–1212.

85. Walsh, P., & Epstein, J. (2000). The oral effects of smokeless tobacco. Retrieved March 27, 2008, from http://www.cda-adc.ca/jcda/vol-66/issue-1/22.html.

86. Bergstrom, J., Keilani, H., Lundholm, C., & Radestad, U. (2006). Smokeless tobacco (snuff) use and periodontal bone loss. *J Clin Periodontol,* 33:549–54.

87. Academy of General Dentistry. (1996). *How many teeth are in that cigarette pack?* Retrieved November 2006, from http://www.agd.org.

88. Rao, L. P., Das, S. R., Mathews, A., Naik, B. R., Chacko, E., & Pandey, M. (2004). Mandibular invasion in oral squamous cell carcinoma. *Int J Oral Maxillofac Surg,* 33:454–57.

89. Frije, J., & Kumar, J. V. (2001, March). Prevention of cancers of oral cavity and pharynx in New York State. *NY State Dent J,* 67:26–30.

90. National Institute on Drug Abuse. (2006, April). *NIDA InfoFacts: Marijuana.* Bethesda, MD: U.S. Department of Health and Human Services, National Institutes of Health.

91. Office of Applied Studies. (2004). *Results from the 2004 National Survey on Drug Use and Health: National findings.* (DHHS Publication No. SMA 05-4061). (Office of Applied Studies NSDUH Series H-27). Rockville, MD: Office of Applied Studies.

92. Darling, M. R., & Arendorf, T. M. (1992). Effects of cannabis smoking on oral health. *Int Dent J,* 42:19–22.

93. Darling, M. R., & Arendorf, T. M. (1993). Effects of cannabis smoking on oral soft tissues. *Community Dent Oral Epidemiol,* 21:78–81.

94. Hashibe, M., Ford, D., & Zhang, A. (2002). Marijuana smoking and head and neck cancer. *J Clin Pharmacol,* 42:103S–107S.

95. Cho, C. M., Hirsch, R., & Johnstone, S. (2005). General and oral health implications of cannabis use. *Aust Dent J,* 50:70–74.

96. Darling, M. R., Arendorf, T. M., & Coldrey, N. A. (1990). Effects of cannabis smoking on oral candidal carriage. *J Oral Pathol Med,* 19:319–21.

97. Seyer, B., Grist, W., & Muller, S. (2002). Aggressive destructive midfacial lesion from cocaine abuse. *Oral Surg Oral Med Oral Pathol Oral Radiol Endod,* 94:465–70.

98. National Institute on Drug Abuse. (2006). *Cocaine abuse and addiction.* (Research Report Series). Rockville, MD: U.S. Department of Health and Human Services, National Institutes of Health, National Institute on Drug Abuse.

99. U.S. Department of Justice, U.S. Drug Enforcement Administration. (2006, August) Cocaine. Retrieved October 2007, from http://www.dea.gov/concern/cocaine.html.

100. National Institute on Drug Abuse. (2006, April). *NIDA InfoFacts: Crack and cocaine.* U.S. Department of Health and Human Services, National Institutes of Health, National Institute on Drug Abuse. Retrieved from http://www.drugabuse.gov/publications/drugfacts/cocaine.

101. Swan, N. (2005). *Brain scans open window to view cocaine's effects on the brain.* U.S. Department of Health and Human Services, National Institutes of Health, National Institute on Drug Abuse. Bethesda, MD. Retrieved November 22, 2006, from http://www.nida.nih.gov/NIDA_Notes/NNVol13N2/Brain.html.

102. Villa, P. D. (1999). Midfacial complications of prolonged cocaine snort. *J Can Dent Assoc,* 65:218–23.

103. Darby, M. L., & Walsh, M. (2003). *Dental hygiene theory and practice.* St. Louis, MO: Elsevier Saunders.

104. Smith, J., Kacker, A., & Anand, V. K. (2002). Midline nasal and hard palate destruction in cocaine abusers and cocaine's role in rhinologic practice. *Ear Nose Throat J,* 81:172–77.

105. Ibsen, O. A. C., & Phelan, J. A. (2000). *Oral pathology for the dental hygienist.* St. Louis, MO: Saunders.

106. Chang, L., Ernst, T., Speck, O., & Grob, C. (2005). Addictive effects of HIV and chronic methamphetamine use on brain metabolite abnormalities. *Am J Psychiatr,* 162:36–69.

107. Richards, J., & Brofeldt. B. (2000). Patterns of tooth wear associated with methamphetamine use. *J Periodontol,* 71:1271–74.

108. Stein, W. (2005, September–October). Rotten times are here again. *Northwest Dent,* 84:10.

109. National Institute on Drug Abuse. (2010, March). *NIDA InfoFacts: Methamphetamine.* U.S. Department of Health and Human Services, National Institutes of Health, National Institute on Drug Abuse. Retrieved from http://www.drugabuse.gov/publications/drugfacts/methamphetamine.

110. Curtis, E. (2006). Meth mouth: A review of methamphetamine abuse and its oral manifestations. *Gen Den,* 54:125–29.

111. Saini, T., Edwards, P., Kimmes, N., Carroll, L. R., Shaner, J. W., & Dowd, F. J. (2005). Etiology of xerostomia and dental caries among methamphetamine abusers. *Oral Health Prev Dent,* 3:189–95.

112. Streff, M., & Pachucki-Hyde, L. (1996). Management of the patient with thyroid disease. *Nurs Clin North Am,* 31:779–96.

113. Thyroid gland disorders. In *Merck manual of medical information: Second home edition.* Whitehouse Station, NJ: Merck Research Laboratories, Chapter 163.

114. Mayo Clinic Staff. (2006). Hyperthyroidism. Retrieved March 27, 2008, from http://mayoclinic.com/health/hyperthyroidism/DS00344.

115. Greene, C. (2005). *Thyroid gland.* World Book Online References Center. World Book, Inc. Retrieved April 1, 2008, from http://www.worldbookonline.com/wb/Login?ed=wb.

116. U.S. National Library of Medicine, National Institutes of Health. Hypothyroidism. In *Medline Plus medical encyclopedia.* Retrieved November 22, 2006, from http://www.nlm.nih.gov/medlineplus/ency/article/000353.htm.

117. Silverton, S. (2003). Endocrine disease. In Greensberg, M., & Glick, M., Eds. *Burket's oral medicine diagnosis and treatment* (19th ed.). Ontario, Canada: BC Decker, 578–91.

118. Sun, L., Davies, T. F., Blair, H. C., Abe, E., & Zaidi, M. (2006). TSH and bone loss. *Ann NY Acad Sci,* 1068:309–18.

Populations with Developmental Disabilities

Elmer E. Gonzalez

OBJECTIVES

After reading this chapter, the student should be able to:

1. Describe the developmental disabilities presented in the chapter.
2. Describe common oral conditions and diseases of patients with developmental disabilities.
3. Describe specific preventive strategies to use with patients with developmental disabilities.
4. Describe the role of the dental provider in treating patients with developmental disabilities.
5. Recognize some of the common medications used by people with disabilities for associated medical conditions.

KEY TERMS

Attention Deficit Hyperactivity Disorder, 457
Autism, 461
Activities of daily living (ADL), 457
Cerebral palsy, 463
Developmental disability, 454
Down syndrome, 464
GERD, 459
Macroglossia, 465
Intellectual disability (ID), 457
People first language
Pica, 471

INTRODUCTION

Typically, a **developmental disability** is defined as a severe, chronic disability attributable to mental or physical impairment that manifests before the age of 22 years. This disability is likely to continue indefinitely, resulting in functional limitations and a need for planned care and treatment.[1,2,3,4]

In the 2001 conference and report on improving lives for those individuals with intellectual disabilities, the U.S. Surgeon General discussed the failure of the health care system to provide reasonable access to quality medical and dental care for those persons.[5] One of the goals of the report was to increase the number of health care providers with appropriate training to treat persons with developmental disabilities. One of the results of recognizing this problem has been action taken by the Commission on Dental Accreditation (CODA). Beginning in 2004, CODA required that students who graduate from an accredited dental or dental hygiene school "must be competent in assessing the treatment needs of patients with special needs."[6] Dental professionals need an understanding of the limits and conditions that could possibly affect patients who have these disabilities. Although all patients must be considered on an individual basis, a basic knowledge of developmental disabilities will help the dental practitioner understand the disability, anticipate some of the challenges that might be encountered, ensure that proper training is been delivered to caregivers, and understand how to effectively treat and prevent diseases in this population (see Table 28–1 ■).

TABLE ■ 28–1 Common Oral Manifestations

Oral Manifestation	Disability	Common Causes	Preventive Strategies
Abfraction	All types	Bruxism and/or repetitive trauma to the area	Use of a night guard to prevent bruxism and behavior modification to avoid repetitive trauma
Angular chelitis		Fungal infection or nutritional deficiency	Good nutrition and vitamin B supplements; antifungal cream to relieve symptoms of fungal condition
Aphthous ulcers (canker sores)	All types	Numerous including toothbrush trauma, physical trauma, stress, acidic fruits	Important to instruct proper brushing techniques and prevent any type trauma to the oral tissues; must be careful with citrus, especially for patients susceptible to or with history of canker sores
Attrition	All types	Several including grinding, repetitive biting on hard materials (nails, ice, spoons, etc.)	Behavioral modification important to prevent major damage to tooth structures; use of a mouth guard for patients able to tolerate it
Candidiasis	All types, especially patients with immuno-competent systems	Weak immune system, cancer treatment, use of steroids, stress	Essential to have nutritional counseling to maintain a well-balanced diet to support immune system
Caries	All types, but patients with DS are not the most susceptible to dental caries	Poor oral hygiene, weak immune system for patients in cancer treatment and with xerostomia, cariogenic diets, and increased cariogenic bacterial count	Optimal oral hygiene, nutritional counseling, and saliva substitutes
Palatoschisis (cleft palate)	ID and X-linked syndromes	Genetics, X-linked ID, other X-linked syndromes major causative agents	Oral hygiene instruction crucial
Microdontia	All types, most commonly in patients with DS	Genetics	None; cosmetic dentistry an option
Macroglossia	Patients with DS	Chromosomal disorders	Important to have oral hygiene instruction, to brush tongue with toothbrush or tongue scraper; can affect patient's ability to eat, speak, breathe
Oligodontia	All types, but genetic syndromes more common	Genetics	Only oral hygiene instruction
Hypodontia	All types, commonly in genetic syndromes such as DS	Genetics	Individualized oral hygiene care plan. Tighter recall and monitoring to prevent periodontal disease from developing or progressing due to malocclusion and risk factors (diabetes, heart disease, poor plaque control, difficult access to perform oral hygiene).
Xerostomia	All types	Medications, smoking, some syndromes, mouth breathing, hyposalivation, radiation therapy, dehydration	Individualized oral hygiene plan including use of saliva substitutes, encourage water consumption, sugar-free gum

TABLE ■ 28–1 (Continued)

Oral Manifestation	Disability	Common Causes	Preventive Strategies
Crowding of teeth	All types	Eruption patterns of permanent teeth affected by retained primary teeth	Oral hygiene instruction, however access might be difficult to some areas due to crowding. Oral hygiene adjuncts and in some cases referral to an orthodontist might be necessary.
Retained primary teeth	All types	Congenital	Oral hygiene instruction, especially because of increased susceptibility to dental caries
Malocclusion	All types, especially DS and CP	Mid-face hypoplasia, missing teeth, retained primary teeth, and trauma resulting in destruction of tooth buds	Oral hygiene instruction and introduction of oral hygiene adjuncts to ease proper cleaning; possible referral to see a specialist (i.e., orthodontist)
Mouth breathing	Common in CP and DS	Restricted airway, enlarged tongue, malocclusions, high-vaulted palate	Saliva substitute not only to alleviate dry mouth but also to prevent caries to some extent; fluoride substitutes
Dry lips	All types	Mouth breathing, medications	Use of lip moisturizer to prevent lip cracks/tears
Recession	All types	Excessive toothbrush pressure, repetitive self-damaging behaviors to the gums, oral trauma	Fluoride treatments to help alleviate sensitivity, possible grafting, use of proper toothbrushing techniques
Periodontitis	All types, common in CP and DS	Poor oral hygiene, mouth breathing, malocclusions, tooth morphology, and systemic conditions such as diabetes	Increased oral hygiene and tighter recall for dental cleanings, use of chlorhexidine or similar mouthwash in short term to decrease inflammation and bacterial count, nonsurgical periodontal therapy if necessary at least once every 2 years
Gingivitis	All types	Poor oral hygiene, mouth breathing	Only instruction inproper and frequent toothbrushing and flossing techniques
Drooling	All types, common in CP and DS	Poor lip and muscle tone, lip incompetence, inability to suction and swallow saliva, enlarged tongue.	Instruction, if patient allows, in how to use the lips and muscles, to suction and swallow saliva, to force their lip into a closed position, salivary gland surgery to stop drooling (educate about its benefits and risks)
Bruxism	All types, common in autism and CP	Coping mechanism, primitive rooting reflex	Important to recommend the use of an occlusal guard to prevent more damage to tooth structure if patient allows and is able to tolerate using the appliance.
High palate	Various syndromes and in DS and CP	Cleft palate, oral anatomy, large tongue, breathing difficulties, narrow high-vaulted palate	Important to keep the area clean during cleanings and dental exams and instruct caregivers how to clean it
Deep fissured tongue	All types, common in CP and DS	Enlarged tongue	Oral hygiene instruction to keep tongue clean from food and bacteria by using tongue scraper or toothbrush
Hairy tongue	All types	Hyperkeratinization of papilla. No specific known factor to contribute to it.	Brushing tongue and keeping it clean
Benign migratory glossitis (geographic tongue)	All types	Unknown	Oral hygiene instruction to keep tongue clean
Tight muscles of mastication	All types	Use as a defense mechanism because of past oral trauma or aversions	Educate caregiver on proper oral hygiene techniques to gain access without causing trauma to oral tissues; have an assistant perform oral hygiene because tightness of lips and cheeks causes access to be very difficult
Mobility	All types	Periodontal disease, trauma	For periodontal disease, keep areas as clean as possible to prevent more bone loss; for trauma, use a splint
g-tube calculus	Commonly seen in patients using g-tubes, with CP, or with high aspiration risk	Lack of mechanical motion (chewing and grinding of food) and brushing	Use of ultrasonic scalers with an assistant to ensure adequate water evacuation with high-volume suction to effectively remove most calculus; stress to caregivers importance of brushing even if patient does not eat; tight recall to control calculus buildup and short appointment time to minimize stress and aspiration risk

(Continued)

TABLE ■ 28–1 (Continued)

Oral Manifestation	Disability	Common Causes	Preventive Strategies
Food pouching	All types	Unknown	Instruct caregivers to use toothettes to remove excess food from the vestibule. Toothettes not to be used as a substitute for tooth brushing.
Fusion	All types	Union of two normally separated tooth germs	No preventative measures other than good oral hygiene and parent/caregiver education
Enamel hypoplasia	All types	Hypocalcification but no specific identifiable causes	Only good oral hygiene
Decalcification	All types	Poor oral hygiene, consumption of carbonated drinks with repeated exposure to tooth enamel	Good oral hygiene, education of patients and caregivers on risks of long-term consumption of carbonated drinks; tight recall; use of fluoride
Short roots	Commonly with DS	Genetic predisposition in patients with DS	Good home care
Germination	All types	Two teeth develop from one tooth bud forming an extra tooth with one root	None other than good oral hygiene and parent/caregiver education
Erosion	All types	Erosion of enamel from acidic foods, drinks, stomach fluids	Dietary counseling, proper oral hygiene, referral to primary care physician to evaluate for GERD, bulimia, etc.
Gingival hyperplasia	Patients with epilepsy	Antiepileptic drugs such as Dilantin in combination with plaque	Proper oral hygiene, shorter recall appointments to decrease inflammatory response of gingival tissues, possible gingivectomy
Tooth fractures	All types, common with CP and seizure disorder	Unsteady gait causing falls; seizures; self-injurious behaviors	Educate patients with seizure disorder and their caregivers on importance of wearing safety helmets

DID YOU KNOW?

The term *intellectual disability*, or individual with an intellectual disability, is the current terminology used instead of *mental retardation* (MR).

Populations who have developmental disabilities can have varying degrees of functional level. In a dental setting, patients from this population considered to be high functioning would be able to respond to the dental provider. For example, this level of function would be moving the head when prompted, relaxing the lips and tongue, and having radiographs taken without assistance. In contrast, patients considered to be low functioning would need the dental team to manipulate all functions for them. These patients might not respond to basic commands or have a conscious swallowing ability.

Although there is no particular guide on how to treat a patient with a developmental disability because each patient is different and no disability manifests in the exact same way, it is important for dental providers to follow a few simple steps when treating these patients.

1. Assess medical, dental, and health history.
2. Take vital signs (i.e., blood pressure, pulse, respirations, oxygen saturation).
3. Communicate clearly with a patient who is able to do so. Otherwise, refer questions to the person's caregiver.
4. Obtain consent for treatment and possible medical stabilization (usually on a yearly basis) from the patient or legal guardian. Do not treat a patient without a signed consent form.
5. Assess the patient for possible complications during dental treatment and utilization of medical stabilization if necessary.
6. If medical stabilization is needed, document clearly the time patient utilized medical stabilization and the purpose for which it was utilized (i.e., a head holder was utilized for patient's safety because of his or her severe head movements). The least amount of time a patient is under medical stabilization the better.
7. Document the patient's tolerance for procedures.
8. Note any complications during treatment (i.e., patient experienced a seizure that lasted for 1 minute).
9. Clearly document the procedures performed and those needed in future appointments.
10. Sign your name and professional title. If using software, type your first initial and last name followed by your professional title.

Many different conditions can be considered a developmental disability if they happened during development or are diagnosed when the person is less than 22 years old. Developmental disabilities include but are not limited to bipolar disorder, fetal

TABLE ■ 28–2   The Five Most Frequent Developmental Disabilities

Condition	Acronym	Prevalence	Treatment[a]
Intellectual disability	ID	Approximately 12/1,000 births	Education, behavioral intervention
Autism spectrum disorders	ASDs	Approximately 1/110 births	Education, social/behavioral interventions
Cerebral palsy	CP	Approximately 3.1/1,000 births	Education, behavioral intervention, therapy (physical, occupational, speech, etc.)
Down syndrome	DS	Approximately 1/800 births	Educational, behavioral intervention
Attention deficit hyperactivity disorder	ADHD	2.1 million of U.S. children ages 5–11 (2007 data)	Education, behavioral intervention

[a]Medications are usually taken to treat comorbid conditions instead of the disability itself.

alcohol syndrome, microcephaly, multiple sclerosis, Prader-Willi syndrome, schizophrenia, spina bifida, traumatic brain injuries, hearing loss, and vision impairment. It is important for providers to recognize that many disabilities do not manifest alone but are accompanied by one or more other disabilities and or complicating factors known as *comorbid* or *coexisting disabilities*.[7] An example of this is a patient who has an intellectual disability as well as a seizure disorder and schizophrenia. Many of the medications these patients take are not to treat the disability itself but the accompanying conditions such as seizures.[3,7]

The five most frequently seen and studied developmental disabilities are intellectual disability, autism spectrum disorders, cerebral palsy, down syndrome, and **attention deficit hyperactivity disorder** (Table 28–2 ■).

INTELLECTUAL DISABILITY

Characteristics and Common Oral Manifestations

Intellectual disability (ID) is a cognitive disability characterized by a below average intelligence quotient (IQ) test in addition to limitations in **activities of daily living (ADL)**.[3,7,8]

Causes of ID

There are several causes of intellectual disability. Chromosomal variations or defective genes are genetic causes of conditions such as Down syndrome. Physical or brain damage at the prenatal, neonatal, or postnatal stage can also be the causative factor.[8,9] Prenatal harm is typically caused by maternal influences such as malnutrition, exposure to excessive radiation, alcohol use resulting in fetal alcohol syndrome (FAS), and drug use.[3,7] In addition, infections in the mother such as rubella and syphilis can also be the cause. It is important to note that although there is some correlation of intellectual disability and certain infectious diseases, with the increase of early intervention, newborn screenings and vaccinations, ID has decreased

significantly.[3] Premature birth, insufficient oxygen, or a birth injury can also cause intellectual disability. Infections such as meningitis, toxins such as lead, a brain tumor, or a traumatic brain injury could cause intellectual disability in the postnatal stage (see Figure 28–1 ■). The earlier an insult occurs during development, the more severe the condition will be at the end.[3,7]

In addition to the causes just mentioned, ID can also be categorized into a variety of causative groups: cultural or familial, multifactor, psychosocial, and diagnosis unknown.[9] For example, a person whose parents have significantly limited intelligence, are indifferent to the child, or have rejected the child can result in intellectual disability. Sensory deprivation can also be implicated as a root of intellectual disability.[9]

Classification of Intellectual Disability

To be diagnosed with intellectual disability, a person must meet three criteria[9]: have a general learning deficiency; be unable to achieve age-appropriate milestones in language, motor, and social areas; and the first two criteria must be recognized during the developmental years, that is, before 18 years of age.[8] In addition to significant impairments in adaptive skills, communication, self-care, home living, use of community resources, self-direction, work, and leisure, a person whose IQ score is two standard deviations below the mean of a normal curve is considered to have intellectual disability. Average IQ is 100 and the standard deviation is 15; thus, two standard deviations below the mean is 70. It is important to note that there is a variance of ± 5 in assessing IQ by most barometric tests; therefore, 2 standard deviations below the mean could range from 65–75[7] (Table 28–3 ■) A person with an IQ score of 70 without the presence of any significant impairment in adaptive skills will not likely be diagnosed as having intellectual disability with an IQ of 70 alone.[7,8]

It has been found that approximately 12 infants of every 1,000 births have an intellectual disability.[10] Although ID could be a stand-alone diagnosis, it is frequently found to correspond

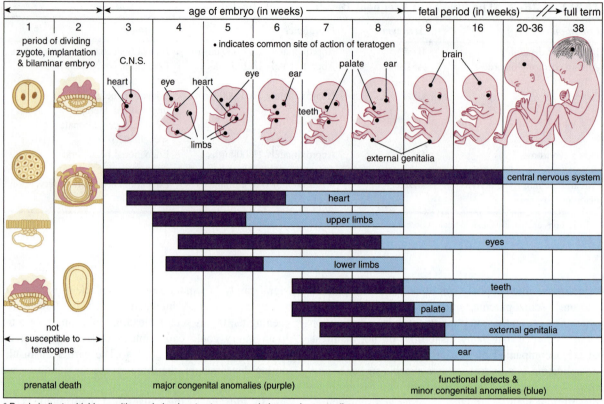

* Purple indicates highly sensitive periods when teratogens may induce major anomalies.

FIGURE ■ 28–1 Gestational diagram of critical periods during human development. http://www.cerebralpalsyinfo.com/CPFetal.html

with other disabilities such as seizure disorders, sensory impairments, psychological and behavioral disorders, and feeding difficulties in addition to the five most frequently seen and studied conditions mentioned earlier.[7,11,12]

Common Physical and Oral Characteristics

The cognitive characteristics of individuals with intellectual disability vary widely.[9] These persons learn visual and auditory discrimination slowly, and they have difficulty with abstract terminology and verbal cues. In addition, they may experience short-term memory deficiencies and difficulty predicting outcomes. These individuals also are easily distracted and may have perseveration habits.[12]

DID YOU KNOW ?

The word **perseveration** occurs when a person uncontrollably repeats a particular response, such as a word, phrase, gesture, or movement despite the absence or cessation of a stimulus.

A person with intellectual disability may have several oral manifestations including an increase in the prevalence of

periodontal diseases related to medications taken, malocclusion (Figure 28–2 ■), supernumerary teeth (Figure 28–3 ■), and poor oral hygiene. Oligodontia, delayed eruption, and enamel hypoplasia are more prevalent in these individuals (Figures 28–4 ■, 28–5 ■. Increases in damaging oral habits such as bruxism,

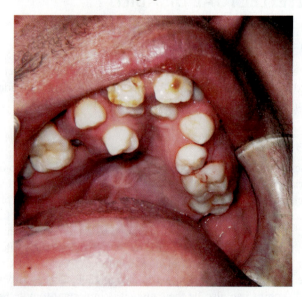

FIGURE ■ 28–2 Individual showing malocclusion of all teeth due to misalignment of tooth buds after cleft palate surgery

(*Source:* Courtesy of Elmer Gonzalez.)

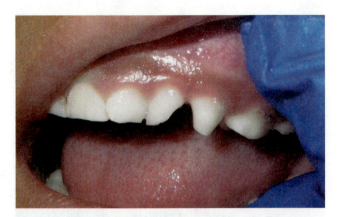

FIGURE ■ **28–3** Supernumerary lateral incisor completely erupted and malpositioned

(*Source:* Courtesy of Elmer Gonzalez.)

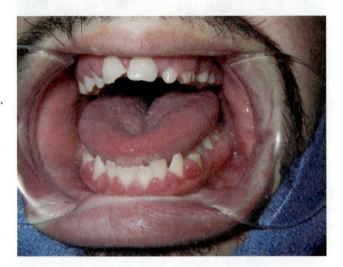

FIGURE ■ **28–4** Enamel hypoplasia seen in retained primary tooth #I

(*Source:* Courtesy of Elmer Gonzalez.)

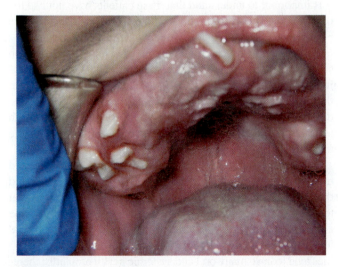

FIGURE ■ **28–5** Delayed eruption seen on a teenage patient with CP and seizure disorder

(*Source:* Courtesy of Elmer Gonzalez.)

impinging, dry/crusty lips, mouth breathing, tongue thrusting, biting lips, enamel erosion as a result of **gastroesophageal reflux disease (GERD)**, and **pica** (see Figures 28–6 ■ and 28–7 ■). See Figure 28–8 ■ showing teeth of a teenage patient with ID with very good oral hygiene.

DID YOU KNOW

Although the *number of untreated caries* is much higher in populations with intellectual disability, the *caries rate* is comparable to that of the general population with intellectual disability.

Intellectual disability cannot be cured with medications because no medications have been found to improve cognitive functioning. Patients with ID who currently take several medications usually take them for other complicating factors or comorbid disabilities, such as autism spectrum disorders (ASDs), attention deficit hyperactivity disorder (ADHD), seizures, or behavioral complications.[7,8]

DID YOU KNOW

Pica is a medical disorder characterized by an appetite for substances not fit as food or of no nutritional value.[12]

Preventive Strategies

Either the individual, caregivers, or both represent the most important strategy for preventive dental care in this population. Parents of children with ID or other disorders often are a great resource for behavioral techniques they use at home and that work well to decrease the individual's anxiety and increased cooperation in different areas of her or his life.[8] Incorporating these techniques can make a difference on how the patient tolerates the overall dental appointment. In addition, stressing the need for regular maintenance appointments and culturally sensitive oral health education is critical when delivering information to patients and caregivers.

The practitioner could use behavioral management techniques, such as tell-show-do and positive reinforcement, which work really well with children and adults who are afraid of the unknown (the dental office). Making the patient's first appointment as pleasant as possible could make the difference for the following recall appointments.[13]

Many patients with disabilities are seen at a hospital setting under general anesthesia because of their maladaptive behavior. When they return to a regular dental office, they usually exhibit the same or worse behavior than they did previously. Several desensitization appointments are needed to have the patient sit in the dental chair and then many more to make the patient

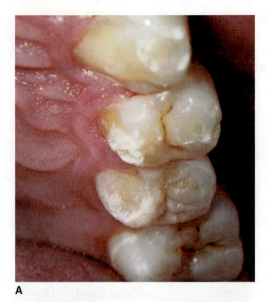

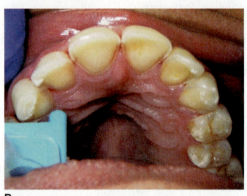

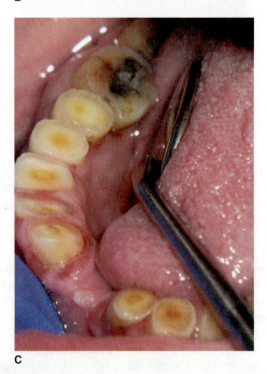

FIGURE ■ 28–6 A. Example of enamel fractures due to excessive tooth grinding, B. Erosion due to GI reflux, C. Severe bruxism.

(*Source:* Courtesy of Elmer Gonzalez.)

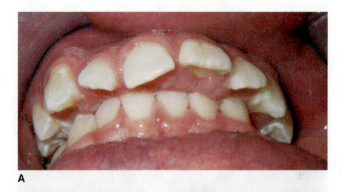

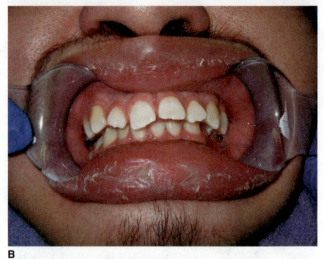

FIGURE ■ 28–7 A. Severe impinging is shown where mandibular teeth impinge onto the palate lingual to maxillary incisors, B. Same patient showing dry/crusty lips

(*Source:* Courtesy of Elmer Gonzalez.)

comfortable to accomplish a prophylaxis. Such behavior management techniques are important for new providers because these techniques require much time and patience from the provider. It is important to understand that these patients have not had the opportunity to learn how to cope with the stress of a dental office because they have usually been seen under general anesthesia.

The number of appointments needed for desensitization sometimes is a barrier because some providers are not willing to invest the necessary time on a single patient. However, the results experienced when a patient responds favorably to desensitization are worth the time spent. By the third or fourth appointment, the provider usually can determine whether the technique is working.

Another important measure is to develop individualized treatment plans that incorporate the individual's abilities and the role of the caregiver not only in the dental office but also at the patient's home; the importance of adequate dental hygiene among all populations, including special populations is crucial to overall well-being.[14] Populations with developmental disabilities tend to have many oral and systemic health problems; therefore, it is necessary to have well-prepared and knowledgeable dental staff to educate caregivers so that they can understand the oral-systemic link and address their patient's oral health needs.

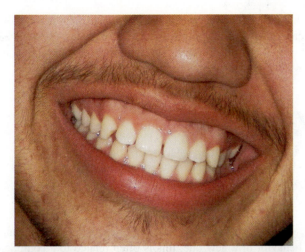

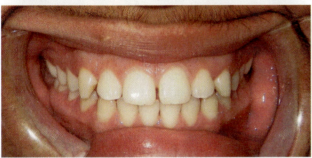

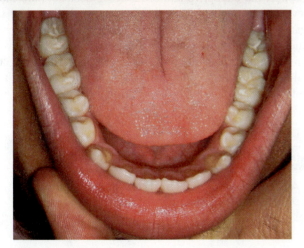

FIGURE ■ 28–8 A,B,C. Teenage patient with optimum oral hygiene

(*Source:* Courtesy of Elmer Gonzalez.)

It is also important to ensure that sufficient use of preventive aids such as fluorides are being used in the office and are recommended to the patient's caregiver(s).

DID YOU KNOW ?

Oligodontia is the absence of one or several teeth. **Anodontia** is characterized by the absence of all teeth. These conditions are commonly seen in people with disabilities.

AUTISM SPECTRUM DISORDERS (ASDS)

Characteristics and Common Oral Manifestations

Autism is a term used to describe a number of neuro developmental disorders commonly known as *pervasive developmental disorder*s (*PDD*), which begin before the age of 3 and last throughout a person's lifetime.[15,16] The symptoms and severity vary widely in people diagnosed with autism spectrum disorders. ASDs are neurodevelopmental disorders characterized by the presence or absence of behaviors in three different areas: social reciprocity, communication, and repetitive behaviors.[7,17] Children diagnosed within the spectrum are affected in different ways, and their disability varies from mild to severe.[15] **Autism** is a diagnosis within the ASDs that affects communication, social/behavioral, and intellectual functioning.[18,19]

Common Causes of ASDs

The causes of ASDs are not clearly specified; however, associations have been made between autism and highly intelligent parents.[7] In addition, a parent with autism or parents who already have a child with autism are more likely to have other children diagnosed within the spectrum.[15] Other possible causes are medications such as valproic acid, and thalidomide taken during pregnancy.[15]

Classification of ASD

Of every 1,000 births in the United States, 3.4 babies will be diagnosed with autism.[20] Current data suggest that in average of 1 in 110 children is diagnosed with autism or other ASDs.[15,16] Some diagnoses within the spectrum include autism, Asperger's disorder, pervasive developmental, childhood disintegrative disorder, and Rett disorder. ASDs are associated with intellectual disability and other conditions such as learning disabilities; epilepsy; tic and sleep disorders; and psychiatric conditions.[7,16,17] Some of the associated conditions with ASDs are treated with behaviorally based therapy and medications; however, medications are used only to treat target symptoms or behaviors not the ASD itself.[7]

Common Physical and Oral Manifestations

A person with autism can appear aloof, distant, or detached and does not respond to common verbal or social cues as expected.[18] Children who are diagnosed with ASDs commonly experience sleep disorders, causing difficulty for family members and caregivers because daytime behavior could be impacted by the patient's sleep patterns.[8] In addition, hyperactivity, inattention, perseveration, and the tendency to become frustrated quickly are common symptoms in children with ASDs.[18] Management of associated disorders and challenging behaviors is best accomplished by using a combination of medications and behavioral therapies. Patients with ASDs are also likely to exhibit externalizing and internalizing behaviors, which are often treated with psychotropic medications. *Externalizing* refers to behaviors such as aggression, impulsivity, agitation, and irritability. *Internalizing behaviors*, on the other hand, include anxiety, depression, perseveration, and behaviors that produce some self-stimulation, such as rubbing hands, picking the skin, and biting lips.[7,8]

Rates of periodontal diseases and caries in persons with autism correspond to those of the general population. As with all persons, a soft food diet high in sugar without proper dental self-care increases the likelihood of caries and periodontal disease. An increase in damaging oral habits, such as bruxism, biting ones' lips, regurgitation, rumination, and pica are also found in patients with autism. These habits may be self-coping mechanisms, exploration, or one of many repetitive behaviors seen in individuals with autism.

DID YOU KNOW ?

Rumination occurs in both animals and humans. In humans, it is known as an eating disorder characterized by the regurgitation of recently ingested food.

Preventive Strategies

When the dental professional provides oral hygiene instruction, the patient's learning level should be assessed to ensure the instruction is being delivered at the appropriate level.[18] This approach helps the individual understand the importance of and need for proper self-care. A person with autism can be sensitive to changes and environment; therefore, consistency and structure in dental appointments and instruction are very important to increase cooperation and prevent overstimulation.

Several appointments are often necessary to help desensitize an anxious patient and accustom him or her to the environment and dental team. In addition, children and adults with ASDs have heightened issues regarding sensitivity to noise, touch, and odors as well as water aversion.[8] In these cases, environmental modifications are usually effective in gaining compliance and cooperation during the dental appointment.

In some cases, the use of medical stabilization devices is necessary to help the patient tolerate the procedure. A papoose board, for example, offers not only the advantage of keeping a moving patient still but, most important, serves as a comforting device for some patients with autism and other ASDs. In some cases, positive reinforcement is all a patient needs to improve behavior.

Although positive reinforcement works well in children with ASDs, educating parents and caregivers on how to reward good behavior is important. Patients with disabilities, especially those with autism, often have unrestricted diets. Parents and caregivers should reinforce good behavior with sugar-free and other healthy foods instead of giving them sweets and sodas and unhealthy snacks. Using healthy reinforces helps not only with improved compliance but most important helps prevent tooth decay and systemic complications (i.e., diabetes, obesity, heart disease). Nonedible rewards, such as going for walks, going to a movie, and having computer time can also be used.

DID YOU KNOW ?

Medical stabilization refers to any type of restraint. It should be utilized for the least amount of time possible and only for patient's safety and comfort.

When a patient with ASD experiences an abrupt change in behavior or a new one, this is often related to a complicating factor of an existing condition.[7,8] Dental providers and parents must be aware of existing behaviors to rule out symptoms causing new behaviors.[8] Some common medical conditions that could exacerbate existing behaviors or cause new ones are dental pain, sinus infections, otitis media and other related ear infections, constipation, stomach aches, headaches, mouth sores, urinary infections, and trauma caused by seizures or self-injurious behaviors.

Often when patients are older, especially during adolescence, the disruptive and challenging behaviors are more prevalent and severe.[8] This presents a new challenge for the treating provider and if behavior becomes a problem, referring patients to a specialized clinic where more behavioral interventions are employed could be necessary to benefit the patients' oral health and ensure their safety and that of the patient and dental team.

DID YOU KNOW ?

A papoose board or any medical stabilization device should only be used for patient's comfort and safety.

The use of a mouth guard should be considered for use by patients who exhibit self-injurious behavior or bruxism as long as the patient is able to tolerate it.

CEREBRAL PALSY

Common Causes, Classification, Characteristics, and Common Oral Manifestations

Cerebral palsy (CP) is a nonprogressive, neuromuscular disorder caused by damage to the immature brain. CP does not refer to a specific disease but to an injury to the brain's motor portion. This injury can be associated with uncontrolled body movements, seizures, balance problems, sensory dysfunction, and intellectual disability.[21–24]

CP is seen in 3.1 of 1,000 births.[10] Maternal diabetes, hypertension, infections such as herpes, Rh factor incompatibility, excess radiation, and drugs taken by the mother also contribute to CP as can oxygen deprivation, birth injury, and prolonged or difficult labor during the prenatal and neonatal stages. Postnatally, trauma, brain tumors, infections such as encephalitis and meningitis, and toxins such as lead and hydrocarbons can be related to CP.[25]

Cerebral palsy is classified according to severity (mild, moderate, or severe), the area of brain involved, and the resultant disorder.[7,24] The common types of CP are spastic, diskinetic, athetoid, ataxic, and mixed.[23,24] Spastic CP is the most common and is further classified according to the limbs affected. *Spastic hemiplegia* refers to one side of the body affected (i.e., right arm and right leg). In the case of right-side hemiplegia, the left side of the brain is involved because the brain controls the opposite side of the body. *Spastic diplegia,* which is most frequently associated with prematurity, affects the legs more that the arms. *Spastic quadriplegia* involves the four limbs of the body in addition to the muscles of the mouth, tongue, pharynx, and trunk. Patients with spastic quadriplegia are more involved medically and often have other coexisting disabilities such as ID, sensory impairments, and seizures. *Diskinetic CP* involves the entire body and is characterized by abnormalities in muscle tone and involuntary muscle contractions. *Ataxic CP* is characterized by abnormalities of movement of the body in relation to space, which is known as *ataxia;* patients with this type can have increased or decreased muscle tone.[7,26] *Mixed CP* is characterized by more than one type of CP (motor pattern) equally without one predominating.

Common Physical and Oral Characteristics

Approximately 50% to 70% of people with CP also have intellectual disability. The remaining individuals have normal or superior intelligence.[7,24] Roughly 30% of people with CP have epilepsy.[24] Most patients with CP have visual, hearing, and speech defects.[22,24] Their speech can be slow because of an inability to control muscles involved in speech and mastication. A swallowing dysfunction can also lead to frequent drooling. Constant involuntary movements and rooting reflex can make eating difficult.[23,27] An inadequate cough reflex can increase choking, coughing, and aspiration.[24]

Preventive Strategies

Periodontal diseases and caries are both more widespread in this population.[23,24] Enamel hypoplasia, mouth breathing, and food retention in the mouth all contribute to the increased rates of periodontal disease and caries.[21,22] In addition, physical constraints of the patient with CP can make proper oral hygiene difficult. For these reasons, the patient or caregiver should use a unique, individualized dental care plan. A wide-handled, powered toothbrush can assist these patients (Figure 28–9 ■). A manual toothbrush with an enlarged handle, elastic cuff, or

small strap attached to the brush could help individuals who do not have a high level of fine muscle control.[28] Modifications shown in Figures 28–10 ■ through 28–12 ■ may be used with manual toothbrushes. A regimen of daily fluoride treatments

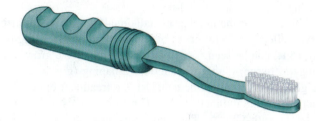

FIGURE ■ 28–9 A wide-handled, grip toothbrush

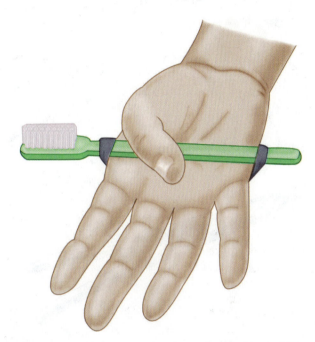

FIGURE ■ 28–10 Toothbrush attached to hand with rubber band

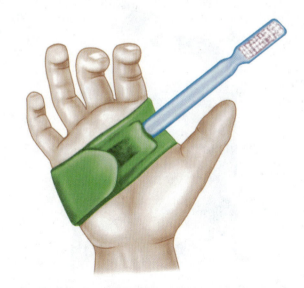

FIGURE ■ 28–11 Toothbrush attached to hand with Velcro

along with individualized, personal, and caregiver-directed plaque control measures, such as the use of a floss threader (Figure 28–13 ■), are some strategies (Figure 28–14 ■) shows an approach of how to sit behind the wheelchair to provide assistance with toothbrushing. These modifications can help reduce the incidence of these oral diseases.

Because of the number of individuals with CP who also have epilepsy, several cases of gingival hyperplasia (Figure 28–15 ■) can be seen.[24,29] In cases with excessive growth of gingival tissue, gingival reduction/reshaping (gingivectomy or gingiviplasty) could be considered a treatment option. An increase in the number of class II malocclusions is found in patients with CP.[23,27] The malocclusion is due to skeletal

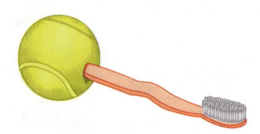

FIGURE ■ **28–12** Toothbrush inserted into tennis ball

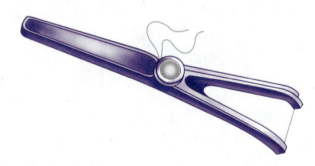

FIGURE ■ **28–13** Dental floss holder

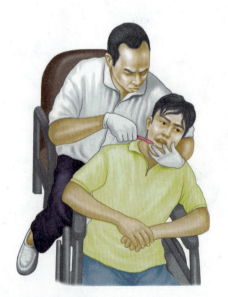

FIGURE ■ **28–14** Sitting behind patient's wheelchair

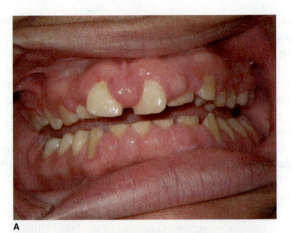

A

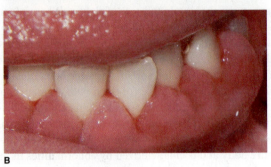

B

FIGURE ■ **28–15** Gingival hyperplasia
(*Source:* Courtesy of Elmer Gonzalez.)

problems, not just tooth misalignment or the common habit of tongue thrusting.[24] The increased rate of temporomandibular joint (TMJ) disorder corresponds with a high rate of bruxism.[23,24,27] Severe bruxism can cause wear of tooth facets, tooth fractures, and possibly pulpal exposure of teeth. The loss of the vertical dimension of the posterior teeth, seen in bruxism, is thought to be a large contributing factor to TMJ problems. The bruxism experienced by patients with CP often is attributed to a primitive rooting reflex. If reasonable for the individual, orthodontics could be considered. Patients with cerebral palsy also tend to have hyperactive bite and gag reflexes.[23] If the gag reflex becomes a problem for the dental provider, keeping the patient in a semiupright position with chin down usually relieves the reflex and allows the practitioner to perform treatment. In cases of CP, a mouthguard could help reduce the effects of the prolonged bruxing and clenching if it is considered to be safe for a patient to wear one. It is also important to note that due to the increased gag reflex (hyper gag) commonly experienced by patients with CP, taking impressions to make a mouthguard is often not possible.

DOWN SYNDROME

Characteristics and Classifications

Down syndrome (DS) is a congenital genetic disorder that occurs in 1 of every 800 births in the United States; the person affected is found to have an extra 21st chromosome.[30–36]

Patients with DS are commonly thought to be happy and loving individuals.

Three types of chromosomal anomalies can lead to Down syndrome. Trisomy 21, which accounts for 95% of cases, results from nondisjunction during meiosis I and can occur during meiosis II. Translocation Down syndrome, which accounts for 4% of cases, occurs when the long arm of an extra chromosome 21 attaches to chromosome 14, 21, or 22. Mosaicism affects 1% of cases; it is characterized from nondisjunction during mitosis of the fertilized egg; in this case, only some have the defect.[7] Medical complications are similar among the three groups of Down syndrome.[7] Nearly all persons with Down syndrome have some level of intellectual disability.

DID YOU KNOW

Trisomy 21 refers to an extra chromosome 21, which results in Down syndrome.

Individuals with Down syndrome have specific orofacial characteristics: a nose with a flat, broad bridge; low-set ears; slanted, almond-shaped eyes; lack of a supraorbital ridge, which contributes to the broad, short head; and absent or reduced maxillary sinuses[34,36,37] (see Figure 28–16 ■).

About 40% of persons with Down syndrome have mitral valve prolapse.[28,33–37] People with Down syndrome have some skeletal malformations that affect their overall oral function. Midface hypoplasia is the most common malformation. As a result of the absent or reduced maxillary sinus, enlarged tongue (macroglossia), underdeveloped midfacial bones, and shortened palate, many with this condition suffer from sleep apnea and underbite[38] (see Figure 28–17 ■). An increase in upper respiratory tract infections is due to an impaired immune system.[33] Signs of Alzheimer's disease and dementia begin around the age of 35.[33,36] Speech, hearing, and vision problems also are common. These patients tend to be below average height, obese, and sexually underdeveloped.[34,36]

Patients with Down syndrome have severe, early onset of periodontal disease attributable to a decreased immune response and xerostomia.[28,29,32] Proper oral hygiene performed at an early age by both the patient and caregivers is imperative. Individuals with Down syndrome experience lower rate of decay compared with the general population,[29] which is attributed to the delayed eruption of the teeth and open proximal contacts. Underdevelopment of the midface gives way to a large number of class III malocclusions (see Figures 28–18 ■ through 28–21 ■).[28,29,32] **Macroglossia** (enlarged tongue) and a fissured, protruding tongue are evident as a result of the forward position of the mandible and slightly opened mouth.[28,32] Variable tooth morphology and short roots can also be present, and increased bruxism is also common among patients with Down syndrome.[32] Other oral manifestations common to this population are congenitally missing teeth and retained primary teeth (Figures 28–18 through 28–22 ■).

Preventive Strategies

Use of fluoride treatments and saliva substitutes could decrease xerostomia for the patient contending with this syndrome. Oral hygiene including dental cleaning in these patients could be

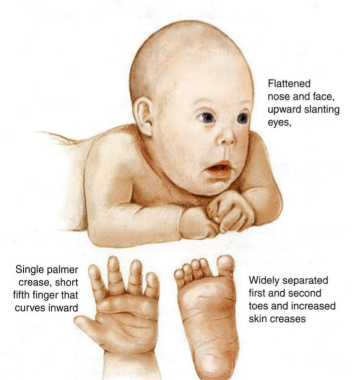

Flattened nose and face, upward slanting eyes,

Single palmer crease, short fifth finger that curves inward

Widely separated first and second toes and increased skin creases

FIGURE ■ **28–16** Physical features of Down syndrome.
(*Source:* The Lucinda Foundation.)

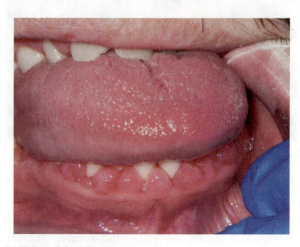

FIGURE ■ **28–17** Macroglossia
(*Source:* Courtesy of Elmer Gonzalez.)

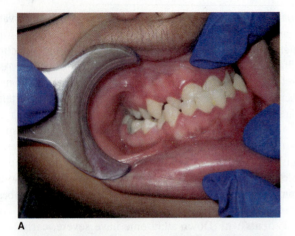

A

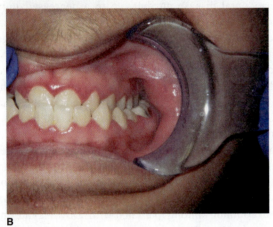

B

FIGURE ■ **28–18** Class III malocclusion

(*Source:* Courtesy of Elmer Gonzalez.)

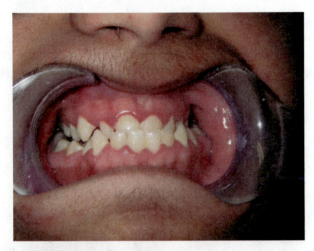

FIGURE ■ **28–19** Class III malocclusion

(*Source:* Courtesy of Elmer Gonzalez.)

challenging because of the enlarged tongue and small ovoid teeth (Figure 28–22 ■). Realization that patients with Down syndrome are many times afraid of the dental chair tilting back is important. Positive reinforcement and assurance is critical with these patients. Proper oral hygiene instruction to parents

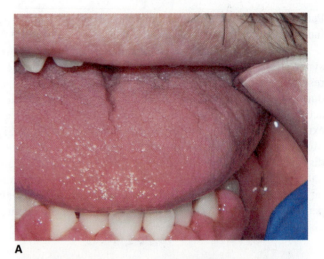

A

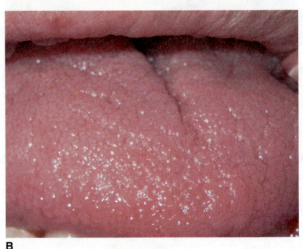

B

FIGURE ■ **28–20** Deep fissured tongue

(*Source:* Courtesy of Elmer Gonzalez.)

and caregivers at an early age and sensitive to cultural values is necessary for better outcomes.

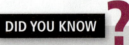

DID YOU KNOW

Although it has been reported that patients with DS have a low incidence of dental caries, without proper oral hygiene, these patients are at the same risk of developing caries as the general population after all teeth have erupted.

In addition, patients take medications at set schedules during the day, and performing oral hygiene after taking medications usually promotes better oral health and decreases the amount of sugars in contact with the teeth. Whenever possible, it is also advisable to instruct parents and caregivers to opt for sugar-free medications.[31] Although no definitive preventive measure can be taken with the anatomic development, educating the patient and caregiver(s) on known oral issues and management strategies is best.

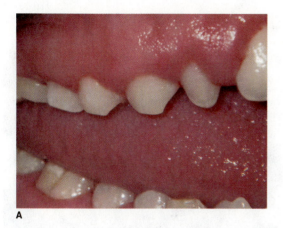

A

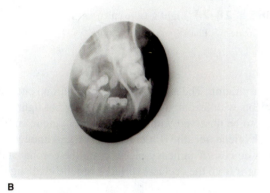

B

FIGURE ■ 28–21 A Congenitally missing #11 and retained #I B. Congenitally missing #28 and 29; retained primary # S,T

(*Source:* Courtesy of Elmer Gonzalez.)

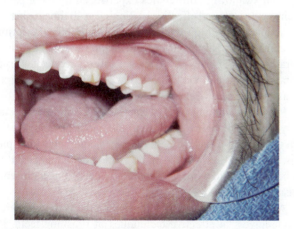

FIGURE ■ 28–22 Small ovoid teeth seen in patients with DS

(*Source:* Courtesy of Elmer Gonzalez.)

ATTENTION DEFICIT AND HYPERACTIVITY DISORDER (ADHD)

Population Statistics and Characteristics

Attention deficit and hyperactivity disorder (ADHD) is one of the most prevalent neurobehavioral disorders of childhood; it affects approximately 2.1 million of school-age children

between the ages of 5 to 11 and 2.4 million between the ages of 12 to 17.[7,8,39] The disorder is characterized by levels of impulsivity, inattention, hyperactivity, and distractibility, causing behavioral problems in school, at home, and in other socially related situations affecting the overall child's[7,8,39] adaptive functioning. Symptoms of ADHD can continue through adolescence and into adulthood.[8,40]

Classification of ADHD

Diagnosis of ADHD is mainly based on ruling out symptoms rather than identifying those related to the condition. Specialists evaluate individuals by collecting questionnaires, conducting interviews, and obtaining rating scales from parents, pediatrician, and teachers. After diagnosis is confirmed, ADHD can be classified in three catergories. First—ADHD predominanty inattentive; in this category, children are easily distracted, have a difficult time following routines, forget things quickly and experience a difficult time staying focused. Second ADHD, predominantly hyperactive/impulsive; children here experience difficulty sitting still, tend to talk a lot and disrupt others. Young children jump, run, climb, and are restless most of the time. If the person also experiences impulsivity then the behavior observed is that of a person constantly interrupting others, grabbing things from people, and speaking out of turn. People who present the hyperactive/impulsive also tend to have more accidents compared to people in the other categories. The third caregory is the ADHD combined where people present symptoms from the first two categories.[39]

The combined type is the most common and studied subtype; a child must have six or more symptoms of both the inattentive an the hyperactive-impulsive type.[7,8,39,40]

Common Physical and Oral Characteristics

ADHD could be a result of other conditions such as traumatic brain injury, premature birth, low birth weight, seizure disorders, and fetal alcohol syndrome.[8,39] Many coexisting conditions, such as learning disabilities, conduct disorders, defiant behavior, anxiety, depression, bipolar disorder, and Tourette syndrome, are identified with ADHD.[8,40]

Children with ADHD have no clear-cut identifiable physical and oral manifestations other than those present in the general population. Poor oral hygiene is seen in those who are less compliant with parents and caregivers. Carious lesions (Figure 28–23 ■) fusion, and supernumerary teeth are comparable to those of the general population.

Preventive Strategies

Patients diagnosed with ADHD might present some challenges in the dental setting. Usually modifying the environment appropriately, establishing routines, and following structured schedules are recommended for a more positive outcome.[8] Scheduling the patient early in the morning and keeping the

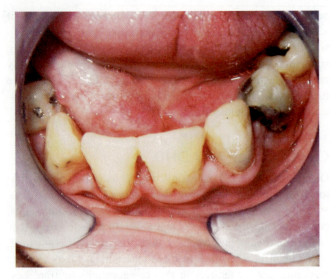

FIGURE ■ 28–23 Fused mandibular incisors
(*Source:* Courtesy of Elmer Gonzalez.)

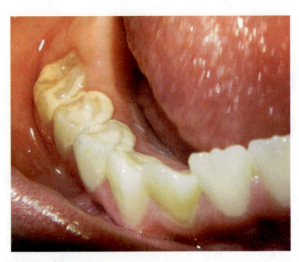

FIGURE ■ 28–24 Light g-tube calculus
(*Source:* Courtesy of Elmer Gonzalez.)

appointment as short as possible is often beneficial, especially for children with hyperactive-impulsive type ADHD.

Behavioral techniques such as tell-show-do and positive reinforcement can be beneficial as long as these are consistent every time and throughout the dental visit. Children should be rewarded for positive behavior whereas negative behavior should be ignored or otherwise used as a way to identify possible causes of discomfort in the dental setting. Oral hygiene instruction (OHI) should be brief and consistent because children with ADHD have minimal attention span and do not stay focused for a long time.

Educating parents and caregivers on the importance of positive reinforcement is crucial. Parents/caregivers should understand that a reward for positive behavior is not candy, soft drinks, or something that might jeopardize the child's oral systemic health but something that interests the child and should be changed every so often to prevent the child from getting bored.

AN OVERLAPPING POPULATION: CHILDREN AND ADULTS WITH GASTROSTOMY TUBES AND ASPIRATION RISK

Many patients from all groups and all disabilities have a gastrostomy tube (g-tube) placed in their stomach. A g-tube is used for many different reasons, including but not limited to aspiration risk, swallowing difficulties, and poor nutrition. The procedure could be either temporary or permanent.

Dental providers encounter many challenges when treating patients who use g-tubes. The fact that the patient is not able to swallow and breathe normally is a complication before treatment starts. Swallowing and breathing difficulties are a problem because patients might not be able to breathe well while instrumenting or using the cavitron. Patients are at increased

risk of aspiration. The amount of calculus buildup encountered on patients with feeding tubes is often heavy but light amounts could also be observed with optimum oral hygiene and tighter dental hygiene recalls (Figure 28–24 ■). Although g-tube calculus comes off in heavy pieces from the coronal surfaces, removing it from the occlusal surfaces is quite challenging.

Preventive Strategies

The use of ultrasonics is often necessary to remove all calculus effectively and quickly; however, the aspiration risk complications and swallowing difficulties experienced by these patients requires extensive and effective suctioning at all times using both the suction and the high-volume evacuation (HVE). Performing a cleaning using only hand instrumentation reduces the risk of aspirating water; however, it does not entirely reduce the risk of aspiration because blood and calculus flakes could be aspirated just as easy as water if proper evacuation is not employed.

Providers working with people with disabilities, especially those with challenging behaviors and medical complications such as aspiration risk, seizure disorders, and behavioral problems, should always work with a certified dental assistant who has been trained to work with these populations as a preventive measure.

A preventive measure for this population is to train parents and caregivers in effective techniques of brushing teeth. It is also important to increase awareness on how aspiration pneumonia could be sometimes prevented by keeping these patients' teeth as plaque and calculus free as possible. Many caregivers/parents are afraid of brushing the patient's teeth because they think that the mechanical removal of plaque in addition to the toothpaste and water on the toothbrush will cause aspiration pneumonia. In order to prevent this, is crucial to instruct parents and caregivers to refrain from using toothpaste because it is not necessary to disturb plaque and remove it from teeth. The only thing necessary to prevent buildup on patients using g-tubes, is a toothbrush and more frequent brushing. Some of these patients have a suction machine at home which should be used to suction debris while brushing. It is helpful to keep in mind that even if these preventive steps are followed, many patients will still present with moderate amounts of calculus, especially on occlusal surfaces due to the lack of chewing and grinding food.

DID YOU KNOW?

Although not reported in the literature, the use of dental sealants for children who use a g-tube could be useful not only to protect against dental caries but also to protect against calculus adhesion and retention on the occlusal surfaces because sealants tend to seal the deep groves and fissures where calculus builds and is retained easily in these patients.

PREVENTIVE OUTREACH FOR PEOPLE WITH DISABILITIES

Considering the link between oral health and total health, optimum dental hygiene is crucial for people's well-being, even more so among populations with systemic conditions such as diabetes and people with physical, mental, and developmental disabilities.[14,41]

Understanding that individuals with developmental disabilities deserve not only to be treated with dignity and respect but also to receive appropriate health care including oral hygiene is crucial.[14] Adequate oral hygiene is important for people with disabilities because a healthy mouth reflects the body's overall well-being[42]; it enables individuals to eat, speak, socialize, and—most importantly—to feel good about themselves.[43]

Answers to Questions Commonly Asked by Caregivers

How long does it take to perform oral hygiene?

Providing oral hygiene for the individuals you care for takes only about 6 minutes: 2 to 3 minutes for brushing and 2 to 3 minutes for flossing, depending on the patient's cooperation and abilities. Performing these tasks consistently on a daily basis could prevent many oral and systemic complications in addition to improving your client's overall health and self-esteem.

Where and when should I brush my client's teeth?

There is no set place to perform oral hygiene and privacy is not a concern for brushing teeth. Your client's teeth should be brushed where he or she feels comfortable. The bathroom is recommended but is not strictly necessary. If your client is more comfortable in the bedroom or living room that is where teeth should be brushed. Adequate lighting must be available to see well inside your client's mouth.

Every individual should have an individualized oral hygiene plan developed in conjunction with a dental professional. It is important to brush your client's teeth at least twice per day for 2 minutes each time. Dental professionals usually recommend brushing once in the morning and once before bedtime; however, when working with an individual who is challenging, assessing the time of day your client cooperates better to brush and floss effectivelyis very important.

Another important aspect to keep in mind is to brush after your client has taken medications. Many medications have high sugar content, which could be very damaging to the teeth. For people who have a swallowing deficit, group homes often use sugary dietary supplements such as Ensure© and various methods to thicken liquids, both of which can put the teeth in danger of developing decay if their teeth are not brushed right after taking medications.

Can I use sponges (Toothettes) instead of a toothbrush?

Although sponges are sometimes used in hospitals, their use is not recommended instead of a toothbrush. Sponges could aid in removing food debris and pouches from an individual's cheek, but the most appropriate way to remove plaque from the teeth and gums is by brushing with a soft-bristle toothbrush.

Do I need to floss my client's teeth?

Yes, teeth should be flossed at least once a day. The time of the day is not important so long as it is done. If behavior is a problem, noting that on the client's notes is important so the issue can be addressed by the individual's team and with the dental professional on your client's next visit.

Should I stop brushing if my client's gums bleed when I brush or floss?

When someone's gums are inflamed and infected, bleeding is likely to occur with any stimulation, especially brushing and flossing. If you notice bleeding while you are brushing your client's teeth, continue to brush gently as recommended. Bleeding should stop after a week or two if you are consistent with your client's oral hygiene. As your client's gums start to heal and inflammation decreases, bleeding will decrease and/or stop.

Bleeding gums generally a sign of gingivitis, which is inflammation of the gums caused by undisturbed plaque buildup and poor oral hygiene; it requires only improved oral hygiene to heal. The best method to care for the problem is to brush and floss.

If you are brushing and flossing your client's teeth as recommended and bleeding persists for more than 7 to 10 days, contact your dental professional for advice and a dental consultation. In addition, if your client is experiencing oral pain, contact the dental professional as soon as possible.

What can I do if my client is difficult to brush and floss?

First make sure that you and your client will be safe when you perform any type of oral hygiene. Working with an individual who has challenging behaviors is of great concern, especially if you are not very familiar with your client. If you are new working with the individual, make sure to have another caregiver help you to brush your client's teeth until she or he has become familiar with you and the oral hygiene procedures.

Often it is helpful to utilize techniques such as the "tell-show-do" approach to help your client understand and see what it is going to be done. Start slowly, and be patient with your client. Introduce the toothbrush, explain what it does, show how to use it, and then it may be helpful to hand it to your client and have her or him show you how to do it. Continue with the floss and follow the same technique. As the procedure becomes familiar, your client should become more cooperative. The key word is consistency, time and time again.

It is always good to give your client positive reinforcement for performing procedures well. In addition, many individuals who have disabilities, especially children and adults who have autism, have difficulties in following a routine; therefore, setting a routine time and place where your client is relaxed could be very comforting and help decrease behavioral concerns.

Do I need to take my client to dental appointments regularly?

You should make sure your client visits his or her dentist once a year for routine examinations and the dental hygienist at least twice per year unless the professional suggests a tighter recall to ensure your client's oral hygiene. Seeing your client's dental professional and performing optimum oral hygiene at home will help your client have a healthy life.

What do I do if my client has false teeth?

Teaching your client to remove the dentures every night before bedtime is important. If the client is capable of brushing his or her own dentures, guide him or her through the process. If the client is unable to do so, you should do the brushing every night. Use of regular toothpaste or no toothpaste at all is acceptable. No bleach or other cleaning solution should be used to clean because the denture the material is delicate and can be damaged easily.

To prevent damage, always line the sink with towels to protect the dentures should you drop them on the sink. After brushing the dentures, make sure to put them in denture solution or water to soak overnight.

My client's jaw gets tired easily when I am brushing his or her teeth; what can I do?

Many people have jaw problems or have difficulty holding their mouth open for a long period of time. To effectively brush your client's teeth, you need to see inside the mouth clearly, but this is difficult if the individual cannot keep his or her mouth open. To assist your client with oral hygiene, use a soft mouth prop approved by the organization where you work. A soft mouth prop serves as a supportive device to help your client keep the mouth open and to assist you providing appropriate oral hygiene.

Should I praise my client with sweets when she or he does well?

Praising your client with sweets, sugary drinks, or cigarettes is not recommended. Sodas have a high content of acid and are not recommended even if they are sugar free. Providing such items could result in compliance but can increase the likelihood the she or he will develop caries and gum disease and can cause the client's overall systemic health to deteriorate, especially by developing diabetes and heart disease. If you really need to offer candy, choose sugar-free products.

Give healthy snacks such as vegetables and fresh fruit. Use other options, such as taking your client for a ride or a walk, as rewards to reinforce positive behavior. Be creative and always consider your client's well-being; after all, you can be your client's best advocate and friend in caring for his or her overall health.

SUMMARY

Although some patients who have developmental disabilities are able to brush their own teeth and can often do so with support and encouragement from dental personnel, intimately involving the patient's primary caregiver in oral hygiene instruction is important. Personalized techniques can be demonstrated and explained to suit each patient's needs. Dental professionals and caregivers may need to alter their methods of performing oral examinations or dental prophylaxis for some patients who have developmental disabilities. See Figure 28–25 ■ for some examples of alternative positioning.

Individuals who have developmental disabilities face many challenges unique to their condition. To provide care that reflects the unique needs of these individuals, the dental team must understand the underlying condition and ensure the patient's comfort and safety before any treatment begins.

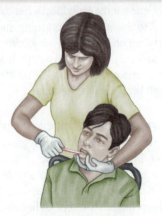

FIGURE ■ 28–25 Caregiver standing behind patient and cradling head to support and perform toothbrushing.

PRACTICAL CONSIDERATIONS

Understanding that people who have disabilities should be treated with dignity and respect is crucial for all dental providers. One way to do this is by utilizing people first language. When speaking to or about a person with a disability, refer to that person using words that identify him or her instead of referring to particular disability they have; they are a human beings, patients, and family members, and should not be referred to using a disability category; refer to people who are elderly, not the elderly. Many people with disabilities have expressed concern because of the negative connotations that refer to them as a category or disease rather than individual human beings. **People first language** puts the person first, the disability second.[44]

Each disability has a unique characteristic and some oral conditions for many people with it. Dental providers must recognize the common conditions but also understand that each patient should be treated on an individual basis without making any assumptions as a result of the patient's disability. For example, a patient with autism is very different from another patient with autism because this particular condition does not have specific common oral manifestations. On the other hand, down syndrome is a condition that has some common oral manifestations, such as short roots, oval small teeth, and congenitally missing teeth.

Best practices for treating patients with disabilities include offering a family-centered care approach. This basically means that consideration of family values, attitudes, and input should guide treatment.[45] In other words, family-centered care is a model in which dental providers and families work together to achieve the same goal or outcome, in this case, the oral health of the patient. Dental providers who are sensitive to families' values and opinions should expect more desired outcomes.

SELF-STUDY QUESTIONS

1. Down syndrome is a common disability caused by teratogens consumed by the mother during the early postnatal period.

   a. Both statements are true.

   b. The first statement is true, but the second is false.

   c. The first statement is false, but second one is true.

   d. Both statements are false.

   Rationale: Down syndrome is caused by a congenital genetic disorder in which chromosome 21 usually has an extra chromosome known as *trisomy 21*.

2. The period during fetal development when teeth are most susceptible to anomalies is between

   a. 4 ½ to 9 weeks

   b. 6 ¾ weeks to full term

   c. 6 ¾ to 16 weeks

   d. 4 ½ weeks to full term

   Rationale: Teeth are more susceptible to teratogens and other changes during weeks 6 ¾ to full term.

3. People first language describes what a person is, not what a person has; in other words, it places the person first and the disability second.

   a. Both statements are true.

   b. The first statement is true, but the second is false.

   c. The first statement is false, but the second is true.

   d. Both statements are false.

   Rationale: Both statements are true because people first language takes into consideration that a disability is part of nature; therefore, individuals with disabilities are first and foremost human beings who have a disability.

4. High risk factors for intellectual disability include prematurity, low birth weight, and low socioeconomic status to mention only some; therefore, infants at risk for ID should not receive early intervention

   a. Both statements are true.

   b. The first statement is true, but the second is false.

   c. The first statement is false, but the second is true.

   d. Both statements are false.

   Rationale: Early intervention is crucial for children at risk or who have a disability. The sooner they receive intervention, the better are the chances to decrease the negative outcomes.

5. Some common oral findings of many disorders including convulsive disorders are:

   a. Dental fractures, oral trauma, and avulsed and missing teeth

   b. Small fingers and toes, short nose, slanted eyes

   c. Gingival hyperplasia (Dilantin)

   d. Both A and C

   Rationale: All of the options are oral findings of developmental disabilities and convulsive disorders except b, which indicates physical characteristics of Down syndrome.

REFERENCES

1. Calderone, J. (1996). *Memorandum: Functional definitions.* Albuquerque, NM: New Mexico Department of Health.

2. National Institutes of Health. *Oral health care for people with developmental disabilities.* Bethesda, MD: National Institutes of Health, National Oral Health Information Clearinghouse.

3. Centers for Disease Control and Prevention. (2011). *Intellectual disability.* Retrieved February 20, 2011, from http://www.cdc.gov/ncbddd/dd/ddmr.htm.

4. Administration for Families and Children, Administration on Developmental Disabilities. (n.d.) *Fact sheet.* Retrieved October 16, 2006, from http://www.acf.hhs.gov/programs/add/.

5. U.S. Public Health Service. (2001). *Closing the gap: A national blueprint for improving the health of individuals with mental retardation. Report of the Surgeon General's conference on health disparities and mental retardation.* Washington, DC: U.S. Government Printing Office.

6. Commission on Dental Accreditation. (2004). Accreditation standards for dental education programs. Standard 2-26. (Adopted July 2004.) American Dental Association.

7. Batshaw, M. L., Pellegrino, L., & Risen, N. J. (2007). *Children with disabilites* (6th ed.). Baltimore, MD: Paul H. Brookes.

8. Charles, J.M. (2010). Dental care in children with developmental disabilities: Attention deficit disorder, intellectual disabilities, and autism. *JDC,* 77:2.

9. Southern Association of Institutional Dentists. (n.d.). *Mental retardation: A review for dental professionals.* (Self-study course, module 1). Retrieved September 28,2012, from http://saiddent.org/admin/images/80769000_1339440193.pdf.

10. Bhasin, T. K., Brocksen, S., Avchen, R. N., & Braun, K. V. (2006, January 18). *Prevalence of four developmental disabilities among children aged 8 years—Metropolitan Atlanta developmental disabilities surveillance program 1996 and 2000.* Retrieved April 1, 2008, from www.cdc.gov.

11. Merriam Webster Online Dictionary. (n.d.). *Mental retardation.* Retrieved March 20, 2011. from http://www.merriam-webster.com/dictionary/Mental%20retardation.

12. U.S. Department of Health and Human Services. (2004, May). *Practical oral care for people with mental retardation* (NIH Publication No. 04-5194). Rockville, MD: U.S. Department of Health and Human Services, National Institute of Dental and Craniofacial Research, National Institutes of Health.

13. Lyons, R. A. (2009). Understanding basic behavioral support techniques as an alternative to sedation and anesthesia. *Spec Care Dentist,* 29:39–50.

14. Reed, R., Broder, H. L., Jenkins, G., Spivack, E., & Janal, M. N. (2006). Oral health promotion among older persons and their care providers in a nursing home facility. *Gerodontology,* 23:73–78.

15. Centers for Disease Control and Prevention. (2012). *Autism spectrum disorders (ASDs).* Retrieved August 7, 2012, from http://www.cdc.gov/ncbddd/autism/index.html.

16. Centers for Disease Control and Prevention. (2012). *Autism speaks. What is autism?* Retrieved August 7, 2012, from http://www.cdc.gov/ncbddd/autism/index.html.

17. Marshall, J., Sheller, B., & Mancl, L. (2010). Caries risk assessment and caries status of children with autism. *Pediatric Dentistry,* 32:69–75.

18. U.S. Department of Health and Human Services. (2004, May). *Practical oral care for people with autism* (NIH Publication No. 04-5190). Rockville, MD: U.S. Department of Health and Human Services, National Institute of Dental and Craniofacial Research, National Institutes of Health.

19. Merriam Webster Online Dictionary. (n.d.). *Autism.* Retrieved March 20, 2011 from http://www.merriam-webster.com/dictionary/autism.

20. National Institute of Mental Health. (n.d.). *Autism spectrum disorders (pervasive developmental disorders).* Retrieved April 1, 2012, from http://www.nimh.nih.gov/health/topics/autism-spectrum-disorders-pervasive-developmental-disorders/index.shtml.

21. Merriam Webster Online Dictionary. (n.d.). *Cerebral palsy.* Retrieved March 20,2012 from http://www.merriam-webster.com/dictionary/cerebral%20palsy.

22. Aswal, S., Russman, B. S., Blasco, P. A., Miller, G., Sandler, A., Shevell, M., & Stevenson, R. (2004). Practice parameter: Diagnostic assessment of the child with cerebral palsy: Report of the Quality Standards Subcommittee of the American Academy of Neurology and the Practice Committee of the Child Neurology Society. *Neurology* 62:851–63.

23. U.S. Department of Health and Human Services. (2004, May). *Practical oral care for people with cerebral palsy* (NIH Publication No. 04-5190). Rockville, MD: U.S. Department of Health and Human Services, National Institute of Dental and Craniofacial Research, National Institutes of Health.

24. Southern Association of Institutional Dentists. (n.d.). *Cerebral palsy: A review for dental professionals.* (Self-study course, module 4). Retrieved September 28,2012 from http://saiddent.org/admin/images/30095700_1339441426.pdf.

25. Obladen, M. (2011). Lame from birth: Early concepts of cerebral palsy. *Journal of Child Neurology,* 26:248–56.

26. Yeargin-allsopp, M. (2011). Distribution of motor types in cerebral palsy: How do registry data compare? *Developmental Medicine and Child Neurology,* 53:197–201.

27. Scheutz, F., & Langeback, J. (1995). Dental care of infectious patients in Denmark. *Community Dent Oral Epidemiol,* 23:226–31.

28. Bhowate, R., & Dubey, A. (2005). Dentofacial changes and oral health status in mentally challenged children. *J Indian Soc Pedodont Prev Dent,* 23:71–73.

29. Fenton, S., Hood, H., Holder, M., May, P., & Mouradian, W. (2003, December). The American Academy of Developmental Medicine and Dentistry: Eliminating health disparities for individuals with mental retardation and other developmental disabilities. *J Dent Edu,* 67:1337–44.

30. National Down Syndrome Society. (n.d.). *Information topics.* Retrieved Septerber 28, 2012, from http://www.ndss.org/Down-Syndrome/Down-Syndrome-Facts/.

31. Shore, S., Lightfoot, T., & Ansell, P. (2010). Oral disease in children with Down syndrome: Causes and prevention. *Community Practitioner,* 83:18–21.

32. Merriam Webster Online Dictionary. *Down syndrome.* Retrieved March 20, 2012 from http://www.merriam-webster.com/dictionary/down%20syndrome.

33. Saenz, R. (1999, January). Primary care of infants and young children with Down syndrome. *Am Fam Physician,* 59:381–90 d.

34. Southern Association of Institutional Dentists. (n.d.). *Down syndrome: A review for dental professionals.* (Self-study course, module 3). Retrieved September 28, 2012, from http://saiddent.org/admin/images/68542000_1339440469.pdf.

35. Waldman, H. B., & Perlman, S. (2002, January). Preparing to meet the dental needs of individuals with disabilities. *J Dent Educ,* 66:82–85.

36. Chung, E., Sung, E., & Sakurai, K. (2004, May). Dental management of the Down and Eisenmenger syndrome patient. *J Contemp Dent Pract,* 5:70–80.

37. U.S. Department of Health and Human Services. (2004, May). *Practical oral care for people with Down syndrome* (NIH Publication No. 04-5193). Rockville, MD: U.S. Department of Health and Human Services, National Institute of Dental and Craniofacial Research, National Institutes of Health.

38. Bauer, D., Evans, C. A., BeGole, E. A., and Salzmann L. (2012). Severity of occlusal disharmonies in Down syndrome. *Int J Dent,* 872367. Retrieved on Sept 28,2012 from http://www .ncbi.nlm.nih.gov/pmc/articles/PMC3426224/.

39. Centers for Disease Control and Prevention. (2010). *Attention deficit hyperactivity disorder (ADHD).* Retrieved March 20, 2012, from http://www.cdc.gov/ncbddd/adhd/facts.html

40. National Institute of Mental Health. (2009). *Attention deficit hyperactivity disorder (ADHD).* Retrieved September 28, 2012, from http://www.nimh.nih.gov/health/publications/ attention-deficit-hyperactivity-disorder/what-conditions-can-coexist-with-adhd.shtml.

41. Akpabio, A., Klausner, C. P., & Inglehart, M. R. (2008). Mothers'/ guardians' knowledge about promoting children's oral health. *J Dent Hyg,* 82:12.

42. Kim, J., & Amar, S. (2006). Periodontal disease and systemic conditions: A bidirectional relationship. *Odontology,* 94:10–21.

43. Dougall, A., & Fiske, J. (2008). Access to special care dentistry, part 4: Education. *Br Dent J,* 205:119–30.

44. Association of University Centers on Disabilities. (2011). *Portrayal of people with disabilities.* Retrieved September 27, 2012, from http://www.aucd.org/template/page.cfm?id=605.

45. St. Jude Children's Research Hospital. *What is patient family centered care?* Retrieved February 21, 2011, from http://www .stjude.org.

46. Critical Periods of Human Development. (2012). Retrieved September 27, 2012, from http://www.cerebralpalsyinfo.com/ CPFetal.html.

Glossary

Abutment teeth: The teeth to which the two ends of a bridge are attached.

Acidogenesis: Acid production.

Aciduric: The ability to thrive in a relatively acidic environment.

Acquired pellicle: The coating of saliva origin that forms on exposed tooth surfaces.

Actinic cheilitis: A precancerous condition on the lip that is due to prolonged exposure to the sun. Sometimes referred to as "farmer's lips" or sailor's lips."

Active immunity: The production of antibodies against a specific agent by the immune system that can be acquired in two ways, by contracting an infectious disease or by receiving a vaccination.

Adhesion: The surface appendage of a bacterium that allows the microbe to attach to receptor sites on the tooth or on other bacteria in the plaque.

Aerobic bacteria: Bacteria that require oxygen for survival.

Ageusia: The loss of taste functions of the tongue, particularly the inability to detect sweetness, sourness, bitterness, and saltiness.

Alimentary tract: The mucous membrane-lined tube of the digestive system through which food passes, in which digestion takes place, and from which wastes are eliminated. It extends from the mouth to the anus and includes the pharynx, esophagus, stomach, and intestines. Also called *digestive tract.*

Alternative restorative technique (ART): The excavation of cavitated carious lesions with hand instruments and restoration of the cavities and associated pits and fissures with a glass ionomer or dental sealant material.

Alveolar crest fibers: The periodontal fibers that attach to the cementum just apical to the cementoenamel junction, run downward, and insert into the alveolar bone.

Alveolar fracture: A fracture of the alveolar bone.

Alveolar mucosa: The mucosa which covers the alveolar bone.

Alveolar process: The thickened ridge of bone that contains the tooth sockets on bones that bear teeth and is also referred to as the alveolar bone.

Alveolar ridge: One of the two jaw ridges either on the roof of the mouth between the maxillary teeth and the hard palate or on the bottom of the mouth behind the mandibular teeth.

Alveologingival fibers: The fibers collected into fiber bundles within the subepithelial connective tissue of the gingival that extend from the crest of the alveolus and insert into the dense irregular collagenous connective tissue of the attached and free gingival.

Alveolus: Sockets in the jaws in which the roots of teeth are held in the alveolar process of maxilla with the periodontal ligament, sometimes referred to as tooth sockets.

Amalgams: A commonly used dental restorative material which is a mixture of mercury with at least one other metal, such as silver, tin, copper, and zinc.

Ameloblasts: Cells which secrete the enamel proteins enamelin and amelogenin, which will later mineralize to form enamel on teeth, the strongest substance in the human body.

Amelogenesis: The formation of enamel on teeth and occurs during the crown stage of tooth development after dentinogenesis, which is the formation of dentin.

Amourphous calcium phosphates: Used in dental products for the remineralization of demineralized tooth surfaces.

Amylase: An enzyme that breaks starch down into sugar and is present in saliva, where it begins the chemical process of digestion.

Anaerobic bacteria: Bacteria that survive only in the absence of oxygen.

Angiogenesis: Process involving the growth of new blood vessels from pre-existing blood vessels.

Angled filaments: Arrangement of toothbrush bristle filaments.

Ankylosis: The fusion of the tooth to the bone, which prevents the tooth from erupting.

Anorexia nervosa: An eating disorder characterized by unrealistic fear of weight gain, self-starvation, and conspicuous distortion of body image.

Anterior: Anatomical location of the front surface, such as the "front teeth."

Antimicrobial mouthwash: A mouthwash with antimicrobial properties.

Apex: Anatomically the "root tip" of the tooth.

Apexification: The process of induced root development or apical closure of the root by hard tissue deposition.

APF, acidulated phosphate fluoride: A type of fluoride used in topical fluoride agents.

Apical fibers: Periodontal fibers located at the root tip surface.

Apical migration: Migration of a periodontal pocket to the root surface, which results in bone loss.

Apical: Toward the root tip surface.

Apices: Pertaining to the area surrounding the root tip surface.

Apoptosis: A form of programmed cell death in multicellular organisms.

Approximal plaque: Plaque biofilm found on interproximal surfaces.

Arrested root caries: Carious lesions on the root surfaces that have stopped the demineralization process and have begun to remineralize.

Arthritis: A group of conditions involving damage to the joints of the body.

Articulating paper: Used to determine where cusps are occluding.

Artificially acquired active immunity: Artificially acquired passive immunity is a short-term immunization by the injection of antibodies that are not produced by the recipient's cells.

Aspartame: A dipeptide that is used as a non-nutritive, noncariogenic sweetener.

Assessment: A thorough analysis of all factors of a patient's or target populations health issues.

Assurance: Something that inspires or tries to inspire confidence.

Asthma: A chronic disease that affects the pulmonary system.

Athletic mouthguard: A thermoplastic oral appliance used to prevent dental trauma.

Attached gingiva: The mucous membrane extending from the muco-gingival fold to the marginal gingival on the facial side of the alveolar process.

Attachment apparatus: The tissues that invest and support the teeth for function including the cementum, periodontal ligament, and alveolar bone.

Autistic: A neural development disorder characterized by impaired social and communication skills.

Automated flossers: A flossing apparatus that is automated, and many patients with difficulty flossing, find automated flossers easier to use.

Autopolymerization: The ability to accomplish polymerization, such as during the dental sealant procedure without the use of a light source, but instead with a chemical catalyst.

Avulsion: The traumatic removal of teeth that may occur during an accident or traumatic event during sport activities.

Baby bottle tooth decay: Dental decay caused by the prolonged use a baby bottle or sippy cup, referred to as nursing bottle decay or more commonly early childhood caries.

Bacteremias: The usually transient presence of bacteria in the blood.

Bacterial biofilm: A biofilm is a structured community of microorganisms encapsulated within a self-developed polymeric matrix and adherent to a living or inert surface.

Bacterial endocarditis: Bacterial infection of the heart.

Bacteriostatic: Having the capability to inhibit the growth or reproduction of bacteria, which is different than bactericidal, which is the capability of killing bacteria.

Bass method: A specific toothbrushing method focusing on supragingival plaque removal.

Battery-powered brushes: Toothbrushes powered by a battery, particularly useful for patients who have difficulty brushing.

B-complex vitamins: Eight water-soluble vitamins that play important roles in cell metabolism.

Behavior management: Techniques used to control behavior issues during dental services.

Behavior modification: A change in behavior due to motivation causing a shift in self-designated goals.

Beta-defensin peptides: The beta-defensins comprise a large family of small cationic antimicrobial peptides widely distributed in plants, mammals, and insects, which display multifunctional properties with implications as potential therapeutic agents.

Bidirectional synergism: Two or more agents working together to produce a result not obtainable by any of the agents independently that can be controlled from either end and can move forward or backward with equal ease without any need to be turned around.

Bidis: A thin, often flavored, South Asian cigarette made of tobacco wrapped in a leaf and secured with colored thread at one end.

Binding agents: Agents that are used to maintain the consistency of a toothpaste and prevent separation of the other additives.

Binge-eating disorder (BED): Individuals with this disorder eat unusually large quantities of food without control over their eating.

Biofilm: A layer of living organisms that can attach to a solid object, for instance moss or seaweed to rocks, or in a dental context, plaque bacteria to the teeth.

Biopsy: The excision (removal) and microscopic examination of tissue suspected of being cancerous.

Bipolar disorder: The category of mood disorders defined by the presence of one or more episodes of abnormally elevated mood, clinically referred to as mania.

Bis-GMA: The abbreviation of the chemical name of the plastic used for sealants. (Bisphenol A-glycidyl methylacrlate).

Bitewing radiograph: A radiograph that shows the crowns of both the maxillary and mandibular teeth on the same film and are used to detect interproximal carious lesions and when taken vertically can also detect bone loss.

Bleeding index: A record of the location of marginal bleeding following gentle probing of the free margin of the gingiva.

Body defense cells: Cells that identify the presence of antigens (foreign bodies), remove the antigens, and/or repair the damage caused by the antigens.

Body Mass Index: BMI. A medical standard for defining obesity.

Body wraps: Blanket-like wraps that fully enfold a young patient to restrain body parts or patient actions during a dental procedure.

Bone marrow transplant: A procedure that transplants healthy bone marrow into a patient whose bone marrow is not working properly.

Brachytherapy: A form of radiotherapy where a radioactive source is placed inside or next to the area requiring treatment, also known as sealed source radiotherapy or endocurietherapy that is commonly used to treat localized cancers of the head and neck.

Bradycardia: A resting heart rate of under 60 beats per minute, though it is seldom symptomatic until the rate drops below 50 beat/min.

Bristles: A part of the toothbrush that is often made from synthetic fibers, although natural toothbrushes are also known in many parts of the world.

Brush biopsy: Computer-assisted analysis of an oral brush test used to evaluate innocuous lesions.

Brushite: A mineral, formula $CaHPO_4 \cdot 2H_2O$.

Buccal salivary glands: Salivary glands located within the buccal mucosa.

Buccal: Of or pertaining to the cheek or facial area.

Buds: The tooth bud, sometimes called the tooth germ, is an aggregation of cells that eventually forms a tooth.

Buffering: The ability to neutralize acidity (of the plaque) by use of alkaline substances.

Bulimia nervosa: Binge eating. Eating a meal, and then resorting to regurgitation to eliminate the stomach contents. Often accompanied by lingual erosion of teeth from stomach acid.

Burnishing: Refers to the damaging result of not removing calculus from the tooth structure but actually allowing it to stay on the tooth surface.

Bidirectional synergism: Meaning that a specific disease may be a risk factor for adverse systemic diseases or conditions.

Calcium bridging: Theory that suggests that cells are held in place within biofilms by a web of polymers, but that proximity to neighboring cells is dependent on calcium bridging and that this may be manipulated to allow increased penetration of therapeutic agents.

Calcium carbonate: Calcium carbonate is a chemical compound with the chemical formula $CaCO_3$.

Calcium: The fifth most abundant element by mass in the human body and a major component of teeth.

Calculus: Calcified deposits on the teeth, formed by the continuous presence of dental plaque biofilm, sometimes called tartar.

Caloric sugar: Sugars containing calories such as sucrose, glucose, fructose, and lactose.

CAMBRA: The acronym used for Caries Management by Risk Assessment. This model bases the planning of caries preventive care and treatment based upon the known risk factors of each patient. Risk levels range from low to moderate or high and servere. Guidelines include specific regimens for each risk category.

Canaliculi: An anatomical term used to describe a small passageway that includes the small channel found in ossified bone.

Cancer: A term for diseases in which abnormal cells divide without control.

Candida albicans: A diploid fungus, which is capable of mating but not of meiosis, and a causal agent of opportunistic oral infections.

Candidiasis: A fungal infection (mycosis) of any of the *Candida* species, can be seen in the oral cavity and is referred to as thrush.

Cannula: A small diameter tip of an irrigator syringe or device that allows a deeper irrigation of a periodontal pocket.

Carbamide peroxide: A commonly used tooth bleaching agent.

Carcinogen: A substance or agent that causes cancer.

Carcinogenesis: Cancer production.

Carcinoma in situ: An early form of carcinoma defined by the absence of invasion of surrounding tissues.

Carcinoma: Malignant neoplasm derived from epithelial tissue.

Carcinomas: Malignancies that originate in the epithelial tissues.

Cardiac arrhythmias: A term for any of a large and heterogeneous group of conditions in which there is abnormal electrical activity in the heart, the heartbeat may be too fast or too slow, and may be regular or irregular.

Caregiver: Members of the family, a friend, or hired personnel who assume responsibility of helping compromised persons.

Caries activity: A level of caries risk as determined by use of laboratory methods, plaque index and other evidence-based evaluations.

Caries risk factors: Specific, measurable characteristics of individual patients that increase their risk of developing caries. Among these factors are diet, salivary flow, tooth morphology and prior caries experience.

Caries: A progressive destruction of any kind of bone structure, including the skull, ribs, teeth, and other bones.

Caries-Activity Indictors (CAI): Evidence-based predictors of the course and outcome of the dental caries process.

Caries-free: Having no presence of carious lesions in the oral cavity.

Cariogenic: Increasing the likelihood that dental caries will develop.

Cariostatic: Acting to halt bone or tooth decay.

Carious lesion: A lesion of demineralized tooth surface.

Catheter: A tube connecting a body cavity with the exterior for purposes of irrigation or drainage.

Cavitated: An incipient lesion in which the surface zone has collapsed over the body of the lesion, thus creating an overt cavity.

Cavitation: Refers to the breakdown of the integrity of the enamel surfaces as they are undermined by the caries process. A "cavity" or hole indicating complete loss of the enamel surface becomes visible on examination.

Cellular immunity: Immunity resulting from a cell-mediated immune response, sometimes called cell-mediated immunity.

Cementoblasts: A biological cell that forms from the follicular cells around the root of a tooth, and whose biological function is cementogenesis, which is the creation of cementum.

Cemento-enamel junction: The junction point between the coronal enamel and the cementum.

Cementum: The surface layer of the root of the tooth.

Cerebral hemorrhage: A subtype of intracranial hemorrhage that occurs within the brain tissue.

Cerebral palsy: An umbrella term encompassing a group of non-progressive, non-contagious conditions that cause physical disability in human development.

Cervical caries: Caries that are located on the cervical surface of the tooth.

Cervical: The area of the tooth in between the crown and the root.

Cetylpyridinium chloride: A cationic quaternary ammonium compound in some types of mouthwashes, toothpastes, etc.

CFUs: Colony-forming units (bacteria). The number of bacterial colonies that are found on a suitable agar after an appropriate period of incubation.

Charters technique: A toothbrushing method that focuses on circular strokes.

Chelating: Binding together.

Chemical activation: A process activated by a chemical means.

Chemical plaque control: The use of antimicrobial mouthrinses to aid in plaque control.

Chemical-cured sealants: Dental sealants that are polymerized by mixing in a chemical catalyst.

Chemicoparasitic theory: Based on the well-established evidence that carious lesions result from the dissolution of mineral salts from tooth tissues by the action of specific acid-producing bacteria in the oral cavity.

Chemotaxis: A response to a chemical signal that initiates the movement of body defense cells to an area of inflammation.

Chemotherapeutic agents: Dental agents used to prevent or maintain dental health.

Chew tobacco: A tobacco product that is placed in the mouth and "chewed" to release the tobacco product, is a risk factor in oral cancer.

Chlorhexidine gluconate: An effective antimicrobial mouthrinse that is effective for suppressing cariogenic and periopathogenic organisms.

Chlorination: The addition of chlorine compounds to water supplies to kill pathogenic bacteria.

Chromosomes: Organized structures of DNA and proteins that are found in cells.

Chronic obstructive pulmonary disease: A disease of the lungs where the airways become narrowed.

Chronic periodontitis: The most common type of periodontal disease that is characterized by progressive loss of the bone and soft tissues that surround and support your teeth.

Clasp brush: A brush used by a patient to clean the clasps of a removable partial denture.

Classical conditioning: Suggests that individuals can become conditioned to specific stimuli to act in a specific way.

Cleft palate: An oral malformation in which there is a lack of union at the midline of the palate, which may involve only a split uvula of the soft palate to a cleft of all structures of the palate and include the upper lip.

Clefting: An area of the gingival margin that becomes clefted in the middle due to aggressive brushing or other reason.

Cocci: Description of a bacterium such as a coccus, or sphere, distinguishes it from bacillus, or rod.

Cognition: Ability to concentrate and think logically.

Col: That portion of the interdental gingiva of molar teeth that is located between the oral and the vestibular papilla.

Collagen: Collagen is the protein for the framework of soft and hard tissues of the body.

Collagenase: The enzyme that attacks collagen.

Colonization: The colonizing of bacteria.

Colorado brown stain: The early designation for severe fluorosis (with brown coloration of teeth) before its etiology was known.

Community water fluoridation: The term used when adding fluoride to a community water supply for the intent to decrease the incidence of dental caries in a community.

Compliance: A willingness of a patient to follow prescribed actions.

Composites: A tooth colored dental restorative material.

Compromised individual: A person with one or more physical, medical, mental, or emotional problems that limit their ability to function.

Concept: After an individual has learned a sufficient number of facts relating to a subject, by reasoning these facts begin to form an overall belief called a concept.

Concussion: The most common and least serious type of traumatic brain injury condition.

Congestive heart failure: A condition in which the heart can't pump enough blood to the body's other organs.

Coronal caries: Caries located on the crown of the tooth.

Coronal: The area around the crown of the tooth.

Cost-effective analysis: A calculation of how much money is saved (or overspent) as a result of some action.

Community Periodontal Index of Treatment Needs (CPITN): A worldwide standardized periodontal needs index based on the severity (pocket depth) exhibited by a population.

Craniofacial disorders: Refers to an abnormality of the face and/or the head.

Crevicular fluid: A tissue fluid that arises from the underlying connective tissue, flows slowly through the gingival crevice into the mouth; its two major functions are to (1) flush out catabolites, and (2) act as a carrier for immune cells and antibodies that bathe (and protect) the four smooth surfaces on every tooth.

Cultural competence: The ability to deliver health care to a diverse group of people from different cultures.

Cultural diversity: The diversity of people from different cultures existing within a population.

Cultural group representation: The balance of cultural group representation within a population.

Cure: Occurs when a disease process terminates with a return to histologic normalcy of all tissues involved. The return to normal can be due to natural body defense mechanisms or because of professional intercession.

Cytokine: A proinflammatory bloodborne agent of the body's immune system.

Daily values: A dietary reference value to help consumers use food label information to plan a healthy overall diet.

Debridement: The mechanical or chemical removal of infectious or necrotic material from an inflamed, or potentially inflamed area.

Defluoridation: The removal of naturally occurring fluoride in a community water supply, when the fluoride above the optimum level.

Dementia: The progressive decline in cognitive function.

Demineralization: The loss of mineral from the tooth because of bacterial acids, acid foods (soft drinks, acid juices, etc.), or even toothbrushing abrasion.

Demographic data: Environment conditions relating to and having an effect on data found in a survey, such as population, socioeconomic status, race, age, unusual environmental conditions.

Dentacult SM and Denticult L: Commercially available test kits that facilitate counting of mutans streptococci and lactobacilli, respectively.

Dental calculus: Mineralization of the deeper portions of plaque.

Dental caries: A carbohydrate modified transmissible localized infection caused mainly by mutans streptococci and lactobacilli.

Dental demineralization: The loss of tooth mineralization caused by dental decay.

Dental hygiene process of care: The steps or protocol used when providing comprehensive dental hygiene treatment.

Dental plaque biofilm: A combination of bacteria, saliva, and complex polysaccharides on the surface of the teeth.

Dental public health: The art and science of preventing and controlling oral disease, with an emphasis on the practice of the dental hygiene sciences.

Dental sealants: A liquid plastic that is placed on pits and/or fissures of tooth surfaces and then hardened to help prevent tooth demineralization.

Dental trauma: Trauma to the oral cavity.

Dentate: With teeth. The opposite is edentulous, i.e., not to have teeth.

Dentifrice: A more scientific, but less used, term for toothpaste.

Dentinal tubules: Tubules present within the dentin.

Dentinoenamel junction: A junction of the dentin and enamel.

Dentition: The teeth, collectively.

Dentogingival fiber: Gingival fibers that are inserted into the dentin.

Dentogingival junction: The junction of the dentin and gingival.

Denture adhesive: A pliable dental product used to hold a dental prosthesis in position.

Denture liner: A resin used to coat the tissue surface of a dental prosthesis to restore or improve the conformation of the prosthesis to improve the retention of the denture.

Depressive disorders: The collective term for mental health disorders of a depressive nature.

Desensitization agent: An therapeutic agent is applied to hypersensitive cementum.

Desquamate: To shed skin cells.

Developmental disability: A diverse group of severe chronic conditions and/or diseases that may cause mental and/or physical disabilities.

Dextrose: Common lay designation of glucose.

Diabetes mellitus: A syndrome characterized by disordered metabolism and abnormally high blood sugar (hyperglycaemia) resulting from insufficient levels of the hormone insulin.

Diagnosis: The process of identifying a medical condition or disease by its signs, symptoms, and from the results of various assessments and diagnostic procedures.

Diastemas: Spaces between the interproximal areas of teeth.

Dietary fluoride supplement schedule: Recommended daily dosage of fluoride supplements, applicable to fluoride drops or tablets.

Dietary guidance: Professional recommendations regarding an individual's nutritional habits.

Dietary Reference Intake (DRIs): A system of recommendations to describe nutritional and dietary needs of individuals.

Differentiation: Involves the degree of alteration of cells from their normal morphology (form) and function.

Diffusion: Diffusion is described as the extension of benefits of community water fluoridation to residents of fluoride-deficient communities.

Digitized radiographs: Producing images of objects by electronically detecting the arrival of x-ray photons transmitted through the object or emitted from it on various media and converting the sensed analog signals to digital signals representing the intensity of x-ray photons at each position.

Dilution: Results from the increased availability of fluoride from multiple sources; therefore, diluting the impact of any one source of fluoride, particularly water.

Disaccharide: A combination of two simple sugars. Example— Glucose + fructose = sucrose.

Disclosing agents: Agents that color dental plaque biofilm so that an individual can clearly see areas of plaque in the mouth, used during patient education.

Disclosing tablet: A tablet that is chewed to mix with saliva and then swished around the mouth to disclose (by red and purple colors) the presence and location of dental plaque on the teeth.

Distal: Away from the midline.

DNA repair: Refers to a collection of processes by which a cell identifies and corrects damage to the DNA molecules that encode its genome.

DNA: Deoxyribonucleic acid (DNA) is a nucleic acid that contains the genetic instructions used in the development and functioning of all known living organisms

Dry storage: A tooth that has been lost due to trauma is not placed in a fluid or solution to keep its structures moist, which affects its ability to be resorbed back into the tooth socket.

Dysgeusia: The distortion or decrease of the sense of taste.

Dysthymia: A mood disorder that falls within the depression spectrum.

Early and Periodic Screening, Diagnosis and Treatment (EPDST): A federal program that mandates that medical and dental services be provided to children from low-income families to receive a dental screening within 12 months of birth.

Early childhood caries: Usually caused by an infant taking milk by bottle as nourishment when hungry, and then retaining the nipple and the milk in the mouth during "sleep time." Can also be caused by "demand" breast-feeding.

Ecchymoses: Blotchy areas of hemorrhage in the skin.

Ecologic niche: The relational position of a species or population in its ecosystem.

Ectodermal dysplasias: Not a single disorder, but a group of syndromes all deriving from abnormalities of the ectodermal structures.

Edema: Swelling and inflammation.

Edentulism: Without teeth.

Efficacy: Having the ability to produce a desired effect.

Elderly: Young elderly, from 65 to 74 years of age; mid-old, 75 to 84; and 85 > oldest old.

Electrocardiogram: A measurement of the electrical activity of the heart as a diagnostic measure.

Electronic periodontal probes: Electronic probes attached to a computer that automatically triggers a measurement of pocket depth when a given pressure on the bottom of the sulcus is encountered.

Embrasure: The interproximal space between two adjacent teeth. Classified as class 1 embrasures that occurs when a soft tissue papilla fills the entire space, type 3 when the papilla is missing, and type 2, intermediate.

Enamaloplasty: Removing demineralized areas of tooth structure and etching and then placing dental sealant material to prevent further dental decay.

Enamel maturation: A period of one or two years after eruption during which time the enamel becomes "fully" mineralized (matured).

Enamel rods: A tightly packed, highly organized mass of hydroxyapatite crystals.

Enamel spindles: Short, linear defects, found at the dentinoenamel junction (DEJ) and extend into the enamel, often being more prevalent at the cusp tips.

Endodontics: The treatment of diseased root canals.

Endogenous origin: Arising from within.

Endoscope: A small probe-like videocamera for examining areas that are not readily available, for visual examination—for example, intranasal examination, colonoscopy, intraoral dental examination.

Endosseous implants: Endosseous means that this type of implant is actually placed in a hole drilled in the bone and then allowed to integrate.

Endothelial cells: The cells lining blood vessels.

End-tuft brush: Small brush head addresses special maintenance concerns including orthodontic bands, implants, and other hard-to-reach areas.

Epidemiologic phase: The phase during which community water fluoridation was studied for its preventive benefit in regard to dental caries.

Epidemiological survey: A controlled study of the origin, presence, extent or consequences of a condition or disease.

Epilepsy: A common chronic neurological disorder that is characterized by recurrent unprovoked seizures.

Epithelial attachment: The junctional epithelial cells that attach the crevicular epithelium to the tooth.

Epithelial dysplasia: A disorder of differentiation of epithelial cells which may regress, remain stable, or progress to invasive carcinoma.

Eruptive period, post-: A short, indefinite period after eruption.

Eruptive period, pre-: Before eruption. It is a period during which teeth are developing.

Erythroleukoplakia: Red and white or "speckled" lesions that are considered premalignant.

Erythroplakia: Red lesions that are considered premalignant.

Essential oil: Any concentrated, hydrophobic liquid containing volatile aroma compounds from plants, which are called aromatic herbs or aromatic plants.

Etchant: An acid (40 to 50%) phosphoric acid that is used to etch the tooth surface to provide more surface area that in turn enhances retention of sealants.

Etiologic agent: Etiologic agents are those microorganisms and microbial toxins that cause disease in humans and include bacteria, bacterial toxins, viruses, fungi, rickettsiae, protozoans, and parasites.

Etiology: The cause of a disease.

Evidence-based decisions: The basing of decisions on verified research evidence that certain signs or symptoms are predictive of certain outcomes. For instance, the finding of a greater number of mutans streptococci poses a greater risk for future caries development than does a low count.

Evidence-based principles: Practice that is based on scientifically sound theories.

Excisional biopsy: A procedure for complete removal of a lump or abnormal area from the skin or other part of the body.

Exfoliate: The natural loss of primary teeth.

Exfoliative cytology: Involves the microscopic examination of cells obtained from tissues.

Exocrine glands: A procedure for complete removal of a lump or abnormal area from the skin or other part of the body that is opposite to endocrine glands, which secrete their products (hormones) directly into the bloodstream (ductless glands) or release hormones (paracrines) that affect only target cell nearby the release site.

Exodontia: Extraction is the term given to a tooth extraction.

Exodontics: The extraction of teeth.

Extra-alveolar time: The time a tooth spends outside of tooth socket such as during dental trauma and subsequent treatment.

Extracellular: Outside of the cell.

Extrinsic stain: A stain that is on the outside of the tooth surface that can be removed.

Extruded teeth: Movement of a tooth in an occlusal or incisal direction.

Facial: Anatomical term inferring of or near the facial area.

Facultative aerobic and anaerobic bacteria: Bacteria that can survive in the presence, or absence of oxygen, respectively.

Filaments: The material that comprises toothbrush bristles.

Filiform: Thin, long papillae "V"-shaped cones that don't contain taste buds but are the most numerous on the tongue.

Fimbria: Small microscopic projections from a bacterial cell wall.

Fine-needle aspiration biopsy: Diagnostic procedure sometimes used to investigate superficial (just under the skin) lumps or masses.

Fissured tongue: A benign condition characterized by deep grooves (fissures) in the dorsum of the tongue.

Fistula: A tissue connection between a subsurface infected area and the surface of a mucosal membrane or skin.

Flap surgery (periodontal diseases): The removal of a sufficient circumferential portion of the marginal gingival to lessen pocket depth and open the subgingival area to self-care preventive procedures.

Fluoridation: The addition of fluoride to public drinking water, most commonly called community water fluoridation.

Fluoride diffusion effect: Also referred to as a "halo effect." It is the caries reduction experienced by individuals not living in a water fluoridated area, but getting its benefits by eating and drinking food processed in an area with optimum water fluoride content. Also, the term applies to those who commute between fluoridated and nonfluoridated communities.

Fluoride mouthrinses: Mouthrinses that contain fluoride.

Fluoride varnish: A varnish material that contains fluoride and is used to treat hypersensitivity or to prevent decay or aid in remineralization of decay in smooth surfaces.

Fluorosis: Cosmetic deviation of enamel in development because of an excessive intake of fluoride during the development periods of the primary and the permanent teeth. Depending on amount of intake, the cosmetic effect ranges from mild veining to a severe brown coloration with a pitting of the enamel.

Fones method: A circular toothbrushing method in which the teeth are in centric occlusion, developed by the founder of dental hygiene, Dr. Alfred C. Fones.

Fossa: A depression or hollow, in general, in a bone.

Frank lesion: Same as cavitated or overt caries lesion.

Free marginal groove: The margin of the free gingival.

Fructose: A simple reducing sugar (monosaccharide) found in many foods.

Functional dentition: Dentition that functions properly.

Fungiform papilla: Mushroom-shaped papillae (projections) on the tongue.

Furcation areas: The space between multi-rooted posterior teeth.

Furcation: The area of the tooth where the roots (of multirooted teeth) are joined.

Gag reflex: A reflex to a tendency to vomit. Often encountered when workers irritate the posterior tongue or palatal area when cleaning the teeth. Also can occur with an obnoxious taste or with some during pregnancy.

Gene polymorphisms: Polymorphism is a genetic variant that appears in at least 1% of a population.

Genes: A locatable region of genomic sequence, corresponding to a unit of inheritance, which is associated with regulatory regions, transcribed regions, and/or other functional sequence regions.

Genome: The whole hereditary information, which is encoded in the DNA or, for some viruses, RNA.

Genomics: The study of an organism's entire genome.

Gestational diabetes: Diabetes acquired during pregancy.

Gingival crevice: The area between the cervical enamel of a tooth and the overlying unattached gingiva.

Gingival crevicular fluid: Fluid that arises from the connective tissue beneath the gingival sulcus that slowly flows through the gingival crevice. Its purpose is to flush debris from the sulcus, and carry defense agents into the oral cavity.

Gingival fibers: The fibers of the gingiva.

Gingival recession: Areas of recession of the gingival that expose the root surface.

Gingival sulcus: Around each tooth there is a collar of approximately 3 millimeters on depth of soft tissue.

Gingivitis: Inflammation and infection of the gingiva caused by dental plaque.

Glass ionomer: A hard plastic with fine incorporated glass powder to resist abrasion. Used for restorations and tried as a sealant substitute.

Glaucoma: An increased intraocular pressure that, unless treated, can lead to blindness.

Glucans: A polysaccharide of D-glucose monomers linked by glycosidic bonds.

Glucosyltransferase: A type of glycosyltransferase, which enables the transfer of glucose.

Goal orientation: An objective than an individual has decided to attain; it may be only a temporary short-term goal or a long-term goal; it may be a temporary short-term goal that is powerful only until attained.

Grading: The prognosis, or forecast of the probable course or outcome of squamous cell carcinoma is determined by a system of grading, which is the determination of the histologic subtype.

Granulocytes: A category of white blood cells characterized by the presence of granules in their cytoplasm.

Granulomas: A nodule consisting mainly of epithelioid macrophages and other inflammatory and immune cells as well as extracellular matrix.

Growth regulation: The regulation of growth.

Guideline: An established and agreed upon method for examining, treating, preventing, and/or monitoring a disease.

Halitosis: Another term for bad breath.

Health disparities: Pertaining to populations within society that have significant rates of disease and health.

Health education: The teaching of health behaviors that bring an individual to a state of health awareness.

Health promotion: The informing and motivating of people to adopt health behaviors.

Health: A state of complete physical, mental, spiritual, emotional and social well-being.

Hematopoietic cell transplantation: The intravenous infusion of autologous or allogeneic stem cells collected from bone marrow, peripheral blood, or umbilical cord blood to reestablish hematopoietic function in patients with damaged or defective bone marrow or immune systems.

Hemidesmosomes: Small stud- or rivet-like structures on the inner basal surface of keratinocytes in the epidermis of skin.

Hemophilia: A rare inherited bleeding disorder that the blood does not clot normally.

Histologic: The study of the microscopic anatomy of cells and tissues.

HIV: Human immunodeficiency virus, usually a predecessor of AIDS.

Homeostasis: Occurs when the body is in normal metabolic balance. Reference to caries: a balance between demineralization and remineralization.

Hopewood House: An orphanage in Australia that demonstrated that in children raised on a good diet, caries is minimal. It also proved that once the children left Hopewood House and its diet, caries again became a problem, proving that the acquired low caries status of the orphanage was not permanent.

Human Genome Project: Probably the greatest health research program of the 20th century. This has been a worldwide research effort to decipher "the molecule of life"—desoxynucleic acid.

Human papillomavirus: A common sexually transmitted disease that is linked to oral cancer.

Humectants: Gives toothpaste its texture as well as retain moisture so that toothpaste does not dry out.

Humeral body defenses: Genetic defense factors found in body fluids.

Hydrogen peroxide: A commonly used tooth bleaching agent.

Hydrophobicity: A repellent to water.

Hydroxyapatite: The basic building crystal in the formation of enamel rods. It is composed of mainly calcium, phosphate, and hydroxyl, but also includes many other trace quantities of up to 30 or 40 elements.

Hyper-: Above normal.

Hypersensitivity: Areas of tooth sensitivity, commonly occurs when roots are exposed.

Hypertension: A medical condition in which the blood pressure is chronically elevated.

Hypo-: Below normal.

Hypoglycemic shock: A decrease in the level of blood glucose (in diabetes mellitus) that can be accompanied by a variety of symptoms from confusion to coma and death.

Hypomineralization: An area of the enamel that is not mineralized.

Hypothyroidism: A condition in which the body lacks sufficient thyroid hormone.

Iatrogenic disease: Disease that is caused by a health provider or health care service.

Idiopathic: An adjective used primarily in medicine meaning arising spontaneously or from an obscure or unknown cause.

Immune response: Any time a foreign substance penetrates the body's defenses, there is a cellular reaction (immune response) to seek out the antigen (foreign substance) and to neutralize or eliminate it.

Immunity: A state of having sufficient biological defenses to avoid infection or disease.

Immunization: The injection, or ingestion of an antigen into the body to cause an enhancement of the body's capability to resist disease.

Immunoglobulins: Play an essential role in the body's immune system.

Implant: A metallic "root" (the implant) that is surgically inserted into the alveolus in the space of a missing tooth. Following healing, a crown is later constructed on the "root."

Incidence: The number of newly diagnosed cases during a specific time period.

Incipient caries lesion: A pre-caries lesion that exists before cavitation. Seen on the enamel as a "white spot." It can be remineralized.

Incisional biopsy: A biopsy in which only a sample of the suspicious tissue is removed for testing.

Inclusiveness: The inclusion of an individual into a community, group, or societal structure.

Infection: The detrimental colonization of a host organism by a foreign species.

Informed patient consent: Before any treatment is commenced, the patient is informed verbally or in writing of all primary and treatment options, costs, and expected results.

Intense sweetener: Considered noncaloric because of their small bulk needed to deliver desired sweetness.

Interdental brushes: Toothbrushes specifically designed for removal of plaque in the interdental area.

Interdental papillae: The gingival peak between closely adjacent teeth.

Interproximal: The area between the mesial and distal surfaces of two adjacent teeth.

Intrinsic stain: A stain that was incorporated in the enamel during development and that cannot be removed without damage to the enamel.

Intrinsic stains: Tooth stains that are inside or intrinsic to the tooth.

Intruded teeth: A tooth that is "pushed" into the bone from trauma.

Iron deficiency anemia: Anemia caused by too little iron.

Irrigator: A small device containing a reservoir for water that is pumped at relatively low velocity to cleanse the interproximal spaces or loosening plaque.

Ischemia: Lack of sufficient blood to a part of the body.

Kaposi's sarcoma: An oral malignancy linked to HIV infection.

Keratin: A family of fibrous structural proteins.

Kyphosis: A curvature of the upper spine.

Labial: Of or pertaining to the area of the lips.

Lactobacilli: An acidogenic bacterial species that is an etiologic microorganism seen at the later stages of the incipient caries lesion.

Lamina dura: The part of the alveolar bone that lines the socket and is a thin layer of dense cortical bone.

Leukoplakia: A white lesion found that is considered premalignant.

Lichen planus: A disorder of the skin and mucous membranes resulting in inflammation, itching, and distinctive skin lesions.

Life span: The maximum of life potentially possible, now considered 120 years-of-age.

Lingual: Anatomical term pertaining to the tongue.

Loss of attachment: Loss of periodontal attachment (LOA) of the tooth to the tooth socket such as in pocketing, bone loss, and/or recession.

Lucency: (As applied to dental radiographs), a darker area on the x-ray indicating demineralization (caries) or the enamel, dentin, or cementum.

Luxation: The dislocation or displacement of a tooth.

Lysozyme: An antibacterial enzyme found in the saliva and other fluids of the body.

Macroglossia: Enlarged tongue.

Malnutrition: Not receiving adequate nutrition.

Malodor, oral: A term used for halitosis or bad breath.

Manifestations: An obvious indication or specific evidence that a disease is present such as a symptom.

Marginal gingival: The margin of the gingiva.

Mastication: Occluding such as when chewing.

Materia alba: Accumulation or aggregation of microorganisms, desquamated epithelial cells, blood cells, and food debris loosely adherent to surfaces of plaques, teeth, gingiva, or dental appliances.

Maxillofacial surgeon: A dental specialist specifically trained as an oral surgeon.

Mechanical plaque control: The use of toothbrushes, dental floss, and irrigators to aid in plaque removal.

Medicament: An agent such as medicine or chemotherapeutic used to treat or prevent a disease or condition.

Menopause: The complete cessation of the female reproductive system.

Mesial: Anatomical term, toward the midline.

Methamphetamine: A street drug that when used frequently can result in "meth mouth."

Milk fluoridation: The addition of fluoride to milk to help reduce dental decay in a population.

Mineralized: The process where a substance is converted from an organic substance to an inorganic substance.

Monomer: A liquid plastic that when mixed with a catalyst, polymerizes to a hard plastic (polymer); or a liquid plastic containing a catalyst that is activated with a light (light cured).

Monosaccharide: A simple sugar, such as fructose, and glucose.

Morbidity: A ratio of sick to a given number of persons per unit time. Example 12: 100,000/year.

Mortality: The number of deaths from a given cause in a population per unit time. Example: 1: 1000 per year.

Motivation: An inner drive of an individual to attain a self-designated goal.

Mucogingival junction: The junction of the mucosa and the attached gingiva.

Mucosal: Pertaining to the mucosa.

Mucositis: An inflammation of a mucous membrane.

Multifactorial disease process: The process in which as several factors must coalesce in order to cause a disease.

Multiple fluoride therapy: The use of multiple forms of fluoride, such as fluoride toothpaste, fluoride mouthrinse, and professional fluoride gels twice a year, to reduce dental decay.

mutans streptococci: A causative cariogenic organism linked to the early stages of an incipient caries lesion.

MyPyramid: Used to guide an individual in healthy nutritional practices.

Neoplasm: Refers to a new growth and describes a cellular proliferation that has exceeded normal growth.

Nitrosamines: Cancer-causing agents found in tobacco products.

Noncarcinogenic: Not a risk factor of cancer.

Noninvasive care: Care that can be administered without damage to the body tissues.

Noninvasive caries: The beginning stages of demineralization.

Nonspecific plaque hypothesis: This concept relates periodontal disease to the overall amount of plaque present, so as the amount of plaque increases, inflammation and disease increase.

Obturator: A specialized maxillary prosthesis constructed to facilitate speech and eating by a cleft palate individual, as well as to prevent food from entering the nasal cavity.

Occlusal surface: Each posterior tooth has five surfaces, mesial, distal, lingual, buccal, and occlusal; the occlusal surface is the biting surface of the posterior teeth.

Octocalcium phosphate: The first mineral laid down for enamel formation before its conversion to hydroxyapatite.

Operant conditioning: The use of consequences to modify the occurrence and form of behavior.

Opportunistic infections: An infection caused by pathogens that usually do not cause disease in a healthy immune system.

Oral cancer: A variety of malignant neoplasms that occur in the mouth and oropharynx.

Oral hairy leukoplakia: A pathology of the associated with Epstein-Barr virus (EBV) and it occurs mostly in people with HIV.

Oral lichen planus: A chronic dermatologic disease that frequently manifests in lesions of the oral mucosa.

Oral-health self-care: Any action taken by an individual to maintain optimum oral health, including carrying out daily mechanical and chemical plaque control regimens as well as complying with recommendations by the dentist or dental hygienist.

Oropharynx: The entire area from the base of the tongue, pharyngeal wall, tonsillar fossae, and soft palate.

Oscillation movement: The movement of a powered toothbrush.

Osteoporosis: A pathology of bone marked with fragility and porosity.

OTC drugs: Drugs sold over-the-counter without a prescription.

Overt caries lesion: A cavity where the undermined enamel has broken down into a cavity, a process called cavitation. Remineralization is not a possibility (at least at this point in time, 2013).

Papillae: 1. The triangular soft tissue that fills the inter-proximal embrasures. 2. The specialized projections from the surface of the tongue that allow reception of different taste sensations.

Passive smoking: Relates to the tobacco smoke inhaled by family members or bystanders who breathe secondhand smoke.

Pasteurization: The heating of a product (usually milk) to a given temperature (often 60°C) for a given time (30 minutes) in order to kill pathogenic bacteria and extend the time before other bacteria become pathogenic.

Patient's explanatory model: A patient's understanding of the cause of illness, what is the expected treatment, the role of the sick individual, and how the illness affects his or her life.

Perfusion: Microvascular blood flow.

Peri-implantitis: Following the placement of an implant, the same meticulous self-care is necessary as with natural teeth. When this care does not materialize, the same infection and apical migration occurs to the epithelial attachment as occurs with periodontitis.

Periodontal abscess: An abscess of the periodontium, which is the result of infection.

Periodontal disease indicators: Signs and symptoms that usually precede the onset of periodontal disease. Also called "markers."

Periodontal ligament: A ligament of the periodontium.

Periodontal pocket: An abnormal deepening of the gingival sulcus marked by an accompanying apical migration of the epithelial attachment.

Periodontium: The four anatomical structures that support the teeth including the gingiva, periodontal ligament, cementum, and alveolar bone.

Permiability (of teeth): The ability of fluids to pass from the surface to the pulp and vice versa.

pH values: A numeric scale ranging from 1 to 14, used to depict the acidity, or alkalinitiy of substances. Values below 7 are considered acidic and those values above are alkaline. A pH value below 5.5 in the oral cavity facilitates the caries process.

Phagocytosis: The envelopment and destruction of an antigen by one of the body defense cells.

Pit-and-fissure caries: Caries located in the pit-and-fissure surfaces of the tooth.

Plaque index: O'Leary's index charts the location of the location of plaque on the teeth. The index of Silness and Löe is much the same with the exception that the status of the adjoining index is also recorded.

Polymerization: The reaction that occurs when the liquid resin sealant, which is a monomer, is met with a catalyst. The chemical bond repeatedly forms, increasing in number and complexity, which is polymerization and results in a harded resin sealant.

Polyol (alcohol sugar): Sweeteners that have an alcohol grouping to each carbon atom of the polyol. Referred to as sugar alcohols, such as sorbitol, mannitol, and xylitol.

Polypharmacy: Excessive multiple usage of medications often seen with senior citizens.

Pontic: The artificial teeth or tooth that are (is) part of the bridge between the abutment teeth.

Potassium nitrate: A commonly used OTC desensitizing agent.

Potassium oxylate: A commonly used OTC desensitizing agent.

Prediction: A clinical decision as to the outcome of a disease process based on professional judgment and evidence-based information.

Predictive value, negative: Probability that the subject will not develop disease.

Predictive value, positive: Probability that the subject will develop disease.

Pregnancy gingivitis: Gingivitis that may occur and can be exacerbated during pregnancy.

Pregnancy granulomas: Pyogenic granulomas that occur during pregnancy.

Prevalence: The number of cases of a disease that are present in a particular population at a given time.

Primary prevention: Employs strategies and agents to forestall the onset of disease, reverse the progress of disease, or arrest the disease process before secondary preventive treatment becomes necessary and can be termed dental hygiene.

Primary preventive dentistry: The preventive aspects of the dental hygiene sciences and emphasize the use of diagnostic and therapeutic modalities to prevent disease.

Prognosis: A synonym for "prediction."

Proliferation: The multiplication of bacteria.

Prophylaxis: A cleaning, including a debridement and polishing of the hard calculus, plaque biofilm and food particles (material alba) from the tooth surfaces.

Prosthesis: An artificial replacement for a lost tooth or teeth such as a bridge or dentures.

PSR (Periodontal Screening and Recording System): Similar to the CPITN, with the exception that it offers suggested treatment to match each level of severity.

Pulpal necrosis: Necrosis of the pulp that does not respond to stimulation.

Punch biopsy: A type of biopsy.

Pyrophosphates: Crystal growth inhibitors that reduce the amount of calculus formed.

Radiation caries: The rampant caries that often occurs because of the destruction of the oral salivary glands that have been in the x-ray beam as a part of cancer treatment.

Re-contouring: When a tooth is lost and replanted, the direct attachment of bone leads to recontouring of the physiologic bone, with the entire root being replaced by bone.

Refractory disease: A disease that does not respond to accepted treatment therapies.

Reimplantation: Reimplanting a lost tooth back into the tooth socket.

Reliability: The degree of stability exhibited when a measurement is repeated under identical conditions.

Remineralization: The addition of minerals to dimimeralized tooth structure.

Remineralization: The replacement of tooth mineral (hydroxyapatite) that has been lost by demineralization. The minerals needed for the remineralization are derived from the saliva (or from man-made products).

Reparative dentin: Morphologically irregular dentin formed in response to an irritant, such as caries, disease, or drilling to prepare a cavity for filling.

Replacement resorption: A process that occurs when the damage to the slow-growing cementoblasts allows osteoblasts to attach areas of bone directly to the root before the cementoblasts can cover the root with cementum. The direct attachment of bone leads to recontouring of the physiologic bone, with the entire root being replaced by bone.

Resting and stimulated salivary flow: Variations in the amount and content of saliva secreted during "resting" periods, when one is not eating or is sleeping versus "stimulated" periods when one is eating foods or drinking liquids.

Risk assessment: A professional judgement on an individual's susceptibility or resistance to disease, based on evidence-based information.

Risk factor: An evidence-based sign, test, or circumstance reliably associated with the onset or progression of a disease process.

Risk: The probability that a harmful or unwanted event will occur.

Root caries: Caries located on the root (cementum) of a tooth, which frequently increases with age due to increased gingival recession, or exposure of root surfaces.

Root resorption: The resorption of root into the alveolar bone.

Root-surface caries: Caries that occur on the root surface.

Rubber tip stimulators: Aids used to remove plaque.

Saccharin: A nonnutritive and noncariogenic artificial sweetener.

Saliva substitutes: Substitutes for saliva used in individuals with xerostomia.

Salt fluoridation: The addition of fluoride to salt in order to reduce dental decay in a population.

Sclerotic dentin: Dentin that has become translucent due to calcification of the dentinal tubules as a result of injury or normal aging.

Screening tests: A rapid examination to identify healthy from unhealthy individuals, and the characteristics that separate them.

Secondary caries: Caries that develop around a restoration.

Secondary prevention: Employs routine treatment methods to terminate a disease process and/or restore tissues to as near normal as possible and can be termed restorative care.

Secondary standard: The Safe Drinking Water Act enacted by Congress in 1986 established primary and secondary standards for natural fluoride levels in public drinking water in the United States.

Sequelae: A pathological condition resulting from a disease, injury, or other trauma.

Sharpey's fibers: A matrix of connective tissue consisting of bundles of strong collagenous fibers connecting periosteum to bone.

Sialogogues: A medicine or substance that stimulates the flow of saliva.

Sialoliths: Calculi occurring in a salivary gland.

Sialorrhea: Drooling or excessive salivation.

Silicas: Agents used in toothpastes.

Smooth-surface caries: Carious lesions found on the smooth surfaces of the tooth.

Snyder test: A colorometric test used to estimate the relative acidogenic potential of salivary lactobacilli.

Social cognitive theory: A theory that focuses on an individual's knowledge acquisition can be directly related to observing others within the context of social interactions, experiences, and outside media influences.

Social learning theory: A theory that focuses on the learning that occurs within a social context.

Sodium citrate: A commonly used OTC desensitizing agent.

Sodium fluoride (NaF): A type of fluoride used in preventive agents.

Sodium lauryl sulfate: A detergent and surfactant found in toothpastes.

Sodium monofluorophosphate: A type of fluoride used in preventive agents.

Soft palate: An anatomical landmark directly behind the hard palate.

Soft ties: Cloth or leather straps use to immobilize uncontrollable body parts resulting from imperfect neuromuscular control.

Sorbitol: A sugar alcohol that occurs in many fruits and berries.

Specific plaque hypothesis: The premise that the presence of pathogens is not enough to initiate disease; the host must also be susceptible to disease.

"Spit" tobacco: A contemptuous term for the habit associated with either chewing tobacco or use of snuff.

Staging system: A system of grading (histological subtype) and staging (clinical extent) of the tumor.

Stannous fluoride: A type of fluoride used in preventive agents.

Stannous: Meaning tin.

Stem cells: Cells found in most multi-cellular organisms that are characterized by the ability to renew themselves through mitotic cell division and differentiating into a diverse range of specialized cell types.

Stephan curve: The relationship between acid levels (pH) at the tooth surface and time following consumption of sugar.

Stillman method: A toothbrushing method that focuses on gingival stimulation.

Stomatitis: Inflammation of the mucous lining of any of the structures in the mouth, which may involve the cheeks, gums, tongue, lips, throat, and roof or floor of the mouth.

striae of Retzius: Incremental growth lines seen in enamel and are results of enamel's development.

Strontium chloride: A commonly used OTC desensitizing agent.

Study model: A model made of dental stone that replicates the dentition.

Subgingival and supragingival plaque: The plaque that is located on the tooth below, and above the gingiva, respectively.

Subgingival: Below the gingival margin.

Subluxated: Having the tooth loosened and possibly malpositioned, but retained in the jaw such as during a trauma.

Substance abuse: Abuse of a substance such as drugs or alcohol.

Substance dependence: Being dependent upon a substance such as drugs or alcohol.

Substantivity: Pertaining to the capacity of an oral antimicrobial agent to continue its therapeutic activity for a prolonged period of time.

Subsurface pellicle: Below the surface acquired pellicle.

Sucrose: A nutritive sweetener and the most commonly used tabletop sweetener, often referred to as sugar.

Sugar alcohols: Commonly used to replace sugar in food.

Sugar discipline: Restricting sugar intake as to decrease chances of decay.

Sugar substitutes: Sweetening agents that are substituted for sugar.

Sulcular epithelium: Epithelium of the sulcus.

Suppuration: Commonly referred to as pus, a purulent discharge from an infected area.

Supragingival: Above the gingival margin.

Sweeteners: Agents used to sweeten food, gum, or toothpastes.

Symbiosis (bacterial): Two or more species of bacteria that mutually support one another.

Symptom: An abnormal function or feeling that is noticed by a patient, indicating the presence of disease.

Synergistic: Systems working together.

Systemic conditions: Conditions that involve many organs or the whole body.

Systemic diseases: Diseases that involve many organs or the whole body.

Systemic fluoride: Systemic fluorides are those that are ingested into the body and become incorporated into forming tooth structures.

Tachycardia: Rapid beating of the heart.

Target population: A specific population that is grouped together because of one or more similarities such as age, gender, ethnicity, living situation.

Taste buds: Small structures on the upper surface of the tongue, soft palate, and epiglottis that provide information about the taste of food and drink.

Tertiary prevention: Employs measures necessary to replace lost tissues and rehabilitation.

Theory of reasoned action: A theory that suggests that a person's behavioral intention depends on the person's attitude about the behavior and subjective norms.

Therapeutic: Having healing powers.

Thickening agents: Agents used to stabilize the toothpaste.

Thixotropic: A thick, viscous gel.

Tobacco cessation programs: Programs aimed at helping smokers or tobacco chewers quit.

Tolerable upper intake: Defined as the maximum level of a total chronic daily intake of a nutrient that is unlikely to pose risks of adverse health effects for almost all individuals in the general population

Toothbrush abrasion: Abrasion of the tooth surface caused by brushing.

Topical fluoride: Applying fluoride to teeth already present in the mouth making them more resistant to demineralization.

Triclosan: A broad-spectrum antibacterial agent used in dental products.

Trismus: As applied to dentistry, difficulty in opening the mouth due to nerve involvement, pain, and/or infection of the masticatory muscles.

Vaccine: The introduction of beneficial agent into the body to enhance the capability of the immune system to challenge and/or eliminate and repair the damage caused by a foreign antigen.

Validity: The reproducible accuracy of a test as a predictive measure.

Value: A strongly held belief of an individual, based on an unknown number of positive or negative concepts, that in turn are based on an unknown number of positive or negative facts.

Vasculitis: Inflammation of blood vessels resulting in the leakage of fluid and the migration of defense cells through the capillary walls.

Vasoconstriction: The narrowing of the blood vessels resulting from contracting of the muscular wall of the vessels.

Vermilion border: The border between the skin of the face and the lip.

Vipeholm: A study conducted in a mental institution in Vipeholm, Sweden. The clients were fed cariogenic snacks at different frequencies, at mealtime, between meals, etc. to see which situation was the most cariogenic.

Virulence: Refers to the degree of pathogenicity of a microbe.

White spot lesion: Describes the early caries process on smooth enamel surfaces, before cavitation occurs, when the decalicified area appears very white relative to surrounding healthy tissue. These lesions are most often seen as extensive white lines across the cervical areas of teeth. These lesions also occur on proximal surfaces, but they are difficult to detect there.

Whitlockite: A rare mineral, a form of calcium phosphate.

Xerostomia: Dry mouth. A lower than normal secretion of saliva (1 ml per minute). A symptom with Sjorgrens disease, also following exposure of the salivary glands to cancer radiation and a common side effect to many types of medication.

Xylitol: A sugar alcohol that is used as a flavoring agent that is both non-cariogenic and anticariogenic.

Index